Clinical Assessment in

RESPIRATORY CARE

The Latest *Evolution* in Learning.

Evolve provides online access to free learning resources and activities designed specifically for the textbook you are using in your class. The resources will provide you with information that enhances the material covered in the book and much more.

Visit the Web address listed below to start your learning evolution today!

▶▶ *LOGIN: http://evolve.elsevier.com/Wilkins/assessment*

Evolve Learning Resources for Wilkins/Sheldon/Krider: *Clinical Assessment in Respiratory Care,* Fifth Edition, offers the following features:

- **WebLinks**
  Links to places of interest on the web specific to respiratory care.

- **Links to Related Products**
  See what else Elsevier has to offer in a specific field of interest.

Think outside the book... *evolve.*

Clinical Assessment in
RESPIRATORY CARE

Fifth Edition

Robert L. Wilkins, PhD, RRT, FAARC
Chairman/Professor
Department of Cardiopulmonary Sciences
School of Allied Health Professions
Loma Linda University
Loma Linda, California

Richard L. Sheldon, MD, FACP, FCCP
Clinical Professor of Medicine
Loma Linda University
Loma Linda, California
Staff Pulmonologist/Intensivist
Beaver Medical Group, LP
Redlands, California
Medical Director, Respiratory Care Program
Crafton Hills Community College
Yucaipa, California

Susan Jones Krider, RN, MS
Assistant Clinical Professor
School of Nursing
Loma Linda University
Administrative Director
Loma Linda International Heart Institute
Loma Linda University and Medical Center
Loma Linda, California

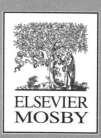

ELSEVIER
MOSBY

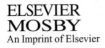

ELSEVIER
MOSBY
An Imprint of Elsevier

11830 Westline Industrial Drive
St. Louis, Missouri 63146

Previous editions copyrighted 1985, 1990, 1995, 2000

International Standard Book Number 0-323-02885-3

Managing Editor: Mindy Hutchinson
Senior Developmental Editor: Melissa K. Boyle
Publishing Services Manager: Melissa Lastarria
Senior Project Manager: Joy Moore
Designer: Paula Ruckenbrod
Seven new illustrations (within Chapters 4 and 5) provided by Stuart Wakefield

Printed in the United States of America.

Last digit is the print number: 9 8 7 6 5 4 3 2 1

To my sister, Dr. Linda Chu,
who has been an inspiration and a great source of
wisdom over the years.

RLW

To Dorothy Sheldon.
She was all a mother should be! And to the new
grandchildren, Riley, Dylan, and the one that is on the way.

RLS

Contributors

Douglas D. Deming, MD
Professor of Pediatrics, Loma Linda University School of
Medicine
Medical Director, ECMO Program
Medical Director, Neonatal Respiratory Care
Loma Linda University Children's Hospital
Loma Linda, California

James R. Dexter, MD, FACP, FCCP
Associate Clinical Professor of Medicine
Loma Linda University
Loma Linda, California
Chairman, Pulmonary, Critical Care and Sleep Medicine
Beaver Medical Group
Redlands, California

Ralph Downey III, PhD
Diplomate, American Board of Sleep Medicine
Director, Loma Linda VA and University Sleep Disorders Center
Associate Professor of Medicine, Pediatrics, and Neurology
Loma Linda University School of Medicine
Loma Linda, California
Adjunct Associate Professor of Psychology
University of California
Riverside, California

Hank Lockridge, RCP, RRT
Assistant Chief Respiratory Therapist
Riverside County Regional Medical Center
Moreno Valley, California

Michael L. Lum, BS, RCP, RRT
Clinical Manager
Department of Respiratory Care
Loma Linda University Medical Center
Loma Linda, California

Judy L. Marcello, RRT, RCP, BA
Pulmonary Lab Coordinator
Beaver Medical Group
Banning, California

Traci L. Marin, MPH, RRT
Training Center Coordinator
Respiratory Therapy Department
Jerry L. Pettis Veteran's Administration Medical Center
Loma Linda, California

Susan L. McInturff, RCP, RRT
Clinical Director
Farrell's Home Health
Bremerton, Washington

Ronald M. Perkin, MD, MA
Professor and Chairman
Department of Pediatrics
Brody School of Medicine at East Carolina University
Greenville, North Carolina

James A. Peters, MD, DrPH, MPH, RD, RRT, LDN, FACPM
President & CEO/Medical Director
Adventist WholeHealth Network
Wyomissing, Pennsylvania

Helen M. Sorenson, MA, RRT, FAARC
Assistant Professor
Department of Respiratory Care
The University of Texas Health Science Center at San Antonio
San Antonio, Texas

Lennard Specht
Assistant Professor
School of Medicine and School of Allied Health Professions
Medical Director, Respiratory Care Program
Loma Linda University
Loma Linda, California

Michael H. Terry, RCP, RRT
Clinical Manager
Department of Respiratory Care
Loma Linda University Adventist Health Sciences Center
Loma Linda, California

Cheryl D. Thomas-Peters, RD, LDN
Practice Administrator/Director of Nutrition
Adventist WholeHealth Network
Wyomissing, Pennsylvania

Reviewers

Steven Bishop, RRT, PhD
Dean of Allied Health
Ozarks Technical Community College
Springfield, Missouri

Regina Clark, MEd, RRT
Respiratory Care Program Director
Northwest Mississippi Community College
Southaven, Mississippi

Lisa M. Johnson, BS, RRT-NPS
Director of Clinical Instruction
Stony Brook University
Stony Brook, New York

Arthur B. Marshak, RRT, RPFT
Director of Clinical Education
Department of Cardiopulmonary Sciences
School of Allied Health Professions
Loma Linda University
Loma Linda, California

Michael R. McCumber, EdD, RRT
Chair, Allied Health
Daytona Beach Community College
Daytona Beach, Florida

J. Kenneth Le Jeune, MS, BSE, RRT, CPFT
Respiratory Education Program Director
University of Arkansas Community College, Hope
Hope, Arkansas

Stanley M. Pearson, RRT, MSEd
Assistant Professor, Respiratory Therapy
Southern Illinois University, Carbondale
Carbondale, Illinois

Preface

The intended audience of this fifth edition is, as in previous editions, respiratory care students. They represent the future providers of respiratory care and they must be skilled at patient assessment to be successful. Practitioners who care for patients with cardiopulmonary disease, such as respiratory therapists, nurses, and physicians will also benefit from reading this text.

The goal of this book continues to be to teach the fundamental and advanced concepts related to assessment of patients with cardiopulmonary disease. This information is critical to master because all patient encounters call for some degree of patient assessment regardless of the setting. The role of respiratory therapists continues to evolve but will always require a keen ability to assess the patient and act accordingly.

The National Board for Respiratory Care (NBRC) puts a major emphasis on patient assessment in both the entry level and advanced practitioner examinations. This fact not only emphasizes the importance of learning patient assessment, but also demands that respiratory care students commit themselves to learning as much as possible in this domain if they are to pass national board examinations. For this reason, this text continues to be a very complete and organized approach to the study of patient assessment.

Those who read and study this text will become more knowledgeable about patient assessment and will be in an ideal position to put these concepts into practice in the clinical setting. This text, however, is no substitute for clinical experience. Actual contact with patients is where the concepts of patient assessment become solidified and the skills described within are developed.

The changes for this fifth edition are numerous. Each chapter has been updated and modified to reflect current medical practice. The chapter on the medical history has now been divided into two chapters: one on interviewing and the medical history, and the other on the symptoms associated with cardiopulmonary disease. The physical examination chapter now includes an overview of evaluating the neurologic system of the patient. While respiratory therapists do not perform detailed examination of the patient's neurologic function, they must understand what the findings indicate and the potential impact on the respiratory system. The clinical laboratory chapter has been heavily revised thanks to the assistance of Dr. James Dexter, a pulmonologist and critical care intensivist in the Southern California area. He did an excellent job of describing how laboratory data are useful in evaluating the patient with lung disease. Many new ECG dysrhythmias and practice strips have been added to the ECG interpretation chapter. The hemodynamic monitoring chapter has been heavily edited, also by Dr. James Dexter, to reflect current practice and to provide a consistent study of arterial pressure, CVP, and pulmonary artery pressure monitoring. Finally, new case studies have been added to many of the chapters to further develop the reader's ability to see how the concepts apply to patient care.

Numerous people come to mind when gratitude is to be expressed related to the completion of this fifth edition. First, we would like to thank the contributors who spent many hours updating their respective chapters. Their expertise is vital to the success of this text. Second, we would like to thank Susan Krider, who did not participate in the current revision because of other obligations, but has spent countless hours in past shaping and writing this book. Her vision of the goals of this book continue to play a key role in making this text what it is. We thank Barbara Parton for secretarial support with this project. Finally, we would like to thank the staff at Elsevier. Melissa Boyle (the developmental editor) and Mindy Hutchison (the managing editor) are committed to excellence and made working on this book enjoyable.

RLW
RLS

Contents

Clinical Assessment in

RESPIRATORY CARE

C H A P T E R

1

Robert L. Wilkins

Preparing for the Patient Encounter

LEARNING OBJECTIVES

Upon completion of this chapter, the reader should be able to accomplish the following:

1. Describe the role of the respiratory therapist in patient assessment.
2. Recognize the purpose(s) of the preinteraction, introductory, initial assessment, treatment and monitoring, and follow-up stages of patient-clinician interaction.
3. Recognize the approximate distances and appropriate activities for proper conduct within the social, personal, and intimate spaces.
4. Recognize the value of the clinician being aware of territoriality.
5. Describe techniques that convey genuine concern during patient-clinician interaction.
6. Describe the general premise of universal precautions and methods by which they are practiced.

CHAPTER OUTLINE

KEY TERMS

diagnostic reasoning	social space
intimate space	territoriality
personal space	

CHAPTER OVERVIEW

The purpose of this chapter is to describe your role as a respiratory therapist (RT) in patient assessment and to help you develop an appropriate bedside manner, which is vitally important to the process of patient assessment. As a bedside clinician, you must be capable of efficient and accurate assessments and must conduct yourself in a professional manner during all patient encounters. This chapter will help you understand some of the important issues related to professionalism at the bedside of patients needing medical care. A professional bedside manner is the foundation on which each assessment and all quality patient care are built.

ROLE OF THE RESPIRATORY THERAPIST IN PATIENT ASSESSMENT

The role of the RT has changed dramatically over the past several decades. Originally, RTs served as equipment technicians who were not expected to evaluate patients or their response to treatment. Today, however, RTs are often called on to assist the physician in the process of diagnostic reasoning (Table 1-1). **Diagnostic reasoning** calls for cognitive skills in communicating, selecting assessment tests, interpreting results, formulating solutions, and evaluating treatment plans. This is known as critical thinking and is a vital part of the modern health care system. All RTs should be able to apply these skills to their daily care of patients with cardiopulmonary disease.

Although the RT does not determine a medical diagnosis, he/she often does help the physician in selected steps of diagnostic reasoning. For example, the patient who suffers from acute dyspnea with exercise may need pulmonary function testing to rule out or identify possible causes. The RT plays a key role in this case and may assist the physician in selecting

Table 1-1	Steps of Diagnostic Reasoning
Steps	**Example**
1. Identify the patient problem(s)	Patient complains of dyspnea
2. Clarify the problem(s)	Dyspnea occurs only during exercise
3. Perform additional assessment procedures	Auscultation reveals wheezing
4. Formulate list of potential causes	Asthma, CHF, bronchitis
5. Obtain specialized test(s)	PFT shows obstructive lung disease
6. Determine potential solution(s)	Bronchodilators before exercise
7. Evaluate solution and monitor patient	Patient states SOB has resolved with bronchodilators

specific tests and in interpreting the results. In addition, the RT is often stationed at the bedside of the hospitalized patient and is in a good position to evaluate his/her response to care. This is particularly true of the ICU patient who is at high risk for complications. For example, the ICU patient who is being mechanically ventilated may suddenly develop acute shortness of breath. The RT must implement his/her patient assessment and critical thinking skills to address the problem. Once potential causes and solutions are identified, the RT should consult with the physician before implementing treatment.

In summary, the role of the RT in patient assessment is important. He/she may be called on to assist the physician in making a diagnosis and must be able to apply assessment and critical thinking skills to acute problems that develop in the hospitalized patient. Critical thinking skills are an important part of the assessment process because they help the RT determine the diagnostic procedures to implement and are needed to make conclusions about the findings.

STAGES OF PATIENT-CLINICIAN INTERACTION

Preinteraction Stage

The majority of patient encounters begin with a review of the patient's chart to identify details such as the name, age, gender, chief complaints, history of present illness (see Chapter 2), and the physician's initial orders. You can use this information when you introduce yourself to the patient and for making an initial assessment of the patient. This stage should take only a few minutes but is well worth the time and effort. Finally, clarify in your mind what your role will be with regard to caring for the patient you are about to encounter.

Introductory Stage

This is the stage in which you enter the patient's room and introduce yourself. Your initial introduction should take place in the social space, which is about 4 to 12 feet from the patient (see later discussion of "Use of Space"). This introduction sets the tone for the rest of the visit. You should introduce yourself by greeting the patient with his/her formal name. This is to be followed by a brief description of the purpose of your visit and your role in caring for the patient during the hospitalization. This type of formal introduction is to be used in most clinical settings. Even the comatose patient unable to respond deserves this type of respect. An exception would be made for the critically ill patient in need of emergency care such as cardiopulmonary resuscitation.

An important part of the introductory phase is the confirmation of patient identification. The most reliable method for verifying the patient identity is to read the identification (ID) bracelet. The patient name and identification number on the bracelet should match the name and number on your paperwork before you begin any formal assessment or treatment.

Before reading the patient's ID bracelet, you should ask the patient for permission to do so. Simply reaching for the ID bracelet may be misinterpreted by the patient and received poorly. It is more appropriate to ask the following question: "May I look at your ID bracelet to make sure I am working with the correct patient?" This conveys to the patient that you respect his/her privacy and you are committed to providing quality patient care.

Many clinicians take a two-step approach to verifying patient identity in the conscious patient. The first step is to use the patient's name and monitor the response. For example, you walk into the room of a patient you believe to be Mr. Carter and begin by saying, "Good morning. Are you Mr. Carter?" If he responds with "Good morning. Yes I am," you have some evidence that he is probably Mr. Carter. This step should supplement and never replace reading the patient's identification bracelet (step 2).

The introductory stage is important in establishing a rapport between you and the patient. A positive rapport is necessary to obtain the patient's cooperation with assessment and treatment procedures. Patients usually appreciate and respond positively to a warm, friendly introduction done in a professional manner. Be careful to avoid overly friendly or jovial statements because they may be irritating to those patients who are depressed or upset as a result of their illness. For example, stating "Isn't it a wonderful day?" to a patient dying from lung cancer is likely to be received poorly. Be friendly, but avoid extremes.

During the introductory phase, look for signs of resistive behavior in the patient. This may be seen as crossed arms, refusal to make eye contact, or very brief responses to your questions. These responses represent clues that the patient is not likely to be cooperative or accepting of your suggestions and may not be listening carefully to your questions and instructions. In such cases you will need to make an extra effort to establish a rapport with the patient and improve communication. Other techniques for establishing a rapport and demonstrating genuine concern are discussed later in this chapter.

Initial Assessment Stage

This stage actually overlaps with the introductory stage because you can easily begin visual inspection of the patient during your introduction. Take time to note the patient's general appearance, attitudes, and responses to your statements and questions as mentioned previously. Formal assessment of the patient with a brief interview regarding chief complaints at admission can now take place (see Chapter 2). The interview is followed in most cases by a brief physical examination to determine the pretreatment status of the patient (see Chapters 4 and 5). Your goal at this point is to determine the condition of the patient and to make sure the prescribed treatment ordered by the physician is appropriate. Occasionally, you may evaluate the patient whose condition has abruptly changed recently and who is now in need of different treatment. In fact, the prescribed treatment may be contraindicated. If you skip the initial assessment stage, you will be blindly following orders that may result in inappropriate and possibly harmful treatment. Contacting the head nurse and the attending physician is necessary when your initial assessment reveals a need for different treatment.

Treatment and Monitoring Stage

After your initial assessment of the patient, you are now ready to administer treatment. During the treatment stage you will need to continue to use your assessment skills to evaluate the effects of the treatment. Occasionally the patient may develop side effects from the treatment, or the therapy may not result in the expected beneficial response. Your ability to identify and document the positive and negative effects of the therapy is crucial to the patient's care. Therapy should be stopped immediately when side effects occur. The respiratory care supervisor, head nurse, and attending physician need to be notified in such cases.

Follow-up Stage

You should take a minute to communicate with the patient once the treatment or bedside procedure is completed. Note any changes in symptoms, attitudes, alertness, and so forth, and document your findings. Let the patient know when you will return and how to contact you if the need arises. Make sure the patient is as comfortable as possible and ask if there is anything you can do to help the patient before exiting the room. This brief stage is useful in developing your rapport with the patient and in building a positive attitude in the patient toward you and your employer.

COMMUNICATING THE ASSESSMENT FINDINGS

After most interactions with the patient you will need to communicate your findings to other members of the health care team. Written documentation in the patient's chart may be sufficient communication if the patient is stable following routine treatment. Verbal communication is also needed when the patient's condition has deteriorated or when the procedure was not tolerated well. You should communicate your findings to the patient's nurse and physician in such circumstances, in addition to writing your findings in the patient's chart. Documentation in the chart should include specific findings as well as the details of who was notified about the patient's change in condition (see Chapter 20).

For example, you enter the room of Mr. Jones to provide treatment for his asthma. On entering the room you note that he appears much more short of breath than usual and his vital signs have deteriorated significantly. The treatment you give him does not seem to be helping. It is imperative that you document and communicate your findings. Verbal discussion with the patient's nurse is a good place to start. Paging the patient's physician to notify him/her of the change in Mr. Jones' condition is also appropriate in such cases. Next you must document the patient's condition in his chart and note who you communicated with about the patient and what was said. If you perceive that the patient's condition is serious, stay with him/her and use your diagnostic reasoning and assessment skills to evaluate the problem and develop potential solutions.

USE OF SPACE

An important, but often overlooked, issue related to interaction with patients is the appropriate use of the space surrounding each patient. Proper use of the three zones described next adds to the professionalism of all bedside clinicians.

Social Space

The social space (4 to 12 feet) is useful for your introduction to the patient and is where you begin to establish rapport (Figure 1-1). At this distance you can see the "big picture" and gain an appreciation for the whole patient and his/her environment. Vocalizations are limited to the more formal issues, and personal questions are to be avoided in this space because others in the room can easily overhear the conversation.

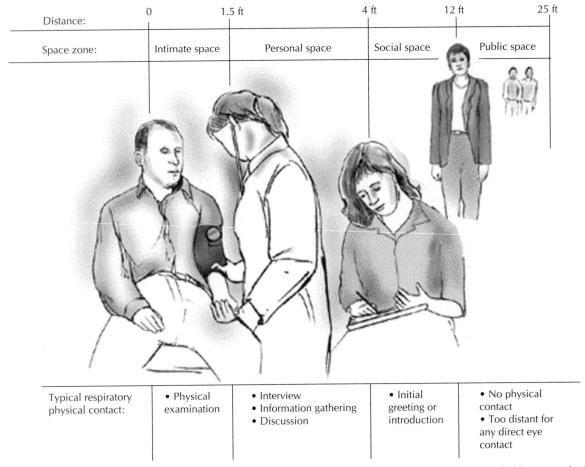

Distance:	0	1.5 ft		4 ft	12 ft	25 ft
Space zone:	Intimate space	Personal space		Social space		Public space

Typical respiratory physical contact:	• Physical examination	• Interview • Information gathering • Discussion	• Initial greeting or introduction	• No physical contact • Too distant for any direct eye contact

Figure 1-1 Illustration of the social, personal, and intimate spaces of the patient needing health care. (From Wilkins RL, Sheldon RL, Krider SJ: Clinical assessment in respiratory care; as redrawn in Hess DR, et al: *Respiratory care: principles and practice,* Philadelphia, 2002, Saunders.)

Personal Space

The personal space (18 inches to 4 feet) is most useful for the interview, especially when more personal questions are to be asked. For example, some patients are uncomfortable when answering questions about their daily sputum production or smoking habits. Answers to such personal questions are more likely to be accurate and detailed when the questions are asked from the personal space. In addition, providing privacy by pulling the bedside curtain may be useful in making the patient feel more comfortable about answering questions. The personal space is best entered only after a rapport with the patient has been established in the social space previously described.

The interview is not only useful for gathering information but also for further development of the rapport between you and the patient. The rapport you have with the patient becomes more important when you invade his/her intimate space, as described below, and when you begin therapeutic procedures. Attention to details regarding your professional appearance is important in the personal space. The patient will often feel more comfortable and confident with you if your appearance is neat, clean, and professional. Appropriate use of eye contact is needed in the personal space, since this will increase the patient's trust in you. (See Figure 1-1.)

Intimate Space

In most cases invasion of the intimate space (0 to 18 inches) is done only after your introduction in the social space and brief interview in the personal space. These initial steps in establishing a rapport with the patient make invasion of the patient's intimate space more comfortable for both of you. In addition, invasion of the intimate space should be preceded by a request for permission to do so. This communicates your respect for the patient as a person and also lets the patient know that he/she has a say in the medical care provided. Permission to invade the patient's intimate space is often obtained simply by requesting permission to listen to breath sounds or check vital signs.

The intimate space is reserved primarily for physical examination of the patient and for therapeutic procedures. Minimal or no eye contact is used in this space. Verbal communication with the patient should be limited to simple questions or brief commands such as, "Please take a deep breath."

Invasion of the patient's intimate space is often met with a variety of responses. Gender, age, race, physical appearance, health status, and cultural background represent a few of the many factors that may influence the comfort level of the patient when you enter the intimate space. Be aware that some patients may respond poorly to your invasion of their space and be prepared to move more slowly and communicate very carefully in such cases.

SIMPLY STATED

The social zone (4 to 12 feet) is for introductions, the personal space (18 inches to 4 feet) for interviewing, and the intimate space (0 to 18 inches) for physical examination.

TERRITORIALITY

Most patients "lay claim" to all items within a certain boundary around their bed. For patients in a private room the boundary will extend to the walls of the room. Removing items from the patient's "territory" should occur only after permission has been obtained. For example, when borrowing a chair from the bedside of Mr. Jones for use at the bedside of Mr. Smith, you should ask Mr. Jones for permission. Although technically the majority of bedside items are owned by the hospital, they temporarily "belong" to the patient while he/she is hospitalized. Being aware of the territoriality issue will improve your bedside manner and may avoid upsetting a patient.

CONFIDENTIALITY

While reviewing the patient's chart and conducting the interview, you will learn about the patient's current and past medical history. This information is private and not for public knowledge. Perhaps the patient has a history of alcohol or drug abuse or has been diagnosed with a sexually transmitted disease. You are responsible for respecting the patient's right to privacy by not sharing such assessment information with others who are not in a position of needing to know the patient's medical history. Violations of patient confidentiality are unethical and may be subject to legal recourse. Most often, violations of patient confidentiality occur in the hospital elevator or cafeteria when a clinician discusses a certain patient with other clinicians while being overheard by visitors. A good rule to follow is to discuss your patient's health status only with other members of the health care team who need to know such information and only in a private report room where visitors are not allowed (Box 1-1). Family members and visitors often ask questions about the patient's diagnosis but should be referred to the attending physician in all cases. This should be done in a way that does not alarm or offend the person asking about your patient. Most people will understand and appreciate an honest response in which you inform them that it is against hospital policy for you to discuss the patient's diagnosis with others.

EXPRESSING GENUINE CONCERN

Working in a hospital setting requires a sincere demonstration of concern or empathy toward your patients. Phony attempts at empathy are easily detected by patients and usually have a very negative effect on the patient's attitude. Expressing empathy can be awkward for some clinicians, especially when they are new to the hospital setting. For this reason several general techniques for expressing genuine concern are listed below. Use them only when you feel comfortable with the technique described. The list represents just a few of the more commonly used techniques. You may discover other techniques by watching more experienced clinicians. Learning to use any of the techniques associated with demonstrating empathy will require practice to become more effective.

Face the Patient Squarely

This simple maneuver, used during all conversations with the patient, tells the patient that he/she has your undivided attention. It suggests that you are interested in what the patient has to say and allows you to better visualize the patient.

Use Eye Contact Appropriately

This represents one of the most important and powerful techniques for demonstrating true concern for the patient. Appropriate use of eye contact conveys your interest in the patient and in his/her comments. Eye contact is particularly important when the patient is speaking to you and when you are asking questions of the patient. Equally important is the avoidance of extremes with eye contact. For example, staring at the patient or out the window during conversation is inappropriate. Looking out the window while the patient is speaking sends a message to the patient that you are not interested in what he/she has to say.

Maintain an Open Posture

An open posture means sitting or standing in a relaxed manner with your arms at your side. This relaxed position creates a more comfortable setting for the patient and represents nonverbal communication that says you accept the patient and want to help. Sitting or standing with your arms crossed sends a signal of unacceptance.

Consider Appropriate Use of Touch

Touch can also be a powerful tool for communicating genuine concern to the patient. It is, however, the most difficult technique to use appropriately. Touch to communicate empathy should only be used in those patients with whom you have established a solid rapport. Even then its use should be reserved for those patients in whom you feel it will be received positively.

Only certain sites on the patient are acceptable for you to touch as an empathic gesture. The patient's hands, arms, or shoulders are acceptable sites for most patients. For example, a gentle pat or squeeze of the patient's shoulder or hand just before exiting the room while reassuring the patient you will return later is an effective way to communicate genuine empathy. Keep in mind that cultural background, gender, age, and so forth are factors that may influence how receptive a patient will be to the use of touch. If you sense that your patient is

BOX 1-1	Ten Golden Rules of Clinical Etiquette

1. **Maintain a professional appearance whenever you come into contact with patients or their families.**
   Dress codes vary among hospitals, clinics, and home care services and also according to the clinician's role. However, whether appropriate dress includes a white laboratory coat, conventional business wear, or a scrub suit, it (and the person in it) should be clean and reasonably neat.
2. **Identify yourself—not only by name but also by role.**
   Always wear a name tag when dealing with patients and explain why you are there. Attending physicians, residents, students, respiratory therapists, nurses, and others use the same medical terms and may dress similarly. Patients may assume that anyone in hospital dress is a doctor, and there can be serious medical, psychological, and even legal consequences if misconceptions are not corrected.
3. **Do not call adult patients by their first names.**
   What may be intended as a means of "breaking the ice" and establishing rapport is perceived by many patients as condescending and insulting. In general, patients older than high school age should be called "Ms," "Miss," "Mrs," or "Mr." Use of a patient's first name requires that person's permission, would generally be considered only after numerous contacts, and would seldom be appropriate on a first encounter.
4. **Respect and preserve the patient's modesty.**
   Draw the curtains. Do not uncover the patient in view of visitors or other patients. Remember that boys and men are often as modest as girls and women.
5. **Do not rest your foot on the bed frame or sit on the patient's bed without permission.**
   Hospitalization renders patients vulnerable in many ways, and such uninvited invasions of their "territory" may cause unnecessary distress.
6. **Do not talk about patients in the elevator (or in the hallways, in the cafeteria, on a bus, or in other public places).**
   Being a health professional allows one access to privileged, personal information that should not be shared, intentionally or unintentionally, with anyone not directly caring for the patient. Offhand remarks heard by family members in the elevator can cause great distress and interfere with clinician-patient relationships. Inappropriate use of such information is not only unethical, but also against the law.
7. **Do not discuss prognosis or other sensitive issues with others in front of the patient.**
   Patients may misinterpret snatches of conversation, or think remarks about another patient apply to them. Such terms as "death," "terminal," and "cancer" are especially upsetting and should be avoided around patients.
8. **Do not argue in front of the patient.**
   Differences of opinion and disciplinary actions should take place well out of patients' earshot. Displays of anger have no place in patient care areas.
9. **Do not criticize the actions of other members of the health care team with or within earshot of the patient.**
   You may not agree with Dr. so-and-so's diagnosis or treatment plan, but to voice this disagreement in front of the patient or family members is harmful to clinician-patient relationships and, indirectly, to the team's effectiveness.
10. **Keep disagreements and criticism out of the patient's chart.**
    Such things should be dealt with one-on-one, in person, and not in the permanent (legal) record.

From Pierson DJ, Kacmarek RM: *Foundations of respiratory care*, New York, 1992, Churchill Livingstone.

demonstrating verbal or nonverbal signs of resistive behavior, touch is probably not likely to be well received.

Be an Active Listener

Listening carefully to what the patient has to say is another technique that communicates true concern. Clues that you are not listening carefully are often demonstrated by repeating questions that you asked just minutes ago or by lack of eye contact when the patient is making statements or asking questions. If the patient senses that you are not listening carefully, you are not likely to get his/her attention when you need it and the patient's responses to your questions will become progressively briefer. In addition, patients often

interpret poor listening as a general lack of concern for their well-being. Active listening takes practice to become proficient. Good eye contact, asking for clarification on certain points, and brief note-taking demonstrate active listening. Active listening can lead to more accurate assessments when all details are noted.

> **SIMPLY STATED**
> Expressing genuine concern for your patient is an important aspect of patient care and is done through the proper use of eye contact, posture, touch, and active listening.

UNIVERSAL PRECAUTIONS

The Centers for Disease Control and Prevention (CDC) (www.cdc.gov) recommends that all clinicians who may come into contact with the body fluids of their patients wear protective gear. This recommendation is based on the fact that it is often not clear which patients are infected with transmittable diseases. As a result, the term *universal precautions* is used for the precautionary measures that clinicians should take to protect themselves against possible exposure to the body fluids of patients.

The assessment process often calls for bedside clinicians to draw blood from the patient or to obtain sputum samples for analysis. Rubber gloves are needed in all situations in which you may contact the blood, saliva, or sputum of your patient. In addition, if splashes or airborne droplets of the patient's body fluids are a possibility, masks and protective eyewear are needed.

Accidental needle sticks with a contaminated needle represent one of the most common ways in which health care workers are exposed to transmissible diseases. For this reason all hospital and clinic workers must be extra careful when handling used needles. Needles should not be recapped, manipulated, or removed from the syringe after use on a patient. Used needles must be discarded into appropriate puncture-resistant containers usually located in all patient care areas. Thorough hand washing before and after each patient contact is equally important in reducing the incidence of transmissible diseases.

REVIEW QUESTIONS

1. The role of the respiratory therapist in patient assessment includes all the following *except*:
   a. Helping the physician select appropriate pulmonary function tests for a specific patient.
   b. Interviewing the patient with dyspnea to determine the effects of treatment.
   c. Interviewing and examining the patient to make a medical diagnosis.
   d. Assisting the physician in interpretation of an arterial blood gas.

2. The preinteraction stage is useful in which of the following ways?
   a. To determine the effect of the therapy
   b. For clarifying the patient's history and your role in the therapy
   c. For establishing rapport with the patient
   d. To allow the patient to evaluate the clinician's abilities

3. What is the appropriate distance of the social space?
   a. 0–18 inches
   b. 18 inches– 4 feet
   c. 4 –12 feet
   d. 6 –18 feet

4. In which of the following spaces is patient introduction properly performed?
   a. Social
   b. Personal
   c. Intimate
   d. All of the above

5. In which of the following spaces is the interview properly performed?
   a. Social
   b. Personal
   c. Intimate
   d. All of the above

6. T   F   Eye contact is appropriate in the intimate space during patient-clinician interaction.

7. In which of the following spaces is rapport best established?
   a. Social
   b. Personal
   c. Intimate
   d. a and b

8. T   F   A clinician who, during the patient encounter, stands with his arms crossed and avoids eye contact is conveying a lack of concern for the patient.

9. Which of the following is useful to express genuine concern for the patient?
   a. Appropriate eye contact
   b. Use of touch
   c. Maintaining an open posture
   d. All of the above

10. T   F   Asking for permission to use an article within the patient's room acknowledges the patient's territorial rights while conveying respect for the patient.

11. T   F   The practice of universal precautions presumes that all patients are potentially infective.

12. Which of the following pieces of personal protective equipment is required when splattering of blood or other body fluids is likely?
    a. Gown
    b. Gloves
    c. Eye shield
    d. All the above

BIBLIOGRAPHY

Barkauskas VH, Stoltenberg-Allen K, Baumann LC, Darling-Fisher C: *Health and physical assessment*, ed 2, St Louis, 1998, Mosby.

Elkin MK, Perry AG, Potter PA: *Nursing interventions and clinical skills*, ed 3, St Louis, 2004, Mosby.

Pierson DJ, Wilkins RL: Clinical skills in respiratory care. In Pierson DJ, Kacmarek RM, editors: *Foundations of respiratory care*, New York, 1992, Churchill Livingstone.

Potter PA, Perry AG: *Fundamentals of nursing*, ed 5, St Louis, 2001, Mosby.

Wilkins RL, Stoller JK, Scanlan C: *Egan's fundamentals of respiratory care*, ed 8, St Louis, 2004, Mosby.

The Medical History and the Interview

LEARNING OBJECTIVES

Upon completion of this chapter, the reader should be able to accomplish the following:

1. Describe the importance of properly obtaining and recording a patient history.
2. Recognize factors that can influence communication between the patient and clinician during the interview.
3. Describe techniques for structuring the interview.
4. Describe the techniques used to facilitate conversational interviewing.
5. Recognize alternative sources that are available for the patient history.
6. Recognize the difference between objective and subjective data.
7. Recognize the components of a complete health history and the type of information found in each section of the history.

CHAPTER OUTLINE

Patient Interview
 Principles of Communication
 Structuring the Interview
 Questions and Statements Used to Facilitate
 Conversational Interviewing
 Alternative Sources for a Patient History
**Cardiopulmonary History and Comprehensive
 Health History**
 Variations in Health Histories
 General Content of Health Histories
 Review of Systems
 Chief Complaint
 History of Present Illness
 Past History
 Family History
 Occupational and Environmental History
**Assessment Standards for Patients with
 Pulmonary Dysfunction**

Susan Jones Krider, RN, MS, contributed this chapter in the previous edition.

KEY TERMS

objective data
pack years
pertinent negative
pertinent positive

signs
subjective data
symptoms

CHAPTER OVERVIEW

The history is the foundation of comprehensive assessment. It is a written picture of the patient's perception of his/her past and present health status and how health problems have affected both personal and family lifestyle. Properly recorded, it provides an organized, unbiased, detailed, and chronologic description of the development of symptoms that caused the patient to seek health care. The history guides the rest of the assessment process: physical examination, x-ray and laboratory studies, and special diagnostic procedures. When skillfully obtained, the history often provides sufficient information for an accurate diagnosis. It has been said that at least 75% of the time an accurate diagnosis can be made after the history has been obtained and before the physical examination begins.

Traditionally, the task of obtaining a patient's complete history has belonged to the physician, and only sections of the history were taken by other members of the health care team. Today, however, complete health histories are taken by nurses and physician assistants. Physical therapists, social workers, dietitians, and respiratory therapists working in rehabilitation, home care, or pulmonary function laboratories complete histories, placing emphasis on information pertaining to their specialty.

Regardless of whether a student or clinician is expected to obtain and write a comprehensive history, each must be able to locate and interpret historical information recorded in the patient's medical record. The information is used with other assessment data to develop or alter a plan of care. In addition, obtaining subjective data—those which the patient reports, feels, or experiences that cannot be perceived by an observer—is an important part of assessing the effects of therapeutic intervention. Those involved in direct patient care obtain subjective data from patients each day through interview and general conversation. The same techniques are used to identify, clarify, and communicate subjective and historical information.

This chapter highlights interviewing principles and the types of questions used in history taking and describes the content of the comprehensive health history, emphasizing specific information needed for assessment of the patient with cardiopulmonary complaints. Chapter 3 discusses the most common cardiopulmonary symptoms.

PATIENT INTERVIEW

Principles of Communication

Communication is a process of imparting a meaningful message. If the receiver does not understand the message, communication has not occurred. Multiple personal and environmental factors affect the way both patients and health care professionals send and receive messages. Figure 2-1 shows the multiple factors that can influence communication during an interview. Attention to the potential effects each of these components may have on communication makes the difference between an effective and an ineffective interview.

Each person brings to an interchange with another individual attitudes and values developed by previous experiences, cultural heritage, religious beliefs, level of education, and self-concept. These internal forces alter the way a message is sent as well as the interpretation of an incoming message. Messages can be sent in a variety of ways and at times without awareness. Body movement, facial expression, touch, and eye movement are all types of *nonverbal communication.* Combined with voice tone, body language (nonverbal communication) frequently says more than words. Since one of the purposes of the interview is to establish a trusting relationship (rapport) with the patient, the interviewer must make a conscious effort to send signals of compassion, empathy, and professionalism.

Messages are also altered by feelings, language barriers (jargon as well as foreign languages), listening habits, comfort with the situation, and preoccupation. Patients experiencing pain or difficulty breathing have a hard time concentrating on the content of an interview until their comfort is restored. The temperature, lighting, noise, and privacy of the environment, to say nothing of the patient's attire (or lack thereof), also contribute greatly to comfort. Patients may communicate their discomfort nonverbally. Sighing, restlessness, looking into space, and avoiding eye contact may be clues that the patient is experiencing physical or psychological discomfort. In one case, a trip to the bathroom may allow communication to be reestablished; in another, changing the current topic of the interview may solve the problem.

One of the most common mistakes made by the interviewer is failing to listen carefully to the patient's answers and questions. Good listening skills require concentration on the task at hand and appropriate eye contact with the patient. Active listening also calls for responding to the patient's comments and questions with appropriate responses that come only with

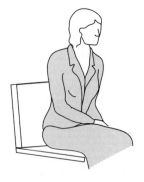

INTERNAL FACTORS

Previous experiences
Attitudes, values
Cultural heritage
Religious beliefs
Self-concept
Listening habits
Preoccupations, feelings

SENSORY/EMOTIONAL FACTORS

Fear
Stress, anxiety
Pain
Mental acuity, brain damage, hypoxia
Sight, hearing, speech impairment

ENVIRONMENTAL FACTORS

Lighting
Noise
Privacy
Distance
Temperature

VERBAL EXPRESSION

Language barrier
Jargon
Choice of words/questions
Feedback, voice tone

NONVERBAL EXPRESSION

Body movement
Facial expression
Dress, professionalism
Warmth, interest

INTERNAL FACTORS

Previous experiences
Attitudes, values
Cultural heritage
Religious beliefs
Self-concept
Listening habits
Preoccupations, feelings
Illness

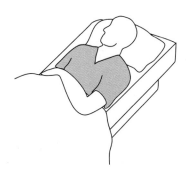

Figure 2-1 Factors that influence communication.

good listening. Patients are quick to identify the interviewer who is not listening and will often interpret this as a lack of empathy.

Structuring the Interview

The ideal interview, whether a 5-minute assessment of therapy or a 50-minute history, is one in which the patient feels secure and free to talk about important personal things. Interviewing is an art that takes time and experience to develop. It is a skill as useful in daily patient care as it is to the person obtaining a comprehensive history. Keeping the following points in mind facilitates an effective interaction with the patient.

1. Your ability to project a sense of undivided interest in the patient is the key to a successful interview and patient rapport.
    *   Review records or new information and prepare equipment and charting materials before entering the room.
    *   Provide for privacy. Don't permit interruptions.
    *   Listen and observe carefully. Avoid worrying about what to say next while the patient is talking. Rather, be attentive and respond to the patient's priorities, concerns, feelings, and comfort.
2. Your introduction establishes your professional role, asks permission to be involved in the patient's care, and conveys your interest in the patient.
    *   Dress and groom professionally.
    *   Enter with a smile and an unhurried manner.
    *   Make immediate eye contact and, if the patient is well enough, introduce yourself with a firm handshake.
    *   State your role and the purpose of your visit, and define the patient's involvement in the interaction.
    *   Call the patient by name. A person's name is one of the most important things in the world to that person; use it to identify the patient and establish the fact that you are concerned with the patient as an individual. Address adult patients by title—Mr., Mrs., Miss, or Ms.—and their last name. Occasionally patients will ask to be called by their first name or nickname, but that is the patient's choice and not an assumption to be made by the health care professional. Keep in mind that by using the more formal terms of address you alert the patient to the importance of the interaction.
3. Professional conduct shows your respect for the patient's beliefs, attitudes, and rights and enhances patient rapport.
    *   Be sure the patient is appropriately covered.
    *   Position yourself so that eye contact is comfortable for the patient. Ideally, patients should be sitting up with their eye level at or slightly above yours, which suggests that their opinion is important too. Avoid positions that require the patient to look directly into the light.
    *   Avoid standing at the foot of the bed or with your hand on the door while you talk with the patient. This may send the nonverbal message that you do not have time for the patient.
    *   Ask the patient's permission before moving any personal items or making adjustments in the room (see Chapter 1).
    *   Remember, the patient's dialogue with you and the medical record are *confidential*. The patient expects, and the law demands, that this information be shared only with other professionals directly involved in the patient's care. When a case is discussed for teaching purposes, the patient's identity should be protected.
    *   Be honest. Never guess at an answer or information you do not know. Remember too that you have neither the obligation nor the right to provide information beyond your scope of practice. Providing new information to the patient is the privilege and responsibility of the attending physician.
    *   Make no moral judgments about the patient. Set your values for patient care according to the patient's values, beliefs, and priorities. Belittling or laughing at a patient for any reason is unprofessional and intolerable.
    *   Expect a patient to have an emotional response toward illness and the health care environment and accept that response. *Listen,* then clarify and teach, but *never argue.* If you are not prepared to explore the issues with the patient, contact someone who is.
    *   Adjust the time, length, and content of the interaction to your patient's needs. If the patient is in distress, obtain only the information necessary to clarify immediate needs. It may be necessary to repeat some questions again later, to schedule several short interviews, or to obtain the information from other sources.
4. A relaxed, conversational style on the part of the health care professional with questions and statements that communicate empathy encourages patients to express their concerns.
    *   Expect and accept some periods of silence in a long or first interview. Both you and the patient need short periods to think out the correct responses.
    *   Close even the briefest interview by asking if there is anything else the patient needs or wants to discuss and tell the patient when you will return.

SIMPLY STATED

A patient interview, whether a short assessment of therapy or an extended history, must allow the patient to feel secure and free to discuss personal things.
*   Dress and act professionally.
*   Project a sense of undivided interest.
*   Use a relaxed conversational style.
*   Respect the patient's beliefs and attitudes.
*   Remember, the patient's conversation with you and the medical record are confidential.

Questions and Statements Used to Facilitate Conversational Interviewing

An interview made up of one direct question followed by an answer and another direct question is mechanical, monotonous, and anxiety producing. This type of interview usually takes longer and acquires less pertinent information than a conversational interview; however, it is a characteristic pattern for people who are anxious about interviewing. A rambling discussion is also inefficient and frustrating. Using a conversational style by mixing the types of questions and responses described below encourages spontaneous descriptions by the patient while giving enough direction to clarify, quantify, and qualify details.

1. *Open-ended questions* encourage patients to describe events and priorities as they see them and thereby help bring out concerns and attitudes and promote understanding. Questions such as "What brought you to the hospital?" or "What happened next?" encourage conversational flow and rapport while giving patients enough direction to know where to start.

2. *Closed questions* such as "When did your cough start?" or "How long did the pain last?" focus on specific information and provide clarification.

3. *Direct questions* can be either open-ended or closed questions and always end in a question mark. Although they are used to obtain specific information, a series of direct questions or frequent use of the word "Why?" can sound intimidating.

4. *Indirect questions* are less threatening because they sound like statements: "I gather your doctor told you to take the breathing treatments every 4 hours." Inquiries of this type also work well to confront discrepancies in the patient's statements: "If I understood you correctly, it is harder for you to breathe now than it was before your treatment."

5. *Neutral questions and statements* are preferred for all interactions with the patient. "What happened next?" and "Tell me more about . . ." are neutral open-ended questions. A neutral closed question might give a patient a choice of responses while focusing on the type of information desired: "Would you say there was a teaspoon, a tablespoon, or a half cup?" By contrast, leading questions such as "You didn't cough up blood, did you?" should be avoided because they imply a desired response.

6. *Reflecting (echoing)* is repeating words, thoughts, or feelings the patient has just stated and is a successful way to clarify and stimulate the patient to elaborate on a particular point. However, overuse of reflecting can make the interviewer sound like a parrot.

7. *Facilitating phrases* like "yes" or "umm" or "I see," used while establishing eye contact and perhaps nodding your head, show interest and encourage patients to continue their story, but this type of phrase should not be overused.

8. *Communicating empathy (support)* with statements like "That must have been very hard for you" shows your concern for the patient as a human being. Showing the patient that you really care about how life situations have caused stress, hurt, or happiness tells the patient it is safe to risk being honest about real concerns. Other techniques for showing empathy were described in Chapter 1.

Alternative Sources for a Patient History

Various factors affect the patient's ability or willingness to provide an accurate history. Age, alterations in level of consciousness, language and cultural barriers, emotional state, ability to breathe comfortably, and the acuteness of the disease process may alter a patient's ability to communicate. For instance, the patient suffering an acute asthma attack or someone just admitted to an intensive care unit may be unable to give even the most brief history. Patients with long-standing chronic disease may have become so accustomed to the accompanying symptoms or their lives may have changed so gradually that they may minimize and even deny symptoms. In such cases family members, friends, work associates, previous physicians, and past medical records often can provide a more accurate picture of the history and progression of symptoms. Keeping these possibilities in mind, most hospital histories begin with a one- or two-sentence description of the current state of the patient, the source of the history, and a statement of the estimated reliability of the historian.

CARDIOPULMONARY HISTORY AND COMPREHENSIVE HEALTH HISTORY

Abnormalities of the respiratory system are frequently manifestations of other systemic disease processes. In addition, alterations in pulmonary function may affect other body systems. Therefore cardiopulmonary assessment cannot be limited to the chest; a comprehensive evaluation of the patient's entire health status is essential. A detailed discussion of all aspects of obtaining and recording such a health history is beyond the scope of this text but has been well covered by other authors (see the Bibliography list at the end of this chapter). This section provides an overview of the content of complete health histories and discusses specifically (in their classic order) chief complaint, history of present illness, past history, family history, and occupational and environmental history.

Variations in Health Histories

Health (medical) histories vary in length, organization, and content depending on the preparation and experience of the interviewer, the patient's age, the reason for obtaining the history, and the circumstances surrounding the visit or admission. A history taken for a 60-year-old person complaining of chronic and debilitating symptoms is much more detailed and complex than that obtained for a summer camp applicant or a school physical. Histories recorded in emergency situations are usually limited to describing events surrounding the patient's immediate condition, with hours and sometimes days before a name, much less a complete history, can be obtained. Nursing histories emphasize the effect of the symptoms on activities of daily living and the identification of the unique care, teaching, and emotional support needs of the patient and family. Histories performed by physicians emphasize making a diagnosis. Since diagnosis and initial treatment may be done before there is time to dictate or record the history, the experienced physician may record data obtained from a combination of the history, physical examination, laboratory tests, and x-ray films rather than the more traditional history outlined in Box 2-1.

General Content of Health Histories

Although variations in recording styles do exist, all histories contain the same types of information.

BOX 2-1   Outline of a Complete Health History

1. **Demographic data** (usually found on first page of chart)
   Name, address, age, birth date, birth place, race, nationality, marital status, religion, occupation, source of referral
2. **Date and source of history,** estimate of reliability of historian
3. **Brief description of patient's condition at time of history or patient profile**
4. **Chief complaint:** reason for seeking health care
5. **History of present illness** (chronologic description of each symptom):
   Onset: time, type, source, setting
   Frequency and duration
   Location and radiation
   Severity (quantity)
   Quality (character)
   Aggravating/alleviating factors
   Associated manifestations
6. **Past history or past medical history**
   Childhood diseases and development
   Hospitalizations, surgeries, injuries, accidents, major illnesses
   Allergies
   Drugs and medications
   Immunizations
   Habits
   General health and sources of previous health care
7. **Family history**
   Familial disease history
   Family history
   Marital history
   Family relationships
8. **Social and environmental history**
   Education
   Military experience
   Occupational history
   Religious and social activities
   Living arrangements
   Hobbies and recreation
   Satisfaction/stress with life situation, finances, relationships
   Recent travel or other event that might affect health
9. **Review of systems** (Figure 2-2)
10. **Signature**

- General background information
- Screening information
- Descriptions of present health status or illness

Background Information

Background information tells the interviewer who the patient is and what types of diseases are likely to develop. It also provides a basic understanding of the patient's previous experiences with illness and health care and the patient's current life situation, including the effect of culture, attitudes, relationships, and finances on health. Knowing the level of education, patterns of health-related learning, past health care practices, and reasons for compliance or noncompliance with past courses of therapy gives insight into patients' ability to comprehend their current health status. This may predict their willingness or ability to participate in learning and therapy. From the free discussion used to obtain background information, the interviewer may also get clues about patients' reliability and possible psychosocial implications of their disease.

Screening Information

Screening information is designed to uncover problem areas the patient forgot to mention or omitted. This information is classically obtained by a head-to-toe review of all body systems but may also be obtained by a review of common diseases or from a description of body functions.

Description of Present Health Status or Illness

This is included in even the briefest histories. Chief Complaint (CC) and History of Present Illness (HPI) are the most commonly used headings, although, Reason for Visit and Current Health Status may be seen in some outpatient records. Since this is the information that most concerns the patient, the interview and recording of the history begins with this information.

Review of Systems

Review of systems (ROS) is a recording of past and present information that may be relevant to the present problem but might otherwise have been overlooked. It is grouped by body or physiologic systems to guarantee completeness and to assist the examiner in arriving at a diagnosis. Figure 2-2 is an example of a review of systems checklist that may be completed by a patient before an interview or by an examiner. It provides for recording both positive and negative responses so that when the documentation is later reviewed, there is no doubt as to which questions were asked. Negative responses to important questions asked at any time during the interview are termed pertinent negatives; affirmative responses are termed pertinent positives.

Experienced examiners usually elicit the review of systems information in conjunction with the system-by-system physical

Have you recently had the following? (Circle "yes" or "no"; if in doubt, leave blank)

General

Tire easily, weakness	yes	no
Marked weight change	yes	no
Night sweats	yes	no
Persistent fever	yes	no
Sensitivity to heat	yes	no
Sensitivity to cold	yes	no

Skin

Eruptions (rash)	yes	no
Change in color	yes	no
Change in hair	yes	no
Change in fingernails	yes	no

Eyes

Trouble seeing	yes	no
Eye pain	yes	no
Inflamed eyes	yes	no
Double vision	yes	no
Wear corrective lenses	yes	no

Ears

Loss of hearing	yes	no
Ringing in ears	yes	no
Discharge	yes	no

Nose

Loss of smell	yes	no
Frequent colds	yes	no
Obstruction	yes	no
Excess drainage	yes	no
Nosebleeds	yes	no

Mouth

Sore gums	yes	no
Soreness of tongue	yes	no
Dental problems	yes	no

Throat

Postnasal drainage	yes	no
Soreness	yes	no
Hoarseness	yes	no

Breasts

Lumps	yes	no
Discharge	yes	no

Cardiorespiratory system

Cough, persistent	yes	no
Sputum (phlegm)	yes	no
Bloody sputum	yes	no
Wheezing	yes	no
Chest pain or discomfort	yes	no
Pain on breathing	yes	no
Shortness of breath	yes	no
Difficulty breathing while lying down	yes	no
Swelling of ankles	yes	no
Bluish fingers or lips	yes	no
High blood pressure	yes	no
Palpitations	yes	no
Vein trouble	yes	no

Digestive system

List average food selection each meal
Breakfast:

Lunch:

Dinner:

Digestive system (cont.)

Change in appetite	yes	no
Difficulty swallowing	yes	no
Heartburn	yes	no
Abdominal distress	yes	no
Belching or excess gas	yes	no
Abdominal enlargement	yes	no
Nausea	yes	no
Vomiting	yes	no
Vomiting of blood	yes	no
Rectal bleeding	yes	no
Tarry stools	yes	no
Dark urine	yes	no
Jaundice	yes	no
Constipation	yes	no
Diarrhea	yes	no
Hemorrhoids	yes	no
Need for laxatives	yes	no

Genitourinary system

Increase in frequency of urination (day)	yes	no
Increase in frequency of urination (night)	yes	no
Feel need to urinate without much urine	yes	no
Unable to hold urine	yes	no
Pain or burning	yes	no
Blood in urine	yes	no
Albuminuria	yes	no
Impotence	yes	no
Lack of sex drive	yes	no
Pain with intercourse	yes	no

Endocrine system

Thyroid trouble	yes	no
Adrenal trouble	yes	no
Cortisone treatment	yes	no
Diabetes	yes	no

Motor system

Muscle cramps	yes	no
Muscle weakness	yes	no
Pain in joints	yes	no
Swollen joints	yes	no
Stiffness	yes	no
Deformity of joints	yes	no

Nervous system

Headache	yes	no
Dizziness	yes	no
Fainting	yes	no
Convulsions or fits	yes	no
Nervousness	yes	no
Sleeplessness	yes	no
Depression	yes	no
Change in sensation	yes	no
Memory loss	yes	no
Poor coordination	yes	no
Weakness or paralysis	yes	no

GYN-OB

Age started menstruating _____
Interval between periods _____
Duration of periods _____
Flow: light   normal   heavy
Pain with periods? _____
Date of last period _____
Pregnancies _____ Births_____
Weight of babies at birth _____

Figure 2-2 Review of systems form that can be completed by patient or examiner.

examination; however, the two must not be confused. The physical examination provides objective data: that which can be seen, felt, smelled, or heard by the examiner, commonly referred to as signs. On the other hand, the review of systems provides subjective data; that which is evident only to the patient and cannot be perceived by an observer or is no longer present for the observer to see and therefore can only be described by the patient. Subjective manifestations of disease are termed symptoms.

Chief Complaint

The chief complaint (CC) is a brief notation explaining why the patient sought health care. It is the answer to such open-ended questions as "What brought you to the hospital?" or "What is bothering you the most?" Each symptom is recorded separately with its duration or date of initial occurrence. Ideally, symptom descriptions are written in the patient's own words. They should not be diagnostic statements, someone else's opinion, or vague generalities. At times, more directed questions such as "Could you describe what you mean by `not enough air'?" or "In what ways don't you feel well?" are necessary to clarify the changes in perceptions or body functions experienced by the patient.

Asking the patient to recount the sequence of symptoms and then closing this section of the interview with a question such as "What else is bothering you?" often elicits problems the patient forgot to mention or was too uncomfortable to mention earlier. Now the interviewer is left with two types of problems: (1) those related to the chief complaint and (2) those that are important to the patient but may have little or no relationship to the present illness. The interviewer must now group the problems and decide how to proceed with the interview. Problems not related to the illness are usually incorporated with an appropriate section of background data when the history is written.

The symptoms relating to the current illness are listed as the CC and then investigated one by one and described in detail under history of present illness. Once written, the CC should express the patient's, not the examiner's, priorities; provide a capsule account of the patient's illness; and guide the collection of the history of present illness.

The symptoms most commonly associated with problems of the cardiopulmonary system include coughing with or without sputum production (*expectoration*), breathlessness (*dyspnea*), chest pain, and wheezing, commonly described as chest tightness. Other symptoms associated with cardiopulmonary problems include coughing up blood (*hemoptysis*), hoarseness, voice changes, dizziness and fainting (*syncope*), headache, altered mental status, and ankle swelling. These symptoms are discussed in the following chapter. Some symptoms such as ankle swelling can also be seen by the examiner; therefore they can be both a sign and a symptom. Common cardiopulmonary signs are discussed in Chapter 3.

Patients with cardiopulmonary problems may also have any of the so-called *constitutional symptoms,* those commonly occurring with problems in any of the body systems. Constitutional symptoms include chills and fever, excessive sweating, loss of appetite (*anorexia),* nausea, vomiting, weight loss, fatigue, weakness, exercise intolerance, and altered sleep patterns. Hay fever, allergies, acute sinusitis, postnasal discharge, and frequent bouts of colds or "flu" are upper respiratory tract symptoms commonly associated with pulmonary disease.

History of Present Illness

The history of present illness (HPI) is the narrative portion of the history that describes chronologically and in detail each symptom listed in the CC and its effect on the patient's life. It is the most difficult portion of the history to obtain and record accurately, but it is the information that guides the physical examination and diagnostic testing to follow. All caregivers should be familiar with the HPI for each of their patients.

Encouraging the patient to talk freely about each problem allows maximal information to be obtained. The patient is first asked to describe the progression of symptoms from the first occurrence to the present. On occasion, patients are unable to recall the first occurrence of the symptom, and the chronologic picture must then be developed by working backward from the most recent event.

Once a rough chronologic picture is outlined, the interviewer obtains a description of each symptom by using an open-ended approach like "Now tell me about your . . . (cough, chest pain, etc.)." Using silence, nonverbal clues (like leaning forward expectantly), and facilitative expressions such as "Yes," "hmm," and "Tell me more about . . . ," or restating or summarizing what the patient just said shows interest and encourages the patient to continue talking. When the patient exhausts the spontaneous description of each symptom, directed questions are used to elicit whatever additional information is necessary. Questions that can be answered with "yes" or "no" and leading questions are avoided. For example, "What brings on your cough?" encourages more accurate information than a question like "The only time you cough is when you first get up in the morning, isn't it?" Since most patients want to please the interviewer, they are likely to agree with a leading question rather than report the specific information needed.

> **SIMPLY STATED**
> Cardiopulmonary symptoms are subjective—known only to the patient—so information about symptoms can be obtained only from the patient. Although initial information can be obtained by having the patient complete a questionnaire, a complete history can be obtained only through questioning the patient.

> **SIMPLY STATED**
> All clinicians who care for patients should be familiar with the history of present illness for each patient treated.

Describing Symptoms

When the patient's descriptions and the interviewer's clarifying questions are complete, the following information should have been gathered for each symptom listed in the chief complaint and each additional symptom identified during the interview:

1. *Description of onset:* date, time, type (sudden or gradual)
2. *Setting:* cause, circumstance, or activity surrounding onset
3. *Location:* where on the body the problem is located and whether or not it radiates
4. *Severity:* how bad it is; how it affects activities of daily living
5. *Quantity:* how much, how large an area, or how many
6. *Quality:* what it is like; character or unique properties such as color, texture, odor, composition, sharp, viselike, throbbing
7. *Frequency:* how often it occurs
8. *Duration:* how long it lasts, constant or intermittent
9. *Course:* is it getting better, worse, or staying the same
10. *Associated symptoms:* symptoms from the same body system or other systems that occur before, with, or following the problem
11. *Aggravating factors:* things that make it worse (a certain position, weather, temperature, anxiety, exercise, etc.)
12. *Alleviating factors:* things that make it better (a change in position, hot, cold, rest, etc.)

Various listings and mnemonic devices have been suggested to help the novice remember all of the information necessary to fully describe a symptom. One such mnemonic device is PQRST (Box 2-2).

Once all the information is collected, it is written in narrative form with a paragraph given to each time division in the chronologic progression of the symptom(s). The left-hand margin of the page or the first few words of each paragraph are used to identify the applicable date or the time period (days, weeks, months, or years) prior to admission (PTA).

By the time each symptom is reviewed in detail, even a novice is usually able to assign the majority of the symptoms to one body system. The pertinent points of the review of systems, personal history, and family history are reviewed for the applicable body system(s). The pertinent negatives as well as positives are recorded. Usually, when writing the review of systems,

---

BOX 2-2	PQRST Mnemonic
P	Provocative/palliative: What is the cause? What makes it better? What makes it worse?
Q	Quality/quantity: How much is involved? How does it look, feel, sound?
R	Region/radiation: Where is it? Does it spread?
S	Severity scale: Does it interfere with activities? (Rate on scale of 1 to 10)
T	Timing: When did it begin? How often does it occur? Is it sudden or gradual?

---

the interviewer puts "see HPI" behind the applicable body system rather than restating data previously recorded.

Past History

The past history, also called the *past medical history,* is a written description of the patient's past medical problems. It may include previous experiences with health care, and personal attitudes and habits that may affect both health and compliance with medical treatment plans. Information recorded in the past history includes a chronologic listing of the following:

1. Illnesses and development since birth
2. Surgeries and hospitalizations
3. Injuries and accidents
4. Immunizations
5. Allergies, including a description of the allergic reactions and effective treatment
6. Medications, both prescribed by a physician and over-the-counter (OTC) drugs, vitamins, and "home remedies"
7. Names of physicians and sources and types of previous health care
8. Habits, including diet, sleep, exercise, and the use of alcohol, coffee, tobacco, and illicit drugs
9. Description of general health

Forms (Figure 2-3) may be used by either the patient or the interviewer to concisely record much of the information just listed. It is important to record the dates of accidents, major illnesses, hospitalizations, and immunizations. If past medical records are needed during the patient's hospitalization, the names and addresses of hospitals and physicians that have provided care to the patient in the past should be recorded.

Disease and Procedure History

For patients with cardiopulmonary complaints, it is important to ask about the frequency and treatment of each of the following diseases: pneumonia, pleurisy, fungal diseases, tuberculosis, colds, sinus infections, bronchiectasis, asthma, allergies, pneumothorax, bronchitis, or emphysema. Because of the close relationship between the heart and the lungs, it is also important to know if the patient has a history of heart attack, hypertension (high blood pressure), heart failure, or congenital heart disease.

Dates and types of heart or chest surgery and trauma should be recorded. Dates and results of tests that assess pulmonary status, including chest x-ray films, bronchoscopy, pulmonary function tests, and skin tests, should also be documented. This respiratory-specific past history information is summarized in the portion of a pulmonary history questionnaire shown in Figure 2-4. Patients' discussion of previous diseases, tests, and treatments gives a good indication of their understanding of the disease process and compliance with medical therapy.

Drug and Smoking History

There is a strong link between the use of illicit drugs and cardiopulmonary problems; however, an honest history of drug abuse is extremely difficult if not impossible for even the most

PERSONAL HISTORY

Birthplace _____ Date _____

Nationality _____ Religion _____

Marital status _____ Health of spouse _____

Occupations_____

_____

Residence past 5 years:_____

Education through _____ grade   Sleep (usual hrs.)_____ Aids to sleep_____

Recreation _____

Exercise _____

Average per day: _____

  Alcohol (type) _____

  Tobacco (type) _____

  Tea, coffee _____

Medicines taken regularly	Reason	Last Dose

PERSONAL PAST HISTORY

Circle "yes" or "no"		Year	Circle "yes" or "no"		Year
Have you ever had:			**Operations**		
Measles	yes no		Tonsils	yes no	
Mumps	yes no		Appendix	yes no	
Whooping cough	yes no		Gallbladder	yes no	
Polio	yes no		Stomach	yes no	
Scarlet fever	yes no		Breast	yes no	
Diphtheria	yes no		Uterus and/or ovary	yes no	
Meningitis	yes no		Prostate	yes no	
Infectious mono	yes no		Hernia	yes no	
Valley fever	yes no		Thyroid	yes no	
Tuberculosis (TB)	yes no		Varicose veins	yes no	
Exposure to TB	yes no		Hemorrhoids	yes no	
Malaria	yes no		Heart	yes no	
Hives	yes no		Other	yes no	
Cancer	yes no				
Venereal disease	yes no		**Injuries**		
Arthritis	yes no		Head	yes no	
Back trouble	yes no		Chest	yes no	
Bronchitis	yes no		Abdomen	yes no	
Pneumonia	yes no		Broken bones	yes no	
Pleurisy	yes no		Back	yes no	
Asthma	yes no		Other	yes no	
Emphysema	yes no		**Allergies (are you allergic to)**		
Rheumatic fever	yes no		Tetanus antitoxin	yes no	
High blood pressure	yes no		Penicillin	yes no	
Heart disease	yes no		Sulfa	yes no	
Anemia	yes no		Other drugs	yes no	
Bleeding tendency	yes no		List _____		
Blood transfusion	yes no		_____		
Hepatitis	yes no		Foods	yes no	
(yellow jaundice)			Cosmetics	yes no	
Ulcer	yes no		Other	yes no	
Hemorrhoids	yes no		**Immunizations**		
Bladder infections	yes no		Smallpox	yes no	
Kidney disease	yes no		Tetanus	yes no	
Hay fever/sinusitis	yes no		Polio, shots	yes no	
Glaucoma	yes no		Polio, oral	yes no	
Nose bleeds	yes no		Other	yes no	

Figure 2-3 Form for recording personal history and personal past history (past medical history).

Please answer by circling "yes" or "no" and provide the specific information.

PAST MEDICAL HISTORY

Have you ever had the following?   **If "yes" give year/specifics**

Asthma	yes no	_____
Allergies	yes no	_____
Frequent colds	yes no	_____
Sinus infections	yes no	_____
Chronic bronchitis	yes no	_____
Emphysema	yes no	_____
Pleurisy	yes no	_____
Pneumonia	yes no	_____
Pneumothorax	yes no	_____
Tuberculosis	yes no	_____
Other lung problems	yes no	_____
Heart trouble of any type	yes no	_____
Chest trauma	yes no	_____
Chest, lung, or heart surgery	yes no	List: _____

Have you ever had any of the following?   **If "yes" give month/year last performed**

Chest x-ray: ever abnormal?	yes no	_____ / _____
TB skin test: ever positive?	yes no	_____ / _____

Have you had any of the following?

Other skin tests	yes no	_____ / _____
Pulmonary function test	yes no	_____ / _____
Bronchoscopy	yes no	_____ / _____
Other pulmonary tests	yes no	_____ / _____

SMOKING HISTORY

Do you currently smoke or use tobacco regularly?   **yes   no**
1. How old were you when you started smoking?   _____
2. For how many years have you smoke regularly?   _____
3. How many cigarettes do you now smoke each day?   _____
4. How many cigars do you now smoke each day?   _____
5. How much pipe tobacco do you now smoke each week?   _____
6. Were there periods when you stopped smoking?   _____
7. How long did you stop smoking?   _____

Have you ever smoked regularly?   **yes   no**
1. How old were you when you started smoking?   _____
2. How many years did you smoke regularly?   _____
3. When did you quit smoking? (month/year)   _____ / _____
4. How many cigarettes did you usually smoke per day?   _____
5. How many cigars did you usually smoke per day?   _____
6. How much pipe tobacco did you smoke per week?   _____

Did you smoke anything other than tobacco?   **yes   no**
What, how much, how often? _____

Does someone smoke in your home or office?   **yes   no**
1. How many years has someone smoked in your home?   _____
2. How many years has someone smoked in your office?   _____

Figure 2-4 Past medical history and smoking sections from a pulmonary history questionnaire.

experienced examiner to obtain. It is often the staff members giving routine daily care who have the first indication that drug abuse may be implicated in the patient's complaints. The patient should be encouraged to share this information honestly with the primary physician so that the best treatment can be obtained as early as possible. Staff members and students must remember that free dissemination of such information is a breach of confidentiality and may result in losing the patient's

trust. Also, concluding too quickly that a drug history is the cause of the patient's problem may result in a missed diagnosis and an improper treatment program.

Because of the strong relationship between smoking and chronic pulmonary diseases, respiratory infections, lung cancer, and cardiovascular diseases, a careful and accurate smoking history is important. It is preferable to ask a patient "What types of tobacco have you used?" rather than "Do you smoke?" Use of pipes, cigars, marijuana, chewing tobacco, or snuff is usually recorded in terms of the amount used daily. The consumption of cigarettes may be recorded in "pack years." The term pack years refers to the number of years the patient has smoked times the number of packs smoked each day. If a patient smoked three packs a day for 10 years, it would be recorded as a 30 pack year smoking history. It is also important to record the age when the patient began to smoke, variations in smoking habits over the years, the type and length of the cigarettes smoked, the habit of inhaling, the number and success of attempts to stop smoking, and the date when the patient last smoked (see Figure 2-4). Members of the health care team have a professional responsibility to educate patients and their family about the harmful effects of smoking and guide them to programs designed to help people stop smoking.

Family History

The purposes of the family history are to learn about the health status of the patient's blood relatives and immediate family, the presence within the family of diseases with hereditary tendencies, and sources of physical, emotional, or economic support or stress within the family structure.

To assess the current health status of the extended family, the patient is asked to describe the present age and state of health of blood relatives for three generations: siblings; parents, aunts and uncles; and grandparents. The resulting information may be recorded in narrative style, drawn schematically as a family tree, or written on a form like the one shown in Figure 2-5. When patients are asked to complete a form before an interview, the responses should be reviewed and notations added as necessary to capture the age and cause of death or current health status for each family member. A notation such as "18 A/W" indicates that the person listed was 18 years old and alive and well on the day the history was recorded.

The health of the current family of a patient who was adopted is important for identification of communicable and environmentally related diseases; however, a history of the patient's true blood relatives is needed to assess genetically transmitted diseases or illnesses with strong familial relationships.

In addition to documenting the current health status of the family members, a review of diseases with strong hereditary or familial tendencies is also performed. Figure 2-5 shows a form that permits either the patient or examiner to record the presence or absence of the most frequently reviewed diseases known to occur in the patient's family (pertinent positives) and those denied by the patient (pertinent negatives).

Patients with cardiopulmonary complaints are asked specifically about the following diseases or problems that have been shown to have a hereditary link with pulmonary disease: chronic allergies, asthma, lung cancer, cystic fibrosis, emphysema, neuromuscular disorders, kyphosis, scoliosis, sleep disturbances and sleep apnea, collagen-vascular diseases (such as lupus erythematosus), alpha$_1$-antitrypsin

Has any blood relative had any of the following?	Circle "yes" or "no"	If "yes," what relationship?
Anemia	yes no	_____
Bleeding tendency	yes no	_____
Leukemia	yes no	_____
Repeated infections	yes no	_____
Crippling infections	yes no	_____
Heart disease	yes no	_____
Chronic lung disease	yes no	_____
Tuberculosis	yes no	_____
High blood pressure	yes no	_____
Kidney disease	yes no	_____
Asthma	yes no	_____
Severe allergies	yes no	_____
Mental illness	yes no	_____
Convulsions or fits	yes no	_____
Migraine headaches	yes no	_____
Diabetes	yes no	_____
Gout	yes no	_____
Obesity	yes no	_____
Thyroid trouble	yes no	_____
Peptic ulcer	yes no	_____
Chronic diarrhea	yes no	_____
Cancer	yes no	_____

	Present Age, or Age at Death	If living, health (good, fair, poor) if deceased, cause of death
Father		
Mother		
Brother or Sisters		
1.		
2.		
3.		
4.		
5.		
6.		
7.		
Children		
1.		
2.		
3.		
4.		
5.		
6.		
7.		

Figure 2-5 Form for recording family history.

deficiency, cardiovascular disorders (such as hypertension, heart attack, heart failure, and congenital abnormalities), diabetes, and obesity. Since exposure to family and friends with infections can also result in pulmonary symptoms, the patient is asked about contact with, or family history of, frequent colds, tuberculosis, influenza, pneumonia, and fungal infections.

Occupational and Environmental History

An occupational and environmental history is particularly important in patients with pulmonary symptoms. The purpose is to elicit information concerning exposure to potential disease-producing substances or environments. Most occupational pulmonary diseases are the result of workers' inhaling particles, dusts, fumes, or gases during the extraction, manufacture, transfer, storage, or disposal of industrial substances (Table 2-1).

However, the hazards of an industrial society are not limited to those working directly with the toxic substances. Other employees working in or near an industrial plant, as well as people living in the surrounding areas, are subject to breathing toxic fumes and dusts. Family members come in contact with contaminated clothing and may develop pulmonary disease years later. Accidental spills of toxic chemicals and gases can endanger and even necessitate evacuation and treatment of large numbers of people.

Although there have been dramatic decreases in exposure to some hazardous materials, exposures to dusts, fumes, and chemicals from indoor as well as outdoor air pollutants con-

Table 2-1   Occupational Lung Diseases

Inhaled Substance	Occupation or Source	Usual Symptoms and Course	Disease Names
Acute Airway or Lung Reactions			
Irritant Gases			
Chlorine, ammonia, sulfur dioxide	Various industries Accidental exposure	Short exposure Eye and airway irritation, productive cough Prolonged exposure Dyspnea, wheezing, pulmonary edema	
Insoluble Gases and Metal Fumes			
Nitrogen dioxide	Filled silos, closed welding spaces, chemical laboratories	Very little airway irritation Headache, shortness of breath, cough, chest tightness, pulmonary edema	Silo-filler's disease
Phosgene	Chemical warfare, heating metals treated with production chlorine and toluene diisocyanate (TDI)	Acute pulmonary edema, pneumonia	
Copper, zinc, iron, nickel, tin, antimony, manganese, magnesium	Welders in closed spaces, mining, electroplating	Fever, malaise, nausea, aching muscles, lasting 2-3 days	Metal fume fever Galvanization Polymer fume fever
Cadmium, mercury, beryllium		Above with acute pulmonary edema and pneumonia	
Acute or Subacute Allergic Reactions			
TDI	Plastic and foam production	Immediate or delayed asthmalike reactions usually occur in sensitive persons but may occur in others; fever, chills, malaise, weight loss, nocturnal wheezing, cough, cyanosis, dyspnea at rest	Hypersensitivity pneumonitis
Proteolytic enzymes (detergents)	Industrial accidents Manufacture of detergents		Extrinsic allergic alveolitis Occupational asthma
Droppings/Feathers			
Pigeons, parakeets, chickens, turkeys	Bird handlers	Acute reactions within 4-8 hours Delayed reactions occur at night after leaving work environment In some cases, chronic disease with fibrosis may develop if repeated exposure continues	Bird fancier's lung, ornithosis Pigeon breeder's lung
Pituitary Extract/Organic Dusts			
Paprika, fishmeal, coffee bean, weevil-infested flour	Workers with specific products		Pituitary-snufftaker's lung Wheat-weevil lung
Cotton, hemp, flax	Textile and farm workers	"Monday fever"	Byssinosis (brown lung)
Fungal spores from moldy hay, straw, grains, malt, or barley, sugar cane (bagasse), mushroom compost, maple bark, logs, wood pulp (Western red cedar)	Agriculture and farm workers Wood and paper mill workers Lumbering	Repeated bouts of pneumonia with symptoms listed and weight loss	Farmer's lung Malt-worker's lung Bagassosis Mushroom-handler's lung Wood/paper mill–worker's lung Maple bark–stripper's lung
Contaminated water	Air conditioners, humidifiers		Air conditioner (humidifier) lung
Drugs and chemicals	Antibiotic, pharmaceutical, chemical manufacture		

Table 2-1	Occupational Lung Diseases—cont'd		
Inhaled Substance	Occupation or Source	Usual Symptoms and Course	Disease Names
Chronic Occupational Lung Diseases			
Crystalline-free silica	Sandblasters in enclosed spaces, manufacture of ceramics and abrasive agents, construction, mines, quarries, foundries: gold, copper, lead, zinc, iron, coal, granite	Acute—1-3 years of intense exposure: shortness of breath, fever, frequent pulmonary infections Chronic—20 years or more of exposure: no symptoms to exertional dyspnea, obstructed breathing, productive cough, reduced exercise tolerance, chest pain, weight loss, hemoptysis with fibrosis 40+ years: infection, cor pulmonale	Silicosis Associated in unknown way with rheumatoid arthritis and scleroderma High incidence of associated tuberculosis and bronchogenic cancer
Coal	Coal miners	Simple: Asymptomatic, cough with smoking Complicated with fibrosis: as just listed with black sputum	Coal-worker's pneumoconiosis Coal-miner's lung
Asbestos	Manufacture of fireproofing and insulation, shipbuilding, automobile mechanics (clutch and brake), demolition workers, fire fighters, living/working near dumps or high-use areas	Extertional dyspnea, clubbing, restricted breathing, crackles at lung bases usually appear before x-ray film changes and cancer symptoms approximately 20 years after exposure	Asbestosis
Other Mineral Dusts			
Fuller's earth, kaolin (China clay), graphite, tin, iron, mixed dusts, tungsten	Quarrying, mining, milling, drying, bagging, and loading minerals Welding and foundries Manufacture of industrial precision instruments	Vary from asymptomatic with dust retention to same as complicated silicosis	Pneumoconiosis Stannosis Siderosis
Beryllium	Nuclear physics, manufacture of electronics, ceramics, x-ray tube windows (in past: fluorescent lights)	Acute Pulmonary edema, pneumonia Chronic granulomatous disease appears years after exposure Dyspnea, dry cough, weakness, weight loss, skin lesions, crackles	Pulmonary granuloma
Paraquat	Agriculture	Inhalation or ingestion may lead to pulmonary fibrosis	

tinue to increase. Outbreaks of work-related illnesses in buildings not contaminated by industrial processes can be traced to these pollutants or simply to an inadequate provision of fresh air with no identifiable contaminant. The terms *tight building syndrome* or *sick building syndrome* are now used to describe these epidemics in which large numbers of employees complain of symptoms, including runny or stuffy nose, eye irritation, cough, chest tightness, fatigue, headache, and malaise.

Reactions to inhalation of toxic substances can occur within minutes to hours (acute) or may take weeks, months, or years to develop. Inhalation of soluble gases such as ammonia, chlorine, or sulfur dioxide causes sufficient upper airway irritation to warn workers of immediate danger. However, metal fumes and insoluble gases like phosgene and nitrogen dioxide are less irritating to the upper airways. Because they may be inhaled for long periods of time with little discomfort, workers are not warned to escape, and more severe pulmonary damage results.

Hypersensitivity reactions may be acute or delayed and often occur in patterns. Shortness of breath, wheezes, or flulike symptoms usually occur within 4 to 8 hours of exposure. However, symptoms may occur only at night and may recur for several nights following a single exposure. In some cases the most severe symptoms occur at the start of the workweek, and tolerance develops as the week progresses. Such a pattern, often termed *Monday fever,* is commonly seen with inhalation of cotton dust. More commonly, allergic reactions worsen with reexposure and decrease during days off. In subacute forms of

BOX 2-3   American Thoracic Society's Nursing Assessment Guide for Adult Patients with Pulmonary Dysfunction

History and Symptoms

Pulmonary Symptoms *

Dyspnea
Cough
Sputum
Hemoptysis
Wheeze
Chest pain (e.g., pleuritic)

Extrapulmonary Symptoms *

Night sweats
Headaches on awakening
Weight changes
Fluid retention
Nasal stuffiness, discharge
Fatigue
Orthopnea, paroxysmal nocturnal apnea
Snoring, sleep disturbances, daytime drowsiness
Sinus problems

Pulmonary Risk Factors

Smoking history
    Type (cigarettes, cigar, pipe)
    Amount per day
    Duration (years)
Childhood respiratory diseases/symptoms
Family history of respiratory disease
Alcohol and chemical substance abuse (e.g., heroin, marijuana, cocaine)
Environmental exposures
    Location (e.g., home, work, region)
    Type (e.g., asbestos, silica, gases, aerosols)
    Duration
Obesity or nutritional depletion
Compromised immune system function (e.g., IGg deficiency, human immunodeficiency virus (HIV) infection, alpha$_1$-antitrypsin deficiency)

Previous History

Pulmonary problems
Treatments
Number of hospitalizations
Medical diagnosis(es)
Immunizations

Self-Management Capacity

Physical Ability (0 to 4 scale, 0 = independent, 4 = dependent)

Lower extremity (e.g., walking, stair climbing)
Upper extremity (e.g., shampooing, meal preparation)

Activities of daily living
    Toileting
    Hygiene
    Feeding
    Dressing
Activity pattern during a typical day
Patient statement re: management of problems
Sensory-perceptual factors (e.g., vision, hearing)

Cognitive Ability

Mental age
Memory
Knowledge about diagnosis, end treatment of pulmonary problems, or risk factors of pulmonary disease
Judgment

Psychosocial-Cultural Factors

Self-concept
    Self-esteem
    Body image
    Role(s), changes
Value system (e.g., spiritual and health beliefs)
Coping mechanisms
    Displaced anger
    Anxiety
    Hostility
    Dependency
    Withdrawal, isolation
    Avoidance
    Denial
    Noncompliance
    Acceptance

Socioeconomic Factors

Social support system
    Family
    Significant others
    Friends
    Community resources
    Government resources
Financial situation/health insurance
Employment/disability

Environmental factors

Home
Community
Worksite
Health care setting (e.g., hospital, nursing home)

Modified from American Thoracic Society Medical Section of the American Lung Association: Standards of nursing care for adult patients with pulmonary dysfunction, *Am Rev Respir Dis* 144:231, 1991.

*Consider onset, duration, character, precipitating, aggravating, and relieving factors of symptoms.

hypersensitivity pneumonitis, symptoms occur insidiously over weeks. Most of the chronic occupational pulmonary diseases (pneumoconioses) take 20 years or more to become symptomatic. Whenever there is a delay in the development of pulmonary symptoms, their relationship to occupational and environmental exposure becomes obscure.

The occupational and environmental history therefore must be more than just a chronologic listing of job titles. Questioning may include the occupation of the patient's father and descriptions of childhood residences. Lung disease caused by the inhalation of asbestos fibers (asbestosis) has been seen in people who lived near shipyards or asbestos dump sites as children and in people whose fathers were asbestos workers. The patient should be queried about location of schools, summer jobs, dates and types of military service, and all subsequent full- and part-time jobs. The precise dates, duration, and activities of each job must be delineated. These include materials and processes involved, amount of workspace and type of ventilation, use of protective devices, cleanup practices, and work going on in adjacent areas.

Work or residence near mines, farms, mills, shipyards, or foundries should be clarified. Sources of possible irritants within the home such as humidifiers, air-conditioning systems, woodpiles, insulation, smoking, paints and glues used for hobbies, and household pets must also be reviewed.

It is important to review the various places a patient has lived or visited for any period of time. Certain fungal infections that involve the respiratory system have strong geographic relationships. Histoplasmosis is particularly common in Ohio, Maryland, the central Mississippi Valley, and the Appalachian Mountains; blastomycosis is found in the southeastern United States, especially Texas and the San Joaquin Valley in California, as well as sections of South America.

When the pulmonary history is written, occupational and environmental histories are usually given specific headings because of the detail recorded. However, in most routine histories this information may be found under general headings such as personal history, social history, psychosocial history, or social-environmental history.

ASSESSMENT STANDARDS FOR PATIENTS WITH PULMONARY DYSFUNCTION

The beginning student may be confused by the fact that the patient's medical record contains more than one style of history done on or about the same date. This occurs in teaching institutions because students and residents see the patient, as well as the attending physician. It also occurs because each of the health care professions is responsible for specifying the scope of practice for its practitioners and monitoring the quality of their performance. As a result, there may be patient histories completed by nursing and several allied health professions in addition to those done by physicians. Some hospitals are moving toward what is termed the *patient history*—one history per patient per admission—which is used and augmented by all the allied health professionals involved in the patient's care, as well as by physicians.

In 1989, the American Thoracic Society adopted specific standards for assessment of adult patients with actual or potential pulmonary dysfunction. These process and outcome standards are used with assessment, goal setting, intervention, and evaluation to ensure that the patient receives an acceptable level of care. The pulmonary history assessment guide from these standards is shown in Box 2-3. Note that in addition to gathering and analyzing the traditional pulmonary history, this assessment includes additional categories that focus on the patient's response to interferences with normal respiratory function, self-management capacity, resources, and knowledge of respiratory medications and treatments. The student will find this document helpful as a tool to review the multiple variables that affect both the quality of care and quality of life for a patient with pulmonary dysfunction.

REVIEW QUESTIONS

1. T F   Nonverbal communication is often more valuable in determining the progress of an interview than verbal communication.

2. T F   Proper diagnosis and treatment are determined to a great extent by the accuracy and detail of the patient's history.

3. During the interview, if the therapist responds to the information provided by the patient with appropriate comments, this is evidence of which of the following?
   a. Non-verbal communication
   b. Active listening
   c. Pertinent positives
   d. Reflecting

4. Proper introduction of yourself to the patient before the interview is useful for all the following *except*:
   a. Establishing your role
   b. Asking permission to be involved
   c. Conveying your sincere interest in the patient
   d. Identifying diagnostic information

5. Which of the following would be examples of techniques used in conversational interviewing?
   a. Using questions such as "What happened next?"
   b. Saying things like "You feel better now, don't you?"
   c. Asking for clarification of a symptom
   d. a and c

6. If a patient cannot provide a medical history and it is obtained from a close relative, this is an example of which of the following?
   a. Family history
   b. Background information
   c. Screening information
   d. Alternative source

7. In what section of the patient history can a detailed description of the patient's current symptoms be found?
   a. Chief complaints
   b. History of present illness
   c. Past medical history
   d. Occupational history

8. Information that is evident only to the patient and cannot be perceived by the observer is known as:
   a. Subjective data
   b. Objective data
   c. Clinical signs
   d. None of the above

9. In what section of the patient's history would you find information about a possible history of exposure to asbestos?
   a. History of present illness
   b. Family history
   c. Occupational history
   d. Past medical history

10. Your patient has a 50 pack/year smoking history. Which of the following is consistent with this history?
    a. He has smoked 2 packs/day for 25 years
    b. He has smoked 1 pack/day for 50 years
    c. He has smoked 5 packs/day for 10 years
    d. Any of the above

11. Subjective manifestations of disease are termed:
    a. Symptoms
    b. Clinical findings
    c. Objective data
    d. Pertinent negatives

12. Your patient has pneumonia and complains of chest pain and cough but denies fever. How would you classify the lack of fever in this case?
    a. Objective data
    b. Pertinent positive
    c. Pertinent negative
    d. Physical exam finding

13. Which of the following is NOT considered a constitutional symptom?
    a. Nausea
    b. Weakness
    c. Chills and fever
    d. Dyspnea

14. The family history may be helpful in diagnosing a patient with which of the following problems?
    a. Acute bronchitis
    b. Cystic fibrosis
    c. Pneumothorax
    d. Pulmonary edema

BIBLIOGRAPHY

Barkauskas VH, Baumann LC, Darling-Fisher CS: *Health and physical assessment*, ed 3, St Louis, 2002, Mosby.

Elkin MK, Perry AG, Potter PA: *Nursing interventions and clinical skills*, ed 3, St Louis, 2004, Mosby.

Seidel HM and others: *Mosby's guide to physical examination*, ed 5, St Louis, 2003, Mosby.

CHAPTER

3

Robert L. Wilkins

Cardiopulmonary Symptoms

LEARNING OBJECTIVES

Upon completion of this chapter, the reader should be able to accomplish the following:

1. For each of the following symptoms, be able to describe causes and common characteristics:
   a. Cough
   b. Sputum production
   c. Hemoptysis
   d. Dyspnea
   e. Chest pain
   f. Dizziness and fainting
   g. Swelling of the ankles
   h. Fever, chills, and night sweats
   i. Headache, altered mental status, and personality changes
   j. Snoring

CHAPTER OUTLINE

Cough
   Causes and Clinical Presentation
   Descriptions
Sputum Production
   Causes and Descriptions
Hemoptysis
   Causes
   Descriptions
   Hemoptysis versus Hematemesis
Shortness of Breath (Dyspnea)
   Subjectiveness of Dyspnea
   Dyspnea Scoring System
   Causes, Types, and Clinical Presentation of
      Dyspnea
   Descriptions
Chest Pain
   Pulmonary Causes of Chest Pain
   Descriptions
Dizziness and Fainting (Syncope)
   Descriptions

Susan Jones Krider, RN, MS, contributed this chapter in the previous edition.

Swelling of the Ankles (Dependent Edema)
   Descriptions
Fever, Chills, and Night Sweats
   Descriptions
   Fever with Pulmonary Disorders
**Headache, Altered Mental Status,
   and Personality Changes**
Snoring
   Incidence and Causes of Snoring
   Clinical Presentation

KEY TERMS

angina	orthopnea
cough	orthostatic hypotension
diaphoresis	paroxysmal nocturnal
dyspnea	dyspnea
edema	phlegm
fever	platypnea
hematemesis	sputum
hemoptysis	syncope
night sweats	treopnea
orthodeoxia	

CHAPTER OVERVIEW

The RT will encounter patients with a variety of symptoms. The primary symptoms associated with cardiopulmonary disorders are cough, sputum production, hemoptysis, shortness of breath (dyspnea), and chest pain. Dizziness and fainting; ankle swelling (peripheral edema); fever, chills, and night sweats; personality changes; and snoring are frequent but less specific complaints. This chapter defines terms associated with these symptoms, briefly discusses causes (etiology), describes normal and abnormal characteristics, and lists related symptoms and diseases for each of the primary symptoms just mentioned. The RT must be familiar with these symptoms and their characteristics in order to ask relevant questions and provide optimal care.

> ## SIMPLY STATED
> Cardiopulmonary symptoms are assessed to determine:
> - The seriousness of the patient's problem
> - The potential underlying cause of the problem
> - The effectiveness of treatment

COUGH

Cough is one of the most common symptoms seen in patients with pulmonary disease. It is a powerful protective reflex arising from stimulation of receptors located in the pharynx, larynx, trachea, large bronchi, and even the lung and the visceral pleura. Coughing can be produced by inflammatory, mechanical, chemical, or thermal stimulation of cough receptors anywhere from the oropharynx to the terminal bronchioles or simply by tactile pressure in the ear canal (Table 3-1).

Impulses generated by stimulation of the cough receptors are carried by efferent pathways of the reflex, primarily the vagus, phrenic, glossopharyngeal, and trigeminal nerves, to the cough center located diffusely in the medulla, separate from the respiratory center. Conduction of the impulses down the efferent pathway of the reflex stimulates the smooth muscles of the larynx and tracheobronchial tree via the vagus nerve and the diaphragm and other respiratory muscles via the phrenic and other spinal motor nerves. The cough mechanism can be divided into three phases:

1. *Inspiratory phase:* Reflex opening of the glottis and contraction of the diaphragm, thoracic, and abdominal muscles cause deep inspiration with a concomitant increase in lung volume accompanied by an increase in the caliber and length of the bronchi.
2. *Compression phase:* Closure of the glottis and relaxation of the diaphragm while the expiratory muscles contract against the closed glottis can generate very high intrathoracic pressures and narrowing of the trachea and bronchi.
3. *Expiratory phase:* Opening of the glottis, explosive release of trapped intrathoracic air, and vibration of the vocal cords and mucosal lining of the posterior laryngeal wall,

which shakes secretions loose from the larynx and moves undesired material out of the respiratory tract.

The cough reflex may be voluntary or involuntary and occurs in everyone from time to time. The efficiency of the cough (force of the airflow) is determined by the depth of the inspiration and amount of pressure that can be generated in the airways. The effectiveness of a cough is reduced if one or more of the following conditions exist:

1. Weakness of either the inspiratory or expiratory muscles
2. Inability of the glottis to open or close correctly
3. Obstruction, collapsibility, or alteration in shape or contours of the airways
4. Decrease in lung recoil as occurs with emphysema
5. Abnormal quantity or quality of mucus production (e.g., thick sputum)

Causes and Clinical Presentation

Cough may be *acute* (sudden onset, usually severe with a short course), *chronic* (persistent and troublesome for more than 3 weeks), or *paroxysmal* (periodic, prolonged, forceful episodes). An acute self-limiting cough is usually due to a viral infection involving the upper airway. It usually resolves in a few days. Chronic persistent cough is most commonly caused by postnasal drip syndrome, followed by asthma, gastroesophageal reflux, chronic bronchitis, bronchiectasis, and other conditions such as left heart failure, bronchogenic cancer, and sarcoidosis. In smokers, chronic cough is usually due to chronic bronchitis. Postnasal drip, asthma, and gastroesophageal reflux account for most chronic coughs in nonsmokers who have a normal chest x-ray and who are not taking angiotensin converting enzyme (ACE) inhibitors. Most patients will have a single cause for their cough; however, in some patients, two or three simultaneous causes may be found for their chronic cough. Frequent, annoying, painful, or persistent cough or cough equivalent, such as throat clearing, is not normal, especially when it is productive.

Cough is not only a symptom of pulmonary problems; it may occur in conjunction with other pulmonary symptoms such as wheezing, stridor, chest pain, and dyspnea. In addition, cough may cause problems. The vigorous muscular activity and high intrathoracic pressures created by chronic forceful cough-

Table 3-1	Possible Causes of Cough Receptor Stimulation
Types of Stimulation	**Possible Causes**
Inflammatory	Infection, lung abscess, drug reaction, allergy, edema, hyperemia, collagen-vascular disease, radiotherapy, pneumoconiosis, tuberculosis
Mechanical	Inhaled dusts
Obstructive	Foreign bodies, aspiration of nasal secretions, tumor or granulomas within or around the lung, aortic aneurysm
Airway wall tension	Pulmonary edema, atelectasis, fibrosis, chronic interstitial pneumonitis
Chemical	Inhaled irritant gases, fumes, smoke
Temperature	Inhaled hot or cold air
Ear	Tactile pressure in the ear canal (Arnold's nerve response) or from otitis media

Modified from Schmidt CO: In Conn HF, Conn RB, editors: *Current diagnosis*, ed 6, Philadelphia, 1980, WB Saunders.

ing may produce a number of complications in addition to fatigue, including torn chest muscles, rib fractures, disruption of surgical wounds, pneumothorax or pneumomediastinum, syncope (fainting), arrhythmia, esophageal rupture, and urinary incontinence.

Descriptions

Cough should be described as *effective* (strong enough to clear the airway) or *inadequate* (audible but too weak to mobilize the secretions), *productive* (mucus or other material is expelled by the cough), or *dry* (moisture or secretions are not produced). Since dry coughs often become productive, a chronologic report of the circumstances surrounding the change and a description of the sputum should be recorded.

The quality, time, and setting in which a cough occurs may also provide some clues to the location and type of disorder (Table 3-2). *Barking* (like a seal bark), *brassy* (harsh, dry), and *hoarse* coughs and those associated with *inspiratory stridor* are usually heard when there is a problem with the larynx (e.g., infection, tumor); *wheezy* coughs (accompanied by whistling or sighing sounds) suggest bronchial disorders; and *chronic productive* coughs are generally indicative of significant bronchopulmonary disease (e.g., chronic bronchitis). *Hacking* (frequent brief periods of coughing or clearing the throat) may be dry and may be the result of smoking, a viral infection, a nervous habit, or difficult-to-move secretions as occur with postnasal drip.

Acute onset or change in a cough is obvious to the patient and family and probably to the interviewer; therefore an accurate history is easily obtained. However, careful inquiry is often required to identify the characteristics of a chronic cough. Because coughing and sputum production are not socially acceptable, patients may deny or minimize their presence or learn to adapt to the extent that they may even be unaware of chronic coughing. Questioning family members or close friends may provide valuable information about the onset, persistence, duration, severity, and factors that precipitate and aggravate the coughing.

SPUTUM PRODUCTION

Sputum is the substance expelled from the tracheobronchial tree, pharynx, mouth, sinuses, and nose by coughing or clearing the throat. The term phlegm refers strictly to secretions from the lungs and tracheobronchial tree. These respiratory tract secretions may contain a variety of materials including mucus, cellular debris, microorganisms, blood, pus, and foreign particles and should not be confused with saliva. The tracheobronchial tree normally secretes up to 100 mL of sputum each day. Sputum is moved upward by the wavelike motion of the

Table 3-2	Terms Used to Describe Cough
Description	Possible Causes
Acute (<3 weeks)	Postnasal drip, allergies, infections especially viral URI, bronchitis, laryngitis
Chronic (>3 weeks) or recurrent (adults)	Postnasal drip, asthma, chronic bronchitis, gastroesophageal reflux, bronchiectasis, COPD, TB, lung tumor, sarcoidosis, ACE inhibitors, left heart failure, habit
Recurrent (children)	Viral bronchitis, asthma, allergies
Dry	Viral infections, inhalation of irritant gases, interstitial lung diseases, pleural effusion, cardiac condition, nervous habit, tumor, radiation therapy, chemotherapy
Dry progressing to productive	Atypical and mycoplasmal pneumonia, AIDS, legionnaires' disease, asthma, silicosis, pulmonary embolus and edema, lung abscess, emphysema (late in disease), smoking
Chronic productive	Bronchiectasis, chronic bronchitis, lung abscess, asthma, fungal infections, bacterial pneumonias, tuberculosis
Inadequate	Debility, weakness, oversedation, pain, poor motivation, emphysema
Paroxysmal (esp. night)	Aspiration, asthma, left heart failure
Barking	Epiglottal disease, croup, influenza, laryngotracheal bronchitis
Brassy or hoarse	Laryngitis, laryngotracheal bronchitis, laryngeal paralysis, pressure on recurrent laryngeal nerve: mediastinal tumor, aortic aneurysm, left atrial enlargement
Inspiratory stridor	Tracheal or mainstem bronchial obstruction, croup, epiglottitis
Wheezy	Bronchospasm, asthma, bronchitis, cystic fibrosis
Morning	Chronic bronchitis, smoking
Afternoon and evening	Exposure to irritants during the day
Associated with position change or lying down	Bronchiectasis, left heart failure, chronic postnasal drip or sinusitis, gastroesophageal reflux with aspiration
Associated with eating or drinking	Neuromuscular disease of the upper airway, esophageal problems, aspiration

ACE, Angiotensin converting enzyme; *AIDS*, acquired immunodeficiency syndrome; *COPD*, chronic obstructive pulmonary disease; *TB*, tuberculosis; *URI*, upper respiratory infection (common cold).

Questions to Ask About
COUGH

Can you describe your cough? How long have you had the cough?

When did the cough start? Did the cough start suddenly? What were you doing when the cough started?

Do you smoke? If so, What do you smoke? How much and for how long? (see previous section on smoking)

Do you cough up sputum or mucus?

Do you usually cough first thing in the morning?

Do you usually cough at other times during the day or night? Does the cough wake you up?

Do you cough on most days? How many months/years have you had this cough?

Do you cough more on a particular day of the week? a particular time of the day? a particular season of the year?

Is the cough worse in any position or when you are in a certain location?

Is the cough associated with eating, drinking, or medications?

Are there any other symptoms associated with the cough like chest pain? wheezing? fever? runny nose? hoarseness? night sweats? weight loss? headache? dizziness? loss of consciousness?

What relieves the cough?

Do you have birds as pets? Do you feed pigeons? Have you recently cleaned a church steeple or other semienclosed space?

Have you ever been exposed to anyone with tuberculosis?

cilia (tiny hairlike structures) lining the larynx, trachea, and bronchi, and it is usually swallowed unnoticed. As previously mentioned, sputum may be difficult or impossible for the patient to describe accurately because of social stigma and lack of awareness. Thus collection and inspection of a sample is often necessary.

Causes and Descriptions

Excessive sputum production is most often caused by inflammation of the mucous glands that line the tracheobronchial tree. Inflammation of these glands occurs most often with infection, cigarette smoking, and allergies.

Sputum should be described as to color, consistency, quantity, time of day, odor, and presence of blood or distinguishing matter. The character may be highly indicative of the underlying disorder (Table 3-3). The amount may vary from scanty (a few teaspoons) to copious (as much as a pint or more), which is seen in chronic bronchial and pulmonary inflammation.

The consistency may be described as thin, thick, viscous (gelatinous), **tenacious** (extremely sticky), or **frothy**. Color depends on the origin and cause of the sputum production. Other descriptions include *mucoid* (clear, thin, may be somewhat viscid as a result of oversecretion of bronchial mucus), *mucopurulent* (thick, viscous, colored, and often in globs with an offensive odor), and blood-tinged. Copious, foul-smelling **(fetid)** sputum that separates into layers on standing and is produced when the patient's position is changed occurs with lung abscess and bronchiectasis.

Morning expectoration implies accumulation of secretions during the night and is commonly seen with bronchitis. Nonpurulent, silicone-like bronchial casts are seen with asthma. Sudden large amounts of sputum production may be indicative of development of a bronchopleural fistula.

Table 3-3 Presumptive Sputum Analysis

Appearance of Sputum	Possible Cause
Clear, colorless like egg white	Normal
Black	Smoke or coal dust inhalation
Brownish	Cigarette smoker
Frothy white or pink	Pulmonary edema
Sand or small stone	Aspiration of foreign material, broncholithiasis
Purulent	Infection, pneumonia caused by:
Apple-green, thick	*Haemophilus influenzae*
Pink, thin, blood-streaked	Streptococci or staphylococci
Red currant jelly	*Klebsiella*
Rusty	Pneumococci
Yellow or green, copious	*Pseudomonas* pneumonia, advanced chronic bronchitis, bronchiectasis (separates into layers)
Foul odor (fetid)	Lung abscess, aspiration, anaerobic infections, bronchiectasis
Mucoid	Emphysema, pulmonary tuberculosis, early chronic bronchitis, neoplasms, asthma
Grayish	Legionnaires' disease
Silicone-like casts	Bronchial asthma
Mucopurulent	As above with infection, pneumonia, cystic fibrosis
Blood streaked or hemoptysis (frankly bloody)	Bronchogenic carcinoma, tuberculosis, chronic bronchitis, coagulopathy, pulmonary contusion or abscess (see Causes of Hemoptysis)

SIMPLY STATED

Chronic sputum production is most often related to irritation or disease of the airways (e.g., asthma, chronic bronchitis).

Questions to Ask About SPUTUM

Do you usually bring up phlegm or mucus from your chest first thing in the morning?

Do you usually bring up phlegm or mucus at other times of the day?

Can you estimate the amount you bring up? About a cup? About a tablespoon?

What color is it? Does it have a foul odor?

Has the sputum changed color recently?

HEMOPTYSIS

Hemoptysis, expectoration of sputum containing blood, varies in severity from slight streaking to frank bleeding. It is an alarming symptom that may herald serious disease and massive hemorrhage.

Causes

Differential diagnosis is complex and includes bronchopulmonary, cardiovascular, hematologic, and other systemic disorders (Box 3-1). A history of pulmonary or cardiovascular disease, cigarette smoking, trauma, aspiration of a foreign body, bleeding disorder, or anticoagulant therapy suggests the possible cause of hemoptysis. Travel to areas where tuberculosis or fungal infections such as coccidioidomycosis or histoplasmosis are prevalent help to identify the underlying disorder.

The site of bleeding may be anywhere in the respiratory tract, including the nose or mouth. The amount and mechanisms of bleeding are varied. Tissues engorged by inflammation or back pressure from heart failure or other cardiac problems may bleed easily and cause frothy pink sputum. Trauma bruises tissue or may tear a vessel. A tumor or granuloma can erode surrounding tissue or the bronchial wall. An infective process can create an abscess in the bronchial tree or lung parenchyma, which can erode into another structure (e.g., bronchopleural fistula) or completely through a vessel wall. If the vessel is an artery, hemorrhage can be sudden, massive, and exsanguinating.

Tuberculosis and bronchiectasis used to be the most common causes of hemoptysis. Erosive bronchitis in smokers with chronic bronchitis now accounts for nearly half of the cases of hemoptysis. Bronchogenic carcinoma is the second most frequent cause. In fact, blood-streaked sputum may be the only hint that bronchogenic cancer has developed in the smoker.

BOX 3-1   Some Causes of Hemoptysis

Frequent Causes of Hemoptysis

Bronchogenic carcinoma
Chronic bronchitis*
Acute bronchitis with severe coughing

Infrequent Causes of Hemoptysis

Pulmonary

Aspiration of a foreign body
Bronchoarterial fistula*
Bronchiectasis*
Broncholithiasis
Deep mycotic infection*
Metastatic carcinoma
Pulmonary abscess*
Pulmonary embolism, infarction
Tuberculosis*
Trauma, pulmonary contusion

Cardiopulmonary

Arteriovenous malformation
Mitral stenosis
Cardiac pulmonary edema
Pulmonary hypertension

Systemic

Coagulation disorders*
Goodpasture's syndrome
Sarcoidosis, Wegener's granulomatosis

Other Pseudohemoptysis

Emesis
Oropharyngeal or nose bleed

*Most frequent causes of massive hemoptysis.

Descriptions

Obtaining a description of the amount, odor, color, and appearance of blood produced as well as the acuteness or chronicity of the bleeding may provide a clue to the source of bleeding. The most common causes of *streaky hemoptysis* are pulmonary infection (chronic bronchitis, bronchiectasis, bacterial pneumonias), lung cancer, and thromboemboli. Small stones or gravel mixed with the sputum and blood suggest broncholithiasis.

Careful evaluation and description of the hemoptysis is crucial, because it can include clots of blood as well as blood-tinged sputum. Coughing up clots of blood is a symptom of extreme importance suggesting serious illness. *Massive hemoptysis* (400 mL in 3 hours or more than 600 mL in 24 hours) is seen with carcinoma of the lung, tuberculosis, bronchiectasis, and trauma. It is an emergency condition associated with possible mortality. Immediate action is required to maintain an adequate airway, and emergency bronchoscopy and surgery may be necessary.

Associated symptoms may also provide a clue to the source of bleeding. Sometimes patients can describe a sensation, often warmth, in the area where the blood originates. Others perceive a bubbling sensation in the tracheobronchial tree followed by expectoration of blood. Hemoptysis associated with sudden onset of chest pain and dyspnea in a patient at risk for venous stasis of the legs must be evaluated for pulmonary embolism and possible infarction. Frothy, blood-tinged sputum associated with paroxysmal cough accompanies cardiac-induced pulmonary edema. Hemoptysis without severe coughing suggests a cavitary lesion in the lung or bronchial tumor.

Hemoptysis Versus Hematemesis

"Spitting up blood," as patients frequently call it, may be confused with blood originating in the oropharynx, esophagus, or stomach. The patient with a nosebleed at night could cough up blood in the morning. The presence of symptoms such as nausea and vomiting, especially with a history of alcoholism or cirrhosis of the liver, may suggest the esophagus or stomach as a source. Conversely, vomiting of blood may sometimes manifest bronchopulmonary bleeding. When bleeding occurs during the night and the blood reaches the oropharynx, it may be swallowed without the patient waking. The swallowed blood may act as an irritant and the patient may vomit early in the morning. Careful questioning and often examination of the bloody sputum are required to distinguish hemoptysis from hematemesis (vomited blood) (Table 3-4). It is important to obtain a detailed sequence of events to determine whether the blood originated in the respiratory tract and was swallowed and then vomited, or the blood was vomited, aspirated, and later expectorated.

SHORTNESS OF BREATH (DYSPNEA)

Shortness of breath (commonly abbreviated as SOB in the medical record) or difficult breathing is the most distressing symptom of respiratory disease and is also a cardinal symptom of cardiac disease. Difficult breathing impairs the ability to work or exercise and may interfere with the simplest activities of daily living like walking, eating, bathing, speaking, and sleeping. In patients with pulmonary disease it is the single most important

Questions to Ask About HEMOPTYSIS

Do you smoke?
Did you start coughing up the blood suddenly?
How long have you noticed the blood?
Do you cough up anything else with the blood? Can you describe what it looks like?
Is the sputum blood-tinged or are there actual clots of blood?
Have there been recurrent episodes of coughing up blood?
What seems to bring on the coughing up of blood? vomiting? coughing? nausea?
Have you felt any unusual sensations in your chest after you cough up the blood? Before you cough up the blood? If yes, Where? Can you tell me how it feels?
Have you had a recent nose bleed?
Have you been involved in a recent accident or had an injury to your chest?
Have you traveled lately?
Have you ever had tuberculosis? Have you been exposed to anyone who has had tuberculosis?
Have you had recent surgery?
Have you had night sweats? shortness of breath? irregular heartbeats? hoarseness? weight loss? swelling or pain in your legs?
Is there a family history of coughing up blood? Are you aware of any bleeding tendency in you or your family?
Do you take any blood thinners? aspirin? If yes: How much? how often? If a woman: Do you take oral contraceptives?

factor limiting their ability to function on a day-to-day basis and is frequently the reason the patient seeks medical care.

Dyspnea (*dys,* difficult; *pnea,* breathing) is a term defined by the American Thoracic Society as a subjective experience of breathing discomfort that consists of qualitatively distinct sensations that vary in intensity.[1] The sensations associated

Table 3-4	**Distinguishing Characteristics of Hemoptysis and Hematemesis**	
Characteristic	Hemoptysis	Hematemesis
History	Cardiopulmonary disease	Gastrointestinal disease
Patient says	Coughed up from lungs/chest	Vomited from stomach
Associated symptoms	Dyspnea, pain or tickling sensation in chest	Nausea, pain referred to stomach
Blood: pH	Alkaline	Acid
Mixed with	Sputum	Food
Froth	May be present	Absent
Color	Bright red	Dark, clotted, "coffee grounds"

with dyspnea range from a slight awareness of breathing to severe respiratory distress and may be mixed with anxiety in severe cases. The sensations experienced by the patient are a product of various factors such as the severity of the physiological impairment and the psychological makeup of the patient.

Subjectiveness of Dyspnea

Dyspnea may be difficult to evaluate because it is so subjective. The sensation of dyspnea is made up of two components:

1. *Sensory input to the cerebral cortex.* Multiple sources of sensory information from mechanoreceptors in the upper airway, thorax, and muscles are integrated in the central nervous system and sent to the sensorimotor cortex in the brain. In general, the sensation of dyspnea is related to the intensity of the input from the thoracic structures and from the chemoreceptors. It varies directly with ventilatory demand such as exercise and inversely with ventilatory capacity. Dyspnea tends to occur if ventilatory demand increases or if ventilatory capacity decreases.

2. *Perception of the sensation.* Perception relies on interpretation of the information arriving at the sensorimotor cortex, and interpretation is highly dependent on the psychological makeup of the person.

A patient's perception of dyspnea may have no relation to the patient's breathing appearance. Remember, dyspnea is subjective—a symptom—what the patient feels. A patient may have labored and rapid breathing and deny feeling short of breath. Conversely, a patient may appear to be breathing comfortably and slowly but may feel breathless. You can never assume that a patient with a rapid respiratory rate is dyspneic. In addition, a patient's complaint of dyspnea must be considered a symptom of a medical problem and must be taken seriously until proven otherwise. In fact, onset of dyspnea may be the first clue to identifying serious problems.

Patients' perceptions of dyspnea vary greatly. A healthy person notices the increased ventilation required to climb stairs or to exercise but expects it and does not interpret it as unpleasant. In fact, the athlete may consider the breathlessness occurring after a sprint to be exhilarating. Patients, on the other hand, may describe the feeling as "breathless," "short-winded," "feeling of suffocation," or a sensation of air hunger at rest or during minimal exercise.

Dyspnea Scoring Systems

A variety of scaling methods have been devised to help quantify dyspnea at a single point in time or to help track changes in dyspnea over time or with treatment. In the clinical setting, patients are frequently asked to rate the severity of a symptom such as dyspnea or pain using a severity scale of 0 to 10. The patient is asked a question such as "On a scale of 0 to 10, how would you rate your shortness of breath when you are resting? Zero means no shortness of breath and ten means the worst or maximum shortness of breath." The patient's response may be recorded simply as "SOB at rest 7/10."

Visual analog scales are straight lines, usually 10 cm long, running from the words "Not Breathless" at one end to "Extremely Breathless" at the other end. The patient marks the line to indicate his or her level of respiratory discomfort. The score is measured as the length of the line between "Not Breathless" and the mark made by the patient. The score may be recorded as 5.5/10 or simply as 5.5 (the 10 is implied).

A *Modified Borg Scale,* such as shown as Table 3-5, also uses a 0 to 10 grading system with descriptive terms to depict the perceived intensity of a symptom such as dyspnea after a specified task. Tools like the frequently used *American Thoracic Society Shortness of Breath Scale* (Table 3-6) specify the degree of dyspnea (slight, moderate, severe, very severe) using descriptive terms as well as a numeric grading system. Questionnaires like the *UCSD Shortness of Breath Questionnaire* (Figure 3-1) have patients rate their shortness of breath while performing a variety of activities of daily living. Other self-administered questionnaires have been developed to include additional items related to speaking,[2] social activities, well-being, and quality of life.[3] No single scale is applicable to all patients or situations.

Causes, Types, and Clinical Presentation of Dyspnea

Dyspnea is most often related to pulmonary or cardiac disease, but it is also seen with hematologic, metabolic, chemical, neurologic, psychogenic, and mechanical disorders. Dyspnea may be described by clinical type as shown in Table 3-7 or the causes of dyspnea may be grouped by body system as listed in Table 3-8.

Attempts to understand the physiologic bases of dyspnea have evolved around several separate concepts, including mechanics of breathing, ventilatory performance, work and efficiency of breathing, oxygen cost, length-tension inappropriateness, chemoreception, and exercise testing. The discussion of each concept and its related disorders is beyond the scope of this text. However, it is helpful to remember that patients with respiratory disorders will complain of dyspnea when any of the following are present alone or in combination:

Table 3-5	Modified Borg Scale for Estimation of Subjective Symptoms
Rating	**Intensity of Sensation**
0	Nothing at all
0.5	Very, very mild/weak
1	Very mild/weak
2	Mild/weak
3	Moderate
4	Somewhat severe/strong
5	
6	
7	Very severe/strong
8	
9	Very, very severe/strong
10	MAXIMAL

Table 3-6	Shortness of Breath Scale	
Degree	Description	Grade
None	No breathlessness except with exercise	0
Slight	Troubled by shortness of breath when hurrying on the level or walking up a slight hill	1
Moderate	Walks more slowly than people of the same age on the level because of breathlessness or has to stop for breath when walking at own pace on the level	2
Severe	Stops for breath after walking about 100 yards or after a few minutes on the level	3
Very severe	Too breathless to leave the house; breathless when dressing or undressing	4

From Muza SR and others: Comparison of scales used to quantitate the sense of effort to breathe in patients with chronic obstructive pulmonary disease, *Am Rev Respir Dis* 141: 909, 1990.

For each activity listed below, please rate your breathlessness on a scale between 0 and 5 when 0 is not at all breathless and 5 is maximally breathless or too breathless to do the activity.
If the activity is one that you do not perform, please give your best estimate of breathlessness.
Your response should be for an average day during the past week.

0 **Not at all**
1
2
3
4 **Severely**
5 **Maximally or unable to do because of breathlessness**

How short of breath do you get:
1. At rest   0 1 2 3 4 5
2. Walking on a level at your own pace   0 1 2 3 4 5
3. Walking on a level with others your age   0 1 2 3 4 5
4. Walking up a hill   0 1 2 3 4 5
5. Walking up stairs   0 1 2 3 4 5
6. While eating   0 1 2 3 4 5
7. Standing up from a chair   0 1 2 3 4 5
8. Brushing teeth   0 1 2 3 4 5
9. Shaving and/or brushing hair   0 1 2 3 4 5
10. Showering/bathing   0 1 2 3 4 5
11. Dressing   0 1 2 3 4 5
12. Picking up and straightening up   0 1 2 3 4 5
13. Doing dishes   0 1 2 3 4 5
14. Sweeping/vacuuming   0 1 2 3 4 5
15. Making bed   0 1 2 3 4 5
16. Shopping   0 1 2 3 4 5
17. Doing laundry   0 1 2 3 4 5
18. Washing car   0 1 2 3 4 5
19. Mowing lawn   0 1 2 3 4 5
20. Watering lawn   0 1 2 3 4 5
21. Sexual activities   0 1 2 3 4 5

How much do these limit you in your daily life?
22. Shortness of breath   0 1 2 3 4 5
23. Fear of "hurting myself" by overexerting   0 1 2 3 4 5
24. Fear of shortness of breath   0 1 2 3 4 5

Figure 3-1 The patient marks the Shortness of Breath Questionnaire (SOBQ) to indicate the severity of shortness of breath experienced during 21 different activities of daily living associated with various levels of exertion and to rate three questions about limitations in his/her daily life. The patient is asked to estimate the degree of shortness of breath anticipated for activities he/she does not perform. The SOBQ is scored by summing the responses across all 24 items to obtain a total score. Scores range from 0 to 120. (Modified from Eakin EG, Resnikoff PM, Prewitt LM, et al: Validation of a new dyspnea measure: the UCSD Shortness of Breath Questionnaire, *Chest* 113[3]:619, 1998.)

1. The work of breathing is abnormally high for the given level of exertion. This is common with narrowed airways as in asthma and when the lung is stiff as in pneumonia.
2. The ventilatory capacity is reduced. This is common when the vital capacity is abnormally low as seen patients with neuromuscular disease.
3. The drive to breathe is elevated beyond normal (e.g., hypoxemia, acidosis, exercise)

Clinical Types of Dyspnea

Research has demonstrated that the physiologic cause of the patient's dyspnea often results in the patient using unique terms to describe their discomfort. The patient with asthma frequently describes dyspnea as "tightness in the chest." Patients with congestive heart failure (CHF) often describe a sensation of "suffocation" or "air hunger." Patients with COPD and interstitial lung disease often complain of "increased effort to breathe," probably because of the increased work of breathing associated with these disorders. These results suggest that dyspnea may vary from patient to patient according to the underlying pathophysiology.[1]

Cardiac- and circulatory-related dyspnea occur primarily when there is an inadequate supply of oxygen to the tissues. In early heart failure, dyspnea is seen primarily during exercise when the decreased pumping power of the heart cannot keep up with the demands created by exercise. The shortness of breath may be accompanied by hyperventilation and be associated with fatigue or a feeling of smothering or sternal compression. In later stages, the lungs become congested with blood and edema, causing an increase in the work of breathing and dyspnea at rest and when lying down. Dyspnea is also associated with anemia and occurs primarily with exertion unless the anemia is extreme. *"Air hunger"* is a grave sign indicating the need for immediate transfusion in the anemic patient.

Psychogenic dyspnea, or panic disorder as it is sometimes called, is a hysterical type of overbreathing that usually presents as breathlessness. The event is not related to exertion, and a precipitating event other than a stress can rarely be identified; testing and physical examination are negative. Hyperventilation is common in patients with panic disorder.

Hyperventilating is breathing at a rate and depth in excess of the body's metabolic need, which causes a decrease in arterial carbon dioxide ($PaCO_2$) and results in a decrease in cerebral

Table 3-7	Clinical Types of Dyspnea	
Dyspnea	Associated With	Associated Signs and Symptoms
Physiologic	Exercise, acute hypoxia (e.g., high altitude) Breathing high concentration of CO_2 in a closed space	Awareness of increased ventilation If space is also devoid of O_2, confusion and unconsciousness may occur before dyspnea warns of danger
Pulmonary *Restrictive*	Pulmonary fibrosis Chest deformities Pleural effusion Pneumothorax	Comfortable at rest Intensely dyspneic when exertion nears patient's limited breathing capacity
Obstructive	Asthma Obstructive emphysema	Increased ventilatory effort Dyspnea at rest Breathing labored and retarded especially during expiration
Cardiac	Heart failure	Orthopnea, paroxysmal nocturnal dyspnea, "cardiac asthma," periodic respiration
Circulatory	Chronic anemia Exsanguinating hemorrhage	Dyspnea only with exertion unless anemia is extreme "Air hunger" a grave sign
Chemical	Uremia (kidney failure)	Dyspnea with severe panting caused by acidosis, heart failure, pulmonary edema, and anemia
Central	Head injury Cerebral lesion	Hyperventilation Intense hyperventilation Sometimes noisy & stertorous Biot's respiration
Psychogenic	Pain-related dyspnea Hysterical overbreathing Sighing dyspnea	Continuous hyperventilation or deep sighing respirations at maximal depth

Table 3-8	Causes of Dyspnea by Body System
System	Common Causes of Dyspnea
Respiratory	Airway obstruction, asthma, COPD, pneumonia, pulmonary embolus, pneumothorax, pulmonary fibrosis, pleural effusion
Cardiac	Congestive heart failure, pericardial effusion, cardiac shunts, valvular lesions
Hematologic	Severe anemia, carbon monoxide poisoning, hemoglobinopathies
Neurologic	Brain tumor, CNS inflammation, increased intracranial pressure, hypertensive encephalopathy, some CVA
Metabolic and endocrine	Toxins, uremia, hepatic coma, thyrotoxicosis, myxedema
Psychiatric	Pain-related dyspnea, severe anxiety, hyperventilation syndrome
Mechanical factors	Chest wall deformities, diaphragmatic paralysis, hepatosplenomegaly, massive ascites, tumors, pregnancy, obesity

CNS, Central nervous system; *COPD*, chronic obstructive pulmonary disease; *CVA*, cerebrovascular accident.

blood flow. Patients with psychogenic dyspnea are usually very anxious and may describe feeling faint or lightheaded with numbness and tingling around their mouth and in their extremities. They may report having visual disturbances. If they continue to hyperventilate, they may pass out.

Acute and Chronic Dyspnea

Dyspnea may be acute or chronic, progressive, recurrent, paroxysmal, or episodic. *Acute dyspnea* in children is most frequently associated with asthma, epiglottitis, croup, and bronchiolitis. In adults the causes are more varied (Box 3-2). Pulmonary embolism should be suspected if the patient is in the postoperative period or has a history of prolonged bed rest, phlebitis, or cardiac arrhythmia. Women who are pregnant or are taking birth control pills are also at higher risk for pulmonary embolism. Asthma, upper airway obstruction, foreign body aspiration, pneumonia, pneumothorax, pulmonary edema, hyperventilation, and panic disorder may also cause acute dyspnea.

BOX 3-2 Common Causes of Acute and Chronic Dyspnea

Acute Dyspnea

Asthma*
Chest trauma
Pleural effusion
Pneumonia
Pulmonary edema
Pulmonary embolism
Pulmonary hemorrhage
Spontaneous pneumothorax
Cardiac pulmonary edema
Acute interstitial lung disease (e.g., hemorrhage, ARDS)
Upper airway obstruction (e.g., aspirated foreign body, laryngospasm)

Chronic Dyspnea

(usually progressive)
Asthma*
CHF, left ventricular failure*
Cystic fibrosis
Pleural effusion
Interstitial lung diseases
Pulmonary vascular disease
Pulmonary thromboembolic disease
Chronic obstructive pulmonary disease
Severe anemia
Psychogenic dyspnea
Hypersensitivity disorders
Chest wall abnormalities (e.g., neuromuscular disease, kyphoscoliosis, diaphragm paralysis)

ARDS, Adult respiratory distress syndrome; *CHF,* Congestive heart failure.
*Asthma and left ventricular failure represent chronic causes of dyspnea with paroxysmal exacerbations.

Chronic dyspnea is almost always progressive. It begins with dyspnea on exertion and over time progresses to dyspnea at rest. Most patients with chronic dyspnea do not seek medical help until their lung disease is very advanced and treatment options are limited. Instead, as their lung disease progresses, they adopt a sedentary lifestyle that requires very little exertion to avoid feeling short of breath.

COPD and chronic CHF are the most common causes of chronic dyspnea in adults. Determining whether the dyspnea is related to the lungs versus the heart can be difficult, especially in older patients. Pulmonary function testing, electrocardiogram, and chest radiographs often prove helpful.

Descriptions

Patients may complain of dyspnea occurring at certain times of the day, in association with a position, or during a specific phase of the respiratory cycle. Inspiratory dyspnea is usually associated with upper airway obstruction, whereas expiratory dyspnea occurs with obstruction of smaller bronchi and bronchioles.

Paroxysmal nocturnal dyspnea (PND) is the sudden onset of difficult breathing that occurs when a sleeping patient is in the recumbent position. It is often associated with coughing and is relieved when the patient assumes an upright position. In patients with CHF, PND usually occurs 1 to 2 hours after lying down and is caused by the gradual transfer of fluid in the lower extremities to the lungs.

Orthopnea is the inability to breathe when lying down. It is often described as two- or three-pillow orthopnea, depending on the number of pillows the patient must use to elevate the upper portion of the body and obtain relief. PND and orthopnea are most commonly associated with left-sided heart failure and occur when reclining causes fluid to collect in the lungs.

Treopnea is dyspnea caused by lying on one side, but that does not occur when the patient turns to the other side. Treopnea is most often associated with disorders of the chest that occur on only one side, such as unilateral lung disease, unilateral pleural effusion, or unilateral airway obstruction.

Platypnea, the opposite of orthopnea, is dyspnea caused by upright posture and relieved by a recumbent position. Orthodeoxia (*ortho,* positional; *deoxia,* decrease of oxygen) is arterial oxygen desaturation (hypoxemia) that is produced by assuming an upright position and relieved by returning to a recumbent position. Orthodeoxia and platypnea are seen in patients with right-to-left intracardiac shunts from congenital heart disease and in patients with venous-to-arterial shunts in the lung related to severe lung disease or chronic liver diseases such as cirrhosis. Simply stated, when these patients are upright, there is an increased amount of blood being shunted from the right side of the heart to the left without being adequately oxygenated. When orthodeoxia is severe, patients experience increasing dyspnea (platypnea) while standing. Orthodeoxia also may occur after a pneumonectomy (removal of a lung). Terms commonly used to describe dyspnea are listed in Table 3-9.

Occurrences of dyspnea should be chronologically recorded, including related symptoms such as coughing, wheezing, pain, position, and exertion. Coughing in conjunction with dyspnea occurs with acute or chronic infection, asthma, aspiration, CHF, COPD, and many of the diffuse lung diseases. Dyspnea with minimal exertion is frequently associated with poor conditioning, inactivity, obesity, and heavy smoking. Shortness of breath during exercise or excitement is also a common complaint associated with chronic severe anemia (e.g., hemoglobin concentration under 6 to 7 g/dL). Table 3-10 lists associated symptoms, precipitating and relieving factors, and characteristics of the dyspnea-related disorders.

The effects of dyspnea on activities of daily living (dressing, eating, sleeping, walking) must be reviewed. Patients with COPD tend to decrease their exercise progressively to prevent being short of breath until their activities of daily living are compromised out of proportion to their actual cardiorespiratory potential. It is essential to gain a picture of the patient's daily habits and routines as well as the physical, emotional, familial, and occupational environment. The potential for relief of the factors contributing to dyspnea should be assessed and recorded.

Table 3-9	Terms Commonly Used to Describe Breathing

Medical Term	Definition
Apnea	Absence of spontaneous ventilation
Dyspnea	Unpleasant awareness of difficulty breathing, shortness of breath, or breathlessness
Eupnea	Normal rate and depth of breathing
Bradypnea	Less than normal rate of breathing
Tachypnea	Rapid rate of breathing
Hypopnea	Decreased depth of breathing
Hyperpnea	Increased depth of breathing with or without an increased rate
Orthopnea	Dyspnea in the recumbent position but not in the upright or semivertical position
Treopnea	Dyspnea in one lateral position but not in the other lateral position
Platypnea	Dyspnea caused by upright posture and relieved by a recumbent position
Orthodeoxia	Arterial oxygen desaturation (hypoxemia) that is produced by assuming an upright position and relieved by returning to a recumbent position
Hyperventilation	Increased alveolar ventilation caused by either an increased rate or increased depth of breathing or both
Hypoventilation	Decreased alveolar ventilation caused by either a decreased rate or decreased depth of breathing or both
Air hunger	A grave sign indicating the need for immediate treatment

Table 3-10	Causes and Characteristics of Shortness of Breath

Cause	Type of Dyspnea	Associated Symptoms	Precipitating and Aggravating Factors	Patient Characteristics	Usual Physical Findings
Acute or Recurrent Dyspnea					
Asthma	Acute dyspnea Episodic	Cough indicates asthmatic bronchitis Dyspnea may be exertional and worse at night	Allergens, noxious fumes, exercise, recumbency, respiratory tract infection Exposure to cold or use of beta blockers	Most common cause of recurrent dyspnea in children	Bilateral wheezing, prolonged expiration ✓
Pneumothorax	Acute onset	Sudden sharp pleuritic pain	Spontaneous, COPD, trauma, cystic fibrosis	Often a prior history of similar episode, may be familial	Decreased or absent breath sounds Tracheal shift if tension pneumothorax
Foreign body aspiration	Acute dyspnea			Most common in children and intoxicated or semiconscious people during eating	Tachypnea, inspiratory stridor, localized or unilateral wheeze, suprasternal retraction with respiration
Pulmonary emboli	Acute onset	Chest pain, faintness, loss of consciousness	Prolonged recumbency, women using birth control pills	Postoperative, phlebitis, postpartum, arrhythmia (esp. atrial fibrillation)	Tachypnea, crackles, low blood pressure, wheezing → pleural friction rub
Pulmonary edema	Acute onset Episodic	Dyspnea on exertion Orthopnea, PND			Gallop rhythm crackles at bases
Hyperventilation and anxiety	Acute dyspnea, "sighing" respirations	Lightheaded, palpitations, paresthesias (esp. around mouth and extremities)	Stress panic	Usually anxious	Signs of anxiety but no signs of dyspnea

Continued

| Table 3-10 | Causes and Characteristics of Shortness of Breath—cont'd |

Cause	Type of Dyspnea	Associated Symptoms	Precipitating and Aggravating Factors	Patient Characteristics	Usual Physical Findings
Acute or Recurrent Dyspnea—cont'd					
Poor physical conditioning	Dyspnea on minimal exertion			Obese, physically inactive	After exercise pulse slows very gradually
Chronic Dyspnea					
Congestive heart failure	Chronic dyspnea with gradual onset, PND	Edema, dyspnea remains long after exercise is stopped	Exercise, recumbency, trauma, anesthesia, shock, hemorrhage, calcium channel blockers or beta blockers	Older patients, nocturnal dyspnea relieved by sitting	Shallow respirations but not necessarily rapid, basilar crackles, jugular venous distention, edema, third heart sound, hepatomegaly
Chronic bronchitis	Dyspnea not necessarily presenting symptom	Persistent, productive cough	Infection exertion	Overweight	Coarse crackles, cyanosis
Emphysema	Progressive, usually no dyspnea at rest	Weak cough	Exertion	Malnourished	Hyperinflated lungs, decreased breath sounds, increased resonance, increased AP chest diameter, use of accessory muscles; at rest

AP, Anteroposterior; *COPD*, chronic obstructive pulmonary disease; *PND*, paroxysmal nocturnal dyspnea.

Questions to Ask About
SHORTNESS OF BREATH

What do you do when you experience breathlessness? Can you continue to do what you were doing or do you have to sit down or lie down? Can you continue to speak?

Does the difficult breathing alter your normal activities during the day? Does it make it hard for you to sleep at night? What makes it better? What makes it worse?

Are you always short of breath or do you have attacks of breathlessness? (The onset of dyspnea may be gradual or sudden or intermittent.)

What relieves the attacks? relaxing? changing location? changing position? taking medication?

Does a body position, time of day, or certain activity affect your breathing?

Do the attacks cause your lips or nail beds to turn blue?

How many stairs can you climb or how may blocks can you walk before you begin to feel short of breath? Do activities like taking a shower, getting dressed, or shopping make you feel short of breath?

(Dyspnea from activity suggests an inefficient breathing mechanism or poor ventilation or perfusion.)

When you feel breathless, do you feel any other symptoms like sweating or cough or chest discomfort?

Do you make any sounds like wheezing or snoring?

Does the shortness of breath seem to be getting better or worse or staying the same?

Have you ever had exposure to asbestos? sandblasting? pigeon breeding?

Have you ever been exposed to anyone with tuberculosis?

Have you ever lived near the San Joaquin Valley in California (coccidioidomycosis)? Midwestern or Southeastern United States (histoplasmosis)?

Table 3-11	Causes and Characteristics of Chest Pain		
Condition	**Location and Characteristics**	**Etiology/Precipitating Factors**	**Associated Findings**
Chest Wall Pain			
Myalgia	Intercostal and pectoralis muscles Localized dull aching Increases with movement Usually long-lasting	Trauma, seizure, nonisometric and isometric exercise, COPD, steroid therapy Persistent severe cough	Usually no visible erythema or ecchymosis with occult trauma
Chondro-ostealgia	Ribs and cartilages, precisely located (chondral pain in sternal area) Increases with pressure to area, movement, respiration, coughing Can be severe and disabling	Trauma (e.g., steering wheel, cardiopulmonary resuscitation), severe coughing, osteoporosis, tumor, myelocytic leukemia, systemic autoimmune disease, Tietze's syndrome, COPD	Rib fractures, chondral dislocations, periostitis, fever with some systemic causes
Neuralgia	Dermatome distribution Superficial tingling to deep burning pain	Thoracic spine disease, metastatic tumor, blunt trauma, herpes zoster (shingles)	Specific changes on x-ray films, fever with infection
Pleuritic and Pulmonary Pain			
Pleuritis (pleurisy)	Pleura, usually well localized Sharp, stabbing, raw, burning Often rapid onset, increased by inspiration, coughing, laughing, hiccuping	Infection/inflammation of pleura, trauma, autoimmune and connective tissue disease	Fever, productive cough, tachypnea, splinting of affected side
Pulmonary embolus, pulmonary infarction	Usually at base of lung, may radiate to abdomen or costal margins Stabbing, sudden onset, increased by inspiration	Immobilization, obesity, pelvic surgery	Symptoms vary with size of embolus Anxiety to panic Dyspnea, tachypnea, tachycardia, coughing with blood-tinged to hemoptic sputum
Pneumothorax	Lateral thorax, well localized Sharp, tearing Sudden onset Increased by inspiration	Interstitial lung disease, bullous emphysema, asthma, idiopathic May follow deep inspiration, Valsalva maneuver, or exercise, or occur at rest	Dyspnea, tachypnea, decreased breath sounds on affected side Mediastinal shift and jugular venous distention if tension pneumothorax develops
Tumors	May be localized or diffuse Constant, sharp, boring, or dull	Invasion of primary or metastatic tumor through parenchyma to parietal pleura, mesothelioma	Symptoms vary with type and location Evidence from x-ray films History of asbestos exposure
Pulmonary hypertension (primary)	Substernal, dull, aching similar to angina Related to stress and exertion	Unknown Seen most commonly in young women	Dyspnea, tachypnea, anxiety, syncope, jugular venous distention
Cardiac Pain			
Angina pectoris	Substernal, may radiate to arms, shoulders, neck, and jaw Tightness or dull, heavy pressure-like pain not related to respiration	Coronary artery blockage or spasm Hot, humid weather, large meals, intense emotion, exertion	Anxiety, feeling of impending doom, dyspnea, sweating, nausea Relieved by nitroglycerin and rest
Myocardial infarction	Substernal, radiating like angina Sudden crushing, viselike pain lasting minutes to hours		As above, diaphoresis, vomiting Not relieved by nitroglycerin or rest

Continued

Table 3-11	Causes and Characteristics of Chest Pain—cont'd		
Condition	Location and Characteristics	Etiology/Precipitating Factors	Associated Findings
Cardiac Pain—cont'd			
Pericardial pain	Substernal or parasternal radiating to neck, shoulder, and epigastrium (rarely to arms) Sharp, stabbing, intermittent Intensified by respiration and lying on left side	Inflammation of pericardium, infection, metastatic tumor, trauma, irradiation, autoimmune diseases	Pericardial friction rub Tachycardia, distended neck veins, paradoxical pulse with tamponade, dyspnea
Mediastinal Pain			
Esophageal	Substernal, retrosternal, epigastric Radiates toward shoulders Deep burning pain Sudden, tearing pain	Esophagitis aggravated by bending over, lying down, smoking, ingestion of coffee, fats, large meals Esophageal spasm Esophageal tear	Regurgitation of sour-tasting acid secretions relieved by antacids or may be relieved by nitroglycerin Hematemesis, shock
Dissecting aortic aneurysm	Tearing midline chest or posterior thoracic pain Sudden onset, may last hours	Blunt trauma, hypertension, inflammatory or degenerative diseases	May have lower blood pressure in legs or one arm, paralysis, murmur of aortic insufficiency, paradoxical pulse, hypertension, shock, death
Tracheobronchitis	Substernal burning discomfort May be referred to anterior chest	Acute viral infections, prolonged cigarette smoking	Cough may or may not be productive May have fever with infection
Other causes	Substernal, retrosternal, epigastric pain or burning Vague tightness to severe crushing	Referred abdominal pain: hiatal hernia, peptic ulcer, gallbladder, acute pancreatitis Hyperventilation syndrome	Symptoms vary with disease Respiratory distress, tachypnea, diaphoresis, numbness of fingers and around mouth Respiratory alkalosis

CHEST PAIN

Chest pain is common in patients with cardiac ischemia (low blood supply to the myocardium) or inflammatory disorders affecting thoracic or abdominal structures—the heart, pleurae, trachea, main airways, chest wall, esophagus, stomach, gallbladder, and pancreas. Because of the complexity of the nerve structure of the chest, pain from other locations can be referred to the chest and pain from the chest may be referred to other sites. For example, pain from indigestion is often referred to the chest. Pain from a dissecting aneurysm of the thoracic aorta may start just below the sternum (anterior substernal location), but then migrates or tears toward the back.

Chest pain is the cardinal symptom of heart disease. In its classic presentation, the "viselike" pain of a heart attack is referred down the arms, most often the left, and may radiate into the shoulder or up into the jaw. This type of chest pain is known as angina and signals a medical emergency; intervention to open a clogged coronary artery and reestablish blood flow to the heart muscle needs to occur within 4 hours of the onset of pain or irreversible damage of the heart muscle occurs. Unfortunately, not all heart pain presents with this classic pic-

ture. In fact, in some people there is only a weak relationship between the severity of the chest pain and the importance of the underlying cause. Therefore *all chest pain must be taken seriously.*

> **SIMPLY STATED**
> Cardiac chest pain is most often located in the center of the chest and may radiate to the arm, jaw, or back.

Chest pain can also occur from musculoskeletal disorders, trauma, drug therapy, indigestion, and anxiety. It can range in character from sharp or stabbing to a vague feeling of heaviness or discomfort. It may be steady or intermittent, mild or acute. It may be caused or aggravated by stress, exertion, deep breathing, coughing, moving, or eating certain foods. The characteristics of the more common causes of chest pain are summarized in Table 3-11. The precise cause of chest pain cannot always be determined by taking a history, but it is usually possible to determine whether the origin is from the chest wall, the pleurae, or viscera, and if emergency care is needed. *History taking is the key to evaluating chest pain.*

Pulmonary Causes of Chest Pain

Chest pain caused by pulmonary disease is usually the result of involvement of the chest wall or parietal pleura (the serous membrane that lines the inner chest wall), both of which are well supplied with pain fibers. The lung parenchyma has no pain receptors. However, acute pulmonary diseases such as pneumonia, lung abscess, and pulmonary infarction often involve the overlying pleura and may induce pleuritic pain. Mediastinitis (inflammation of mediastinal structures) causes retrosternal, aching, oppressive sensations that may be severe. Chronic disorders of the large airway, such as tracheal or bronchial tumors or ulcers, usually do not cause pain. But the inflammation of tracheobronchitis may induce substernal discomfort that changes to a tearing, rasping, sharp, substernal pain with coughing.

Pleuritic pain, often described as inspiratory pain, is the most common symptom of disease causing inflammation of the pleura (pleurisy). It is sharp, often abrupt in onset, and severe enough to cause the patient to seek medical help (often within hours of onset). It increases with inspiration, a cough, a sneeze, a hiccup, or a laugh. Pleuritic pain is usually localized to one side of the chest, frequently the lower, lateral aspect. It may be only partially relieved by splinting and pain medication. Pleuritic pain increases with pressure and movement but not to the same degree as pain originating from the outer chest wall. In contrast, the lung parenchyma and the visceral pleura that cover the lungs are relatively insensitive to pain; therefore, pain with breathing usually indicates involvement of the parietal pleura.

Chest wall pain may originate from the intercostal and pectoral muscles, ribs, and cartilages, or stimulation of a neural pathway (neuralgia) anywhere along a dermatome (skin area innervated by a particular spinal cord segment). It is usually described as a well-localized, constant aching soreness that increases with direct pressure on the area of tenderness and with any arm movement that stretches the thoracic muscles.

Descriptions

The patient's body language as well as his/her descriptive terms give clues about the cause of chest pain. Patients with pleuritic pain may be bent to the side, taking shallow breaths, and holding their chest to decrease the amount of movement. They describe their pain as "sharp," "stabbing," "raw," or "burning," progressing to "excruciating" when they breathe or laugh. A patient with chest wall pain may complain of aching pain or soreness at a specific site and will pull away from being touched. Esophageal pain may be described as "knotlike," or "like a big bubble trapped inside," or "burning." Patients with spontaneous pneumothorax or dissecting aortic aneurysm may describe the pain as excruciating "tearing" or "knifelike."

Patients with heart pain *(angina)* will frequently hold a clenched fist over their sternum as they describe the pain as "aching," "squeezing," "pressing," or "viselike." Their pain is worse with exercise and may prevent them from performing physical activity. The pain may diminish with rest. Patients with this type of chest pain must be evaluated by a physician.

Pain is a purely subjective symptom. The perception of pain varies not only with the source of pain, but also with previous experience, culture, personality traits, amount of rest, and emotional implications of the pain. Since chest pain varies from relatively benign neuromuscular skeletal pain (the most common) to life-threatening angina (caused by a decreased blood supply to the heart muscle), the interviewer must be careful to obtain an accurate and impartial history. The following characteristics must be reviewed in detail: onset, location, radiation, frequency, duration, severity, precipitating and relieving factors, and specific descriptions (e.g., tearing, stabbing, dull, sharp, crushing, burning). Clues to locating the source of chest pain include a history of trauma, surgery, or muscle strain; local tenderness; swelling; and relationship to inhaling, coughing, position, and activity.

Questions to Ask About CHEST PAIN

Where is the pain?

Did the pain start suddenly? gradually? Is it more severe now than when it started?

Have you ever had a pain like this before? What medicine did you take to relieve the pain?

How would you describe the pain? [let the patient describe the character of the pain in his/her own words; if unable to give a description then use suggestions of descriptive words] *aching? throbbing? knifelike? sharp? constricting? sticking? burning? dull? shooting? tearing?*

How long have you had the pain?

Do you have recurrent episodes of pain? How often do you get the pain? How long does the pain last?

What makes the pain worse? breathing? lying flat? moving your arms or neck?

Is the pain associated with coughing? shortness of breath? palpitations? coughing up blood? nausea or vomiting? leg pain? dizziness? weakness? headache? muscle fatigue?

Does the pain occur at rest? exercise? while sleeping? with stress? after eating?

What do you do to make it better?

Have you ever had a heart attack? Has anyone in your family had heart disease? at what age?

Have you had a recent respiratory infection? Do you have pulmonary disease?

Have you had trauma to your chest? a hip or leg fracture? been involved in an accident?

What medications are you taking? Have you recently changed the dose or how you take them?

Do you take any other type of drugs? cocaine?

DIZZINESS AND FAINTING (SYNCOPE)

Syncope is a temporary loss of consciousness caused by reduced blood flow and therefore a reduced supply of oxygen and nutrients to the brain. Reduced cerebral blood flow may be localized (as in cerebral thrombosis, embolism, or atherosclerotic obstruction) or generalized as occurs with obstruction to blood flow from the heart, cardiac arrhythmias, and hypovolemia (decreased available blood volume). Pulmonary causes of syncope include pulmonary embolism or hypertension (obstruction of blood flow from the right heart), prolonged bouts of coughing (tussive syncope), and low levels of blood oxygen (hypoxia) or carbon dioxide (hypocapnia). Holding one's breath following a deep inspiration (Valsalva maneuver) results in high intrathoracic pressure and decreased venous return to the heart. Causes of syncope are listed in Box 3-3. While some of these causes of syncope are not associated with poor long-term outcomes, others can be serious problems.

Descriptions

The activity that preceded syncope and the position of the patient give clues to the causes of syncope. Primary pulmonary hypertension and some cardiac causes are associated with syncope during exercise. An irregular heart rhythm or palpitations before syncope suggest cardiac arrhythmia as the cause.

Vasovagal syncope, or "common dizziness and fainting," is the most usual type of syncope and results from a loss of peripheral venous tone. It can occur with all forms of physical and emotional stress including (but not limited to) pain; venipuncture; prolonged standing, especially in hot weather; and anxiety. Special attention must be given to careful review of all parts of the history and to the physical examination to rule out the organic causes of syncope.

Orthostatic hypotension is an excessive drop in blood pressure on assuming a standing position. In normal individuals, standing suddenly causes pooling of blood in the venous capacitance vessels of the legs and trunk, but compensatory mechanisms in the autonomic system maintain blood pressure and the blood supply to the brain. When portions of the reflex arc are impaired by disease processes, drugs, or an inadequate blood volume, these homeostatic mechanisms may be inadequate for restoring the lowered blood pressure. If the patient stands suddenly, the adaptive reflexes do not compensate fast enough and there is a sudden drop in blood pressure. The patient will experience dizziness, blurring vision, profound weakness, and syncope. Orthostatic hypotension is suggested when a patient reports fainting after suddenly getting up from a chair or after rising suddenly from bed in the middle of the night to run to answer the telephone. Medications that affect vascular tone or vascular volume can lead to orthostatic hypotension. Elderly patients are more prone to orthostatic hypotension because of dehydration.

Carotid sinus syncope is associated with a hypersensitive carotid sinus and is seen more commonly in the aged population. Whenever a patient with carotid sinus syncope wears a tight shirt collar or turns the neck in a certain way, there is an increased stimulation of the carotid sinus. This slows the pulse rate and causes a sudden fall in systemic pressure, resulting in syncope.

Cough (tussive) syncope is the transient loss of consciousness following severe coughing. It occurs most commonly in middle-aged men with underlying COPD who are outgoing and

BOX 3-3   Causes of Syncope

Circulatory Control Abnormalities

Drugs (very common)
Vasovagal syncope
Orthostatic hypotension
Hypovolemia
Carotid sinus hypersensitivity
Autonomic failure

Cardiopulmonary Abnormalities

Valvular and myocardial disease
    Prosthetic valve dysfunction
    Aortic stenosis
    Mitral valve prolapse
    Pulmonary stenosis
    Pulmonary embolism
    Hypertrophic obstructive cardiomyopathy
    Acute myocardial ischemia/infarction
Inadequate cardiac filling
    Coughing, Valsalva maneuver
    Atrial myxoma
Cardiac arrhythmias
    Sick sinus syndrome
    Atrioventricular block
    Supraventricular tachycardia
    Ventricular tachycardia
    Wolff-Parkinson-White syndrome
    Long Q-T syndrome

Metabolic Conditions

Hypoxia
Hypocapnia
Hypoglycemia
Intoxication

Neurologic Conditions

Neurovascular disease
Convulsive disorders
Generalized seizures
Transient ischemic attack

Psychological Conditions

Hysterical fainting
Panic attacks

moderately obese and have a great appetite for food, alcohol, and smoking. It rarely occurs in women. The cough may be chronic and is usually dry and unproductive. Typically there is a "tickle" in the patient's throat precipitating a coughing paroxysm; then the patient's face becomes red, vision dims, the eyes become fixed, and the patient suddenly loses consciousness. The attacks usually last only a few seconds, but the patient may fall or slump in a chair since the muscles relax completely. Some patients have reported more than 20 episodes a day. Cough syncope is usually a benign symptom, and patients return to their previous activity with little recall of the episode. However, deaths and serious injury have been reported when the syncope occurred while driving.

A precise description of the syncopal event should include a description of the preceding events as well as coexisting symptoms, including dyspnea, nausea, neurologic events, angina (chest pain), and palpitations or irregular heartbeat. A careful interview of witnesses (if available) and ambulance personnel can be extremely helpful. In addition, a detailed review of medications and medical history, including known neurologic or heart disease, arrhythmia, pacemaker placement, or known sudden death of a family member, will provide clues to the cause of the syncope.

Questions to Ask About
DIZZINESS & FAINTING

What do you mean when you say you were dizzy? felt faint? Did you lose consciousness?

What were you doing just before you fainted? Did you have any warning that you were going to faint?

Have you had recurrent fainting spells? If so, How often do you have these attacks?

What position were you in when you fainted?

Was the fainting preceded by any other symptom? nausea? chest pain? palpitations? confusion? numbness? hunger? cough?

SWELLING OF THE ANKLES (DEPENDENT EDEMA)

Edema is soft-tissue swelling resulting from an abnormal accumulation of fluid. It may be generalized *(anasarca)*, may appear only in dependent body areas (feet and ankles in ambulatory patients, sacral area in patients on bed rest), or may be limited to a single extremity or organ (such as pulmonary edema). Edema is associated with kidney disease, liver disease, cardiac and pulmonary disease, and obstruction of venous or lymphatic drainage of an extremity.

Peripheral (dependent) edema caused by pulmonary disease occurs when the disease process causes narrowing of the capillaries in the lung, requiring the right ventricle to generate higher and higher pressures to move blood through the lungs. Gradually the overworked right ventricle becomes enlarged and unable to pump all its blood through the lungs, which results in a damming effect that causes the venous system to become engorged with blood. Because of the high pressure in the veins, fluid is pushed out into the tissues. At first, the edema is seen only in the dependent (lower) areas of the body. When the patient has been standing or sitting, the edema is seen in the feet and ankles and is relieved by rest and elevation of the legs. Because patients on bed rest have their legs elevated at near heart level, *dependent edema* accumulates in the sacral area (back hip area) or at the side of the hip in patients who prefer to lie on their side.

As right heart failure worsens, dependent edema is no longer relieved by rest or changing position and congestion occurs in the abdominal organs as well as the extremities and dependent areas of the body. As the liver becomes congested *(hepatomegaly)*, the patient may also complain of pain just below the ribs on the right side *(right upper quadrant pain)*. Edema of the bowel and *ascites* (collection of fluid in the abdomen) cause complaints of anorexia, nausea, and sometimes vomiting. Patients may also complain of slowed healing and even skin breakdown in the edematous areas.

Bilateral peripheral or dependent edema suggests pulmonary hypertension, heart failure, or venous insufficiency. *Unilateral peripheral edema* (edema in only one extremity) is most frequently caused by some type of venous obstruction in that extremity. This can occur because of constrictive clothing, jewelry, or wound dressings that surround the extremity and compress venous return. It may also be a danger sign suggesting a deep vein thrombosis (blood clot).

Descriptions

Patients may report that when they press on their swollen ankles or when they remove their shoes and socks, they notice a depression that remains in their feet or ankles. When compression of an edematous area produces a depression that does not fill immediately, *pitting edema* is present. In the medical history, pitting edema is usually described in general terms such as "the patient denies pitting edema" or "the patient reports pitting edema in both ankles that remains for at least 5 minutes after leg elevation." When the history and physical examination are reported together, pitting edema may be recorded using the scale shown in Table 3-12.

Peripheral edema is a sign and a symptom. The examiner may find edematous ankles that the patient had not noticed. The presence of edema is such an important factor that the history of the edema should be traced. Precipitating and alleviating factors and associated symptoms should be documented with the history of present illness.

Questions to Ask About
SWELLING OF THE ANKLES

When did you first notice the swelling? Where else does it occur?

Does it occur only when you have been standing or sitting for a long time? or is it present when you first get up in the morning? How does it change throughout the day?

If you press on the swelling, does it leave a fingerprint in the tissue? How long does the indentation remain?

What happens to the swelling when you sit with your legs elevated?

What makes it worse? What makes it better?

Is the swelling associated with any other activities such as exercise or when you eat food that has a lot of salt?

Do you have any other symptoms when you have the swelling? [use the following suggestive cues when the patient is unable to answer] like cough? difficulty breathing? pain?

Table 3-12	Pitting Edema Scale	
Scale	Degree	Refill
1+ Trace	Slight	Rapid
2+ Mild	0-0.6 cm (0-1/4 in)	10-15 seconds
3+ Moderate	0.6-1.3 cm (1/4-1/2 in)	1-2 minutes
4+ Severe	>1.3 cm (>1/2 in)	>2 minutes

FEVER, CHILLS, AND NIGHT SWEATS

Normal body temperature *(euthermia)* varies between 97° and 99.5° F (36° and 37.5° C) orally and is 1° to 2° F (0.5° to 1° C) higher in the late afternoon than in the early morning. This normal change of temperature during the day is known as the *diurnal variation*. Body temperature is also affected by age (higher in infants), exercise (increases to as high as 100° F during exertion and returns to normal within 30 minutes), excitement, sudden changes in environmental temperature, digestion, technique and route of measurement (about 1° F higher rectally and about 1° F lower axillary), and use of medications containing antipyretics (drugs that decrease temperature).

Descriptions

Fever *(hyperthermia, pyrexia)* is an elevation of body temperature above the normal range resulting from disease. Fever may be described as *sustained* (continuously elevated, varying little more than 1° F during a 24-hour period), *remittent* (continuously elevated with wide, usually diurnal, variations), *intermittent* (daily elevation with a return to normal or subnormal between spikes), or *relapsing* (recurring in bouts of several days interspersed with periods of normal temperature). Terms used to describe fever are listed in Table 3-13.

Fever is a nonspecific symptom and may be caused by multiple factors including a hot environment; dehydration (inadequate fluid volume in the body); reactions to chemical substances, drugs, or protein breakdown; damage to the heat-regulating center in the hypothalamus; infection; malignant neoplasms; connective tissue disease; and a variety of diseases (Table 3-14). In some patients a cause is never found, thus the term *fever of unknown origin* (FUO).

Fever is a concern for two important reasons. First, it often signifies that disease is present. The patient with fever should be evaluated for evidence of infection or other causes. Secondly, fever causes an increase in the metabolic rate of the patient that is proportional to the degree temperature elevation. This is of little consequence to the patient with a healthy cardiopulmonary system but may represent a major problem to the patient with chronic lung or heart disease. As the body temperature elevates, the demand for oxygen at the tissues increases. Additionally, the demand for removal of carbon dioxide increases with fever. As a result, the patient with chronic cardiopulmonary disease is at higher risk for respiratory failure when significant fever is present.

Table 3-13	Terms Used to Describe Fever
Fever, pyrexia	Abnormally high body temperature
High-grade fever	>101°F (38.2° C) orally
Low-grade fever	99.5°-101°F (37.5°-38.2° C) orally
Intermittent fever	Daily elevation with a return to normal or subnormal between spikes
Remittent fever	Continuously elevated with wide, usually diurnal variations
Relapsing fever	Recurring in bouts of several days interspersed with periods of normal temperature
Hyperthermia	Elevation of core body temperature above normal
Mild hyperthermia	99°-102° F (37.2°-38.9° C)
Moderate hyperthermia	102°-105° F (38.9°- 40.6° C)
Critical hyperthermia	>105° F (>40.6° C); medical emergency
Malignant hyperthermia	Core body temperature increases 2° F (1° C) every 15 min; occurs in people with an inherited predisposition to the condition
Fever of unknown origin	Fever >101° F that has occured several times in the past 3 to 4 weeks with no known cause
Hypothermia	Temperature that is below the normal range

Fever is usually accompanied by many other constitutional symptoms such as vague aching, malaise (vague discomfort, uneasiness), irritability, increased heart rate (9 to 10 beats per minute for each 1° F of elevation), and, if high enough, confusion, delirium, or convulsions. A rapidly increasing fever may be accompanied by chills and shivering or even *rigors* (bone-shaking, teeth-rattling chills) as peripheral vasoconstriction occurs to conserve heat.

Normally humans increase sweat production about threefold with their diurnal drop in temperature at night. However, when the temperature falls abruptly, as occurs with intermittent fever, sweat production may increase fivefold to eightfold, resulting in diaphoresis. When this profuse sweating occurs at night, soaking the bed clothes, it is clinically significant and is termed night sweats. Night sweats are common in patients with lymphoma, tuberculosis, and some types of pneumonia.

Fever with Pulmonary Disorders

Since fever is the most common manifestation of infection, it is usually assumed to be caused by an infectious process until proven otherwise. Pulmonary infections, including lung abscess, empyema (infection within the pleural space), tuberculosis, and pneumonia, are accompanied by fever in most patients. Acute bacterial infections are usually accompanied by shaking chills, although the occurrence of a single rigor followed by sustained fever suggests pneumococcal pneumonia.

Table 3-14	Common Causes and Characteristics of Fever		
Type	Nature of Fever Nature of Patient	Associated Symptoms	Precipitating Factors Physical Findings
Acute			
Upper Respiratory Infections			
Viral	Usually <101.5° F orally	Signs of URI, may be systemic	Cough, oropharynx infected
	Any age	symptoms	Exposure to URI
Bacterial	Often high fever, >101° F	Marked signs of URI, few systemic	Pharyngotonsillar exudate
	More common in children	symptoms	Pulmonary findings
			Children are restless
Other Viral Syndromes			
Influenza	Usually mild fever	Muscle aches	Minimal
	Any age		
Gastroenteritis	Any age	Nausea, vomiting, cramps, diarrhea	
Urinary tract infection	Often high fever with chills	Backache	Costovertebral angle tenderness
	Adults more common	Urinary frequency and urgency	Positive urinalysis
Bacterial sepsis	Often high fever	Chills	
Factitious fever	Usually >105° F, can be low grade	No weight loss	Disparity between rectal or oral and urine
	Associated with health care	Pulse rate not proportional	temperature
		to fever	May be emotionally disturbed
Drug reaction	Often high fever, acute or chronic	Occasional rash	Fever abates when drug discontinued
	Taking prescription or OTC medications		
Chronic			
Infectious mononucleosis	Usually low grade	Fatigue	Enanthema, fever, pharyngitis, splenomegaly, adenopathy (especially postcervical)
	Teenagers, young adults		
Tuberculosis	Usually low grade		Chest findings
	More common in diabetics		Positive TB test and chest x-ray
Hepatitis	Usually low grade	Fatigue, jaundice, anorexia	Hepatomegaly, jaundice, liver tender to palpation
	More common in intravenous drug users		

OTC, Over-the-counter; *URI*, upper respiratory infection.

Remittent fever is seen with mycoplasmal pneumonia, legionnaires' disease, and acute viral respiratory infections.

It cannot be assumed that the patient does not have an infection because there is no fever. Patients vary greatly in the degree of fever accompanying a disease process. Patients taking high doses of steroids and other drugs that can be used as immunosuppressants may have no fever in the presence of a massive infection. In addition, patients with a compromised immune system (e.g., leukemia, AIDS, etc.) may have minimal fever despite the presence of severe infection.

Fever, like swelling and wheezing, can be a sign or a symptom. Once the temperature is taken during the physical examination, it is clearly evident when fever is present. However, many patients report fever or chills and fever but have never taken their temperature. It is important to clarify why patients think they have a fever and, if the temperature was taken, to document the route and the patient's technique. The patient should be asked to present any temperature charts that have been made and to describe the pattern of the fever and the accompanying symptoms.

When a cause for fever is not readily apparent, careful attention should also be given to the history of travel, recre-

SIMPLY STATED

In the patient with lung disease, fever usually, but not invariably, signifies infection. However, it cannot be assumed that the patient does not have an infection because there is no fever. Patients taking high doses of steroids and immunosuppressants may have no fever in the presence of massive infection.

ation, occupation, and exposure to toxins or carriers of infectious diseases. All drugs used, including OTC medications, vitamins, and illicit drugs, should be listed, since many drugs, including antibiotics and blood products, can cause drug-related fever.

HEADACHE, ALTERED MENTAL STATUS, AND PERSONALITY CHANGES

Some patients with pulmonary disease complain of headache. When patients cannot get adequate oxygen into their blood, as

Questions to Ask About
FEVER, CHILLS, AND NIGHT SWEATS

How long have you had fever? How did you measure your temperature? What readings did you get?

Has there been any pattern to the fever? Did it start gradually or suddenly? Did it rise then disappear, then reappear?

Have you had other symptoms with the fever such as chills, headache, fatigue, cough, diarrhea, or pain?

Has your neck felt swollen? Have you had a sore throat or earache?

Do you have pain when you take a deep breath or cough? Where is the pain?

Have you had an infection recently? Can you recall a recent exposure to someone who may have had an infection?

Have you had a recent wound? How did it heal? Is the area still painful?

Have you traveled to an area where you may have been bitten by a tick? insect? spider? animal?

Have you been exposed to high temperatures for a prolonged period of time such as playing sports or working out in the heat? How long were you out in the heat? How much water did you drink while you were working? playing?

Have you had any unusual physical or emotional stress lately? injury? anesthetic? surgery? blood transfusion?

Have you taken any new medications in the last few weeks?

Are you taking thyroid medication? antidepressants? amphetamines or diet pills? medications that keep you from sweating? [anticholinergics, phenothiazines, MAO inhibitors]

Have you ever been told that you have pneumonia?

happens with lung disorders, or when the amount of oxygen in the inspired air is low (as at high altitude), the amount of oxygen available to the brain is decreased *(cerebral hypoxia)* and headache can occur. As the carbon dioxide level in the blood increases, the cerebral arterial vessels dilate, causing vascular headaches with throbbing pain over the entire head. Because hypercapnea worsens during sleep in patients with pulmonary disorders, early-morning headaches may be the first indication that the patient is retaining abnormally high amounts of carbon dioxide. If the hypercapnea persists, headaches may be present throughout the day.

As cerebral hypoxia and hypercapnea increase, progressive changes occur in the patient's mental status. Thought processes and memory deteriorate, the mind wanders, and the patient is easily distracted. Headaches, tremors, uncontrolled movements, hallucinations, and nightmares may occur. If the hypercapnea continues, alertness is affected, progressing to drowsiness, disorientation, stupor, then coma.

SIMPLY STATED
Early morning headache may be the first indication that the patient is retaining abnormally high amounts of carbon dioxide.

Personality changes are not uncommon with advanced pulmonary disorders. The patient may complain of forgetfulness or inability to concentrate. On the other hand, the family may report the patient is depressed, anxious, irritable, demanding, or denying the disease process and refusing to follow the treatment regimen. When chronic lung disease develops from occupational hazards, the patient may be hostile and embittered. Such personality changes may be due to chronic hypoxia or stress or result from the chronic use of certain medications.

As chronic pulmonary disease progresses, lifestyle options are decreased for the patient and family. Choices of work, play, and even places to live become more limited, and dependency on others increases. Patients must use more of their limited energy to breathe and perform the basic tasks of everyday living. Fear of acute respiratory failure, coughing up of blood, another hospitalization, and the possibility of death are always present. As a result, it is not uncommon for patients to deny their illness and refuse to cooperate with treatment, use the illness to demand attention, or channel all of their concerns to the illness and use it as a threat to control others.

However, sudden personality changes or alterations in mental status are indicative of an acute problem. Although such changes are nonspecific and may be seen with neurologic or cardiac disease or intoxication, they also result from decreased levels of oxygen and increased levels of carbon dioxide in the blood. A patient with chronic pulmonary disease who experiences an additional insult such as trauma, surgery, unusual stress or exertion, pneumothorax, or inhalation of pollutants may be stressed beyond the ability to adequately oxygenate and remove carbon dioxide from the blood. The patient may have a total change of personality and then deteriorate in a matter of hours. A patient who has been resting quietly and becomes restless deserves the same thorough investigation that would be carried out for the patient who becomes less responsive.

SIMPLY STATED
Sudden personality changes or alteration in mental status are indicative of an acute problem. The patient who suddenly becomes restless deserves the same thorough investigation as the patient who becomes less responsive.

SNORING

Snoring is often a benign symptom that is reported by the patient's spouse. It can be a symptom of serious concern when it is accompanied with periods of apnea during sleep. Patients with this combination must be evaluated for obstructive sleep apnea (OSA) (see Chapter 18).

Incidence and Causes of Snoring

Snoring occurs in about 5% to 10% of children and 10% to 30% of adults.[4-6] In children, snoring occurs equally in boys and girls,[7] but in adults it occurs about twice as often in males. The peak incidence of snoring occurs at ages 50 to 59 years in adult males and at ages 60 to 64 years in women.[8]

Snoring is caused by excessive narrowing of the upper airway with breathing during sleep. Some narrowing of the hypopharynx is normal with sleep and is the result of muscle relaxation. Excessive narrowing is common when obesity causes a build-up of redundant tissue in the airway. For this reason, obesity is one of the most common causes of snoring and OSA. Enlarged tonsils, a large tongue, a short thick neck, nasal obstruction,[9] a large soft palate,[10] abuse of alcohol or sleeping pills, and anatomical defects of the upper airway are possible precipitating factors in selected patients. In addition, snoring is influenced by sleeping position because gravity influences the position of the tongue and lower jaw. In the supine position, the lower jaw and tongue tend to flop back into the hypopharynx. Thus, snoring increases in the supine position and is reduced in the lateral or prone position.

Patients who snore most often have inspiratory snoring. Inspiratory snoring is common because the upper airway tends to narrow naturally during each inspiratory effort as air rushes through. Factors that result in narrowing of the upper airway, therefore, become more of an issue on inspiration. The addition of sleep to the picture further complicates the problem when the upper airway support muscles relax. In addition, the greater the inspiratory effort, the greater the drop in pressure within the upper airway and the more narrow the airway becomes.

The patient with *habitual* snoring snores each night and often snores loudly. The *occasional* snorer most often snores only when he/she is excessively tired, has used alcohol or a sleeping medication, or when sleeping in the supine position.

Clinical Presentation

Patients with snoring and OSA will also complain of excessive daytime sleepiness (EDS). If EDS is not present in the patient who snores, the snoring may be of relevance only to those who try to sleep nearby. The EDS associated with OSA is related to the poor quality of sleep that occurs. Upper airway narrowing increases with effort to breathe and eventually results in total obstruction and apnea. The apnea continues until the patient arouses somewhat (fragmenting the sleep) and the upper airway muscle tone increases in response to the arousal. The patient then is able to breathe until the deeper stage of sleep returns and the pattern cycles again. These cycles may occur hundreds of times each night of sleep. The result is a night of poor quality sleep in which the deeper stages are not sustained. The patient awakens feeling fatigued and experiences daytime sleepiness.

The excessive sleepiness often results in serious consequences such as occupational accidents,[11] motor vehicle accidents,[12-14] loss of employment, and social dysfunction. In many cases, there is no association between the daytime sleepiness and the snoring by the patient, the family, or the patient's family physician. Poor daytime concentration, bedwetting, impotence, high blood pressure and other complicating factors are seen especially in more severe cases.

> **SIMPLY STATED**
> Patients with loud snoring and excessive daytime sleepiness should be evaluated for obstructive sleep apnea.

REVIEW QUESTIONS

1. Which of the following factors may lead to a weak cough?
   a. Reduced lung recoil
   b. Bronchospasm
   c. Weak inspiratory muscles
   d. All the above

2. A cough described as being persistent for more than 3 weeks would be called which of the following?
   a. Acute
   b. Paroxysmal
   c. Chronic
   d. Nocturnal

3. Which of the following problems is associated with hemoptysis?
   a. Tuberculosis
   b. Lung carcinoma
   c. Pneumonia
   d. All of the above

4. A patient's complaint of breathlessness or air hunger would be defined as which of the following?
   a. Hemoptysis
   b. Wheezing
   c. Dyspnea
   d. Cyanosis

5. What term is used to describe shortness of breath in the upright position?
   a. Orthopnea
   b. Platypnea
   c. Eupnea
   d. Apnea

6. T   F   Dyspnea may vary from patient to patient depending on the underlying pathophysiology.

7. Which of the following is not associated with causing dyspnea?
   a. An increase in the work of breathing
   b. A decrease in the ventilatory capacity

c. An increase in the drive to breathe
d. An increase in lung compliance

8. What term is used to describe difficult breathing in the reclining position?
   a. Apnea
   b. Platypnea
   c. Orthopnea
   d. Eupnea

9. T   F   Chest pain associated with inspiration is termed pleuritic.

10. Which of the following may cause syncope?
    a. Severe coughing
    b. Pulmonary embolism
    c. Hypovolemia
    d. All the above

11. Which of the following is (are) true regarding dependent edema caused by lung disease?
    a. It is caused by pulmonary vasodilation.
    b. Accompanying hepatomegaly may be present.
    c. It is caused by acute systemic hypertension.
    d. All of the above.

12. Chronic pulmonary hypertension may lead to which of the following clinical findings?
    a. Pedal edema
    b. Inspiratory crackles
    c. Hepatomegaly
    d. a and c

13. Which of the following is associated with night sweats?
    a. Pneumonia
    b. Congestive heart failure
    c. Asthma
    d. Interstitial pulmonary fibrosis

14. In what decade of life is snoring most likely to be present in adult males?
    a. 20 to 29 years
    b. 30 to 39 years
    c. 40 to 49 years
    d. 50 to 59 years

REFERENCES

1. ATS Statement on dyspnea. *Am J Respir Crit Care Med* 159:321-340, 1999.
2. Lee L and others: Evaluation of dyspnea during physical and speech activities in patients with pulmonary diseases. *Chest* 113:625-628, 1998.
3. Juniper EF and others: Measuring quality of life in asthma. *Am Rev Respir Dis* 147:832, 1993.
4. Corbo GM and others: Snoring in 9- to 15-year-old children: risk factors and clinical relevance. *Pediatrics* 108:1149-1154, 2001.
5. Enright PL: Prevalence and correlates of snoring and observed apneas in 5,201 older adults. *Sleep* 19:529-530, 1996.
6. Teculescu D and others: Who are the "occasional" snorers? *Chest* 122:562-568, 2002.
7. Lu LR, Peat JK, Sullivan CE: Snoring in preschool children: prevalence and association with nocturnal cough and asthma. *Chest* 124(2):587-593, 2003.
8. Larrson LG: Gender differences in symptoms related to sleep apnea in a general population and in relation to referral to sleep clinic. *Chest* 124:204-211, 2003.
9. Young T, Finn L, Palta M: Chronic nasal congestion at night is a risk factor for snoring in a population-based cohort study. *Arch Intern Med* 161:1514-1519, 2001.
10. Teculescu D and others: Prevalence of habitual snoring in a sample of French males. Role of "minor" nose-throat abnormalities. *Respiration* 68:365-370, 2001.
11. Lindberg E, Carter N, Janson C: Role of snoring and daytime sleepiness in occupational accidents. *Am J Respir Crit Care Med* 164:2031-2035, 2001.
12. Teran-Santos J, Jimenez-Gomez A, Cordero-Guevara J: The association between sleep apnea and the risk of traffic accidents. *N Engl J Med* 340:847-851, 1999.
13. Lloberes P: Self-reported sleepiness while driving as a risk factor for traffic accidents in patients with obstructive sleep apnea syndrome and in non-apneic snorers. *Respir Med* 94:971-976, 2000.
14. Young T: Sleep-disordered breathing and motor vehicle accidents in a population-based sample of employed adults. *Sleep* 20:608-613, 1997.

CHAPTER
4

Robert L. Wilkins

Vital Signs

LEARNING OBJECTIVES

Upon completion of this chapter, the reader should be able to accomplish the following:

1. Recognize the four classic vital signs and the value of monitoring their trends.
2. Identify the clinical significance of abnormal sensorium.
3. Recognize what the Glasgow Coma Scale is useful for assessing and its predictive value in terms of patient outcome.
4. Recognize the normal values of the following vital signs and common causes of deviation from normal in the adult:
   a. Pulse
   b. Respiratory rate
   c. Blood pressure
   d. Temperature
5. Recognize the following issues related to body temperature measurement:
   a. Types of devices commonly used
   b. Factors affecting the accuracy of devices
   c. Common sites and temperature ranges of those sites for measurement
6. Describe how fever affects the following:
   a. Oxygen consumption and carbon dioxide production
   b. Respiratory rate
   c. Pulse
7. Define the following terms:
   a. Fever
   b. Tachycardia
   c. Bradycardia
   d. Pulsus paradoxus
   e. Pulsus alternans
   f. Tachypnea
   g. Bradypnea
   h. Systolic blood pressure
   i. Diastolic blood pressure
   j. Hypertension

k. Hypotension
l. Pulse pressure
m. Posture hypotension

8. Recognize the technique, common sites for palpation, and characteristics to evaluate for the pulse.
9. Describe the technique for determining respiratory rate and blood pressure.
10. Recognize how hypotension affects perfusion and tissue oxygen delivery.
11. Recognize the factors that cause erroneously elevated blood pressure measurements.
12. Identify the mechanism by which pulsus paradoxus is produced.

CHAPTER OUTLINE

Susan Jones Krider, RN, MS, contributed this chapter in the previous edition.

KEY TERMS

bradycardia

bradypnea

diastolic blood pressure

fever

hypertension

hypotension

postural hypotension

pulse pressure

systolic blood pressure

tachycardia

tachypnea

CHAPTER OVERVIEW

The previous two chapters focused on subjective data—those which are perceived by the patient. We now turn our attention to objective data—those which are measured. Although subjective data are important, objective data are factual information that are not influenced by patient opinion or feelings. Therefore it is most often relied on to make important clinical decisions. This chapter focuses on *vital signs*—the most frequently measured objective data for monitoring vital body functions and often the first and most important indicator that the patient's condition is changing. Vital signs are used for the following purposes:

- To determine the relative status of vital organs, including the heart, blood vessels, and lungs
- To establish a *baseline* (a record of initial measurements against which future recordings are compared)
- To monitor response to surgery, treatments, and medication
- To observe for trends in the health status of the patient
- To determine the need for further evaluation, diagnostic testing, or intervention

SIMPLY STATED

Patients' knowledge of their condition, as well as their concerns, must be considered vital information and never passed off as simply emotions.

OBTAINING VITAL SIGNS AND CLINICAL IMPRESSION

The four classic vital sign measurements are *temperature, pulse, respirations,* and *blood pressure*. Although they are not always listed as vital signs, the patient's *height* and *weight, level of consciousness* and *responsiveness (sensorium),* and the caregiver's *general clinical impression* are also important observations often included with the vital signs assessment.

Patients who have intravenous (IV) or arterial lines and traumatic or surgical wounds have catheter insertion sites, wounds, and extremity checks performed as part of "routine vitals." Pulse oximetry with continuous heart rate and electrocardiogram (ECG) monitoring are becoming a part of the standard vital signs package in some areas.

FREQUENCY OF VITAL SIGNS MEASUREMENT

The frequency of vital signs measurement depends on the condition of the patient; the nature and severity of the disorder; and the procedures, surgery, or treatments being performed. A baseline measurement should be taken on admission, at the beginning of each shift, before any treatment or procedure, and any time the patient's condition changes. Routine vitals on non–intensive care hospitalized patients are most commonly recorded every 4 to 6 hours (beginning of shift and midshift). Vital signs associated with respiratory care treatments are usually recorded before and after the treatment and occasionally at a midpoint during the treatment to evaluate possible side effects and effectiveness of the treatment.

After surgery or certain procedures, vital signs are measured more frequently to ensure the patient's safety (usually every 15 minutes for 2 hours, then every 30 minutes for 1 to 2 hours, then hourly until the patient is stable). The physician's order in the chart is often written as "Vitals q15m × 8, q30m × 4, qh until stable, then routine." Of course, vital signs should always be monitored and recorded as often as necessary for the safety of the patient. If the patient's condition changes unexpectedly or the patient suddenly comments about "not feeling well," vital signs should be measured immediately by the person closest to the patient.

SIMPLY STATED

Vital signs should be monitored and recorded as often as necessary for the safety of the patient.

TRENDS IN THE VITAL SIGNS

A single vital sign measurement gives information about the patient at that moment in time. Each measurement may be evaluated to see whether it is high or low compared with the normal value for the patient's age; however, an isolated measurement does not provide much information about what is normal for the individual patient or how the patient is changing or responding to therapy over time. To evaluate whether an individual patient has "normal" vital signs, you must understand what is "normal" for the patient's age and disease. Sometimes chronic disease or treatment modalities cause expected alterations in heart rate, respiratory rate, blood pressure, or temperature, which changes what is "normal" for an individual patient. If you doubt a finding, repeat the measurement and be sure the patient's position and your technique are correct for the parameter you are measuring. If you still doubt the measurement or if you think the patient may be getting into trouble, get help.

A series of vital sign measurements over time establishes a *trend* and is far more important clinically than any single measurement. Each time vital signs are measured, they should be compared with several previous measurements. Sometimes the patient's condition may be changing slowly, and comparison with one or two previous measurements does not indicate the trend, whereas comparison over an entire shift or 24 hours of vital signs may indicate clearly that the patient is slowly deteriorating. Because the trend of vital signs is so important, many physicians insist that vital signs on hospitalized patients be recorded on a multiple-day graph.

> **SIMPLY STATED**
> To evaluate whether a patient has "normal" vital signs, you must understand what is "normal" for the patient's age, disease, and environment.
> A vital sign measurement is only as accurate as the technique used to obtain it.

COMPARING VITAL SIGNS INFORMATION

Information about the probability that a patient is experiencing or may be developing a particular problem is obtained by comparing changes in vital signs and other signs and symptoms. For example, patients who are not maintaining adequate blood oxygen levels develop specific changes in general appearance, level of consciousness, heart and respiratory rates, and blood pressure. Table 4-1 lists these common signs of developing *hypoxemia* (partial pressure of arterial oxygen [PaO_2] < 60 mmHg).

In the field of medicine, this comparison of multiple signs and symptoms to arrive at the patient's diagnosis is called *differential diagnosis*. Of course, it takes time for the beginning student to learn all these relationships, but remember, the difference between the novice and expert clinician is not just knowledge, it is also the ability to assess and compare multiple types of subjective and objective data over time and to identify patterns and relationships in an individual patient. The key to expert assessment of vital signs at the bedside is to be constantly aware and to look for change:

- *Look* at the patient: Watch facial expressions, body movements, coordination, position, color, skin, and effort to breathe or move.
- *Listen* to the patient: Hear words, tones, sounds, rhythms, patterns, silence, feelings, and fears.
- *Touch:* Feel moisture, temperature, change in temperature, muscle and skin tone, resistance, and quality of pulses.
- *Reassess and analyze:* Collect information in a timely manner, compare it with normal values for the patient and the disease process, and mentally update this information whenever you are around the patient. Validate its accuracy. Does the information make sense? Is something wrong with the picture?
- *Trend, trend, trend:* What has changed about the patient? How has the patient changed? Why has he/she changed? What has not changed? Why? What does it mean? Does the change indicate a need for immediate action?

> **SIMPLY STATED**
> The key to expert assessment of vital signs at the bedside is to be constantly aware: look, listen, touch, question, validate, reassess, analyze, and trend.

HEIGHT AND WEIGHT

Height and weight are routinely measured as part of the physical examination and usually as part of every outpatient appointment. For hospitalized patients, the admitting height and weight is either obtained and recorded when the patient goes to

Table 4-1	**Signs of Hypoxemia Assessed During Vital Signs Measurement**
Vital Signs Measurement	Sign
General clinical presentation	Impaired coordination or cooperation
	Cool extremities* (can be felt while taking the heart rate and blood pressure)
	Diaphoresis (profuse sweating)
Sensorium (level of consciousness)	Decreased mental function
	Impaired judgment, confusion
	Loss of consciousness
	Decreased pain perception
Respiration	Increased rate and depth of breathing
	Difficulty breathing, use of accessory muscles
Heart rate	Tachycardia
	Arrhythmia (irregular heart rate), especially during sleep
Blood pressure	Increased blood pressure initially

*Temperature of the extremities, as well as diaphoresis, can be felt at the time the heart rate and blood pressure readings are obtained.

preadmitting testing service (PATS) or by the admitting nurse; thereafter, weight is usually measured every day or two. If there is a question of either dehydration or fluid overload, *fluid intake and output* (I & O) and weight may be recorded each shift until the patient's fluid balance is stable. Because weight is often used to calculate medication doses, the weight may be recorded in kilograms (1 kg = 2.2 lb) on the patient's medication record rather than on the vital signs record. Scales and measurement standards should be selected in sizes and styles appropriate for the age of the patient and should be calibrated regularly to ensure their accuracy.

GENERAL CLINICAL PRESENTATION

General observation begins the moment you first see the patient and continues throughout the examination and care. The patient's general appearance gives clues to the level of distress and severity of illness, as well as information about the patient's personality, hygiene, culture, and reaction to illness. This first step may dictate the order of care or physical examination. If the patient is in distress, the priority is to evaluate the problem in the most efficient and rapid way possible and to intervene or locate someone who can assist the patient. A more complete examination can be performed when the patient is more stable. Some visual signs of distress include the following:

- *Cardiopulmonary distress* is suggested by labored, rapid, irregular, or shallow breathing that may be accompanied by coughing, choking, wheezing, dyspnea, chest pain, or a bluish color (cyanosis) of the oral mucosa, lips, and fingers. The patient with cardiopulmonary distress often speaks in short, choppy sentences because of severe dyspnea.
- *Anxiety* is recognized by restlessness, fidgeting, tense looks, and difficulty communicating normally and may be accompanied by cool hands and sweaty palms.
- *Pain* is suggested by drawn features, moaning, shallow breathing, guarding (protecting the painful area), and refusal to deep breathe or cough.
- *Bleeding and loss of consciousness* are signs of extreme distress that require immediate intervention.

When a patient is not in acute distress, this initial observation provides an opportunity to see the patient as a whole person. Using all your senses—hearing, smelling, seeing, touching, and perception—during this head-to-toe inspection gives information about the patient's apparent age, state of health, body structure, nutritional status, posture, motor activity, physical and sensory limitations, and mental acuity. It helps you assess the reliability of the patient as an historian. It also helps you know what type of assistance and teaching the patient may need.

A written description of these initial observations helps others involved in the patient's care know how to plan care and relate to the patient's needs. Usually, these descriptive statements are written in language everyone can understand (e.g., "J.C. is a cooperative, alert, well-nourished, 43-year-old man who appears younger than his stated age and exhibits no indica-

tion of distress. He shows no signs of acute or chronic illness and is admitted for . . ."). You may occasionally find that more specific terms for body types have been used in the written physical examination report. Box 4-1 lists and defines some of those terms.

A statement is usually made in the documentation of the patient's general appearance about the apparent age of the patient relative to his/her stated age. Patients who appear much older than their stated age often suffer from chronic illness such as heart disease, diabetes, or chronic pulmonary disease. For example, the patient with chronic obstructive pulmonary disease often appears older than his/her stated age.

LEVEL OF CONSCIOUSNESS (SENSORIUM)

Evaluation of the patient's level of consciousness is a simple but important task. Adequate cerebral oxygenation must be present for the patient to be conscious, alert, and well oriented. The conscious patient also should be evaluated for orientation to time, place, and person. This is referred to as evaluating the patient's *sensorium* or mental status. The alert and well-oriented patient, whose orientation to time, place, and person is accurate, is said to be "oriented $\times$ 3," and the sensorium is considered normal.

BOX 4-1	Terms Used to Describe Body Types
Ectomorphic:	Slight development, body linear and delicate with sparse muscular development
Endomorphic:	Soft, roundness throughout the body; large trunk and thighs with tapering extremities
Mesomorphic:	Preponderance of muscle, bone, and connective tissue, with heavy hard physique of rectangular outline (between endomorphic and ectomorphic)
Sthenic:	Average height; well-developed musculature, wide shoulders, flat abdomen; oval face
Hypersthenic:	Short, stocky, may be obese; shorter, broader chest; thicker abdominal wall; rectangular-shaped face
Hyposthenic:	Tall, willowy, musculature poorly developed; long, flat chest; abdomen may sag; long neck; triangular face
Asthenic:	Exaggeration of hyposthenic body type
Cachectic:	Profound and marked malnutrition; wasting; ill health
Debilitated:	Weak, feeble, lack of strength (with weakness and loss of energy)
Failure to thrive:	Physical and developmental delay or retardation in infants and children; seen in children with illness but more often in children with psychosocial or maternal deprivation

Questions to Ask Yourself About
THE CLINICAL PRESENTATION

Questions to ask yourself while doing this portion of the examination include:
- What is the general appearance and attitude of the patient?
- Is the patient in distress?
- How is the patient responding?
- Are there abnormalities in the patient's face or movements?
- Does the patient have any motor or sensory limitations?
- Will this patient require assistance, safety precautions, or teaching?

treatment plan is often adjusted according to the evaluation of sensorium.

Glasgow Coma Scale

Many systems for evaluating the patient's level of consciousness have been developed. One assessment tool that allows for objective evaluation based on behavioral response of the patient is the Glasgow Coma Scale (Table 4-2). This scale can be used to monitor trends in the patient's neurologic condition over several days. A person with normal consciousness would obtain a score of 14.

The Glasgow Coma Scale has been the gold standard for assessing the neurologic function of patients who have been sedated, have received anesthesia, have suffered head trauma, or are near coma; however, it has limited ability to predict patient outcome.

An abnormal sensorium and a loss of consciousness may occur when cerebral perfusion is inadequate or when poorly oxygenated blood is delivered to the brain. As cerebral oxygenation deteriorates, the patient initially is restless, confused, and disoriented. If tissue hypoxia continues to deteriorate, the patient eventually becomes comatose. An abnormal sensorium also may occur as a side effect of certain medications and in drug overdose cases. Deterioration of the patient's sensorium often indicates the need for mechanical ventilation in the presence of acute respiratory dysfunction.

Evaluation of the patient's sensorium helps determine not only the status of tissue oxygenation but also the ability of the patient to cooperate and participate in treatment. Patients who are alert and oriented can take an active role in their care, whereas those who are disoriented or comatose cannot. The

SIMPLY STATED

An abnormal sensorium may be caused by inadequate oxygenation of the brain resulting from respiratory or cardiac failure.

TEMPERATURE

Normal body temperature for most people is approximately 98.6° F (37° C), with a normal range from 97.0° to 99.5° F and daily variations of 1° to 2° F (Table 4-3). The body temperature usually is lowest in the early morning and highest in the late afternoon. Most metabolic functions occur optimally when

Table 4-2	**Glasgow Coma Scale—Record of Patient Recovering from Coma**							
	Score		**Day**				
			1	2	3	4	5
Eye-opening response	Spontaneous opening	4					X
	To verbal stimuli	3				X	
	To pain	2	X	X	X		
	None	1					
Most appropriate verbal response	Oriented	5					X
	Confused	4					
	Inappropriate words	3				X	
	Incoherent	2		X	X		
	None	1	X				
Most integrated motor response (arm)	Obeys commands	5				X	X
	Localizes pain	4		X	X		
	Flexion to pain	3					
	Extension to pain	2	X				
	None	1					
TOTAL SCORE			5	8	8	11	14

From Malasanos L, Barkauskas V, Stoltenberg-Allen K: *Health assessment*, ed 4, St Louis, 1990, Mosby.

Questions to Ask Yourself About
LEVEL OF CONSCIOUSNESS

Asking yourself questions such as these while obtaining vital signs will help you assess the patient's sensorium:

- Is the patient conscious? If the patient is medicated, can he/she be aroused easily?
- Is the patient responding and is the response appropriate for the stimulus?
- Is the patient alert?
- Is the patient oriented to person, place, and time?
- Can the patient see, hear, and sense touch?
- Is the patient restless, fidgety, or easily distracted?
- Has the patient's responsiveness or behavior changed?

body temperature is within the normal range. Temperature elevation to between 99° and 100° F occurs normally during exercise and takes approximately 15 minutes to return to normal following exercise. In women, normal temperature increases approximately 1° F during ovulation and during the first 4 months of pregnancy.

Body temperature is maintained in the normal range by balancing heat production with heat loss. If the body had no ability to rid itself of the heat generated by metabolism, the body temperature would rise rapidly. The hypothalamus plays an important role in regulating heat loss and can initiate peripheral vasodilation and sweating in an effort to dissipate body heat.

The respiratory system also helps in the removal of excess heat through ventilation. When the inhaled gas is cooler than the body temperature, the airways warm the gas to body temperature. This warming and subsequent exhalation with each breath aids in removing excess body heat. When the inhaled gas is heated to near body temperature before inhalation, this heat loss mechanism is not functional.

Fever

An elevation of body temperature above normal (*hyperthermia*) can result from disease or from normal activities such as exercise.

When the temperature is elevated from disease, this elevation is called fever, and the patient is said to be *febrile*. Terms used to describe fever and its patterns are described in Chapter 3.

Fever most often results from infection somewhere in the body. Infection in the respiratory system can occur in the sinuses, airways, or lungs. However, fever can occur when infection is not present as a side effect of certain medications, with aspiration pneumonitis, and following a blood transfusion. However, infection is most likely to be the cause of the fever when the body temperature exceeds 102° F.[1]

It is important to remember that not all patients with an infection develop a fever. Some patients are unable to generate a significant fever despite the presence of major infection. Patients with an inadequate immune system are most prone to this finding.

A fever results in an increase in the metabolic rate of the body functions and produces an increase in oxygen consumption and carbon dioxide production by the body tissues. For every 1° C elevation of body temperature, oxygen consumption and carbon dioxide production increase approximately 10%.[2] The demand for an increase in the oxygen supply to the tissues and removal of carbon dioxide must be met by an increase in circulation and ventilation. Examination of the febrile patient often reveals increased heart rate and breathing rate. For the patient with significant cardiac or pulmonary disease, the increased demand on these systems may represent an intolerable stress.

Hypothermia

When the body temperature is below normal, *hypothermia* exists. Hypothermia is not common but can occur in persons with severe head injuries that damage the hypothalamus and in persons suffering from exposure to cold environmental temperatures. When the body temperature is below normal, the hypothalamus initiates shivering in an effort to generate energy and vasoconstriction to conserve body heat.

Because hypothermia reduces oxygen consumption and carbon dioxide production by the body tissues, the patient with hypothermia usually has slow and shallow breathing and a reduced pulse rate. Mechanical ventilators in the control mode may need significant adjustments in the depth and rate of delivered tidal volumes as the body temperature of the patient varies above and below normal.

Table 4-3	Normal Temperature Values by Site and Time Requirements for Accuracy When Using a Glass Thermometer			
		Normal Temperature Ranges		
Site		Fahrenheit	Celsius	Time Required
Oral		97.0°-99.5°	36.5°-37.5°	3-5 min*
Axillary		96.7°-98.5°	35.9°-36.9°	9-11 min
Rectal		98.7°-100.5°	37.1°-38.1°	2-4 min
Ear		Expected to be very close to rectal if measured correctly		2-3 sec

*Wait 15 minutes after eating or drinking.

Measurement of Body Temperature

Body temperature is most often measured at one of four sites: the mouth, ear, axilla, or rectum. Rectal temperatures accurately reflect actual body core temperature but are difficult to obtain in most patients. Feeling the skin temperature to determine elevation of temperature is not reliable, because skin temperature varies depending on the body's need to store or release heat, the ambient temperature, and the adequacy of blood circulation to the area.

Temperature is recorded in degrees Fahrenheit (° F) or degrees Celsius (° C) depending on the policies and equipment in each practice setting. Formulas for converting temperature between Fahrenheit and Celsius and an abbreviated conversion table are shown below.

$$° F = (° C \times 9/5) + 32$$
$$° C = (° F - 32) \times 5/9$$

Temperature normals vary with the site and method of temperature measurement. When glass thermometers are used, accuracy depends on the length of time the thermometer is allowed to register (see Table 4-3). Electronic thermometers can accurately measure the temperature in approximately 30 seconds or less, provided the probe is positioned correctly and the device is correctly calibrated. To trend temperature over time, the same site and same device must be used for each temperature measurement.

Rectal Measurement

Rectal temperatures are used for patients who are comatose, in intensive care, or confused. The average normal rectal temperature is 99.5° F (37.5° C). A minimum of 2 minutes is required for the glass thermometer to register an accurate rectal temperature. Rectal temperatures are often a few tenths of a degree higher than core temperature.[3]

Axillary Measurement

The axillary method is safe for infants and small children who do not tolerate rectal temperatures. It is the method of choice for neonates, because it approximates their core temperature and avoids injury to the rectal tissues. In adults, axillary temperature measurement assesses peripheral or skin temperature rather than core temperature and has poor correlation to other forms of temperature measurement in febrile adults. Average normal axillary temperature in adults is 97.7° F (36.5° C), approximately 1° F lower than oral temperature and 2° F lower than rectal temperature. It can take up to 11 minutes to obtain an axillary temperature in an adult and approximately 5 minutes in a child. For these reasons, axillary temperature is rarely assessed in the adult.

Oral Measurement

Oral temperature measurement is the most convenient and acceptable method for awake adult patients. This method should not be used with infants, comatose patients, or orally intubated patients. Average normal oral temperature in adults is 98.6° F (37° C). Proper placement of the thermometer tip into the posterior sublingual pocket on either side of the mouth is essential, because the temperature in other parts of the mouth may vary as much as 1.7° C. A 10- to 15-minute waiting period is required if a patient has ingested hot or cold liquid or has been smoking. A glass mercury thermometer requires 3 to 5 minutes to register but may take as long as 7 minutes.

The oral temperature is not affected significantly by oxygen administration via nasal cannula, simple mask, or Ventimask. Therefore it is not necessary to remove the oxygen or take rectal temperatures in patients receiving oxygen via cannula or mask to obtain accurate oral temperature readings. Heated aerosol or cool mist by face mask may alter oral temperature slightly but probably not enough to alter clinical decisions.

Tympanic (Ear) Measurement

Tympanic infrared thermometry uses a handheld probe placed in the ear canal to detect infrared emissions from the surfaces of the tympanic membrane and ear canal. No direct contact is made with the tympanic membrane. The temperature is digitized by a computer processor and displayed on a liquid crystal screen in less than 3 seconds. The first ear thermometer was introduced to the U.S. market in 1986 after two decades of use in the aerospace industry.[4] This method has the advantage of being fast, clean, and noninvasive and avoids the embarrassment and time delays associated with the classic forms of temperature measurement. It is commonly used in pediatric outpatient offices and emergency departments around the country. However, there are concerns about its accuracy and use in the hospital setting.

One end of the ear canal is immersed in the body near the tympanic membrane and the other end is exposed to the outside, with a temperature gradient of 0.5° to 1.0° C or more down the canal. Temperature is warmest at the tympanic membrane where it is within several tenths of a degree of core body temperature. The ear canal of an adult is an elliptical S-shaped tube approximately 3 cm long with varied size and shape. Because the otoscope-like probe is placed in the outer part of the ear canal and has a relatively wide-view angle through a curved ear canal, the probe detects both the tympanic membrane temperature and ear canal temperature. The computer processor then uses a mathematical formula to adjust for these temperature differences. Different companies use different mathematical equations, so ear temperature measurement also varies slightly by manufacturer.[5,6]

Multiple studies have been performed in different populations and age groups to evaluate correlations with other types of temperature measurement.[7-11] The effects of examiner technique,[12] ambient temperature changes,[13] middle ear infection, and the influence of wax[14] and exudate in the ear have also been evaluated; results have been mixed. It is clear that there is not 100% equivalence between the temperatures in the ear canal and those in other body sites; however, there is a significant correlation between ear and rectal, oral, and core temperatures.[3] In

Question to Ask Yourself About
TEMPERATURE

To ensure the accuracy of the temperature measurement, ask yourself the following questions:

- What type of thermometer was used?
- What site was used: oral, axillary, rectal, or tympanic?
- Was an appropriate amount of time used to obtain the temperature for the method of measurement?
- Had the patient just had a treatment, food, liquid, medication, or other event that could alter the accuracy of the measurement?
- Was the patient observed during temperature measurement? Is there any reason to believe that an elevated temperature was "facticious fever?"
- What is the time of day? Is the temperature highest in the late afternoon and lowest in the early morning, as expected?

most cases, ear temperature measurements run a few tenths of a degree below core temperature.

SIMPLY STATED

A body temperature higher than 102° F usually indicates infection.

PULSE

The pulse rate should be evaluated for rate, rhythm, and strength. Normal pulse rate varies with the age and status of the patient. As shown in Table 4-4, the younger the patient, the faster the pulse rate. The normal pulse rate for adults is 60 to 100 beats/min and is regular in rhythm.

A pulse rate exceeding 100 beats/min in an adult is termed tachycardia. Common causes of tachycardia include anxiety, fear, exercise, fever, high ambient temperature, low blood pressure, anemia, reduced arterial blood oxygen levels, and certain medications such as bronchodilators.

A pulse rate lower than 60 beats/min is termed bradycardia. This is less common but can occur when the heart is diseased, as a side effect of certain medications, or in well-conditioned athletes who typically have resting pulse rates in the fifties. Irregularity of the pulse suggests *arrhythmias,* which are discussed in Chapter 10.

The amount of oxygen delivered to the tissues depends on the ability of the heart to pump oxygenated blood. The amount of blood pumped through the circulatory system (cardiac output) is a function of heart rate and stroke volume (volume of blood ejected with each contraction of the ventricle). When the oxygen content of the arterial blood falls below normal, usually from lung disease, the heart tries to compensate

Table 4-4	Pulse and Respiratory Rates Referred to Age	
Age	Pulse (beats/min)	Respiratory Rate (breaths/min)
Newborn	90-170	35 to 45-70 with excitement
1 year	80-160	25-35
Preschool	80-120	20-25
10 years	70-110	15-20
Adult	60-100	12-20
Athlete	≅50	12-20

by increasing cardiac output to maintain adequate oxygen delivery to the tissues. An increase in cardiac output is accomplished by an increase in heart rate in most persons. For this reason, the heart rate is important to monitor in patients with lung disease.

Measurement of Pulse Rate

The radial artery is the most common site for evaluation of the pulse. The patient's arm and wrist should be relaxed, with the hand at or below heart level. If the patient's wrist is held above the level of the heart, the pulse may be difficult to obtain. The pads of the examiner's index and middle fingers are placed lightly over the patient's pulse point and then compressed until the maximal pulsation is felt (Figure 4-1). The thumb is not used, because pulsations from the artery in the examiner's thumb can be confused with the patient's pulse. The rhythm and strength of pulse are evaluated, the pulse rate is evaluated, then the pulse rate is counted.

Other common sites available for assessment of the pulse include the brachial artery, the femoral artery, and the carotid artery. When the blood pressure is abnormally low, the more centrally located pulses, such as the carotid pulse in the neck and femoral pulses in the groin, can be identified more easily than the peripheral pulse.

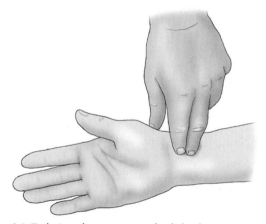

Figure 4-1 Technique for assessment of radial pulse.

Ideally, the pulse rate is counted for a full minute to evaluate rate, rhythm, and volume accurately. When the pulse is regular and rhythm and volume are normal, the pulse rate may be counted for 15 seconds and multiplied by 4 or counted for 30 seconds and multiplied by 2. However, if any irregularity is felt, the pulse is counted for a full minute. The pulse rate, or heart rate as it is called on some vital signs records, is always recorded as beats per minute.

Pulse Rhythm and Pattern

The rhythm of the pulse is the relative equality of the intervals between beats. The rhythm can be described as regular, regularly irregular, or irregularly irregular. A *regularly irregular* rhythm is a pulse with an irregularity that occurs in a definite pattern (e.g., beat, beat, pause, beat, beat, pause). *Bigeminy* is a rhythm coupled in pairs. *Trigeminy* is a rhythm grouped as three beats and a pause. An *irregularly irregular* pulse has no pattern.

When the rhythm is very irregular, it may be necessary to count the heart rate using a stethoscope placed over the heart (auscultation). During very irregular heart rhythms, some heartbeats cannot generate a strong enough pulse wave to be felt in the peripheral pulse. The difference between the number of auscultated beats and peripheral pulse beats is termed the *pulse deficit*. Irregular pulse rhythms are best evaluated by an ECG and may indicate the need for continuous ECG monitoring (see Chapter 10).

The volume of the pulse is assessed by how the artery feels as the blood flows through it with each beat. The volume of the pulse can be described as bounding, full, normal, weak, thready, or absent. A normal pulse is easy to feel, does not fade in and out, and is not easily obliterated by finger pressure. A *bounding* pulse is a full pulse that is difficult to depress with the fingertips. A *weak, thready,* or feeble pulse has a low volume and can be compressed easily. An absent pulse cannot be felt.

There are slight variations in numeric systems used to describe pulses; some scales are 0 to 3, others are 0 to 4, and some rating systems add plus signs (+). Because of this variation, it is important to clarify which scale is used in each healthcare facility. Two commonly accepted grading systems for pulse volume are shown later. *If the preferred grading system is not indicated on the charting forms, it is better to use the descriptive terms for pulse volume.*

The fullness of the pulse can be reduced for many reasons, including an arterial blood clot, atherosclerosis, diabetes mellitus, dehydration, or any other condition that would cause the blood flow through the artery to decrease.

Spontaneous ventilation may influence the strength of the pulse. When the patient's pulse strength decreases with spontaneous inhalation, it is referred to as *pulsus paradoxus. Pulsus alternans* is an alternating succession of strong and weak pulses and usually is not related to respiratory disease. These concepts are described in more detail in the discussion of blood pressure later in this chapter.

Questions to Ask Yourself About PULSE

To ensure the accuracy of the pulse rate, ask yourself the following questions:
- What is the pulse rate? rhythm? quality?
- Has the patient been doing something that might raise the pulse temporarily? Is the patient usually anxious at this time?
- Should I take the pulse again later when the patient is resting?
- If the pulse is irregular, did I count it for a full minute?
- Does the pulse vary with respirations?
- How does the current measurement compare with previous measurements.

SIMPLY STATED
An irregular pulse should be counted for a full minute to determine heart rate accurately.

RESPIRATORY RATE

Respiratory rates vary by age and condition of the patient. Table 4-4 gives reference ranges for patients of various ages. A respiratory rate of 40 breaths/min is unusual, and greater than 60 breaths/min is abnormal at any age. If carefully measured, respiratory rate is a sensitive and reasonably specific marker of acute respiratory disease.

Tachypnea is the term used to describe respiratory rates above normal. Rapid respiratory rates may occur as the result of exercise, atelectasis, fever, reduced arterial blood oxygen content, metabolic acidosis, anxiety, and pain. Tachypnea in the postoperative patient is common when significant fever develops or when the lungs partially collapse (atelectasis) as a side effect of the surgery. Atelectasis causes the lungs to become stiffer than normal, and the patient adopts a breathing pattern that is made up of rapid and shallow breaths as a compensatory mechanism. The degree of atelectasis determines the degree of tachypnea in such cases.

A slow respiratory rate, referred to as bradypnea, is uncommon but may occur in patients with head injuries or hypothermia, as a side effect of certain medications such as narcotics, and in patients with drug overdose.

Along with rate, the pattern and depth of breathing should be assessed. Other medical terms used to describe respiratory rate and depth are listed in Table 4-5. Evaluation of specific respiratory patterns is described in Chapter 5. Intermittent breathing, flaring nostrils, external sounds (e.g., crowing, wheezing, stridor), intercostal and sternal retractions, and use of accessory muscles when breathing are all indications that the patient is in acute distress and requires immediate intervention (see Chapter 5).

Table 4-5	Terms Commonly Used to Describe Breathing Patterns
Medical Term	**Definition**
Apnea	Absence of spontaneous ventilation
Eupnea	Normal rate and depth of breathing
Bradypnea	Less than normal rate of breathing
Tachypnea	Rapid rate of breathing
Hypopnea	Decreased depth of breathing
Hyperpnea	Increased depth of breathing with or without an increased rate
Sighing respiration	Normal rate and depth of breathing with periodic deep and audible breaths
Intermittent breathing	Irregular breathing with periods of apnea

Measurement of Respiratory Rate

The respiratory rate is counted by watching the abdomen or chest wall move in and out with breathing. With practice, even the subtle breathing movements of the healthy person at rest can be identified easily. In some patients, the examiner may need to place his/her hand on the patient's abdomen to identify the breathing rate.

Never ask the patient to "breathe normally" while you are assessing the rate of respiration. When individuals think about their breathing, they often voluntarily change their breathing rate and pattern. A better technique is to observe the patient's chest as you finish counting the radial pulse and evaluate the respirations while still holding the wrist. The patient will not be aware that you stopped counting the pulse, so voluntary changes in breathing usually do not occur. When the respiratory rate is regular, counting the number of respirations in 30 seconds and multiplying the number by 2 provides an accurate respiratory rate. The depth and pattern of breathing should also be assessed and recorded with the respiratory rate.

Questions to Ask Yourself About
RESPIRATORY RATE

To ensure the accuracy of the respiratory rate, ask yourself the following questions:
- What is the respiratory rate? Regularity? Pattern?
- What is the depth of respiration?
- Are accessory muscles used for respiration?
- Did the patient's awareness that respirations were being counted alter the rate or pattern of respiration?
- Did I count the rate for a full minute if the rate was unusually fast, slow, or irregular?
- How does this current respiratory rate compare with previous measurements?

SIMPLY STATED
The respiratory rate should be assessed without the patient being aware of the assessment.

BLOOD PRESSURE

Arterial blood pressure is the force exerted against the walls of the arteries as the blood moves through the arterial vessels. Arterial systolic blood pressure is the peak force exerted during contraction of the left ventricle. Diastolic blood pressure is the force occurring when the heart is relaxed.

Blood pressure is recorded with the systolic pressure listed over diastolic pressure: 120/80 mm Hg.

Pulse pressure is the difference between systolic and diastolic pressures. Normal pulse pressure is 35 to 40 mm Hg. When pulse pressure is less than 30 mm Hg, the peripheral pulse is difficult to detect.

Arterial blood pressure is determined by the force of left ventricular contraction, the peripheral vascular resistance, and the blood volume. The normal values for blood pressure change with age, as shown in Table 4-6. The normal range for systolic pressure in adults is 90 to 130 mm Hg, with 120 mm Hg the average. Normal diastolic pressure ranges from 60 to 85 mm Hg, with 80 mm Hg the average.

Optimal blood pressure with respect to cardiovascular risk is a systolic pressure less than 120 mm Hg and a diastolic pressure less than 80 mm Hg. However, unusually low blood pressure should be evaluated for clinical significance.

A blood pressure persistently higher than 140/90 mm Hg is termed hypertension. Persistent pressures above this level are associated with an escalating risk for development of heart, vascular, and renal diseases. Risk increases progressively: the higher the blood pressure and number of concurrent risk factors, the more advanced the degree of target organ damage. Although hypertension is one of the major modifiable risk factors for stroke, coronary heart disease, congestive heart failure, and

Table 4-6	Average Blood Pressure by Age	
Age	Average Blood Pressure (mm Hg)	90th Percentile (mm Hg)
Infant	84/52	104/66
3-5 years	94/52	110/70
6-10 years	98/62	114/70
11-13 years	106/66	124/84
14-19 years	108/64 (girls)	126/82 (girls)
	116/68 (boys)	136/85 (boys)
20+ years	120/80 (90/60 to 140/90)	

Data from Update on the 1987 Task Force Report on High Blood Pressure in Children and Adolescents: *Pediatrics* 98(4 Pt 1): 649-658, 1996; and Pealo D and others: *Circulation* 88:2460-2470, 1993.

Table 4-7   **Classification of Blood Pressure and Hypertension for Adults (18+ Years) with Follow-up and Treatment Recommendations**

Category	Systolic Blood Pressure (mm Hg)	Diastolic Blood Pressure (mm Hg)	Follow-up and Treatment Recommendations	≤1 Risk Factor, No Diabetes, No Cardiac Disease* or Target Organ Disease†	Diabetes, Cardiac Disease,* or Target Organ Disease†
Optimal	<120	<80			
Normal	<130	<85	Recheck in 2 years		
High-normal	130-139	85-89	Recheck in 1 year	Lifestyle modification	Drug therapy
Hypertension * ‡					
Stage 1 (mild)	140-159	90-99	Confirm within 2 months	Lifestyle modification	Drug therapy
Stage 2 (moderate)	160-179	100-109	Obtain care within 1 month	Drug therapy	Drug therapy
Stage 3 (severe)	≥180	≥110	Obtain care within 1 week	Drug therapy	Drug therapy
Stage 4 (very severe)	≥210	≥120	Obtain care immediately	Drug therapy	Drug therapy

Modified from the Sixth Report of the Joint National Committee on Prevention, Detection, Evaluation and Treatment of High Blood Pressure, *Arch Intern Med* 157:2413–2446, 1997.

*Cardiac disease: angina, prior myocardial infarction or cardiac surgery, left ventricular hypertrophy, heart failure.

Cardiac risk factors: smoking, diabetes mellitus, dyslipidemia, gender (men; postmenopausal women), age >60 years or family history of cardiovascular disease (women <65 years or men <55 years).

†Target organ disease: stroke, transient ischemic attack, peripheral arterial disease, nephropathy, retinopathy.

‡Based on an average of two or more blood pressures taken at two different times when not taking antihypertensive medication and when not acutely ill. When systolic and diastolic pressures fall in different categories, the higher category should be selected.

peripheral vascular disease, it is estimated that approximately half of those affected are not aware of their hypertension. Table 4-7 lists adult blood pressure and hypertension classifications with current recommendations for follow-up and treatment.[15]

Although hypertension is a common problem in the United States and around the world, the exact cause in most cases is not known. Hypertension most often occurs when either the contractility of the heart or the peripheral vascular resistance is abnormally increased. In most cases of hypertension, the cause is complex and involves many factors including genetics, environment, diet, smoking history, body habitus, and stress level. In addition, the presence of select disorders such as obstructive sleep apnea may cause chronic hypertension.[16]

Hypotension is defined as blood pressure less than 90/60 mm Hg in adults. It may occur as the result of peripheral vasodilation, left ventricular failure, or low blood volume. Perfusion of vital body organs may be significantly reduced with hypotension. Without adequate circulation, oxygen delivery to the tissues is impaired, and tissue hypoxia occurs. Adequate pressure and perfusion must be reestablished to prevent organ failure.

Changes in posture may produce abrupt changes in the arterial blood pressure, especially in the hypovolemic patient. Normally, when the patient moves from the supine to the sitting position, blood pressure changes very little, but when hypovolemia or vasodilation is present, blood pressure may fall significantly when the patient sits up; this is referred to as postural hypotension.

Measurement of Blood Pressure

The most common technique for measuring arterial blood pressure uses a sphygmomanometer (an occluding cuff, stethoscope, and manometer). This technique measures blood pressure indi-

rectly by determining the pressure required to collapse the artery in an arm or leg (Figure 4-2). The cuff is applied to the extremity, usually the upper arm, and inflated. When the pressure in the cuff exceeds the systolic blood pressure, blood flow through the artery is occluded and the pulse can no longer be felt. When the cuff is gradually deflated, blood flow in the artery resumes and the pulsations can be felt, heard with a stethoscope, or sensed by a flow probe or sensor. The cuff pressure at the time the blood flow resumes is used as the systolic arterial pressure.

The blood pressure cuff consists of an inflatable rubber bladder encased in a nondistensible cuff. Blood pressure cuffs are made in many different sizes to accommodate various sizes and ages of patients. Some of the most commonly used sizes are listed in Table 4-8. The bladder inside the cuff can be removed for cleaning or repair, so it is important to ensure that the correct size bladder is inside the cuff. Selection of the proper size cuff and bladder is essential to obtain an accurate pressure reading. The length of the bladder should be long enough to cover 80% of the distance around the arm in an adult and 100% of the arm circumference of a child. Overlapping the end of the bladder in children does not produce an error in the measurement. Using too wide a bladder produces a pressure that is lower than actual pressure. Using a bladder that is too narrow or too short results in overestimation of the blood pressure. The error of overestimation is greater, so if the correct size cuff is not available, a larger cuff should be selected.

Auscultatory Blood Pressure Measurement

The auscultatory method of pressure measurement uses the stethoscope to listen for the sounds produced by the arterial pulse waves (Korotkoff sounds) when blood flow in the artery

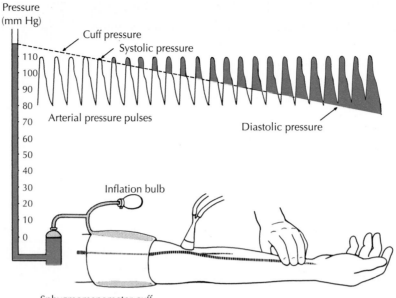

Figure 4-2 When the pressure within the sphygmomanometer cuff is increased above arterial blood pressure, the arteries under the cuff are occluded and no pulse can be palpated at the wrist. As the cuff pressure is gradually released, the systolic peaks of pressure finally exceed cuff pressure, and blood spurts into the arteries below the cuff, producing palpable pulses at the wrist. The sudden acceleration of blood below the cuff produces vibrations that are audible through a stethoscope. The pressure in the mercury manometer at the time the pulse is heard or felt indicates systolic pressure. As cuff pressure is diminished, the sounds increase in intensity and then rather suddenly become muffled at the level of diastolic pressure where the arteries remain open throughout the entire pulse wave. At still lower pressures, the sounds disappear completely when laminar flow is reestablished. (Modified from Rushmer RF: *Cardiovascular dynamics,* ed 3, Philadelphia, 1970, WB Saunders.)

Table 4-8	Acceptable Bladder Dimensions (in cm) for Arms of Different Sizes*		
Cuff	Bladder Width (cm)	Bladder Length (cm)	Arm Circumference Range at Midpoint (cm)
Newborn	3	6	≤6
Infant	5	15	6-15[†]
Child	8	21	16-21[†]
Small adult	10	24	22-26
Adult	13	30	27-34
Large adult	16	38	35-44
Adult thigh	20	42	45-52

Reproduced with permission from Perloff D and others: AHA Medical/Scientific Statement: Human Blood Pressure Determined by Sphygmomanometry. Copyright © 2001, American Heart Association.

*There is some overlapping of the recommended range for arm circumferences in order to limit the number of cuffs; it is recommended that the larger cuff be used when available.

[†]To approximate the bladder width:arm circumference ratio of 0.40 more closely in infants and children, additional cuffs are available.

resumes. As the pressure is reduced during deflation of the occluding cuff, the Korotkoff sounds change in quality and intensity. The five phases of this change are characterized in Table 4-9.

The pressure at which the first sound is heard corresponds to the systolic pressure. There has been debate over whether to use the muffling or disappearance of the sounds as the diastolic pressure. As of the 1993 American Heart Association consensus meeting, Phase V, disappearance of sounds, is used as the diastolic pressure. In small children and pregnant women or others with high cardiac output or vasodilation, sounds are often heard at levels far below those at which muffling occurs, sometimes very near 0 mm Hg. Therefore it was recommended that Phase IV be used as the diastolic pressure for children younger than 13 years. Recent reanalysis of the pediatric blood pressure database has shown that Phase V can be used for most children, as well as for adolescents and adults.[17] When there is a large discrepancy between muffling and disappearance of sounds, both pressures should be recorded (e.g., 110/60/30 mm Hg).

Occasionally, the Korotkoff sounds disappear during Phases II or III and reappear as the cuff pressure decreases. The period of silence is call the *auscultatory gap* and is most common in older patients with high blood pressure. To ensure that the true systolic pressure is not missed, the examiner should inflate the cuff until the palpated arterial pulse is occluded, and both the Phase I pressure and the reappearance pressure should be recorded (e.g., 160/130/70 mm Hg). It is possible to have both an auscultatory gap and a gap between Phases VI and V, in which case all four pressures are recorded (e.g., 170/130/80/40 mm Hg).

The technique for obtaining an auscultatory blood pressure as specified in the sixth edition of the American Heart Association's recommendations for indirect measurement of arterial blood pressure[18] is included in Box 4-2. The student is encouraged to obtain a copy of the recommendations and to check periodically for updates.

Table 4-9 Korotkoff Sounds and Characteristics

Korotkoff Sounds	Characteristic	Pressure Measured
Phase I	First appearance of clear, repetitive, tapping sounds; coincides approximately with the reappearance of a palpable pulse	Systolic pressure
Phase II	Sounds are softer and longer, with the quality of an intermittent murmur	Auscultatory gap may occur
Phase III	Sounds become crisper and louder	Auscultatory gap may occur
Phase IV	Sounds are muffled, less distinct, and softer	Diastolic pressure in pregnant women, patients with high cardiac outputs or peripheral vasodilation, and some small children
Phase V	Sounds disappear completely	Diastolic pressure in adults and children

BOX 4-2 Technique for Measurement of Human Blood Pressure by Sphygmomanometry and Auscultation

The intent and purpose of the measurement should be explained to the subject in a reassuring manner, and every effort should be made to put the subject at ease.

The sequential steps for measuring the blood pressure in the upper extremity, as for routine screening and monitoring purposes, should include the following:

1. Have paper and pen at hand for immediate recording of the pressure.
2. Seat the subject in a quiet, calm environment with his/her bare arm resting on a standard table or other support so that the midpoint of the upper arm is at the level of the heart.
3. Estimate by inspection or measure with a tape the circumference of the bare upper arm at the midpoint between the acromion and olecranon process (between the shoulder and elbow) and select an appropriately sized cuff. The bladder inside the cuff should encircle 80% of the arm in adults and 100% of the arm in children younger than 13 years. If in doubt, use a larger cuff. If the available cuff is too small, this should be noted.
4. Palpate the brachial artery and place the cuff so that the midline of the bladder is over the arterial pulsation, then wrap and secure the cuff snugly around the subject's bare upper arm. Avoid rolling up the sleeve in such a manner that it forms a tight tourniquet around the upper arm. Loose application of the cuff results in overestimation of the pressure. The lower edge of the cuff should be 1 inch (2 cm) above the antecubital fossa (bend of the elbow), where the head of the stethoscope is to be placed.
5. Place the manometer so that the center of the mercury column or aneroid dial is at eye level and is easily visible to the observer and the tubing from the cuff is unobstructed.
6. Inflate the cuff rapidly to 70 mm Hg, and increase by 10–mm Hg increments while palpating the radial pulse. Note the level of pressure at which the pulse disappears and subsequently reappears during deflation. This procedure, the *palpatory method,* provides a necessary preliminary approximation of the systolic blood pressure to ensure an adequate level of inflation when the actual, auscultatory measurement is made. The palpatory method is particularly useful to avoid underinflation of the cuff in patients with an auscultatory gap and overinflation in those with very low blood pressure.
7. Place the earpieces of the stethoscope into the ear canals, angled forward to fit snugly. Switch the stethoscope head to the low-frequency position (bell). The setting can be confirmed by listening as the stethoscope head is tapped gently.
8. Place the head of the stethoscope over the brachial artery pulsation, just above and medial to the antecubital fossa but below the lower edge of the cuff, and hold it firmly in place, making sure that the head makes contact with the skin around its entire circumference. Wedging the head of the stethoscope under the edge of the cuff may free up one hand but results in considerable extraneous noise.
9. Inflate the bladder rapidly and steadily to a pressure 20 to 30 mm Hg above the level previously determined by palpation, then partially unscrew (open) the valve and deflate the bladder at 2 mm/sec while listening for the appearance of the Korotkoff sounds.
10. As the pressure in the bladder falls, note the level of the pressure on the manometer at the first appearance of repetitive sounds (Phase I), at the muffling of these sounds (Phase IV), and when they disappear (Phase V). While the Korotkoff sounds are audible, the rate of deflation should be no more than 2 mm per pulse beat, thereby compensating for both rapid and slow heart rates.
11. After the last Korotkoff sound is heard, the cuff should be deflated slowly for at least another 10 mm Hg, to ensure that no further sounds are audible, and then rapidly and completely deflated, and the subject should be allowed to rest for at least 30 seconds.
12. The systolic (Phase I) and diastolic (Phase V) pressures should be immediately recorded, rounded off (upward) to the nearest 2 mm Hg. In children, and when sounds are heard nearly to a level of 0 mm Hg, the Phase IV pressure should also be recorded. All values should be recorded together with the name of the subject, the date and time of the measurement, the arm on which the measurement was made, the subject's position, and the cuff size (when a nonstandard size is used).
13. The measurement should be repeated after at least 30 seconds, and the two readings averaged. In clinical situations, additional measurements can be made in the same or opposite arm, in the same or an alternative position.

Errors in Blood Pressure Measurement

Causes of arterial blood congestion above the cuff that result in erroneously high cuff pressure measurements include the following (see Table 4-9 and Figure 4-3):

- Too narrow a cuff
- Cuff applied too tightly
- Cuff applied too loosely (when the loose bladder is inflated, the edges rise, so the portion pressing on the artery has a tourniquet effect)
- Excessive pressure placed in the cuff during measurement
- Inflation pressure held in the cuff
- Incomplete deflation of cuff between measurements

A low pressure reading is obtained if the cuff is too wide; however, this produces errors in the range of 3 to 5 mm Hg rather than the 40–mm Hg error often obtained when using too narrow a cuff.

Erroneous diastolic pressures occur when pressure is maintained on the artery so that laminar flow is not reestablished. Because turbulent flow can be heard, muffling or disappearance of sound may not occur. Causes include applying the cuff too tightly and pressing the stethoscope too tightly over the artery. Static electricity, ventilators, extraneous room sounds, and the presence of an auscultatory gap may also cause erroneous cuff measurements.

Effects of the Respiratory Cycle on Blood Pressure

Systolic blood pressure usually decreases slightly (by 2 to 4 mm Hg) with normal inhalation. This decrease in systolic blood pressure is more significant during a forced maximal inhalation. When the systolic pressure drops more than 10 mm Hg during inhalation at rest, a definite abnormality exists; this is termed *paradoxical pulse*. Paradoxical pulse, also called *pulsus paradoxus*, occurs in various circulatory and respiratory conditions such as asthma and cardiac tamponade. The most probable mechanism responsible for this fluctuation in blood pressure centers around the negative intrathoracic pressure created by the respiratory muscles during inhalation. The negative intrathoracic pressure encourages venous blood to return to the right ventricle and discourages arterial blood flow out of the left ventricle. The increased venous return to the right ventricle during inspiration increases the right ventricular filling pressures, which causes the interventricular septum to distend toward the left ventricle. This results in reduced left ventricular filling, reduced stroke volume, and decreased systolic blood pressure simultaneous with inhalation.

The fluctuation in systolic blood pressure with breathing can be identified most accurately with a sphygmomanometer; however, if the pulse can be felt to wane with inspiration in several accessible arteries, paradoxical pulse is probably present. To confirm and quantify the presence of paradoxical pulse, a blood pressure cuff is used. The cuff is inflated until no sounds are heard with the stethoscope bell over the brachial artery, and then it is gradually deflated until sounds are heard on exhalation only. The cuff pressure then is reduced slowly until sounds are heard throughout the respiratory cycle. The difference between the systolic pressure heard only during expiration and systolic pressure heard throughout the respiratory cycle indicates the degree of paradoxical pulse. A reading in excess of 10 mm Hg is significant.

Pulsus paradoxus is commonly seen in patients with restrictions around their heart such as cardiac tamponade, constrictive pericarditis, or restrictive cardiomyopathy. It may also occur in patients with severe pulmonary disease such as acute asthma.

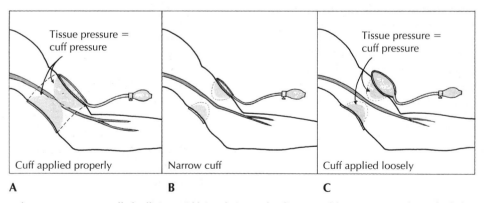

Figure 4-3 A, When a sphygmomanometer cuff of sufficient width in relation to the diameter of the arm is properly applied, the tissue pressure around deep arteries under the cuff equals cuff pressure. However, pressure under the edge of the cuff does not penetrate as deeply as that under the center of the cuff. **B,** A cuff that is too narrow in relation to the diameter of the limb does not transmit its pressure to the center of the limb. Under these conditions, the cuff pressure must greatly exceed arterial pressure to produce complete occlusion of the artery, and erroneously high systolic and diastolic pressures are read from the mercury manometer. **C,** If a cuff of sufficient width is applied too loosely, it becomes rounded before exerting pressure on the tissues and produces the same sort of error as a narrow cuff produces. (From Rushmer RF: *Cardiovascular dynamics,* ed 3, Philadelphia, 1970, WB Saunders.)

Questions to Ask Yourself About
BLOOD PRESSURE

To ensure the accuracy of the blood pressure reading, ask yourself the following questions:
- Is the correct cuff size being used? Is the cuff applied correctly?
- Is the arm in the standard position when the blood pressure is measured?
- Is the same arm used as was used in previous measurements? Which arm has higher blood pressure?
- If using a mercury column or gauge, is it at eye level?
- Has the patient been in the same position long enough to obtain a stable reading?
- Does the blood pressure change when the patient changes position from supine or sitting to standing?
- Does the patient complain of symptoms such as dizziness when changing position?
- Are things occurring in the environment that would artificially alter the patient's blood pressure?
- If the blood pressure is high, does it decrease if measured again in a few minutes?

SIMPLY STATED
Hypotension occurs when the left ventricle is weak, the blood volume is reduced, or vasodilation is excessive. These problems can occur as a side effect of certain medications (e.g., beta-blockers, diuretics).

REVIEW QUESTIONS

1. T   F   Abnormal sensorium can be caused by reduced blood flow and/or oxygenation to the brain.

2. Which of the following is not included in the measurement of vital signs?
   a. Pulse
   b. Respiratory rate
   c. Urinary output
   d. Blood pressure

3. T   F   Fever is defined as an increase in body temperature above normal resulting from disease.

4. Which of the following changes is consistent with a fever?
   a. Decreased respiratory rate
   b. Increased pulse rate
   c. Decreased oxygen consumption
   d. All of the above

5. Which of the following methods of temperature measurement is recommended for neonates?
   a. Oral
   b. Axillary
   c. Rectal
   d. Ear

6. What is the normal value of the resting pulse rate in the adult?
   a. 30-60 beats/min
   b. 60-100 beats/min
   c. 80-120 beats/min
   d. 100-150 beats/min

7. T   F   The normal value for the resting respiratory rate in an adult is 6-10 breaths/min.

8. T   F   Resting pulse and respiratory rates for neonates and children are normally higher than for adults.

9. Which of the following causes tachycardia in the adult?
   a. Hypothermia
   b. Hypoxemia
   c. Hypertension
   d. Polycythemia

10. Which of the following arterial sites is the most common for evaluating the pulse in the adult patient?
    a. Pedal
    b. Temporal
    c. Radial
    d. Femoral

11. Which of the following causes tachypnea in the adult?
    a. Hypothermia
    b. Narcotic overdose
    c. Metabolic acidosis
    d. Hyperoxia

12. Which of the following causes an erroneously high blood pressure measurement?
    a. Inflation pressure held in the cuff between measurements
    b. Use of blood pressure cuff that is too wide
    c. Not enough pressure used in the cuff during measurement
    d. a and b

13. T   F   Hypotension reduces perfusion and tissue oxygen delivery.

14. The peak pressure in the arteries is known as
    a. Pulse pressure.
    b. Diastolic pressure.

c. Systolic pressure
d. None of the above

15. A decrease in the intensity of the palpated pulse during inhalation is a definition of which of the following?
   a. Abdominal paradox
   b. Pulse pressure
   c. Pulsus paradoxus
   d. Pulsus alternans

16. What is the normal range for pulse pressure?
   a. 10-20 mm Hg
   b. 20-25 mm Hg
   c. 30-50 mm Hg
   d. 35-40 mm Hg

17. If a patient experiences syncope upon moving from the supine to the upright position, what is the likely cause?
   a. Left ventricular failure
   b. Postural hypotension
   c. Excessive vasoconstriction
   d. Pulsus paradoxus

REFERENCES

1. Cunha BA: Fever in the critical care unit, *Crit Care Clin* 14:1-14, 1998.
2. Manthous CA, Hall JB, Olson D: Effect of cooling on oxygen consumption in febrile critically ill patients, *Am J Respir Crit Care Med* 151:10-14, 1995.
3. Schmitz T, Bair N, Falk M: A comparison of five methods of temperature measurement in febrile intensive care patients, *Am J Crit Care* 4:286-292, 1995.
4. O'Hara GJ, Phillips DB: Method and apparatus for measuring internal body temperature utilizing infrared emission, US Patents 4602642, (1986), and 4790324, (1988).
5. Erickson RS, Meyer LT: Accuracy of infrared ear thermometry and other temperature methods in adults, *Am J Crit Care* 3:40-54, 1994.
6. Pontious SL and others: Accuracy and reliability of temperature measurement in the emergency department by instrument and site in children, *Pediatr Nurs* 20:58-63, 1994.
7. Nobel JJ: Infrared ear thermometry, *Pediatr Emerg Care* 8:54-58, 1992.
8. Davis K: The accuracy of tympanic temperature measurement in children, *Pediatr Nurs* 19:267-272, 1993.
9. Erickson RS, Yount ST: Comparison of tympanic and oral temperatures in surgical patients, *Nurs Res* 40:90-93, 1991.
10. Milewski A, Ferguson KL, Terndrup TE: Comparison of pulmonary artery, rectal, and tympanic membrane temperatures in adult intensive care unit patients, *Clin Pediatr* 30(4 Suppl):13-16, 1991.
11. Talo H, Macknin ML, Medendorp SV: Tympanic membrane temperatures compared to rectal and oral temperatures, *Clin Pediatr* 30(4 Suppl):30-33, 1991.
12. Pransky SM: The impact of technique and conditions of the tympanic membrane upon infrared tympanic thermometry, *Clin Pediatr* 30(4 Suppl):50-52, 1991.
13. Zehner WJ, Terndrup TE: The impact of moderate ambient temperature variance on the relationship between oral, rectal, and tympanic membrane temperatures, *Clin Pediatr* 30(4 Suppl):61-64, 1991.
14. Hasel KL, Erickson RS: Effect of cerumen on infrared ear temperature measurement, *J Gerontol Nurs* 21:6-14, 1995.
15. The sixth report of the Joint National Committee on prevention, detection, evaluation and treatment of high blood pressure, *Arch Intern Med* 157:2413-2446, 1997.
16. Shamsuzzaman AS, Gersh BJ, Somers VK: Obstructive sleep apnea: Implications for cardiac and vascular disease. *JAMA* 290:1906-1914, 2003.
17. Update on the 1987 Task Force Report on High Blood Pressure in Children and Adolescents: A Working Group Report from the National High Blood Pressure Education Program. National High Blood Pressure Education Program Working Group on Hypertension Control in Children and Adolescents, *Pediatrics* 98(4 Pt 1):649-658, 1996.
18. Perloff D and others: Human blood pressure determination by sphygmomanometry, *Circulation* 88:2460-2470, 1993.

CHAPTER 5

Robert L. Wilkins
Lennard Specht

Fundamentals of Physical Examination

LEARNING OBJECTIVES

Upon completion of this chapter, the reader should be able to accomplish the following:

1. Recognize the four components of the physical examination.
2. Recognize the importance of reviewing the history of present illness before performing a physical examination.
3. Recognize the significance of the following during examination of the head and neck:
   a. Nasal flaring
   b. Cyanosis
   c. Pursed-lip breathing
   d. Changes in pupillary size in response to light
   e. Deviated tracheal position
   f. Jugular venous distention
4. Describe the correct method for measuring jugular venous pressure and expected normal findings.
5. Recognize the topographic position of the following:
   a. Thoracic cage landmarks (suprasternal notch, sternal angle [angle of Louis], vertebral spinous processes [C7 and T1])
   b. Lung fissures (oblique [major] and horizontal [minor])
   c. Tracheal bifurcation anteriorly and posteriorly
   d. Right and left diaphragm anteriorly and posteriorly
   e. Lung borders
6. Define the following terms used to classify thoracic configuration during inspection of the chest:
   a. Pectus carinatum
   b. Pectus excavatum
   c. Kyphosis
   d. Scoliosis
   e. Kyphoscoliosis
   f. Barrel chest
   g. Flail chest
7. Define the following terms used to describe breathing pattern during inspection of the chest:
   a. Apnea
   b. Biot's breathing
   c. Cheyne-Stokes breathing
   d. Kussmaul's breathing
   e. Apneustic
   f. Paradoxical breathing
   g. Asthmatic

8. Identify the breathing patterns associated with restrictive and obstructive lung disease.
9. Recognize the clinical significance of accessory muscle usage and retractions and bulging.
10. Define the following terms and recognize their significance:
    a. Abdominal paradox
    b. Respiratory alternans
    c. Peripheral cyanosis
    d. Central cyanosis
    e. Hoover's sign
11. Identify the clinical significance of peripheral versus central cyanosis.
12. Identify causes of increased and decreased tactile fremitus.
13. Identify causes of decreased thoracic expansion as assessed during chest palpation.
14. Recognize a description of subcutaneous emphysema and its clinical significance.
15. Identify causes of increased and decreased resonance during percussion of the lung.
16. Describe the four basic parts of a stethoscope and their uses.
17. Recognize the proper technique for auscultation of the lungs.
18. Recognize the four characteristics of breath sounds that should be evaluated during auscultation.
19. Define the following terms used to describe lung sounds and the mechanisms responsible for producing the sounds:
    a. Tracheal
    b. Bronchovesicular
    c. Vesicular (normal)
    d. Diminished/absent
    e. Harsh/bronchial
20. Define the following terms used to describe abnormal (adventitious) lung sounds and the mechanisms responsible for producing the sounds:
    a. Crackles (rales)
    b. Wheezes
    c. Stridor
    d. Pleural friction rub

21. Recognize qualifying adjectives that can be used to describe lung sounds and the importance of using these qualifying adjectives.
22. Recognize the significance of the following auscultatory findings:
    a. Monophonic wheeze
    b. Polyphonic wheezes
    c. Stridor
    d. Late inspiratory crackles
    e. Inspiratory and expiratory crackles
    f. Pleural friction rub
23. Define egophony and bronchophony and the causes of each condition.
24. Recognize the topographic location of the apex and base of the heart during examination of the precordium.
25. Define point of maximal impulse, its normal location, and the factors that may cause it to shift to the right or left.
26. Recognize the best location for auscultating sounds produced by the aortic, pulmonic, mitral, and tricuspid valves.
27. Recognize what produces the first (S_1), second (S_2), third (S_3), and fourth (S_4) heart sounds.
28. Describe what is meant by a "gallop rhythm" and what it signifies.
29. Recognize factors that increase or decrease the intensity of the heart sounds.
30. Recognize the clinical significance of a loud P_2 heard during auscultation of the heart.
31. Describe the factors that cause systolic and diastolic heart murmurs.
32. Recognize the components of a neurologic examination and identify the implications of various abnormalities.
33. Define key terms related to the neurologic examination: coma, persistent vegetative state, decerebrate and decorticate posturing, doll's eyes, and oculocephalic reflex.
34. Define hepatomegaly and recognize its significance in the cardiopulmonary patient.
35. Define the following and recognize their significance during examination of the extremities:
    a. Digital clubbing
    b. Cyanosis
    c. Pedal edema
    d. Capillary refill
    e. Peripheral skin temperature

CHAPTER OUTLINE
Examination of the Head and Neck
Head
Eyes
Neck
Lung Topography
Imaginary Lines
Thoracic Cage Landmarks
Lung Fissures
Tracheal Bifurcation

Diaphragm
Lung Borders
Examination of the Thorax
Inspection
Palpation
Percussion of the Chest to Assess Resonance
Auscultation of the Lungs
Examination of the Precordium
Review of Heart Topography
Inspection and Palpation
Auscultation of Heart Sounds
Neurologic Examination
Anatomy and Physiology
Assessment of the Central Nervous System
Assessment of the Peripheral Nervous System
Examination of the Abdomen
Examination of the Extremities
Clubbing
Cyanosis
Pedal Edema
Capillary Refill
Peripheral Skin Temperature
Summary

KEY TERMS

abdominal paradox	heave
acrocyanosis	hepatomegaly
ascites	Hoover's sign
attenuation	loud P_2
barrel chest	miosis
bronchial breath sounds	mydriasis
bronchophony	nystagmus
bulging	oculocephalic reflex
central cyanosis	pedal edema
clubbing	peripheral cyanosis
coma	persistent vegetative
crackles	state
cyanosis	point of maximal impulse
decerebrate posturing	precordium
decorticate posturing	ptosis
diplopia	respiratory alternans
doll's eyes	retractions
egophony	stridor
flail chest	subcutaneous emphysema
gallop rhythm	vesicular breath sound
harsh breath sounds	wheeze

CHAPTER OVERVIEW

Physical examination is the process of examining the patient for the physical signs of disease. It is an inexpensive way to obtain immediate and pertinent information about the patient's health status. The four basic components of the physical examination are *inspection, palpation, percussion,* and *auscultation.*

The patient initially is examined to help determine the correct diagnosis. Once a tentative diagnosis is made, subsequent examinations are valuable in monitoring the patient's hospital course and evaluating the results of treatment. Each examination should be modified according to the patient's history and the purpose of the assessment. Through experience, the examiner learns which of the techniques described in this chapter should be used in any situation. Each examination should be performed in a quiet, well-lighted room, and the examiner should avoid exposing the patient to unnecessary discomfort.

The skills described in this chapter are not difficult to learn; however, proficiency is attained only with practice. The beginner first should practice the skills on healthy persons to improve technique and, more importantly, to obtain an appreciation for normal variations. Abnormalities can be detected only by examiners who have developed an understanding of normal body functions for comparison.

This chapter emphasizes the techniques of examination used in assessment of the patient with cardiopulmonary disease. Because cardiopulmonary disease may indirectly alter other body systems, examination of the whole patient is important. The techniques used in examination of the thorax and other body systems for the abnormalities often associated with respiratory disease are reviewed. The typical order in which the initial physical examination is performed and recorded is presented in Box 5-1. See Chapter 4 for a complete discussion of the initial impression and assessment of the vital signs.

BOX 5-1 **Typical Format for Recording the Physical Examination**

Initial Impression

Age, height, weight, and general appearance

Vital Signs

Pulse rate, respiratory rate, temperature, and blood pressure

HEENT (Head, Ears, Eyes, Nose, and Throat)

Inspection findings

Neck

Inspection and palpation findings

Thorax

Lungs: inspection, palpation, percussion, and auscultation findings

Heart: inspection, palpation, and auscultation findings

Abdomen

Inspection, palpation, percussion, and auscultation findings

Extremities

Inspection and palpation findings

A review of the patient's history of present illness and past medical history before examination is helpful, especially if the examiner was not involved in acquiring the patient's medical history. This review gives the examiner insight into the expected physical examination findings and suggests the techniques to emphasize.

EXAMINATION OF THE HEAD AND NECK

Head

An examination of the head should first identify the patient's facial expression. This may help determine whether the patient is in acute distress or is experiencing physical pain. The facial expression can also help evaluate alertness, mood, general character, and mental capacity. Abnormalities produced by respiratory disease include nasal flaring, cyanosis, and pursed-lip breathing. Nasal flaring is identified by observing the external nares flare outward during inhalation. This occurs especially in neonates with respiratory distress and indicates an increase in the work of breathing.

Cyanosis may be detected, especially around the lips and oral mucosa, when respiratory disease results in reduced oxygenation of the arterial blood. Cyanosis is a bluish cast to the skin that clinically may be difficult to detect, especially in a poorly lighted room and in patients with dark-pigmented skin. The presence of cyanosis is strong evidence that tissue oxygenation may be less than optimal; further investigation (e.g., arterial blood gas analysis) is indicated. The absence of cyanosis does not indicate that tissue oxygenation is adequate, because a sufficient hemoglobin concentration must exist before cyanosis can be identified (see inspection for cyanosis later in this chapter).

Patients with chronic obstructive pulmonary disease (COPD) may use pursed-lip breathing during exhalation. This technique often is taught to patients and may even be used by patients who have not had instruction on its benefits. Some patients naturally begin to pucker their lips during exhalation to provide a slight resistance to the exhaled breath. This resistance provides a slight backpressure in the airways during exhalation and prevents their premature collapse.

Eyes

The pupillary reflexes are evaluated as part of the neurologic examination. Cranial nerves II and III must be intact for normal pupillary reflexes to be present. If the pupils are equal in size, round, and reactive to light and accommodation, the physician may simply write PERRLA (Pupils Equal, Round, Reactive to Light and Accommodation) in the patient's chart. Head trauma, tumors, central nervous system disease, and certain medications can cause abnormal findings. Brain death, catecholamines, and atropine can cause the pupils to become dilated and fixed (mydriasis). Atropine is a common medication used during cardiopulmonary resuscitation, and its administration minimizes the use of assessing pupillary reflexes as a measure of the patient's neurologic status. Parasympathetic stimulants and opiates can cause pinpoint pupils (miosis).

Examination of the eyelids is useful when the examiner suspects disease of the cranial nerves. Drooping of the upper lid (ptosis) may be an early sign of disease involving the third cranial nerve. Congenital defects, cranial tumors, and neuromuscular diseases such as myasthenia gravis may cause ptosis. Ptosis may be an early warning sign of respiratory failure when a descending neuromuscular disease such as myasthenia gravis is occurring. Neuromuscular diseases affecting the cranial nerves also may result in blurred or double vision (diplopia) and involuntary, cyclic movement of the eyeballs known as nystagmus.

Neck

Inspection and palpation of the neck are of value in determining the tracheal position, estimating the jugular venous pressure (JVP), and identifying whether the patient's accessory muscles are in use. Normally, the trachea is located centrally in the neck when the patient is facing forward. The midline of the neck can be identified by palpation of the suprasternal notch at the base of the anterior neck. The midline of the trachea should be directly below the center of the suprasternal notch.

The trachea may be shifted from midline with unilateral upper lobe collapse (atelectasis), pneumothorax, pleural effusion, or lung tumors. The trachea shifts toward the collapsed lung but away from the pneumothorax, pleural effusion, or lung tumor. Abnormalities in the lower lung fields may not shift the trachea unless the defect is severe.

The JVP is estimated by examining the level of the column of blood in the jugular veins. JVP reflects the volume and pressure of the venous blood in the right side of the heart. Both the internal and external jugular veins can be assessed, although the internal jugular is most reliable. Persons with obese necks may not have visible neck veins, even with distention.

In the supine position, the neck veins of a healthy person are full. When the head of the bed is elevated gradually to a 45-degree angle from horizontal, the level of the column of blood descends to a point no more than a few centimeters above the clavicle with normal venous pressure. With elevated venous pressure, the neck veins may be distended as high as the angle of the jaw, even when the patient is sitting upright (Figure 5-1). The degree of venous distention can be estimated by measuring the distance the veins are distended above the sternal angle. The sternal angle has been chosen universally, because its distance above the right atrium remains nearly constant (approximately 5 cm) in all positions. With the head of the bed elevated to a 45-degree angle, venous distention greater than 3 to 4 cm above the sternal angle is abnormal (Figure 5-2).

Exact quantification of the jugular pressure in terms of centimeters above the sternal angle is difficult and probably exceeds the accuracy needed for most observers. A simple grading scale of *normal, increased,* and *markedly increased* is acceptable.

The level of jugular venous distention may vary with breathing. During inhalation, the level of the column of blood may

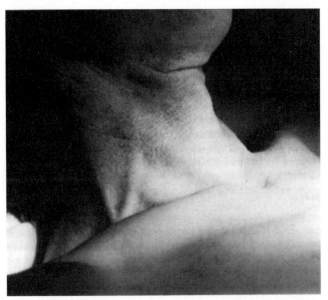

Figure 5-1 Photograph of jugular venous distention. (From Daily EK, Schroeder JP: *Techniques in bedside hemodynamic monitoring,* ed 4, St Louis, 1981, Mosby.)

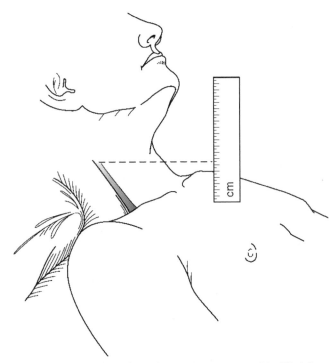

Figure 5-2 Estimation of jugular venous pressure. (Modified from Malasanos L, Barkauskas V, Stoltenberg-Allen K: *Health assessment,* ed 4, St Louis, 1990, Mosby.)

descend toward the thorax and return to the previous position with exhalation. For this reason, JVP should always be estimated at the end of exhalation.

The most common cause of jugular venous distention is right-sided heart failure. Right-sided heart failure may occur secondary to left-sided heart failure or chronic hypoxemia.

Hypoxemia initiates pulmonary vasoconstriction and increases the resistance to blood flow through the pulmonary vasculature, increasing the workload of the right ventricle. Persistent lung disease with hypoxemia may result in right-sided heart failure and jugular venous distention. Jugular venous distention also may occur with hypervolemia and when the venous return to the right atrium is obstructed by tumors in the mediastinum.

SIMPLY STATED

Jugular venous distention most often is the result of right-sided heart failure. Right-sided heart failure occurs with chronic left-sided heart failure or when chronic hypoxemic lung disease is present.

Contraction of the sternomastoid muscle in the neck is an indication that the patient's work of breathing is increased. It is a common finding in patients with airway obstruction and is discussed in the section on chest inspection.

The attending physician often examines the patient's neck for enlarged lymph nodes (*lymphadenopathy*) during the initial examination. Lymphadenopathy is a common finding in patients with respiratory infections, and the lymph nodes usually are tender. Nontender lymphadenopathy may be caused by malignancy or human immunodeficiency virus (HIV).

The carotid pulse in the neck is palpated to evaluate the strength of the left ventricular contraction and the condition of the aortic valve. Heart disease that results in poor left ventricular contraction causes the carotid pulse to become weak. Stenosis of the aortic valve also causes a weak carotid pulse along with a systolic murmur (see Examination of the Precordium). An incompetent aortic valve that causes regurgitation of blood back into the left ventricle results in a pulse that rises sharply and has a narrow summit and then a sudden descent. This is called a *water-hammer pulse.* The left and right carotid pulses must not be palpated simultaneously, because this may significantly reduce blood flow to the brain.

The strength of the pulse at any location is described on a scale of 0 to 4, where

0 = Absent, not palpable
1 = Diminished, barely palpable
2 = Expected normal amplitude
3 = Full and stronger than expected
4 = Bounding

LUNG TOPOGRAPHY

Understanding how the lungs are situated within the chest is vital when preparing to perform an accurate physical assessment of the respiratory system. Topographic (surface) landmarks of the chest are helpful in identifying the location of underlying structures and describing the location of abnormalities.

Imaginary Lines

On the anterior chest, the midsternal line divides the chest into two equal halves. The left and right midclavicular lines parallel the midsternal line and are drawn through the midpoints of the left and right clavicles, respectively (Figure 5-3).

The midaxillary line divides the lateral chest into two equal halves. The anterior axillary line parallels the midaxillary line and is situated along the anterolateral chest. The posterior axillary line is also parallel to the midaxillary line and is located in the posterolateral chest (Figure 5-4).

Three imaginary vertical lines are drawn on the posterior chest. The midspinal line divides the posterior chest into two equal halves. The left and right midscapular lines parallel the midspinal line and pass through the inferior angles of the scapulae in the relaxed upright patient (Figure 5-5).

Thoracic Cage Landmarks

On the anterior chest, the suprasternal notch is located at the top of the manubrium and can be located by palpation of the depression at the base of the neck. Directly below this notch is the sternal angle, which is also called the *angle of Louis.* The sternal angle can be identified by palpating down from the suprasternal notch until the ridge between the gladiolus and the manubrium is identified. This important landmark is visible in most persons. The second rib articulates with the top of the gladiolus at this point (Figure 5-6). Rib identification on the anterior chest can now be accomplished with this as a reference point. It is recommended that ribs be counted to the side of the sternum, because individual costal cartilages that attach the ribs to the sternum are not identified as easily near the sternum.

On the posterior chest, the spinous processes of the vertebrae are useful landmarks (Figure 5-7). The spinous process of the seventh cervical vertebra (C7) usually can be identified by having the patient extend the head and neck forward and slightly down. At the base of the neck, the most prominent spinous

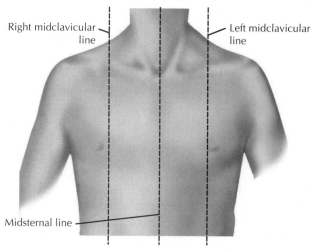

Figure 5-3 Imaginary lines on anterior chest wall. (From Wilkins RL, Stoller JK, Scanlan CL: *Egan's fundamentals of respiratory care,* ed 8, St Louis, 2003, Mosby.)

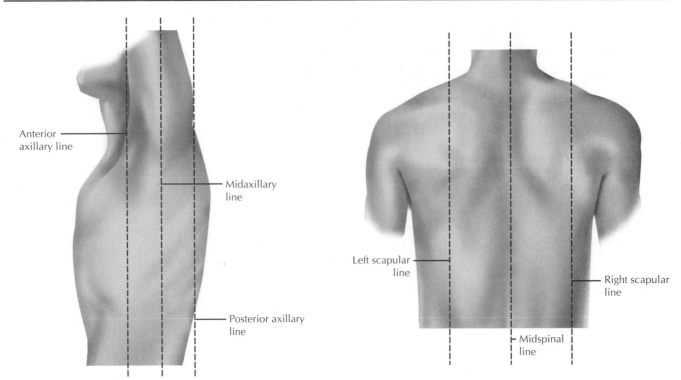

Figure 5-4 Imaginary lines on lateral chest wall. (From Wilkins RL, Stoller JK, Scanlan CL: *Egan's fundamentals of respiratory care*, ed 8, St Louis, 2003, Mosby.)

Figure 5-5 Imaginary lines on posterior chest wall. (From Wilkins RL, Stoller JK, Scanlan CL: *Egan's fundamentals of respiratory care*, ed 8, St Louis, 2003, Mosby.)

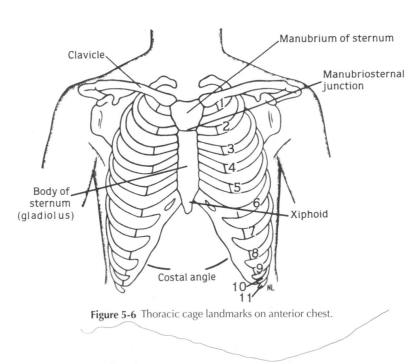

Figure 5-6 Thoracic cage landmarks on anterior chest.

process that can be visualized and palpated is C7. The spinous process just below C7 belongs to the first thoracic vertebra (T1). The scapular borders also can be useful landmarks on the posterior chest. With the patient's arms raised above the head, the inferior border of the scapula approximately overlies the oblique fissure that separates the upper from the lower lobes on the posterior chest.

Lung Fissures

Between the lobes of the lungs are the interlobar fissures. Both lungs have an oblique fissure that begins on the anterior chest at approximately the sixth rib at the midclavicular line. This fissure extends laterally and upward until it crosses the fifth rib on the lateral chest in the midaxillary line and continues on the posterior chest to approximately T3 (Figures 5-8 and 5-9).

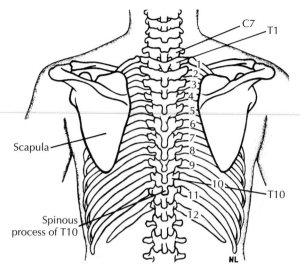

Figure 5-7 Thoracic cage landmarks on posterior chest.

The right lung also has a horizontal fissure that separates the right upper lobe from the right middle lobe. The horizontal fissure extends from the fourth rib at the sternal border around to the fifth rib at the midaxillary line. The left lung rarely has a horizontal fissure.

Tracheal Bifurcation

On the anterior chest, the carina is located approximately beneath the sternal angle and on the posterior chest at approximately T4 (Figure 5-10).

Diaphragm

The diaphragm is a dome-shaped muscle that lies between the thoracic and abdominal cavities and moves up and down during normal ventilation. At the end of a tidal expiration, the right dome of the diaphragm is located at the level of T9 posteriorly and the fifth rib anteriorly. On the left, the diaphragm comes to rest at the end of expiration at T10 posteriorly and the sixth rib anteriorly. The right hemidiaphragm is usually a little higher anatomically than the left hemidiaphragm because of the placement of the liver.

Lung Borders

Superiorly on the anterior chest, the lungs extend 2 to 4 cm above the medial third of the clavicles. The inferior borders on the anterior chest extend to approximately the sixth rib at the midclavicular line and to the eighth rib on the lateral chest wall. On the posterior chest, the superior border extends to T1, and the inferior border varies with ventilation between approximately T9 and T12 (see Figure 5-9).

EXAMINATION OF THE THORAX

Inspection

Visual examination of the chest is of value in assessing the thoracic configuration and the pattern and effort of breathing. For inspection to be adequate, the room must be well lighted and the patient should be sitting upright. If the patient is too ill to sit up, the examiner must roll the patient carefully onto one side to examine the posterior chest. Male patients should be stripped to the waist. Female patients should be given some type of drape to prevent possible embarrassment from exposure of their breasts.

Thoracic Configuration

The normal adult thorax has an anteroposterior diameter less than the transverse diameter. The anteroposterior diameter normally increases gradually with age and prematurely increases in

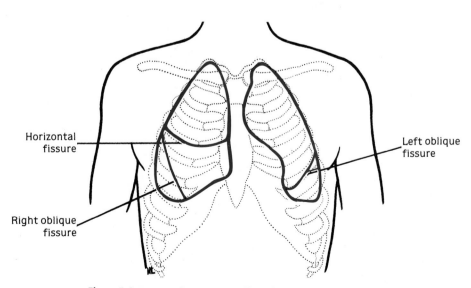

Figure 5-8 Topographic position of lung fissures on anterior chest.

patients with COPD. This abnormal increase in anteroposterior diameter is called barrel chest, and it is commonly seen in patients with emphysema. When the anteroposterior diameter increases, the ribs lose their normal 45-degree angle of slope in relation to the spine and become horizontal (Figure 5-11).

Other abnormalities of the thoracic configuration include the following:

Pectus carinatum: Sternal protrusion anteriorly

Pectus excavatum: Depression of part or all of the sternum, which can produce a restrictive lung defect

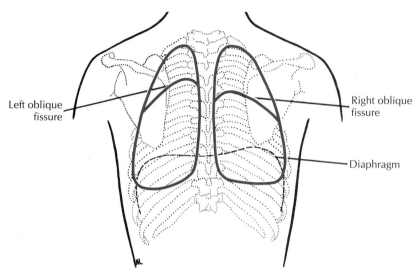

Figure 5-9 Topographic position of lung fissures on posterior chest.

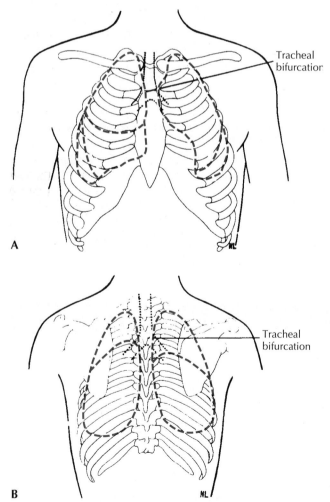

Figure 5-10 Topographic position of tracheal bifurcation and lung borders on anterior chest **(A)** and posterior chest **(B).**

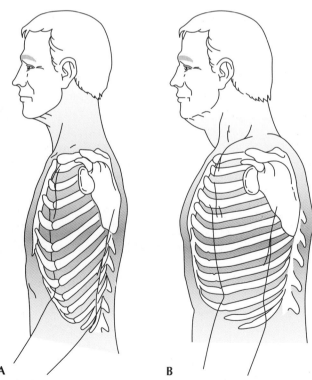

Figure 5-11 A, Patient with normal thoracic configuration. **B,** Patient with increased anteroposterior diameter. Note contrasts in angle or slope of ribs and development of accessory muscles. (Redrawn from Malasanos L, Barkauskas V, Stoltenberg-Allen K: *Health assessment,* ed 4, St Louis, 1990, Mosby.)

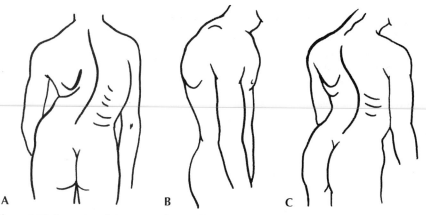

Figure 5-12 Examples of chest cage abnormalities. **A,** Scoliosis. **B,** Kyphosis. **C,** Kyphoscoliosis.

Kyphosis: Spinal deformity in which the spine has an abnormal anteroposterior curvature (Figure 5-12)

Scoliosis: Spinal deformity in which the spine has a lateral curvature (see Figure 5-12)

Kyphoscoliosis: Combination of kyphosis and scoliosis; may produce a severe restrictive lung defect as a result of poor lung expansion (see Figure 5-12)

Severe trauma to the chest cage can result in fractures of the ribs and sternum. Abnormal configuration of the thoracic cage may result, especially if multiple ribs are broken. A section of the rib cage may move paradoxically with breathing when multiple ribs are fractured at more than one site. The paradoxical motion is seen as a sinking inward of the affected region with each spontaneous inspiratory effort and an outward movement with subsequent exhalation. This paradoxical motion of the affected rib cage is called flail chest.

Breathing Pattern and Effort

The healthy adult at rest has a consistent rate and rhythm of ventilation. The effort of breathing is minimal on inhalation and passive on exhalation. Men typically breathe with the diaphragm, causing the stomach to move slightly outward during inhalation. Women tend to use a combination of intercostal muscles and the diaphragm, producing more chest wall movement than men. Table 5-1 describes the abnormal patterns of breathing.

Changes in the patient's breathing pattern can provide important clues to the type of respiratory problem present. Patients with restrictive lung disease (reduced lung volumes) typically breathe with a rapid and shallow pattern. The more severe the loss of lung volume, the more rapid the respiratory rate. Acute obstruction of intrathoracic airways, as occurs with asthma, results in a prolonged exhalation time. The approximate inspiratory/expiratory (I/E) ratio can be determined by timing the two phases of breathing. Normal I/E ratio is approximately 1:1. With more severe cases of airway obstruction, the I/E ratio may be 1:3 or 1:4. Acute upper airway obstruction, as occurs with croup or epiglottitis, often results in a prolonged inspiratory time.

SIMPLY STATED

The patient's breathing pattern often provides strong clues to the underlying pathologic condition. Rapid and shallow breathing suggests a loss of lung volume, a prolonged expiratory time indicates intrathoracic airway obstruction, and a prolonged inspiratory time indicates upper airway obstruction.

Table 5-1	Abnormal Breathing Patterns	
Pattern	Characteristics	Causes
Apnea	No breathing	Cardiac arrest
Biot's	Irregular breathing with long periods of apnea	Increased intracranial pressure
Cheyne-Stokes	Irregular type of breathing; breaths increase and decrease in depth and rate with periods of apnea	Diseases of central nervous system, congestive heart failure
Kussmaul's	Deep and fast	Metabolic acidosis
Apneustic	Prolonged inhalation	Brain damage
Paradoxical	Portion or all of chest wall moves in with inhalation and out with exhalation	Chest trauma, diaphragm paralysis
Asthmatic	Prolonged exhalation	Obstruction to airflow out of lungs

Any respiratory abnormalities that increase the work of breathing may cause the accessory muscles of breathing (scalene and sternomastoid) to become active during breathing at rest. This is common in acute and chronic diffuse airway obstruction, acute upper airway obstruction, and disorders that reduce lung compliance.

Significant increases in the effort of breathing cause large swings in pleural pressure. As a result, the skin overlying the chest cage may sink inward between the ribs during inspiration and bulge outward during exhalation, when the work of breathing is increased. Inward depression of the skin during inspiration is known as retractions. Retractions may be seen between ribs (intercostal), below the ribs (subcostal), or above the clavicles (supraclavicular).

The opposite movement of the skin during exhalation is known as bulging. Obesity and muscular chest walls prevent retractions and bulging from occurring unless the abnormality is severe.

The diaphragm may be nonfunctional in patients with spinal injuries or neuromuscular disease and severely limited in patients with COPD. When this occurs, the accessory muscles of breathing become active, even at rest. The respiratory accessory muscles may also become active during acute airway obstruction. However, its absence does not rule out the possibility that severe airway obstruction is present.

In patients with emphysema, the lungs lose their elastic recoil and become hyperinflated. This results in the diaphragm assuming a lower, less functional position. The accessory muscles must assist ventilation by raising the anterior chest in an effort to increase thoracic volume. Significant use of the accessory muscles of breathing at rest is a sign of more severe chronic obstructive lung disease.

Normally, the abdomen moves gently outward with inspiration and inward with exhalation. When the diaphragm becomes fatigued, the accessory muscles of breathing attempt to maintain ventilation by becoming more active. As the accessory muscles contract in an effort to cause gas to flow into the lung, negative intrathoracic pressure causes the diaphragm to be pulled upward and the abdomen to sink inward during inspiration. This is known as abdominal paradox, which is an important finding that occurs with paralysis or fatigue of the diaphragm. Diaphragm fatigue is common in patients with COPD, especially during weaning from mechanical ventilation. Abdominal paradox may be accompanied by respiratory alternans. Respiratory alternans consists of periods of breathing using only the chest wall muscles alternating with periods of breathing entirely by the diaphragm. It is not as common as abdominal paradox but also is an indication that the diaphragm is fatigued. Not all patients with diaphragm dysfunction develop abdominal paradox or respiratory alternans, but when these clinical signs are present, they indicate significant inspiratory muscle fatigue.

COPD patients with severe hyperinflation have a low, flat diaphragm with limited mobility. Contraction of the flattened diaphragm pulls the lateral margins of the chest wall inward during each inspiratory effort. This abnormal movement of the lateral chest wall during breathing in COPD patients with severe hyperinflation is known as Hoover's sign.

Patients with brain injury may have an abnormal pattern of breathing. The pattern of breathing often proves useful in determining the degree of brainstem function. This is discussed later in the chapter under neurologic examination.

Inspection for Central Cyanosis

Central cyanosis is present when the patient's trunk or oral mucosa is cyanotic. This occurs when the lungs are not oxygenating the blood adequately or when congenital heart disease causes venous blood to be shunted into the arterial system without passing through the lungs. Central cyanosis is an indication that tissue oxygenation may not be adequate and that further investigation is needed (e.g., arterial blood gas analysis). Cyanosis is apparent only when a significant amount of reduced (deoxygenated) hemoglobin is present. In patients with anemia, cyanosis is not detected until advanced oxygenation problems are present.

SIMPLY STATED
Central cyanosis indicates respiratory failure or cyanotic heart disease. Further investigation is needed.

Palpation

Palpation is the act of touching the chest wall in an effort to evaluate underlying lung structure and function. Palpation is performed to evaluate vocal fremitus, estimate thoracic expansion, and assess the skin and subcutaneous tissues of the chest. Palpation is used in selected patients to confirm or rule out suspected problems suggested by the history and initial physical examination.

Vocal Fremitus

The term vocal fremitus refers to the vibrations created by the vocal cords during phonation. These vibrations are transmitted down the tracheobronchial tree and through the alveoli to the chest wall. When these vibrations are felt on the chest wall, they are called tactile fremitus.

During the assessment of tactile fremitus, the patient is directed to repeat the word ninety-nine while the examiner systematically palpates the thorax. The examiner can use the palmar aspect of the fingers or the ulnar aspect of the hand as illustrated in Figure 5-13. If one hand is used, it should be moved from one side of the chest to the corresponding area on the other side. The anterior, lateral, and posterior chest wall should be evaluated.

The vibrations of tactile fremitus may be increased, decreased, or absent. Increased fremitus results from the transmission of the vibration through a more solid medium. The normal lung structure is a combination of solid and air-filled tissue. Any condition that tends to increase the density of the lung, such as the consolidation of pneumonia, results in an increased intensity of fremitus. If the area of consolidation is

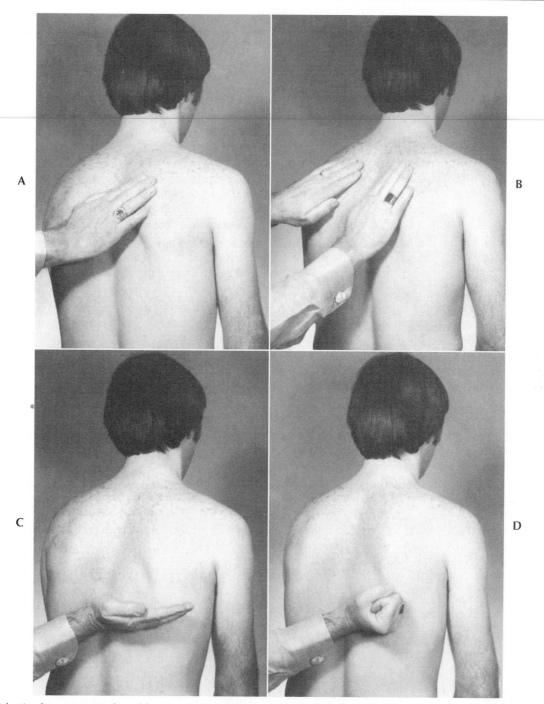

Figure 5-13 Palpation for assessment of vocal fremitus. **A,** Use of palmar surface of fingertips. **B,** Simultaneous application of fingertips of both hands. **C,** Use of ulnar aspect of hand. **D,** Use of ulnar aspect of closed fist. (From Prior JA, Silberstein JS: *Physical diagnosis: The history and examination of the patient,* ed 6, St Louis, 1982, Mosby.)

not in connection with a patent bronchus, fremitus will be absent or decreased.

A reduced tactile fremitus is often present in patients who are obese or overly muscular. In addition, when the pleural space lining the lung becomes filled with air (pneumothorax) or fluid (pleural effusion), the vocal fremitus is reduced significantly or is absent.

The lungs become hyperinflated, with a significant reduction in the density of lung tissue, in patients with emphysema. In this situation, the vocal vibrations from the larynx transmit poorly through the lung tissue, resulting in a bilateral reduction in tactile fremitus. The bilateral reduction in tactile fremitus is more difficult to detect than the unilateral increase in fremitus associated with lobar consolidation. The causes of abnormal tactile fremitus are summarized as follows:

Increased
    Pneumonia
    Lung tumor or mass
    Atelectasis

Decreased

   Unilateral

      Bronchial obstruction with mucous plug or foreign object

      Pneumothorax

      Pleural effusion

   Diffuse

      COPD

      Muscular or obese chest wall

The passage of air through airways contaminated with thick secretions may produce palpable vibrations called *rhonchial fremitus.* Rhonchial fremitus often is identified during inhalation and exhalation and may clear if the patient produces an effective cough. It often is associated with a coarse, low-pitched sound that is audible without a stethoscope.

Thoracic Expansion

The normal chest wall expands symmetrically during deep inhalation. This expansion can be evaluated on the anterior and posterior chest. Anteriorly, the examiner's hands are placed over the anterolateral chest with the thumbs extended along the costal margin toward the xiphoid process. On the posterior chest, the hands are positioned over the posterolateral chest with the thumbs meeting at approximately T8 (Figure 5-14). The patient is instructed to exhale slowly and completely while the examiner's hands are positioned as described. When the patient has exhaled maximally, the examiner gently secures the tips of his/her fingers against the sides of the chest and extends the thumbs toward the midline until the tip of each thumb meets at the midline. The patient is then instructed to take a full, deep breath. The examiner should make note of the distance each thumb moves from the

midline. Normally, each thumb moves an equal distance of approximately 3 to 5 cm.

Diseases that affect expansion of both lungs cause a bilateral reduction in chest expansion. This is seen commonly with neuromuscular diseases and COPD. A unilateral (one-sided) reduction in chest expansion occurs with respiratory diseases that reduce the expansion of one lung or a major part of one lung. This may occur with lobar consolidation, atelectasis, pleural effusion, and pneumothorax.

Skin and Subcutaneous Tissues

The chest wall can be palpated to determine the general temperature and condition of the skin. When air leaks from the lung into subcutaneous tissues, fine beads of air produce a crackling sound and sensation when palpated. This is called subcutaneous emphysema.

Percussion of the Chest to Assess Resonance

Percussion is the act of tapping on a surface in an effort to evaluate the underlying structure. Percussion of the chest wall produces a sound and a palpable vibration useful in the evaluation of the underlying lung tissue. The vibration created by percussion penetrates and thus evaluates the lung to a depth of 5 to 7 cm below the chest wall.

The technique most often used in percussion of the chest wall is called *mediate* or *indirect percussion.* The examiner places the middle finger of the left hand (if the examiner is right-handed) firmly against the chest wall parallel to the ribs with the palm and other fingers held off the chest. The tip of the middle finger on the right hand or the lateral aspect of the right thumb strikes the finger against the chest near the base of the

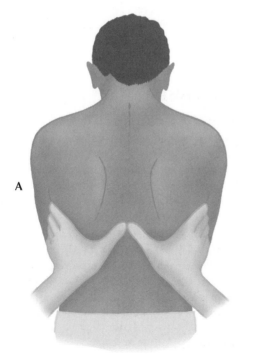 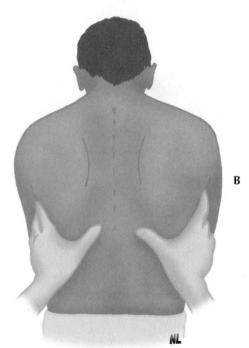

Figure 5-14 Estimation of thoracic expansion. **A,** Exhalation. **B,** Maximal inhalation. (From Wilkins RL, Stoller JK, Scanlan CL: *Egan's fundamentals of respiratory care,* ed 8, St Louis, 2003, Mosby.)

terminal phalanx with a quick, sharp blow. Movement of the hand striking the chest should be generated at the wrist and not the elbow or shoulder (Figure 5-15).

The percussion note is clearest if the examiner remembers to keep the finger on the chest firmly against the chest wall and to strike this finger and immediately withdraw. The two fingers should be in contact for only an instant. As examiners gain experience in percussion of the chest, the feel of the vibration created becomes as important as the sound in the evaluation of lung structures.

Percussion Over Lung Fields

Percussion of the lung fields should be performed systematically, testing comparable areas on both sides of the chest consecutively. Percussion over the bony structures and breasts of the female patient is not of value and should be avoided. The examiner can ask the patient to raise his/her arms above the shoulders, which helps move the scapulae laterally and minimizes interference with percussion on the posterior chest wall.

The sounds generated during percussion of the chest are evaluated for intensity (loudness) and pitch. Percussion over normal lung fields produces a moderately low-pitched sound that can be heard easily. This sound is best described as *normal resonance*. When the percussion note is louder and lower in pitch than normal, the resonance is said to be *increased*. Percussion may produce a sound with characteristics just the opposite of resonance, referred to as *dull* or *flat*. This sound is high pitched, short in duration, and not loud. It is simply described as *decreased resonance*.

Clinical implications

By itself, percussion of the chest is of little value in making a diagnosis. When the percussion note is considered along with the history and other physical findings, it may contribute significantly. Any abnormality that tends to increase the density of the lung tissue, such as the consolidation of pneumonia, lung tumors, or alveolar collapse (atelectasis), results in a loss of resonance and a dull percussion note over the affected area. Percussion over pleural spaces filled with fluid, such as blood or water, also results in decreased resonance.

An increase in resonance is detected in patients with hyperinflated lungs. Hyperinflation can occur as a result of acute bronchial obstruction (asthma) and chronic bronchial obstruction (emphysema). When the pleural space contains large amounts of air (pneumothorax), the percussion note increases in resonance over the affected side.

> **SIMPLY STATED**
> Increased resonance to percussion indicates excessive air trapped in the pleural space or lung; decreased resonance to percussion indicates fluid in the pleural space or consolidation of the lung.

Unilateral abnormalities are easier to detect than are bilateral abnormalities, because the normal side provides an immediate comparison. The decreased resonance heard from percussion over consolidation is a distinct sound that is easier to detect than the subtle increase in resonance associated with hyperinflation or pneumothorax.

Percussion of the chest has limitations that are often clinically important. Abnormalities of the lungs are difficult to detect if the patient's chest wall is obese or overly muscular. Abnormalities that are small or more than 5 cm below the surface are not likely to be detected during percussion of the chest. Percussion to assess lung resonance is not performed routinely on most patients. However, it is useful in selected situations such as in the acutely ill patient suspected of having tension pneumothorax.

Diaphragmatic Excursion

The range of diaphragm movement may be estimated by percussion and is assessed best on the posterior chest wall (Figure 5-16). For the examiner to estimate diaphragm movement, the patient first is instructed to take a deep, full inspiration and to hold it. The examiner then determines the lowest margin of resonance by percussing over the lower lung field and moving downward in small increments until a definite change in the percussion note is detected. The patient then is instructed to exhale maximally, holding this position while the percussion procedure is repeated. The examiner should work rapidly to prevent the patient from becoming short of breath. The normal diaphragmatic excursion during a deep breath is approximately 5 to 7 cm. The range of diaphragm movement is less than normal in certain neuromuscular diseases and in patients with severe pulmonary hyperinflation.

The exact range of movement and position of the diaphragm is difficult to determine by percussion. This probably is because

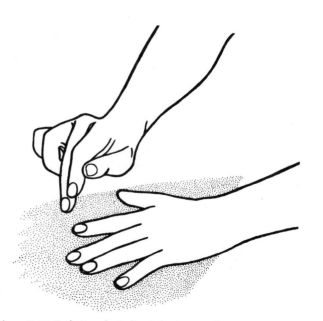

Figure 5-15 Technique for indirect chest percussion.

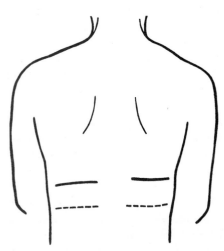

Figure 5-16 Assessment of diaphragmatic excursion by percussion. Horizontal lines indicate position of diaphragm at maximal inhalation *(dashed line)* and exhalation *(solid line)*.

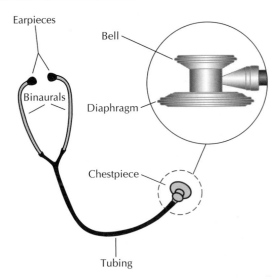

Figure 5-17 Acoustic stethoscope. (From Wilkins RL, Stoller JK, Scanlan CL: *Egan's fundamentals of respiratory care*, ed 8, St Louis, 2003, Mosby.)

the diaphragm is a dome-shaped muscle with the center of the dome 15 cm beneath the surface of the posterior chest. Percussion can only approximate the position and degree of movement of the diaphragm.

Auscultation of the Lungs

Auscultation is the process of listening for sounds produced in the body. Auscultation over the thorax is performed to identify normal or abnormal lung sounds. Careful assessment of the patient's lung sounds is useful in making the initial diagnosis and evaluating the effects of treatment. A stethoscope is used during auscultation for better transmission of sounds to the examiner. The room must be as quiet as possible whenever auscultation is performed.

Stethoscope

The stethoscope includes four basic parts: a bell, a diaphragm, tubing, and earpieces (Figure 5-17). The bell detects a broad spectrum of sounds and is of particular value in listening to low-pitched heart sounds. It is also valuable in auscultation of the lungs in certain situations, such as in the emaciated patient whose rib protrusion restricts placement of the diaphragm flat against the chest. The bell piece should be pressed lightly against the chest when the examiner is attempting to auscultate low-frequency sounds. If the bell is pressed too firmly against the chest wall, the skin will be stretched under the bell and may act as a diaphragm, filtering out certain low-frequency sounds.

The diaphragm piece is used most often in auscultation of the lungs, because most lung sounds are high frequency. It is also useful in listening to high-frequency heart sounds. The diaphragm piece should be pressed firmly against the chest so that external sounds are not heard.

The ideal tubing should be thick enough to exclude external noises and should be approximately 25 to 35 cm (11 to

16 inches) in length. Longer tubing may compromise transmission of lung sounds, and shorter tubing often is inconvenient in reaching the patient's chest.

The stethoscope should be examined regularly for cracks in the diaphragm, wax or dirt in the earpieces, and other defects that may interfere with the transmission of sound. It should be wiped with isopropyl alcohol regularly to prevent a buildup of microorganisms.[1-2]

Technique

The patient should be sitting upright in a relaxed position when possible. The patient is instructed to breathe a little deeper than normal with the mouth open. Inhalation should be an active process and exhalation passive. The bell or diaphragm is placed directly against the chest wall to eliminate clothing as a factor in most cases. However, a thin gown or shirt/blouse probably offers little interference[3] and may make the female patient more comfortable during the procedure. The tubing should not be allowed to rub against any objects, because this may produce extraneous sounds. Auscultation of the lungs should be systematic, including all lobes on the anterior, lateral, and posterior chest. It is recommended that examiners begin at the bases, compare side with side, and work toward the lung apices. The examination begins at the lung bases, because certain abnormal lung sounds (described later) that occur primarily in the dependent lung zones may be altered by several deep breaths. The examiner should listen to at least one full ventilatory cycle at each position on the chest wall. Auscultation over the neck is useful whenever upper airway narrowing may be present.

Four characteristics of breath sounds are to be identified. First, the pitch (vibration frequency) is identified. Second, the amplitude or intensity (loudness) is noted. Third, the examiner listens for the distinctive characteristics. Fourth, the duration of inspiratory sound is compared with that of expiration. The acoustic characteristics of breath sounds can be illustrated in

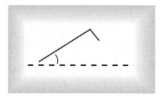

Figure 5-18 Diagrammatic representation of normal breath sound. Upstroke represents inhalation, downstroke represents exhalation, length of upstroke represents duration, thickness of stroke represents intensity, and angle between upstroke and horizontal line represents pitch. The example in this figure illustrates a normal vesicular breath sound. (From Wilkins RL, Stoller JK, Scanlan CL: *Egan's fundamentals of respiratory care*, ed 8, St Louis, 2003, Mosby.)

breath sound diagrams (Figure 5-18). Examiners must have a clear understanding of the characteristics of the normal breath sounds described in Table 5-2 to identify subtle changes that may signify respiratory disease.

Terminology

In healthy persons, the sound heard over the trachea has a loud, tubular quality called a **tracheal** breath sound. Tracheal breath sounds are high-pitched sounds with an expiratory component equal to or slightly longer than the inspiratory component.

A slight variation to the tracheal breath sound is heard around the upper half of the sternum on the anterior chest and between the scapulae on the posterior chest (Figure 5-19). This is not as loud as the tracheal breath sound, is slightly lower in pitch, and has equal inspiratory and expiratory components. It is called a *bronchovesicular* breath sound.

Auscultating over the lung parenchyma of a healthy person yields a soft, muffled sound. This is called a vesicular breath sound or *normal* breath sound and is lower in pitch and intensity (loudness) than the bronchial breath sound. The vesicular sound is difficult to hear and is heard primarily during inhalation with only a minimal exhalation component (see Table 5-2).

Respiratory disease may alter the intensity of normal breath sounds heard over the lung fields. A slight variation in intensity is difficult to detect even for experienced clinicians. Breath sounds are described as diminished when the intensity decreases and *absent* in extreme cases. Breath sounds are described as harsh when the intensity increases. Harsh breath sounds may have an expiratory component equal to the inspiratory component and are described as bronchial breath sounds in such cases.

Abnormal lung sounds produced by the movement of air in the lungs are called *adventitious* sounds. Most adventitious lung sounds (ALS) can be classified as either continuous or discontinuous sounds. Continuous lung sounds are defined as those having a duration longer than 25 msec. (This definition is derived from recording and spectral analysis of lung sounds. Examiners are not expected to time the lung sounds.) Discontinuous lung sounds are characteristically intermittent, crackling, or bubbling sounds of short duration.

Table 5-2	Characteristics of Normal Breath Sounds				
Breath Sound	Pitch	Intensity	Location		Diagram of Sound
Vesicular or normal	Low	Soft	Peripheral lung areas		⁀
Bronchovesicular	Moderate	Moderate	Around upper part of sternum, between scapulae		⋀
Tracheal	High	Loud	Over trachea		⋀

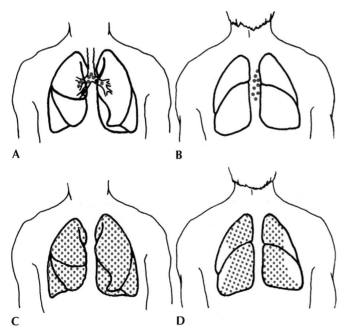

Figure 5-19 Location on chest wall where normal bronchovesicular and vesicular breath sounds are heard. **A,** Anterior bronchovesicular. **B,** Posterior bronchovesicular. **C,** Anterior vesicular. **D,** Posterior vesicular. (From Wilkins RL, Hodgkin JE, Lopez B: *Fundamentals of lung and heart sounds*, ed 3, St Louis, 2004, Mosby.)

> **SIMPLY STATED**
>
> Lung sounds are classified in two basic categories: breath sounds and adventitious lung sounds. The breath sounds are the normal sounds of breathing, and the adventitious lung sounds are the abnormal sounds superimposed on the breath sounds.

Experts have debated for many years the terms to use in the description of ALS. The term *rales* has a long, evolving history that has resulted in it most recently being applied to discontinuous ALS. However, its popularity has diminished recently in certain groups of clinicians following introduction of the term crackles. This newer term may be better suited for documenting discontinuous ALS, because it has onomatopoietic appeal and lacks the confusing history associated with the term *rales*.

The term wheeze is used to describe the musical sounds heard from the chest of the patient with intrathoracic airway obstruction (e.g., asthma). Wheezes are classified as continuous ALS and are easily recognized in most cases.

Low-pitched, continuous ALS have been described in the past with the term *rhonchi*. Like the term *rales,* the term *rhonchi* has a confusing history and has been applied to more than one type of abnormal lung sound. For this reason, there may be an advantage to abandoning the term. For the remainder of this text, the term *crackles* is used for discontinuous ALS and the term *wheeze* is used for continuous ALS.

> **SIMPLY STATED**
>
> The term *crackles* should be used for discontinuous adventitious lung sounds and the term *wheeze* for continuous adventitious lung sounds.

Another continuous sound, heard primarily over the larynx and trachea during inhalation when upper airway obstruction is present, is known as stridor. This is a loud, high-pitched sound that often may be heard without the aid of a stethoscope. Stridor is readily recognized by most clinicians.

Because there is a lack of standardization of lung sound terminology among clinicians, authors of other publications may use different terms to describe abnormal lung sounds. Table 5-3 provides a list of alternative terms that may be used by others.

When abnormal lung sounds are identified, their location and specific characteristics should be noted. Abnormal lung sounds may be high or low pitched, loud or faint, scanty or profuse, and inspiratory or expiratory (or both). The timing during the respiratory cycle should also be noted (e.g., late inspiratory). The examiner must pay close attention to these characteristics of abnormal lung sounds, because they help determine the functional status of the lungs. The importance of using appropriate qualifying adjectives to describe abnormal lung sounds is further emphasized in the following paragraphs.

Table 5-3	Recommended Terminology for Lung Sounds and Other Terms Used	
Recommended Term	Classification	Other Terms Used
Crackles	Discontinuous	Rales Crepitations
Wheezes	High-pitched, continuous	Sibilant rales Musical rales Sibilant rhonchus
	Low-pitched, continuous	Sonorous rales Rhonchi

Mechanisms and Significance of Lung Sounds

The exact mechanisms responsible for the production of normal and abnormal lung sounds are not understood in detail. However, there is enough agreement among investigators to allow a general description. This knowledge should give you a better understanding of the lung sounds often heard through a stethoscope.

Normal breath sounds

Lung sounds heard over the chest of the healthy person are generated primarily by turbulent flow in the larger airways. Turbulent flow creates audible vibrations in the airways, producing sounds that are transmitted through the lung and the chest wall. As the sound travels to the lung periphery and the chest wall, it is altered by the normal lung. Normal lung tissue acts as a low-pass filter, which means it preferentially passes low-frequency sounds. This filtering effect can be demonstrated easily by listening over the periphery of the lung while a subject speaks. The muffled voice sounds are difficult to understand because of the filtering properties of the normal lung. The alteration of sounds that travel through the lung is known as attenuation. Attenuation accounts for the characteristic differences between bronchial breath sounds heard directly over larger airways and vesicular sounds heard over the periphery of the lung.

Normal vesicular lung sounds are at least partly produced locally in the underlying lobe being auscultated. This implies that normal breath sounds heard over a specific lobe indicate airflow into that lobe.

> **SIMPLY STATED**
>
> All normal breath sounds are produced primarily by turbulent flow in the airways. The peripheral lung units normally are silent.

The stability of normal breath sounds over time has been studied. Results indicate that normal vesicular breath sounds remain very stable from one day to the next in healthy persons with regard to pitch and amplitude.[4] This suggests that significant changes in the pitch or loudness of breath sounds in the patient breathing with a similar pattern over time is not normal, and further investigation is indicated.

Auscultation for normal breath sounds following intubation is common practice. This is performed in an attempt to confirm that the tube is placed properly in the trachea and not in the esophagus. The finding of bilateral vesicular breath sounds is strong evidence that the tube is in the trachea. Confirmation by a chest film is recommended, because the breath sounds may be difficult to hear in some patients, and air entering the esophagus may be misinterpreted as breath sounds in some patients.

Abnormal bronchial breath sounds

Bronchial breath sounds may replace the normal vesicular sound when the lung increases in density, as occurs in atelectasis and pneumonia. When the normal air-filled lung becomes consolidated, the attenuation of sound is reduced, and similar sounds are heard over large upper airways and the consolidated lung (Figure 5-20).

Diminished breath sounds

Diminished breath sounds occur when the sound intensity at the site of generation (larger airways) is reduced or when the sound transmission properties of the lung or chest wall are reduced. The intensity of sound created by turbulent flow through the bronchi is reduced with shallow or slow breathing patterns. Obstructed airways (e.g., mucus plugs) and hyperinflated lung tissue increase attenuation of breath sounds through the lungs. Air or fluid in the pleural space and obesity reduce the transmission of breath sounds through the chest wall.

In patients with chronic airflow obstruction, the intensity of vesicular breath sounds often is reduced significantly throughout all lung fields. This is primarily the result of airflow limitation.[5] Poor sound transmission through hyperinflated lung tissue, as occurs with emphysema, may contribute to the identification of reduced breath sounds (see Figure 5-20).

SIMPLY STATED

Diminished breath sounds are produced by shallow breathing or when the turbulent flow sounds of the larger airways are not transmitted through the lung or chest wall. This attenuation of breath sounds is increased with mucus plugging or pleural effusion that absorbs or reflects sound.

Wheezes

Wheezes are generated by the vibration of the wall of a narrowed or compressed airway as air passes through at high velocity (Figure 5-21). The diameter of an airway may be reduced by bronchospasm, mucosal edema, or foreign objects. The pitch of the wheeze is independent of the length of the airway but is related directly to the degree of airway compression. The tighter the compression, the higher the pitch. Low-pitched continuous sounds often are associated with the presence of excessive sputum in the airways. A sputum flap vibrating in the airstream may produce low-pitched wheezes that clear after the patient coughs.

When wheezes are identified, certain characteristics should be noted. Examiners should identify the pitch and intensity and

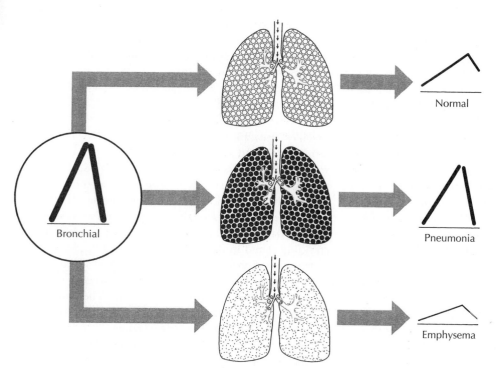

Figure 5-20 Examples of how the normal bronchial breath sound is altered as it passes through normal *(top)*, consolidated *(middle)*, and emphysematous *(bottom)* lung tissue.

Normal

Pneumonia

Emphysema

Bronchial

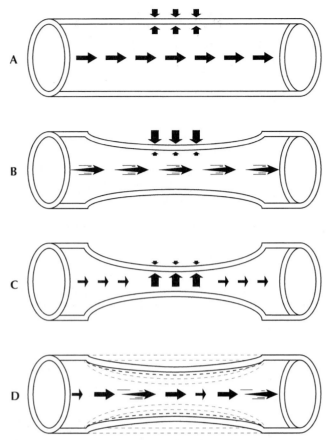

Figure 5-21 Proposed mechanism for wheezing. **A,** Normal airway, where internal and external airway wall pressures are equal. **B,** Slight narrowing of the airway, which causes an increase in the velocity of airflow and a decrease in the lateral wall pressure inside the airway relative to the outside. **C,** Greater narrowing of the airway to the point that forward flow is inhibited and lateral wall pressure increases relative to outside pressure. **D,** Fluttering of the airway walls between position of **B** and **C.**

the portion of the respiratory cycle occupied by the wheezing.[6,7] Improvement in the patient's airway caliber with bronchodilator therapy often results in a decrease in pitch and intensity of the wheezing and in a reduction in the portion of the respiratory cycle occupied by wheezing. For example, before treatment the patient may have loud, high-pitched wheezing that is heard during inspiration and expiration. After bronchodilator therapy, the wheezing may decrease in pitch and intensity and be heard only during the later part of exhalation. Because the intensity of wheezing is related to the flow, loud wheezing indicates that air movement is occurring, whereas soft wheezing may occur with fatigue and the onset of respiratory failure. The examiner must never rely solely on changes in the intensity (loudness) of wheezing in assessing the patient's response to therapy.

Wheezing may be polyphonic (having several different musical notes) or monophonic (having a single note). Polyphonic wheezing is limited to exhalation, and its many different musical notes begin and end simultaneously. They indicate that multiple airways are obstructed, as in asthma. Monophonic wheezes may be single or multiple, with each one indicating

obstruction of a bronchus. When multiple monophonic wheezes are present, the different notes often begin and end at different times and so overlap. The illusion of widespread airway obstruction results from the transmission of a few loud notes to most areas of the chest wall. A single monophonic wheeze indicates obstruction of a single airway. This may be present in the patient with an airway tumor that is partially obstructing a major airway or with aspiration of a foreign object. The clinician who hears a monophonic wheeze over the patient's chest should also auscultate over the patient's neck. If the wheeze is heard loudest over the neck, the upper airway is the source of the sound.

Stridor

Stridor is produced by mechanisms similar to those of wheezing. Rapid airflow through a narrow site of the upper airway causes the lateral walls to vibrate and produce a high-pitched sound often heard without a stethoscope. The diameter of the upper airway is most often narrowed because of infection, as in croup or epiglottitis, or with inflammation following extubation. Stridor is most often heard during inhalation, because the upper airway tends to narrow with significant inspiratory efforts. It may also be heard during inhalation and exhalation when the upper airway obstruction is severe and fixed (airway opening does not vary with breathing). This is seen in patients with laryngeal tumor.

Stridor is a life-threatening sign that indicates ventilation may be compromised. The patient with stridor should be monitored closely, and equipment and personnel needed to perform emergency intubation or tracheostomy should be nearby. The simultaneous presentation of stridor and cyanosis is a particularly ominous sign, because the cyanosis probably is the result of hypoxemia caused by hypoventilation. Like wheezing, stridor can occur only when significant airflow is present through the site of obstruction. As a result, the lack of stridor should never be interpreted as a sign of a healthy upper airway in the patient with a history or other clinical findings consistent with upper airway abnormalities.

Crackles

Crackles often are produced by the movement of excessive secretions or fluid in the airways as air passes through. In this situation, crackles usually are coarse and heard during inspiration and expiration. They often clear if the patient coughs, and they may be associated with rhonchial fremitus.

Crackles also occur in patients without excess secretions when collapsed airways pop open during inspiration. The crackling sound in this situation is caused by the explosive equalization of pressure between the collapsed airways and the patent airways above. Airway closure may occur in peripheral bronchioles or in more proximal bronchi. The source of the crackles in this situation may be suggested by certain characteristics described in the following paragraphs.

Larger, more proximal bronchi may close during expiration when there is an abnormal increase in bronchial compliance or if the retractive pressures around the bronchi are low. In this situation, crackles usually occur early in the inspiratory phase and are called *early inspiratory crackles* (Figure 5-22). Early inspiratory crackles are usually few in number but may be loud or faint. They often are transmitted to the mouth and are not silenced by a cough or change in position. They occur most often in patients with COPD, as in chronic bronchitis, emphysema, and asthma, and may indicate that a more severe airway obstruction is present.

Peripheral alveoli and airways may close during exhalation when the surrounding intrathoracic pressure increases. Crackles produced by the sudden opening of peripheral airways usually occur late in the inspiratory phase and are called *late inspiratory crackles* (Figure 5-23). They are more common in the dependent regions of the lungs, where the gravitational stress predisposes the peripheral airways to collapse during exhalation. They are often identified in several consecutive respiratory cycles, producing a recurrent rhythm. They may clear with changes in posture or if the patient performs several deep inspiratory maneuvers. Coughing or maximal exhalation by the patient may produce the reappearance of late inspiratory crackles. Patients with respiratory disorders such as atelectasis, pneumonia, pulmonary edema, and fibrosis that reduce lung volume (restrictive disorders) are most likely to have the late inspiratory type of crackles (Table 5-4).

> ### SIMPLY STATED
> Wheezing indicates intrathoracic airway obstruction, whereas late inspiratory crackles suggest atelectasis or other conditions of the lung that cause a loss of lung volume.

Pleural friction rub

A *pleural friction rub* is a creaking or grating type of sound that occurs when the pleural surfaces become inflamed and the roughened edges rub together during breathing. It may be heard only during inhalation but often is identified during both phases of breathing. Pleural rubs often sound similar to coarse crackles but are not affected by coughing. Pleural rubs are not commonly encountered in the clinical setting and for this reason often are not identified correctly when present. The intensity of pleural rubs may increase with deep breathing.

Voice Sounds

If inspection, palpation, percussion, or auscultation of the patient's chest suggests any respiratory abnormality, vocal resonance may be useful. Vocal resonance is produced by the same mechanism as vocal fremitus, described earlier. The vibrations created by the vocal cords during phonation travel down the tracheobronchial tree and through the peripheral lung units to the chest wall. The patient is instructed to repeat the words *one, two, three,* or *ninety-nine* while the examiner listens over the chest wall with the aid of a stethoscope, comparing side with side.

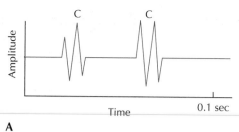

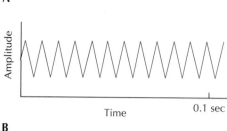

Figure 5-22 Time-expanded waveforms demonstrating inspiratory crackles **(A)** and expiratory polyphonic wheezes **(B).** (Modified from Wilkins RL et al: Lung sound terminology used by respiratory care practitioners, *Respir Care* 34:36, 1989.)

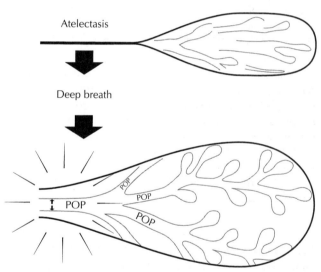

Figure 5-23 Proposed mechanism for late inspiratory crackles. Peripheral airways pop open when inspiratory effort is sufficient to overcome the forces causing the atelectasis.

The normal, air-filled lung tissue filters the voice sounds, resulting in a significant reduction in intensity and clarity. Pathologic abnormalities in lung tissue alter the transmission of voice sounds, resulting in either increased or decreased vocal resonance.

An increase in intensity and clarity of vocal resonance is called bronchophony. Bronchophony occurs as a result of an increase in lung tissue density, as in the consolidation of pneumonia, and is the result of the better transmission of vocal vibrations through consolidation. Bronchophony is easier to detect when it is unilateral and is often associated with bronchial breath sounds, dull percussion note, and increased vocal fremitus.

Table 5-4	Application of Adventitious Lung Sounds		
Lung Sounds	Possible Mechanism	Characteristics	Causes
Wheezes	Rapid airflow through obstructed airways caused by bronchospasm, mucosal edema	High-pitched; most often occur during exhalation	Asthma, congestive heart failure, bronchitis
Stridor	Rapid airflow through obstructed airway caused by inflammation	High-pitched; often occurs during inhalation	Croup, epiglottitis, postextubation
Crackles			
Inspiratory and expiratory	Excess airway secretions moving with airflow	Coarse and often clear with cough	Bronchitis, respiratory infections
Early inspiratory	Sudden opening of proximal bronchi	Scanty, transmitted to mouth; not affected by cough	Bronchitis, emphysema, asthma
Late inspiratory	Sudden opening of peripheral airways	Diffuse, fine; occur initially in the dependent regions	Atelectasis, pneumonia, pulmonary edema, fibrosis

Vocal resonance is reduced in similar lung abnormalities that result in reduced breath sounds and decreased tactile fremitus. Hyperinflation of lung parenchyma, pneumothorax, bronchial obstruction, and pleural effusion reduce the transmission of vocal vibrations through the lung or chest wall, producing decreased vocal resonance.

When the spoken voice increases in intensity and takes on a nasal or bleating quality, it is called egophony. Egophony may be identified over areas of the chest where bronchophony is present. The exact reason for this change in voice-sound character is unknown. It is identified most easily by having the patient say *e-e-e*. If egophony is present, the *e-e-e* is heard with the stethoscope over the peripheral chest wall as *a-a-a*. Egophony usually is identified only over an area of compressed lung above a pleural effusion.

Whispering pectoriloquy

Whispering pectoriloquy may be a helpful physical finding, especially in patients with small or patchy areas of lung consolidation. The patient is instructed to whisper the words *one, two, three* while the examiner listens over the lung periphery with a stethoscope, comparing side with side. Whispering creates high-frequency vibrations that are filtered out selectively by normal lung tissue and normally heard as muffled, low-pitched sounds. However, when consolidation is present, the lung loses its selective transmitter quality and the characteristic high-pitched sounds are transmitted to the chest wall with clarity over the affected region.

EXAMINATION OF THE PRECORDIUM

As mentioned previously, chronic diseases of the lungs may and often do cause abnormalities in other body systems. Recognition of these abnormalities is helpful in identifying respiratory disease and in quantifying its severity. Because of the close working relationship between the heart and lungs, the heart is especially at risk for developing problems secondary to lung disease. The techniques for physical examination of the chest wall overlying the heart (precordium) include inspection, palpation, and auscultation. Percussion is of little or no value in the examination and is omitted. For the sake of convenience, most clinicians perform the examination of the precordium simultaneously with the examination of the lungs.

Review of Heart Topography

The heart lies between the lungs within the mediastinum and is situated so that the right ventricle is more anterior than the left ventricle. The upper portion of the heart consists of both atria and commonly is called the *base of the heart.* The base lies directly beneath the upper-middle portion of the gladiolus (sternum). The lower portion of the heart, which consists of the ventricles, is called the *apex.* The apex points downward and to the left, extending to a point near the midclavicular line, and usually lies directly beneath the lower left portion of the gladiolus and near the costal cartilage of the fifth rib (Figure 5-24).

Inspection and Palpation

The purpose of inspecting and palpating the precordium is to identify any normal or abnormal pulsations. Pulsations on the precordium are affected by the thickness of the chest wall and the quality of the tissue through which the vibrations must travel. The normal apical impulse is produced by the thrust of the contracting left ventricle and usually is identified near the midclavicular line in the fifth intercostal space. This systolic thrust may be felt and visualized in many healthy persons; it may be called the point of maximal impulse (PMI).

Right ventricular hypertrophy, a common manifestation of chronic lung disease, often produces a systolic thrust (heave) that is felt and may be visualized near the lower left sternal border. The palmar aspect of the examiner's right hand is placed over the lower left sternal border for identification. Right ventricular hypertrophy may be the result of chronic hypoxemia, pulmonary valve disease, or pulmonary hypertension.

In patients with chronic pulmonary hyperinflation (emphysema), identification of the apical impulse is more difficult. The increase in anteroposterior diameter and the alteration in lung tissue contribute to poor transmission of the vibrations of systole to the surface of the chest. Therefore in patients with pulmonary emphysema, the intensity of the PMI often is reduced or not identifiable.

The PMI may shift to the left or right with shifts in the mediastinum. Pneumothorax or lobar collapse often shifts the mediastinum, resulting in a shift of the PMI toward the lobar collapse but usually away from the pneumothorax.

Patients with emphysema and low, flat diaphragms may have the PMI located in the epigastric area.

The second left intercostal space near the sternal border is called the *pulmonic area* and is palpated in an effort to identify accentuated pulmonary valve closure. Strong vibrations may be felt in this area with pulmonary hypertension (Figure 5-25).

Auscultation of Heart Sounds

Normal heart sounds are created primarily by the closure of the heart valves. The first heart sound (S_1) is produced by the sudden closure of the mitral and tricuspid valves (often called the *atrioventricular valves* or *AV valves*) during contraction of the

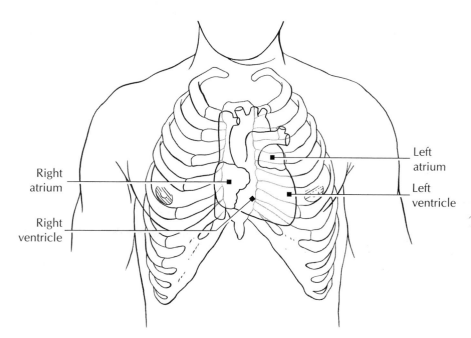

Figure 5-24 Topographic position of the heart.

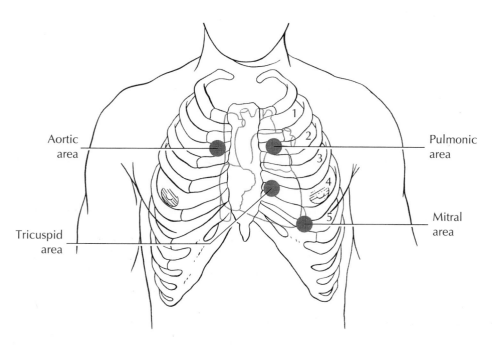

Figure 5-25 Position on the chest where each heart valve is best auscultated. Note that the stethoscope chest piece is placed between the ribs to better hear the underlying heart sounds and to avoid interference by bony structures.

ventricles. When systole ends, the ventricles relax and the pulmonic and aortic valves (semilunar) close, creating the second heart sound (S_2). Because the left side of the heart has a significantly higher pressure created during systole, closure of the mitral valve is louder and contributes more than the closure of the tricuspid valve to S_1 in the healthy person. For the same reason, closure of the aortic valve usually is more significant in producing S_2.

Whenever the two AV valves do not close simultaneously, a split S_1 is heard. Slight splitting of S_1 is normal; however, significant splitting usually indicates heart disease. Defects in the electrical conduction system of the heart, such as bundle branch block, cause the two ventricles to lack synchrony during systole.

Splitting of S_2 occurs when the semilunar valves (pulmonic and aortic) do not close simultaneously. A narrow splitting of S_2 is often related to the effects of spontaneous breathing on blood flow into the heart. The splitting of S_2 is increased during inhalation because of the decrease in intrathoracic pressure, which improves venous return to the right side of the heart and further delays pulmonic valve closure. The splitting in this situation decreases or disappears on exhalation. Wide splitting of the second heart sound is usually a sign of disease and is seen with bundle branch block, pulmonary embolism, and right-sided heart failure.[8]

A third heart sound (S_3) may be identified early in diastole. S_3 is thought to be produced by rapid ventricular filling immediately after systole. The rapid distention of the ventricles causes the walls of the ventricles to vibrate briefly and produce a sound of low intensity and pitch. It is best heard over the apex with the bell of the stethoscope. It is normal in young healthy children and is called *physiologic S_3* in this situation. However, in patients older than 40 years of age and especially in those with a history of heart disease, an S_3 is usually a sign of disease. S_3 usually indicates a ventricular abnormality (e.g., myocardial infarction) or some condition in which ventricular filling is increased.

A fourth heart sound (S_4) also may be identified during diastole. S_4 occurs late in diastole just before S_1. S_4 is produced by active filling of the ventricles from atrial contraction just before systole. It may occur in healthy persons but most often is considered a sign of heart disease. A fourth heart sound indicates diminished ventricular compliance with increased resistance to filling as occurs with systemic hypertension, ischemic heart disease, aortic stenosis, and acute mitral valve regurgitation. Most patients with an acute myocardial infarction have an S_4 if a sinus rhythm is present as seen on the electrocardiogram (see Chapter 10). The patient with an S_4 is often incorrectly thought to have a split S_1, because the timing of S_4 is normally very close to the first heart sound (Figure 5-26).

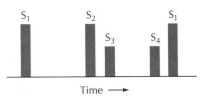

Figure 5-26 Timing of the first, second, third, and fourth heart sounds.

A gallop rhythm is an abnormal condition in which a third or fourth heart sound is present. The spacing of the heart sounds results in a unique sequence of sounds that resembles the gallop of a horse. A gallop rhythm suggests that the left or right ventricle is being overdistended during diastole. When an S_3 or S_4 is present and it originates in the right ventricle, it is best heard at the left sternal border near the apex. When the S_3 or S_4 originates in the left ventricle, it is best heard at the midclavicular line over the apex of the heart.

Auscultation of the heart sounds may identify alterations in the loudness of S_1 or S_2. A reduction in the intensity of the heart sounds may be the result of cardiac or extracardiac abnormalities. Extracardiac factors include alteration in the tissue between the heart and the surface of the chest. Pulmonary hyperinflation, pneumothorax, and obesity make identification of both S_1 and S_2 difficult. S_1 and S_2 intensity may also be reduced when the force of ventricular contraction is poor, as in heart failure, or when valvular abnormalities exist.

Pulmonary hypertension increases intensity of S_2 as a result of more forceful closure of the pulmonic valve; this is called an increased or loud P_2. A loud P_2 is a common finding in patients with pulmonary hypertension and cor pulmonale. An increased P_2 is identified best over the pulmonic area of the chest (see Figure 5-25). A loud aortic valve component (loud A_2) is commonly heard in patients with systemic hypertension. The best location to auscultate each heart valve is presented in Figure 5-25.

> **SIMPLY STATED**
> A loud pulmonic component to the second heart sound is called a *loud P_2* and suggests pulmonary hypertension.

Cardiac murmurs are identified whenever the heart valves are incompetent or stenotic. Murmurs usually are classified as either systolic or diastolic. Systolic murmurs are produced by an incompetent AV valve or a stenotic semilunar valve. An incompetent AV valve allows a backflow of blood into the atrium, usually producing a high-pitched whooshing noise simultaneously with S_1. A stenotic semilunar valve produces a similar sound, created by an obstruction of blood flow out of the ventricle during systole.

Diastolic murmurs are created by an incompetent semilunar valve or a stenotic AV valve. An incompetent semilunar valve allows a backflow of blood into the ventricle simultaneously with or immediately after S_2. A stenotic AV valve obstructs blood flow from the atrium into the ventricles during diastole and creates a turbulent murmur.

A murmur may also be created by rapid blood flow across normal valves. In summary, murmurs are created by a backflow of blood through an incompetent valve, forward flow through a stenotic valve, and rapid flow through a normal valve.

Auscultation of heart sounds usually is performed at the same time the lung sounds are identified when indicated. The bell and diaphragm pieces of the stethoscope are used. The diaphragm is most useful for higher-frequency sounds such as S_1, S_2, and systolic murmurs. The bell is best used for low-frequency sounds such as gallops (S_3 and S_4) and diastolic murmurs. The heart sounds may be easier to identify if the patient leans forward or lies on the left side, because anatomically this moves the heart closer to the chest wall. When the peripheral pulses are difficult to identify, auscultation over the precordium may be an easier method of identifying the heart rate.

NEUROLOGIC EXAMINATION

A neurologic examination is performed by the attending physician when a brain or spinal cord injury is suspected. Because these injuries often affect the patient's respiratory system and the ability of the patient to cooperate with respiratory care procedures, the respiratory therapist must be familiar with this examination. The neurologic examination is often brief if initial interactions with the patient are normal (e.g., the patient responds appropriately to verbal stimuli) and the patient has no symptoms suggesting neurologic disease. A more extensive examination is performed when abnormalities are suspected and may involve the expertise of a neurologist to examine the patient and recommend therapy.

A large variety of evaluation procedures are available to determine the status of the brain and spinal cord. Many of the procedures are simple and can be performed by any healthcare provider (e.g., assessing level of consciousness [LOC]). Other procedures are more complex and should be performed only by those trained in neurology. A discussion of the complete neurologic examination is beyond the scope of this chapter; however, this section of the chapter describes the procedures that most closely relate to the patient with cardiopulmonary disease.

Anatomy and Physiology

To perform or understand a neurologic assessment, the examiner needs a basic understanding of anatomy and physiology of the neurologic system. The neurologic system is made up of two major parts: the central and peripheral nervous systems. The central nervous system is made up of the brain and spinal cord (Figure 5-27), whereas the peripheral nervous system is composed of the 12 cranial nerves and the 31 spinal cord nerves. The brain consists of three parts: the cerebrum, which contains two hemispheres; the brainstem (midbrain, pons, and medulla); and the cerebellum.

The cerebrum is the largest part of the brain and is made up of many different sections, each of which controls a specific intellectual or motor function. Lesions in the cerebrum can lead to a wide variety of abnormalities in functions such as moving body parts, LOC, ability to speak and write, emotions, and/or memory.

The brainstem is of particular importance to the respiratory therapist, because this is where breathing is regulated and controlled. In addition, the brainstem contains reflex centers for certain cranial nerve functions such as pupillary contraction in response to light. Lesions in the brainstem can cause a wide range

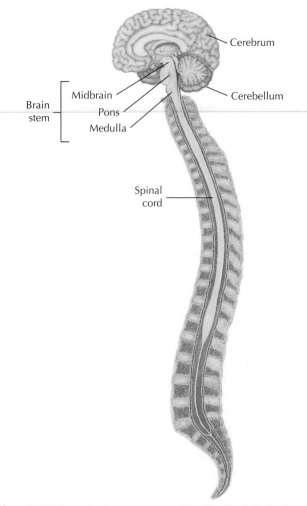

Figure 5-27 The central nervous system. Details of both the brain and the spinal cord are seen in this figure. (From Thibodeau GA, Patton KT: *Anatomy and physiology*, ed 5, St Louis, 2003, Mosby.)

of breathing problems from hyperventilation to apnea (see subsequent discussion) and a loss of pupillary response to light.

The cerebellum is believed to control equilibrium, muscle tone, and coordinated muscle movements. Lesions in the cerebellum cause characteristic symptoms such as loss of muscle coordination, tremors, and disturbances in gait and balance.

The spinal cord lies within the center of the vertebral bodies and extends from the base of the brain down to the level of the first lumbar vertebra. It spans a distance of approximately 45 cm in the average adult. It serves the purpose of connecting the brain to the various parts of the body for motor and sensory function.

The spinal cord is an oval cylinder that has two tapering bulges; one in the cervical region and one in the lumbar region. Two sets of nerve fibers project from both sides of the spinal column at 31 locations along the spine. The two nerve fibers on each side (one anterior and one posterior) come together before exiting the spinal column to form a single spinal nerve that is part of the peripheral nervous system (see subsequent discussion). The posterior nerve fiber comprising the dorsal nerve root carries sensory information into the spinal cord. The anterior nerve fiber comprising the ventral nerve root conducts motor impulses out of the spinal cord. Lesions in the anterior or posterior nerve roots cause a loss of sensory or motor function in the related area. Damage to the spinal cord can lead to dysfunction of all motor and sensory function at and below the site of injury (e.g., injury high in the spinal cord may affect sensory and motor function of upper and lower body parts, whereas injury low in the spinal cord will affect only the lower part of the body).

Assessment of the Central Nervous System

Level of Consciousness (LOC)

One of the most important procedures used to evaluate function of the central nervous system is assessing the LOC. Assessment of LOC begins when you first encounter the patient. Is he/she awake, alert, and interacting with the environment around him/her? A neurologically healthy patient will be awake and interacting with those around him/her unless he/she is asleep. If a healthy patient is asleep, he/she can be easily aroused to an awake, alert state. A patient who cannot be aroused from a sleeplike state (eyes are closed) is said to be in a coma. The patient who is not able to be aroused, but whose eyes are open, is said to be in a persistent vegetative state. This indicates irreversible brain damage. Breathing may not be affected if the brainstem is unaffected by the injury.

When a patient is not alert and responsive, additional assessments may help clarify the degree of neurologic dysfunction. One of the most commonly used instruments for quantifying neurologic impairment is the Glasgow Coma Scale (see Table 4-2). This scale relies on assessments in three areas: eye movements, verbal responses, and motor responses. The scale varies from 15 (normal) to 3 (completely unresponsive). It is easy to perform and readily reproducible but is poorly suited for patients who have impaired verbal responses. Common examples of impaired verbal abilities include aphasia, hearing loss, and orotracheal intubation.

Using the Glasgow Coma Scale, the examiner assesses the patient by verbal exchange and visual inspection of the patient. A brief conversation with a responsive patient establishes his/her degree of verbal responsiveness. Patients who are well oriented during conversation are given a 5 in this category. Patients who are unresponsive are scored at 0. Those who are verbally responsive but not well oriented are given a score somewhere between 0 and 5 depending on their verbal responses.

If the patient does not have spontaneous movements of the eyes or limbs, or does not have a verbal response, the examiner should attempt to arouse the patient with a loud voice, such as calling his/her name. If the patient is still unresponsive after verbal stimuli, a response to pain can be assessed by firmly rubbing the patient's sternum with your knuckles.

The response to pain varies depending on the level of neurologic function. Normally, pain causes the patient to attempt to remove the source of the pain and/or to withdraw from the painful stimulation. If the cerebral cortex is not functioning, there is a withdrawal from painful stimuli in a predictable and

reflexive manner. If the dysfunction extends to high in the brainstem, pain induces flexion of the muscles. This reaction is seen when the arms, wrists, and fingers flex over the chest while the legs extend and internally rotate. This is called decorticate posturing. Dysfunction high in the pons or midbrain may cause decerebrate posturing. This is seen as extension and internal rotation of the arms and legs (Figure 5-28).

Assessment of Brainstem Function

The reasons for a patient having decreased level of consciousness can be grouped into two basic categories: a generalized dysfunction (e.g., drug overdose) or an abnormality in a specific area of the brain. When an abnormality that affects a local area of the brain causes loss of consciousness, it usually does this by putting pressure on the brainstem. When pressure is applied to the brainstem, brainstem functions are lost in a predictable sequence. The loss of function starts from the top of the midbrain and extends sequentially down through the medulla (Table 5-5).

The patient's breathing pattern may reveal the level of brainstem function in the neurologically impaired patient. **Cheyne-Stokes breathing** is seen as a repeated pattern of apnea followed by slow shallow breathing increasing in intensity until the patient is breathing rapidly and deeply. The breathing pattern lessens in intensity slowly until the patient again has apnea. The pattern is continually repeated and indicates that the highest level of brainstem function is the mid-midbrain. A patient with involuntary hyperventilation takes obviously deep and rapid breaths. This indicates that the highest level of function is the pons. **Ataxic breathing** is seen as an irregular and unpredictable breathing pattern and indicates that all brain function above the medulla is absent.

Pupillary response is judged by briefly passing a bright light in front of both open eyes while carefully watching the iris in both eyes for movement. Any visible change in the pupils' size is noted. The pupillary response may be affected by medications the patient is taking. For example, atropine causes the pupils to

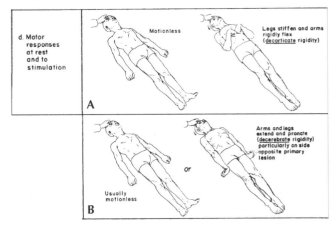

Figure 5-28 A, Decorticate posturing. **B,** Decerebrate posturing. (From Plum F, Posner JB: *Diagnosis of stupor and coma,* Philadelphia, 1980, Oxford University Press.)

Table 5-5	Sequence of Loss of Brainstem Function			
Highest Level of Brainstem Function	Breathing	Oculocephalic Reflex	Pupils	Pain Response
High Midbrain	Normal	Normal	Normal	Withdrawal
Mid-Midbrain	Cheyne-Stokes	Present	Small but reactive	Decorticate
Pons	Hyperventilation	Minimal	Mid-fixed	Decerebrate
Medulla	Ataxic	None	Mid-fixed	None

dilate and not respond to light. Such findings in the patient taking atropine do not suggest neurologic problems.

The oculocephalic reflex is tested by watching the response of the eyes to a back-and-forth movement of the head. The eyes are opened and the head is placed in a neutral position so that the patient is looking straight up. The head is then moved rapidly but gently to one side and then the other. If a person is completely normal, he/she will look around at objects in the room. If a patient has complete brainstem function but the cerebral cortex is not functioning, the eyes will be looking straight ahead (up) when the head is in the neutral position. When the head is turned to one side, the eyes will remain looking up for a few seconds and then will slowly drift to the side the head is tilted until the eyes again are looking straight ahead in the direction the head is tilted. These findings will be repeated as the head is returned to the neutral position and when the head is turned toward the opposite side. When the eyes remain looking in the original direction and slowly drift to a new position, the oculocephalic reflex is present. When the brainstem is not functioning down through the level of the pons, the oculocephalic reflex is absent. The absent oculocephalic reflex is seen as the head is turned from side to side and the eyes remain fixed in the head, looking straight ahead. The eyes appear immovable just as a doll's eyes that are painted onto the doll's head. This finding is sometimes referred to as "doll's eyes."

SIMPLY STATED
The pattern of breathing in the patient with brain injury provides clues to the level of brainstem function. Ataxic breathing (unpredictable breathing) indicates that all brain function above the medulla is absent, and the patient is essentially brain dead.

The patient's response to pain is also an indicator of brainstem function as mentioned before. Table 5-5 summarizes the responses to pain associated with the level of brainstem function.

Assessment of Spinal Cord Function

Evaluation of spinal cord function is performed by using a variety of sensory and motor function tests. The physician may check reflexes in the arms and legs, apply muscle strength tests, and evaluate the patient's response to painful stimuli to assess the function of the spinal cord and the anterior and posterior nerve roots. In many cases, this evaluation is not able to detect the exact location of the lesion when abnormalities are present. For example, weakness in the right hand could be the result of damage to the spinal nerve associated with the right hand or could be related to the associated anterior nerve root. Further testing may be needed to identify the exact location of the defect in such cases.

Assessment of the Peripheral Nervous System

Evaluation of Spinal Nerves

Thirty-one pairs of spinal nerves are connected to the spinal cord. Each pair has no specific name but rather is numbered according to the level of the vertebral column at which they exit the spinal column. There are eight cervical nerve pairs (C1 to C8), twelve thoracic nerve pairs (T1 to T12), five lumbar nerve pairs (L1 to L5), five sacral nerve pairs (S1 to S5), and one coccygeal pair of spinal nerves. All spinal nerves contain both motor and sensory fibers and are called **mixed** nerves for this reason. Each has the ability to provide sensory input to the brain (e.g., feel pain) and the ability to cause muscle movement (e.g., extend the arm on command).

Two spinal nerves important for respiratory function are the right and left phrenic nerves that innervate the diaphragm to control breathing. The phrenic nerves arise from the cervical spine roots of C2 to C4. Damage to this portion of the spinal cord or both phrenic nerves can result in complete paralysis of the diaphragm and dependence on mechanical ventilation for life.

The spinal nerves are evaluated by using a combination of tests. Sensory evaluation is performed by having the patient respond to stimuli at a specific location. For example, damage to the C1 nerve pairs causes a loss of sensation over the back of the head, front of the neck, and parts of the shoulder. In addition, the physician evaluates spinal nerves by testing a variety of reflexes. The most familiar example of this type of procedure is the patellar reflex check. This is performed by tapping on the patellar tendon while the patient dangles his/her legs over the edge of the examining table. Normally, the lower leg jerks forward when this reflex is intact. The reflex is scored on a scale of 0 to +4. A score of 0 indicates no response, +1 indicates reduced response, +2 is normal, and +3 and +4 indicate increased response. Abnormalities in the patellar reflex indicate lesions in the L2 to L4 spinal nerves, the anterior or posterior nerve roots, or the spinal cord itself.

Evaluation of the Cranial Nerves

As stated previously, there are 12 cranial nerves. These nerves are connected to the undersurface of the brain, with most coming from the brainstem (Figure 5-29). Each nerve is named according to its distribution or function (Table 5-6). Some of the cranial nerves are sensory only, some are motor only, and others have both functions. Those that have both functions allow sensory input to the brain for interpretation and control of muscles for function.

The cranial nerves are evaluated by using a combination of sensory and motor function tests. Each nerve is tested according to whether it is sensory, motor, or both. Sensory nerves are exposed to a specific sensation. For example, cranial nerve I (olfactory) is evaluated by testing the patient's sense of smell. Motor function is tested by asking the patient to respond to commands. For example, cranial nerve III (oculomotor) is evaluated by checking the ability of the patient's eyes to follow the physician's finger as it is slowly moved around in front of the patient's face.

Cranial nerve IX is especially important to the respiratory therapist. It is called the **glossopharyngeal nerve,** and it controls a variety of functions. It controls the muscles of swallowing that are needed to prevent aspiration. This function of cranial nerve IX is evaluated by testing the patient's gag reflex. This is performed by gently inserting a tongue depressor into the back of the throat. If the gag reflex is intact, the patient will gag. A negative response suggests that the patient may be prone to aspiration and need intubation to protect the lungs. Cranial nerve IX also has a branch that extends to the carotid sinus and plays a major role in the control of blood pressure.

EXAMINATION OF THE ABDOMEN

An in-depth discussion of the abdominal examination is beyond the scope of this text; however, the abnormalities associated with respiratory disease are reviewed.

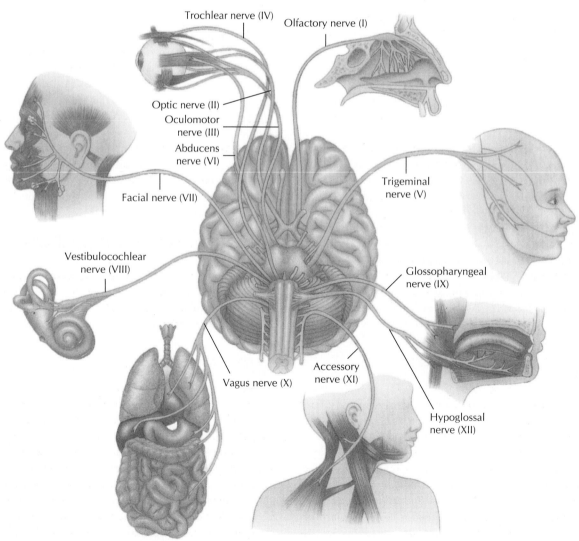

Figure 5-29 The cranial nerves. Ventral surface of the brain showing attachment to the cranial nerves. (From Thibodeau GA, Patton KT: *Anatomy and physiology,* ed 5, St Louis, 2003, Mosby.)

Table 5-6	Names, Numbers, and Functional Classifications of Cranial Nerves*	
Name	Number	Functional Classification
Olfactory	I	Sensory
Optic	II	Sensory
Oculomotor	III	Motor
Trochlear	IV	Motor
Trigeminal	V	Mixed
Abducens	VI	Motor
Facial	VII	Mixed
Vestibulocochlear	VIII	Sensory
Glossopharyngeal	IX	Mixed
Vagus	X	Mixed
Accessory	XI	Motor
Hypoglossal	XII	Motor

From Thibodeau GA, Patton KT: *Anatomy and physiology*, ed 5, St Louis, 2003, Mosby.
*The first letter of the words in the following sentence are the first letters of the name of the cranial nerves, in the correct order. Many anatomy students find that using this sentence, or one like it, helps in memorizing the names and numbers of the cranial nerves. It is "On 'Old Olympus' Tiny Tops, A Friendly Viking Grew Vines And Hops." The functional classification of each cranial nerve can be remembered by using this sentence: "Some Say 'Marry Money,' But My Brothers Say 'Bad Business, Marry Money.'" In this sentence, S indicates *sensory*, M indicates *motor*, and B indicates *both sensory* and motor (mixed).

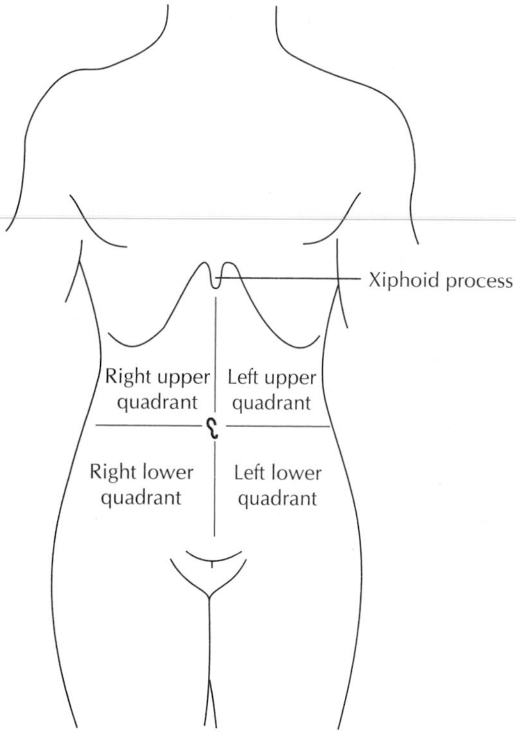

Figure 5-30 Division of the abdomen into quadrants. (Modified from Prior JA, Silberstein JS: *Physical examination: The history and examination of the patient*, ed 6, St Louis, 1982, Mosby.)

The abdomen should be inspected and palpated for evidence of distention and tenderness. Abdominal distention may cause impairment of the diaphragm and contribute to respiratory failure. It may also inhibit the patient from coughing and deep breathing, both of which are extremely important in preventing respiratory complications in the postoperative patient.

Palpation and percussion are used on the right upper quadrant (Figure 5-30) of the abdomen in an effort to estimate the size of the liver. An enlarged liver may be found when chronic right-sided heart failure has occurred as a consequence of chronic respiratory disease. Any respiratory disease that results in a reduction of the oxygen level in the blood causes pulmonary vasoconstriction. If this occurs over a period of months or years, the right ventricle becomes enlarged and fails to pump blood effectively. The venous blood flow returning to the right ventricle is reduced, and engorgement of major veins and organs may occur. The hepatic vein that empties into the inferior vena cava may become engorged in this situation, and the liver may increase in size. This is called hepatomegaly.

To identify hepatomegaly, the examiner locates the superior and inferior borders of the liver by percussion. Normally, the liver spans approximately 10 cm at the midclavicular line. If the liver extends more than 10 cm, it is considered enlarged.

Hepatomegaly may be accompanied by the collection of serous fluid in the peritoneal cavity known as ascites. Ascites most often results from interference with venous return to the right side of the heart, as occurs in heart failure. Cirrhosis of the liver, depletion of plasma proteins, and sodium retention are common contributing factors. Severe ascites may restrict diaphragm movement, as mentioned earlier, and contribute to the onset of respiratory failure.

EXAMINATION OF THE EXTREMITIES

Respiratory disease may result in numerous abnormalities, identified during inspection of the extremities. These abnormalities include digital clubbing, cyanosis, and pedal edema. Each is discussed briefly.

Clubbing

Clubbing of the digits is a significant manifestation of cardiopulmonary disease. The mechanism responsible for clubbing is not known, but it is often associated with a chronic cardiopulmonary disease. It is identified most commonly in patients with cyanotic congenital heart disease, bronchogenic carcinoma, COPD, cystic fibrosis, and bronchiectasis.

Clubbing is characterized by a painless enlargement of the terminal phalanges of the fingers and toes. It requires years to develop. As the process of clubbing advances, the angle of the fingernail to the nail base advances past 180 degrees, and the base of the nail feels spongy. The profile view of the digits allows easier recognition of clubbing (Figure 5-31).

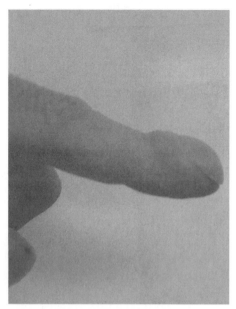

Figure 5-31 Lateral view of digital clubbing of the index finger.

Cyanosis

Examination of the digits should identify the presence or absence of cyanosis in any patient suspected of having cardiopulmonary disease. The transparency of the fingernails and skin covering the digits allows cyanosis to be detected initially in this area. The presence of cyanosis in the digits (peripheral cyanosis or acrocyanosis) indicates that the blood flow is not optimal. The patient with peripheral cyanosis resulting from poor perfusion also has extremities that are cool to the touch. Tissue oxygenation may be compromised in such situations.

> **SIMPLY STATED**
> The ability to see cyanosis depends on the lighting in the room and the patient's hemoglobin level. Reduced hemoglobin concentration in the blood prevents visible cyanosis even if hypoxemia is present.

Pedal Edema

Pedal edema may be a manifestation of chronic lung disease. Because hypoxemia produces pulmonary vasoconstriction, the right ventricle must work harder than normal whenever significant hypoxemia exists. This chronic workload on the right ventricle may result in right ventricular hypertrophy and poor venous blood flow return to the heart. When the venous return to the right side of the heart is reduced, the peripheral blood vessels engorge, resulting in an accumulation of fluid in the subcutaneous tissues of the ankles, called pedal edema. The ankles most often are affected, because they naturally are maintained in a gravity-dependent position throughout the day. The edematous tissues pit (indent) when pressed firmly with the fingertips. The severity of edema usually is characterized by the examining physician using a scale of 1+ to 4+, with 1+ indicating slight edema and 4+ indicating severe edema. Pitting edema should be evaluated for the level of occurrence above the ankle in an effort to quantify the degree of right-sided heart failure. For example, pitting edema occurring at a level well above the knee is much more significant than pitting edema around the ankles only.

> **SIMPLY STATED**
> Pedal edema may occur in patients with chronic lung disease that has resulted in cor pulmonale or chronic right-sided heart failure.

Capillary Refill

Capillary refill is assessed by pressing firmly for a brief period on the fingernail and identifying the speed at which the blood flow returns. When cardiac output is reduced and digital perfusion is poor, capillary refill is slow, taking several seconds to appear. In normal persons with good cardiac output and digital perfusion, capillary refill should take less than 3 seconds.

Peripheral Skin Temperature

When the heart does not circulate the blood at a sufficient rate, compensatory vasoconstriction occurs in the extremities to shunt blood toward the vital organs. The reduction in peripheral perfusion results in a loss of warmth in the extremities. Palpation of the patient's feet and hands may provide general information about perfusion. Cool extremities usually indicate inadequate perfusion.

Actual extremity temperature can be compared with room temperature. The extremity should be at least 2° C warmer than room temperature (unless room temperature is equal to or greater than body temperature). When there is less than 2° C difference, perfusion is reduced; a 0.5° C difference indicates that the patient has serious perfusion problems.

SUMMARY

Physical examination of the patient with cardiopulmonary disease is performed to determine the cause and severity of the patient's problem. It is also performed to evaluate the effects of treatment. The patient's chest is typically inspected, palpated, percussed to evaluate resonance, and auscultated. Other body systems are evaluated to determine possible complications of the cardiopulmonary disease. Once these procedures are complete and the medical history is considered, a clinical picture develops. This clinical picture often identifies a somewhat precise assessment of the patient; however, additional laboratory tests, chest radiographs, and pulmonary function testing may be needed to further determine the exact cause of the findings. These topics are addressed in following chapters.

REVIEW QUESTIONS

1. Which of the following is *not* a typical component to physical examination?
   a. Inspection
   b. Palpation
   c. Auscultation
   d. Interviewing

2. Which of the following may cause an increased jugular venous distention?
   a. Chronic hypoxemia
   b. Left-sided heart failure ✓
   c. Right-sided heart failure
   d. All of the above

3. T F Atelectasis, if large enough, may cause tracheal deviation away from the affected side.

4. T F JVP is measured vertically from the sternal angle with the head of the bed at a 45-degree angle.

5. Pursed-lip breathing is most often seen in patients with which of the following diseases?
   a. Pulmonary fibrosis
   b. COPD ✓
   c. Pneumonia
   d. Congestive heart failure

6. What spinous process is most prominent with the patient sitting and with his/her head bent forward?
   a. T1
   b. C1
   c. C7
   d. S3

7. At which of the following topographic locations is the bifurcation of the trachea located on the anterior chest?
   a. Over the upper part of the manubrium
   b. At the sternal angle
   c. Fourth rib at the sternum
   d. Under the xiphoid process

8. The minor (horizontal) fissure begins at which of the following locations on the anterior chest?
   a. Second rib at the sternal border
   b. Fourth rib at the sternal border
   c. Sixth rib at the sternal border
   d. None of the above

9. "An inward depression of the sternum" describes which of the following thoracic configurations?
   a. Kyphosis
   b. Pectus excavatum
   c. Flail chest
   d. Barrel chest

10. T F Scoliosis is an **S**-shaped (lateral) curvature of the spine.

11. Which of the following best describes an apneustic breathing pattern?
   a. Prolonged exhalation
   b. Prolonged inhalation
   c. Deep and fast
   d. Lack of breathing

12. T F Restrictive lung disease is typified by a rapid and shallow breathing pattern.

13. T F Intercostal retractions indicate an increased work of breathing.

14. Which of the following breathing patterns is associated with narrowing of intrathoracic airways?
   a. Prolonged inspiratory time
   b. Prolonged expiratory time
   c. Rapid and shallow
   d. Rapid and deep

15. Which of the following indicate(s) diaphragmatic fatigue?
   a. Paradoxical pulse
   b. Abdominal paradox
   c. Respiratory alternans
   d. b and c

16. Which of the following causes an increased tactile fremitus?
   a. Atelectasis
   b. Pleural effusion
   c. Emphysema
   d. Obesity

17. Which of the following causes a bilateral decrease in chest expansion?
   a. Lung tumor
   b. Pneumothorax
   c. COPD
   d. Pleural effusion

18. Which of the following causes an increased resonance to percussion of the chest?
   a. Lobar consolidation
   b. Pneumothorax

c. Pleural effusion

d. Atelectasis

19. (T) F   The diaphragm portion of a stethoscope is used to listen to high-frequency sounds such as those over the lungs.

20. Normal tracheal breath sounds are produced by which of the following mechanisms?
    a. Turbulent airflow through large airways
    b. Filtered sounds through lung tissue
    c. Passage of air through secretions
    d. Passage of air through narrowed airways

21. Which of the following terms is used to describe discontinuous ALS?
    a. Wheeze
    b. Crackles
    c. Rhonchi
    d. Stridor

22. The finding of late inspiratory crackles on auscultation of a patient might indicate which of the following?
    a. Atelectasis
    b. Pulmonary fibrosis
    c. Bronchospasm
    d. a and b

23. T (F)   Polyphonic wheezes arise from varying degrees of obstruction of a single bronchus.

24. Which of the following ALS is commonly heard from the patient with upper airway obstruction?
    a. Polyphonic wheezing
    b. Fine inspiratory crackles
    c. Coarse inspiratory and expiratory crackles
    d. Inspiratory stridor

25. Which of the following is the normal topographic location of the PMI?
    a. Third intercostal space at the anterior axillary line
    b. Fourth intercostal space at the anterior axillary line
    c. Fifth intercostal space at the midclavicular line
    d. Sixth intercostal space at the midsternal line

26. Which of the following locations is best for auscultating the mitral valve?
    a. Third intercostal space at the anterior axillary line
    b. Fourth intercostal space at the anterior axillary line
    c. Fifth intercostal space at the midclavicular line
    d. Sixth intercostal space at the midsternal line

27. T (F)   The first (S_1) heart sound is produced as a result of aortic and mitral valve closure.

28. T (F)   A gallop rhythm is present when the third or fourth heart sound is heard on auscultation and usually indicates an atrial distention abnormality during diastole.

29. Which of the following may cause an increased P_2 component of the second heart sound?
    a. Pulmonary hypertension
    b. Pulmonary embolism
    c. Cor pulmonale
    d. All of the above

30. What procedure is one of the most important for assessing central nervous system function?
    a. Deep tendon reflexes
    b. Level of consciousness
    c. Pupillary response to light
    d. Response to painful stimuli

31. What cranial nerve controls the muscles of swallowing to prevent aspiration?
    a. Cranial nerve III
    b. Cranial nerve V
    c. Cranial nerve IX
    d. Cranial nerve XII

32. (T) F   Clubbing of the digits may be seen with cyanotic congenital heart disease.

REFERENCES

1. Bernard L and others: Bacterial contamination of hospital physicians' stethoscopes, *Infect Control Hosp Epidemiol* 20:626-628, 1999.
2. Nunez S and others: The stethoscope in the emergency department: A vector of infection? *Epidemiol Infect* 124:233-237, 2000.
3. Wilkins RL and others: Does auscultating through the patient's gown make a difference in the perceived intensity of the vesicular breath sound? *Respir Care* 45:1004, 2000 (abstract).
4. Mahagnah M, Gavriely N: Repeatability of measurements of normal lung sounds, *Am J Respir Crit Care Med* 149: 477-481, 1994.
5. Schreur HJ, Sterk PJ, Vanderschoot J: Lung sound intensity in patients with emphysema and in normal subjects at standard airflows, *Thorax* 47:674-679, 1992.

6. Baughman RP, Loudon RG: Quantification of wheezing in acute asthma, *Chest* 86:718-722, 1984.

7. Baughman RP, Loudon RG: Lung sound analysis for continuous evaluation of airflow obstruction in asthma, *Chest* 88:364-368, 1985.

8. Fauci AS and others: *Harrison's principles of internal medicine,* ed 14, New York, 1998, McGraw-Hill.

Seidel HM and others: *Mosby's guide to physical examination,* ed 5, St Louis, 2003, Mosby.

Tilkian AG, Conover MB: *Understanding heart sounds and murmurs,* ed 4, St Louis, 2001, Mosby.

Wilkins RL, Hodgkin JE, Lopez B: *The fundamentals of lung and heart sounds,* ed 3, St Louis, 2004, Mosby.

BIBLIOGRAPHY

Barkauskas VH, Baumann LC, Darling-Fisher CS: *Health and physical assessment,* ed 3, St Louis, 2002, Mosby.

C H A P T E R

6

Robert L. Wilkins
James R. Dexter

Clinical Laboratory Studies

LEARNING OBJECTIVES

Upon completion of this chapter, the reader should be able to accomplish the following:

1. Identify the components that make up the formed elements and plasma of the blood.
2. Define blood serum and describe how it is obtained.
3. Recognize the normal values and significance of the following hematology laboratory tests:
   a. White blood cell count
   b. White cell differential
   c. Red blood cell count
   d. Hematocrit
   e. Hemoglobin
   f. Erythrocyte indices (mean cell volume, mean cell hemoglobin, mean cell hemoglobin concentration)
   g. Reticulocyte count
   h. Sedimentation rate
   i. Platelet count
   j. Coagulation studies (bleeding time, activated partial thromboplastin time, prothrombin time)
4. Define the terms *leukocytosis* and *leukopenia* and recognize common causes of each.
5. Recognize the causes for the following white cell abnormalities:
   a. Neutrophilia
   b. Neutropenia
   c. Eosinophilia
   d. Lymphocytosis
   e. Lymphocytopenia
   f. Monocytosis
6. Identify the effect that AIDS and AIDS-related complex have on the ratio of T-helper to T-suppressor cells.
7. Define leukemia and myeloproliferative disorders.
8. Define left shift in terms of the white blood cell differential and its clinical significance.
9. Define anemia and the most common causes of anemia.
10. Identify the potential effect anemia has on oxygen-carrying capacity and tissue oxygenation.
11. Define primary, secondary, and relative polycythemia and identify how polycythemia affects blood oxygen transport and myocardial work.
12. Recognize the normal values and significance of abnormalities for each of the following chemistry laboratory tests:
    a. Electrolytes
    b. Anion gap
    c. Sweat electrolyte concentration
    d. Blood urea nitrogen and creatinine
    e. Enzymes (aspartate aminotransferase, alanine aminotransferase, alkaline phosphatase, acid phosphatase, lactic dehydrogenase, creative kinase, amylase, lipase)
    f. Glucose
    g. Protein (immunoglobulins, albumin)
    h. Lipids (triglycerides, cholesterol, high-density and low-density lipoproteins)
13. Identify the therapeutic level for theophylline and factors that affect its metabolism and clearance.
14. Define the following medical microbiology terms:
    a. Normal flora
    b. Gram stain
    c. Culture
    d. Sensitivity
15. Recognize the type of organism a Ziehl-Neelsen stain is used to identify.
16. Recognize the methods for obtaining a fresh and uncontaminated sputum sample.
17. Identify the factors involved in the macroscopic (gross) sputum examination.
18. Identify the characteristic appearance of the sputum from a patient with bronchiectasis.
19. Identify the microscopic criteria used to determine whether a sputum sample is reliable.
20. Recognize the significance of sputum eosinophilia.
21. Recognize some of the organisms responsible for producing pneumonia and the most common cause of bacterial pneumonia.
22. Identify the indications and method of performing a bronchoalveolar lavage.

Linda W. Chu, MD, contributed to this chapter in the previous edition.

23. Identify the significance of the following during pleural fluid examination:
    a. Increased pleural fluid amount
    b. Milky pleural fluid
    c. Hemorrhagic pleural fluid
    d. Low protein content (less than 3 g/dL)
    e. High protein content (more than 3 g/dL)
    f. High pleural fluid lactic dehydrogenase
24. Identify the significance of the following tests performed during a urinalysis:
    a. Specific gravity
    b. pH
    c. Protein content
    d. Glucose concentration
    e. Ketones
    f. Bilirubin
    g. Blood
    h. Urobilinogen
    i. Nitrates
    j. Sedimentary constituents
25. Describe or identify the purpose of histologic and cytologic examinations.
26. Identify the malignant tumors responsible for producing most primary lung cancers.
27. Recognize the types of pulmonary samples that can be examined cytologically.
28. Recognize the following regarding skin testing:
    a. Diseases diagnosed
    b. Procedures for testing
    c. Significance and causes of anergy
    d. Use of the purified protein derivative
    e. When a purified protein derivative is considered positive
    f. Effect of the bacille Calmette-Guérin vaccine on purified protein derivative

CHAPTER OUTLINE
Hematology
Complete Blood Cell Count
    White Blood Cells
    Red Blood Cells
    Platelet Count
    Coagulation Studies
Chemistry
    Electrolyte Concentrations
    Blood Urea Nitrogen and Creatinine
    Enzymes
    Glucose
    Proteins
    Lipids
    Tumor Markers
    Drug Monitoring
Microbiology
    Examination of Pulmonary Secretions
    Bronchoalveolar Lavage
    Pleural Fluid Examination

Urinalysis
Histology and Cytology
Skin Testing

KEY TERMS

anemia	leukocytosis
anergy	leukopenia
basophilia	lymphocytopenia
blasts	lymphocytosis
cytology	macrocytic
eosinophilia	macrophage
erythrocytes	microcytic
glucosuria	monocytosis
hemostasis	neutropenia
hyperchloremia	neutrophilia
hyperglycemia	normoblasts
hyperkalemia	polycythemia
hypernatremia	polycythemia vera
hypoalbuminemia	pseudoneutropenia
hypochloremia	pseudoneutrophilia
hypoglycemia	reticulocytes
hypokalemia	serum
hyponatremia	spurious polycythemia
left shift	thrombocytes
leukocytes	

CHAPTER OVERVIEW

The modern clinical laboratory consists of a formidable array of equipment and offers a vast number of studies. Most hospitalized patients with respiratory disease undergo many laboratory tests, and it is important for respiratory therapists to have a basic understanding of at least the commonly ordered tests. This chapter attempts to provide that understanding. Although the emphasis is on interpreting laboratory data in patients with respiratory disease, most of the concepts described are applicable to any patient.

Most laboratory tests are performed using peripheral venous blood from the patient. Many other types of body fluids or secretions, including sputum, pleural fluid, cerebrospinal fluid, urine, feces, and sweat, are also used for various tests.

The blood consists of two major components: the formed elements and the plasma. The formed elements are composed of three types of cells: white blood cells (leukocytes), red blood cells (erythrocytes), and platelets (thrombocytes). These formed elements are made in the bone marrow from stem cells (Figure 6-1). The plasma contains numerous substances including electrolytes, clotting factors, immunologic factors, proteins, lipids, and hormones; almost every substance the cells use must be transported by the plasma. Plasma from which the clotting factors have been removed (by allowing the blood sample to clot, centrifuging, and then removing the residual fluid) is known as serum.

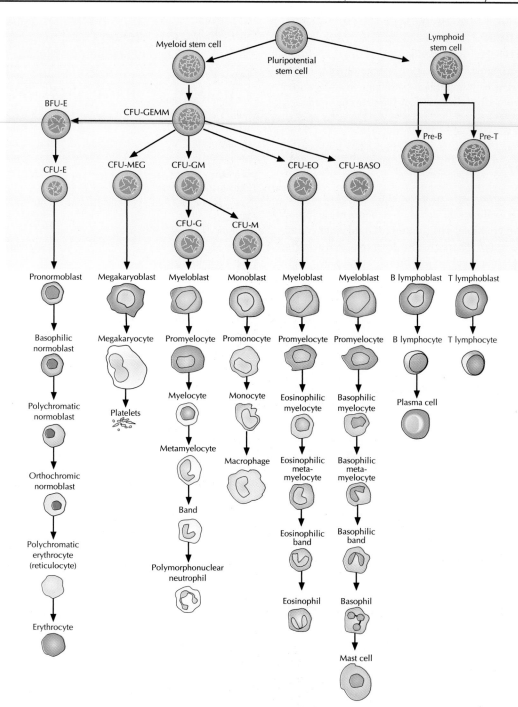

Figure 6-1 Maturation of blood cells: the hematopoietic "tree." The maturation of different blood cells is regulated by various cytokines. *CFU,* Colony-forming unit; *G-CSF,* granulocyte colony–stimulating factor; *GM-CSF,* granulocyte-macrophage colony–stimulating factor; *IL,* interleukin; *M-CSF,* macrophage colony–stimulating factor. (From Carr J, Rodak B: *Clinical hematology atlas,* ed 2, St Louis, 2005, WB Saunders.)

Evaluating laboratory test results requires an understanding of a few basic principles relating to statistical analysis. Normal values usually are expressed as ranges constructed to include 95% of the normal population (two standard deviations). Each laboratory must determine its own normal values using its particular equipment and methods. Therefore the normal values mentioned in this chapter are typical of many laboratories but not absolute national values.

It is possible to obtain a normal test result for a patient who has the disease that a laboratory test is designed to detect. Similarly, it is possible for healthy patients to have abnormal test results. Therefore laboratory tests must always be evaluated in light of other clinical findings and should be regarded as supplemental information. Correlation of clinical findings with laboratory test results leads to more appropriate diagnosis and treatment.

Most large clinical laboratories are divided into sections, with all of the tests relating to a particular area being performed in one section. This chapter is subdivided according to the common sections found in most laboratories: hematology, chemistry, microbiology, and urinalysis. Surgical pathology (histology) and cytology are also described, because they relate to the evaluation of pulmonary specimens.

HEMATOLOGY

Hematology laboratory tests are divided into two main categories. Tests that evaluate the cellular elements of the blood include the complete blood cell count (CBC), platelet count, and reticulocyte count. There are also tests that evaluate the proteins in the plasma involved in forming blood clots; these tests fall into the general category of coagulation and include the prothrombin time (PT) and its international normalized ratio (INR), activated partial thromboplastin time (APTT), and bleeding time. Platelets are also involved in the general function of coagulation.

COMPLETE BLOOD CELL COUNT

The CBC includes counting the number of white blood cells (WBCs) and identifying the different types of white cells present (the white cell differential). Next, the number of red blood cells (RBCs) is determined. Finally, the RBCs are evaluated for their size and hemoglobin (Hb) levels (red cell indices). The counting of RBCs and WBCs usually is done electronically by a machine, whereas the determination of the different types of WBCs is performed either visually (manually) by a technologist or, in larger laboratories, by automated cell counters. Typical normal values are listed in Table 6-1. The following discussion focuses on WBCs and the differential first and then shifts to focus on RBCs and the red cell indices.

White Blood Cells

The WBCs are circulating blood cells that contain a nucleus. Their primary role is fighting infection. Cell counting machines measure the total number of WBCs and the various types of WBCs present. WBCs normally represent several populations of cells (e.g., neutrophils, eosinophils) that function as part of the body's immune system in fighting various bacterial, viral, or parasitic infections. When abnormalities in the WBC count are present, the WBC differential is needed to determine which cell type is responsible for the abnormality.

WBC Differential

The WBC differential of the CBC was traditionally performed by examination of a blood smear by a technologist but now is most often performed by machine and reviewed by a technologist only when abnormal. For this examination to be performed manually, a drop of whole blood is smeared in a thin layer on a

Table 6-1	Normal Values for the Complete Blood Cell Count Tests	
Test	Normal Values
Red Blood Cell Count	
Men	$4.6\text{-}6.2 \times 10^6/mm^3$
Women	$4.2\text{-}5.4 \times 10^6/mm^3$
Hemoglobin	
Men	13.5-16.5 g/dL
Women	12.0-15.0 g/dL
Hematocrit	
Men	40%-54%
Women	38%-47%
Erythrocyte Index	
Mean cell volume	80-96 μm^3
Mean cell hemoglobin	27-31 pg
Mean cell hemoglobin concentration	32%-36%
White Blood Cell Count	4500-11,500/mm³
Differential of White Blood Cells	
Segmented neutrophils	40%-75%
Bands	0%-6%
Eosinophils	0%-6%
Basophils	0%-1%
Lymphocytes	20%-45%
Monocytes	2%-10%
Platelet Count	150,000-400,000/mm³

glass slide; stained, most commonly by a stain known as Wright's stain; and then examined under the microscope. One hundred WBCs are counted and classified according to cell type. WBCs normally seen in the peripheral blood are neutrophils (segmented and band forms), eosinophils, basophils, lymphocytes, and monocytes.

Neutrophils, eosinophils, and basophils are included in the general category of granulocytes. The differential count defines the percentage of the total WBCs made of each cell type. An increase or decrease in the number of a particular cell type may be either absolute or relative. For example, if the total WBC count is elevated and the neutrophils are increased, the lymphocytes may make up a smaller than usual percentage of the WBCs. However, the total absolute number of lymphocytes may be normal. This represents a relative decrease in lymphocytes associated with an absolute increase in neutrophils. To determine the absolute cell count, multiply the total WBC count by the differential count or by the percentage for the particular cell type of interest (Table 6-2).

Neutrophils are also known as *polymorphonuclear neutrophilic leukocytes* and *segmented neutrophilic granulocytes*. Neutrophils usually constitute 40% to 75% of the blood's WBCs. A band is a less mature neutrophil in which the nucleus has not yet segmented. Bands normally make up 0% to 6% of the WBCs but increase dramatically with severe infection. In various abnormal conditions, the more immature cells may be seen: the metamyelocyte, myelocyte, promyelocyte, and myeloblast. (For the normal sequence of granulocyte maturation occuring in the bone marrow, see Figure 6–1.) Neutrophils contain enzymes that destroy bacteria and other invaders. They also are capable

Table 6-2	Normal Absolute and Relative Values for Differential of WBCs	
Cell Type	Relative Value (%)	Absolute Value*
Neutrophils	40-75	1800-7500
Eosinophils	0-6	0-600
Basophils	0-1	0-100
Lymphocytes	20-45	900-4500
Monocytes	2-10	90-1000

*Based on a normal white blood cell range of 4500 to 10,000 and using the following equation:

Absolute value = Relative value × Total WBC.

BOX 6-1   Causes of Neutrophilia

Pathologic

Bacterial infections
Inflammatory responses
    Burn injuries
    Snake bites
    Parasitic infection

In Response to Medications

Corticosteroids
Lithium

Physiologic (Pseudoneutrophilia)

Physical or emotional stress

of phagocytosis (engulfment of bacteria and other foreign material). The interpretation of WBC count and differential is described later in this chapter.

SIMPLY STATED
White blood cells come in five different types, the most common of which is the neutrophil. It is the major line of defense against bacterial infections.

Neutrophils are produced in the bone marrow where they are stored in large numbers. Days later, they are released into the circulating blood where they spend a short time (approximately 6 to 12 hours) before passing into the tissues where they perform their primary function and die soon after. Normally, the life span of a neutrophil is approximately 10 days from the stage of myeloblast in the bone marrow to its death in the tissues. The neutrophil, under normal conditions, spends most of its mature life in the bone marrow pool waiting to be called into service to fight inflammation or infection. The neutrophil spends a shorter time in the bone marrow pool when significant infection is present.

Once neutrophils pass into the circulating blood, they are continuously and rapidly exchanged between two intravascular pools, the *circulating* and *marginated* pools. The circulating pool represents neutrophils that are freely circulating in the bloodstream. Neutrophils in this pool are counted in the CBC. The marginated pool represents a large number of neutrophils that are adhering to the walls of the blood vessels. The marginated neutrophils are not counted in the CBC. Neutrophils shift from one pool to the other based on physiologic conditions. For example, physical or emotional stress causes a sudden release of catecholamines that liberates a large number of the marginated neutrophils and results in what is called a pseudoneutrophilia. The actual number of neutrophils in the intravascular pool does not change with pseudoneutrophilia.

Pseudoneutropenia occurs when a large number of the neutrophils in the circulating pool shift to the marginated pool (Box 6-1). The actual number of neutrophils in the intravascular pool is not decreased with pseudoneutropenia.

Eosinophils are a type of granulocyte with large granules that stain bright red, whereas basophils have large granules that strongly take up the basic stain (dark blue to purple). The function of both cell types is not completely understood; however, they appear to have complementary interactions in allergic reactions. Eosinophils also help defend the body against parasitic infestations. Eosinophils normally constitute 0% to 6% of WBCs, whereas basophils are less plentiful at 0% to 1%.

Lymphocytes are particularly important in the body's defense against viral, tuberculosis (TB), and fungal infections. Two major types of lymphocytes exist: T cells involved in cell-mediated immunity and B cells involved in antibody production (see Figure 6-1). The types appear similar on a blood smear. Lymphocytes normally make up 20% to 45% of circulating WBCs, with most of the circulating peripheral lymphocytes being T cells.

The separation and counting of T cells and B cells can be done only with special studies. The studies identify the type of cell present by using monoclonal antibodies that react with the surface antigen unique to either the T or B cells. T lymphocytes also can be separated into subcategories known as *helper* and *suppressor cells*. The helper or inducer cells provide help in antibody production and other immune responses and are identified by a unique surface antigen known as *CD4*. They are sometimes called *T4 cells*. The suppressor cells play a role in suppressing or dampening immune responses. These cells have the unique antigen CD8, and are called *T8 cells*. CD4 counts provide important information about the severity and prognosis of patients with acquired immunodeficiency syndrome (AIDS). (See discussion of lymphocytopenia below.)

Monocytes are the largest WBC normally seen and constitute 2% to 10% of leukocytes in the peripheral blood. In tissue, the monocyte is known as a macrophage. The primary function of the monocyte is phagocytosis of organisms and other foreign material invading the body.

White Blood Cell Abnormalities

Leukocytosis is an abnormal increase in the WBC count. An abnormal decrease in the WBC count is known as leukopenia.

Abnormalities in the WBC count can be defined more specifically by referring to the exact cell type that is increased or decreased using similar terminology. For example, an increase in neutrophils is called neutrophilia or a **neutrophilic leukocytosis,** and a decrease is called neutropenia. Increases in the cell counts may be *primary* (a result of uncontrolled proliferation of cells in the bone marrow) or *secondary* (a result of stimulation of the bone marrow secondary to other diseases or disorders). Similarly, decreases in cell counts may be caused by either primary bone marrow failure or increased destruction and use of the cells peripherally. Bone marrow failure can occur as a side effect of various drugs and disorders (secondary) or as a result of unknown causes (primary or idiopathic).

Neutrophilia is a common response to inflammation and infection (see Box 6-1). Thus it is a common finding in patients with bacterial pneumonia. Certain drugs and chemicals (e.g., epinephrine, steroids) also cause neutrophilia. When the bone marrow is stimulated to release neutrophils at a rate faster than it can produce them, it releases them at increasingly more immature stages. Under these circumstances, increased numbers of the young cells, usually bands, appear in the peripheral blood. This is called a left shift. When the stimulus is severe, even younger cells may be seen. The degree of the left shift and the severity of the neutrophilia usually correlate with the severity of the infection.

SIMPLY STATED

Significant leukocytosis with a left shift (increase in bands) indicates the bone marrow is attempting to respond to infection.

Pseudoneutrophilia occurs when marginated neutrophils are shifted to the circulating pool and are counted in the CBC. This type of neutrophilia is typically transient, lasting only a matter of hours. It is most common in the patient experiencing sudden stress (e.g., in the child who is fearful of needles and who is undergoing an arterial blood gas draw). The neutrophilia in this case does not show a spike in the number of immature neutrophils as is often seen when the neutrophilia is the result of infection.

Eosinophilia or eosinophilic leukocytosis (increase in eosinophils) is often seen in allergic states and parasitic infestations. Patients with extrinsic types of asthma often have eosinophilia, but it can also be seen in certain skin (e.g., eczema) and gastrointestinal disorders. Basophilia (increase in basophils) is associated with many of the same disorders that cause eosinophilia and myeloproliferative disorders.

Lymphocytosis (increase in lymphocytes) typically is seen in viral infections, especially infectious mononucleosis. In addition, the lymphocytes in these disorders often are enlarged and have a characteristic appearance referred to as *atypical.* Lymphocytopenia (decrease in lymphocytes) is seen in trauma and acute infection. Lymphocytopenia is an important feature of human immunodeficiency virus (HIV) infection, the virus that causes AIDS. Furthermore, there is alteration of the ratio of T4-helper (CD4) to T8-suppressor (CD8) cells in patients with active disease or AIDS-related complex. Normally, the helper cells predominate, with the normal ratio being 2:1 to 3:1. This ratio is reduced in patients with AIDS, and the severity of the reduction is progressive, correlating with the progression of disease.

Monocytosis (increase in monocytes) is characteristic of chronic infections, including TB, syphilis, typhoid fever, and subacute bacterial endocarditis. Monocytosis is also seen in "preleukemia" and other malignancies (Table 6-3). Monocytosis in patients with TB is believed to indicate active disease. Monocytosis is also seen in inflammatory reactions to tissue destruction such as in surgical trauma and certain tumors.

Neutropenia may occur with decreased bone marrow production or with increased destruction of the cells with severe infection (Box 6-2). One of the most common causes of neutropenia is cancer therapy. Chemotherapy prevents effective cell reproduction, which is needed in rapidly growing cancer cells. However, hematopoietic cells in the bone marrow are among the most rapidly dividing normal cells in the human body and are particularly susceptible to chemotherapy. These cells eventually develop into both RBCs and WBCs. Thus chemotherapy causes the circulating WBCs to decrease. Usually, the tolerance of the bone marrow determines the maximal dosage of chemotherapy.

Viral infections may cause a neutropenia by causing some of the neutrophils in the circulating pool to shift to the marginated pool. Thus they are not counted in the CBC. This type of neutropenia is typically more transient.

SIMPLY STATED

Neutropenia is often a sign of a serious health problem and usually occurs with either decreased bone marrow production or increased destruction of neutrophils in the tissues.

Leukemias and Myeloproliferative Disorders

Leukemias and myeloproliferative disorders are primary malignancies (uncontrolled proliferations) involving bone marrow

---

BOX 6-2   Causes of Neutropenia

Decreased Neutrophil Production

Chemotherapy
Bone marrow disease
Cancers affecting the bone marrow

Increase in Neutrophil Destruction

Overwhelming bacterial infection
Certain bacterial infections
Some viral infections

Pseudoneutropenia

Viral infections
Hypothermia

Table 6-3	Types of Leukocytosis	
Cell Type	Causes of Increase	Appropriate Term
Neutrophil	Bacterial infection, inflammation	Neutrophilia
Eosinophil	Allergic reaction, parasitic infection	Eosinophilia
Lymphocyte	Viral infection	Lymphocytosis
Monocyte	Chronic infections, TB, malignancies	Monocytosis
Basophil	Myeloproliferative disorders	Basophilia

cells. Leukemia implies a proliferation of a specific type of WBC (usually either lymphocytic or granulocytic) and may be either acute or chronic. Myeloproliferative disorders encompass a spectrum of diseases resulting from an abnormality of the *stem cell* (the precursor of all bone marrow cells) and often are associated with a proliferation of more than one type of cell. Myeloproliferative disorders may have a variable blood picture as the disease progresses, and they sometimes terminate as an acute leukemia.

In acute leukemia, there is a tremendous proliferation of very immature cells known as blasts. These blasts quickly replace all other cells in the bone marrow and the peripheral blood and may cause a rapid death of the patient. WBC counts may be high, with a differential showing predominantly blasts. The RBCs and platelets usually are decreased. Acute lymphocytic leukemia usually occurs in young children, whereas acute granulocytic or myelogenous leukemia most often occurs in young adults. Pure monocytic leukemia is rare and usually occurs in adults. Acute granulocytic (myelogenous) leukemia often has features of both myeloid and monocytic leukemia, because both myeloid and monocytic cells arise from a common precursor cell (see Figure 6-1).

Chronic leukemias result from a slower proliferation of more mature cells, and even without treatment, the patient may live for years. Chronic lymphocytic leukemia is the most common type of leukemia and usually occurs in elderly people. The WBC count may be high, but the differential shows a preponderance of mature lymphocytes. Only late in the disease are other cells decreased. Chronic granulocytic leukemia (CGL) often occurs in middle-age adults. There is a high WBC count caused mainly by granulocytes in various stages of maturation. Platelets often are increased, and there is progressive anemia. CGL often terminates in acute leukemia, known as *blast crisis*, and is included among the myeloproliferative disorders.

Other myeloproliferative disorders include polycythemia vera, myelofibrosis with myeloid metaplasia, erythroleukemia, and essential thrombocythemia. Myelofibrosis begins with a proliferation of granulocytes and megakaryocytes (the cells that make platelets) in the marrow, but fibrous tissue eventually replaces the marrow cells. The patient may have high or low WBC counts depending on the stage of the disease. Erythroleukemia is a rare disorder, more like an acute leukemia

involving both WBC and RBC precursors. Essential thrombocythemia primarily involves megakaryocytes, with increased platelets in the peripheral blood.

Red Blood Cells

RBCs are produced in the bone marrow by maturation of nucleated cells known as normoblasts. Under normal circumstances, as the normoblasts mature, the nuclei become smaller and darker, and the cytoplasm acquires a red color as a result of the development of Hb. Before the red cell is released from the bone marrow to circulate in the peripheral blood, the nucleus is lost. RBCs have a life span of approximately 120 days.

Normal RBCs assume the shape of a biconcave disk to facilitate their primary function of carrying oxygen (Figure 6-2). Mature RBCs (erythrocytes) are made up largely of Hb, which imparts to blood its normal red color when carrying oxygen. The RBC count is reported in number of cells per cubic millimeter or per liter (see Table 6-1 for normal values). Without a normal RBC count, the ability of the blood to transport oxygen is reduced significantly. However, a normal RBC count does not guarantee a normal Hb level or oxygen-carrying capacity.

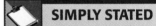

SIMPLY STATED

Red blood cells act as carriers of hemoglobin, which is needed to transport oxygen throughout the body.

Hematocrit (Packed Cell Volume)

Hematocrit is the ratio of red cell volume to that of whole blood. Hematocrit can be determined by centrifuging whole blood so that the blood cells settle and then by determining the percentage or fraction of the total blood volume occupied by the RBCs (Figure 6-3). It is calculated electronically in most laboratories.

Hemoglobin

Hb is the protein that carries oxygen to the tissues; it is the major component of RBCs. Hb is also important in maintaining acid-base balance by acting as a buffer and by carrying carbon dioxide (CO_2) from the tissues to the lungs. The Hb molecule consists of two portions: the heme group, of which iron is a vital constituent, and the protein, or globin chains. Each RBC contains between 200 and 300 million Hb molecules.

Red Blood Cell Indices

Three erythrocyte indices are measured or calculated. They indicate the cell size, Hb content, and Hb concentration and are known, respectively, as *mean cell volume* (MCV), *mean cell Hb* (MCH), and *mean cell Hb concentration* (MCHC). In addition to these three classic indices, the modern electronic counters used today provide an additional index known as *red cell distribution*

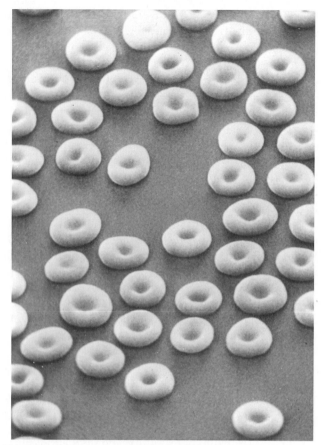

Figure 6-2 Normal red blood cells. (From Rodak B: *Hematology,* ed 2, St Louis, 2002, WB Saunders.)

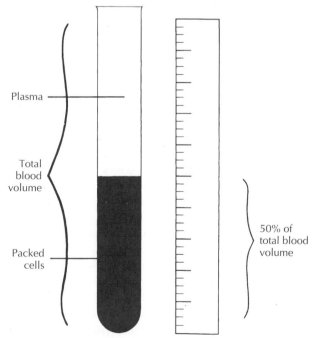

Figure 6-3 Determination of hematocrit from centrifuging blood sample. Packed cell volume is half total blood volume; therefore hematocrit is 50% in this example.

width (RDW). The RDW is a measure of the variation in red cell size, with higher numbers being seen when there is significant variation in cell size. The values are useful in the evaluation and classification of anemias (disorders with decreased RBCs). Interpretation of the RBC indices is described in the following section.

Red Blood Cell Abnormalities

Anemia is a decrease in the RBC count, Hb, and hematocrit. When anemia is present and the MCV, MCH, and MCHC are abnormally low, the anemia is known as a microcytic, **hypochromic** anemia (i.e., the red cells are smaller than normal and contain a lower than normal amount of Hb). When anemia is present and the indices are normal, the anemia is said to be **normocytic, normochromic** anemia. If anemia is present and the RBCs are larger than normal, (increased MCV), the anemia is known as macrocytic. Anemias may be caused by blood loss, increased destruction of RBCs, or decreased production of RBCs. Severe anemia reduces the oxygen-carrying capacity of the blood and may result in dyspnea and tissue hypoxia if the circulatory system is unable to compensate with increased circulation.

The most common type of anemia worldwide is the result of iron deficiency. In the United States, this typically occurs when there is chronic blood loss and the iron contained in the RBCs leaves the body instead of being recycled. In developing countries, iron deficiency often is the result of a dietary deficiency. With low iron levels, the bone marrow produces small RBCs with a small amount of Hb, and the RBC indices are microcytic and hypochromic. An increased RDW is especially typical of iron-deficiency anemia (as opposed to thalassemia) and is reported to be a very sensitive (but not very specific) indicator of that disease.

Anemia is also commonly the result of chronic disease and aging that cause the bone marrow to produce an inadequate amount of RBCs. The resulting anemia is often normochromic and normocytic in such cases.

Macrocytic, hypochromic anemia is most often caused by either folate or vitamin B_{12} deficiency. Low folate or B_{12} levels result in bone marrow production of very large RBCs with low concentration of Hb.

Hb may be converted to an inactive form through oxidation, denaturation, or other chemical reaction. The most common forms of inactive Hb are carboxyhemoglobin (HbCO) methemoglobin (metHb), and sulfhemoglobin. HbCO is formed when carbon monoxide binds to Hb. Carbon monoxide has an affinity for Hb that is 210 times that of oxygen, causing a functional anemia. It also shifts the oxyhemoglobin curve to the left, so oxygen is not released to the tissues. Cigarette smoking can result in HbCO levels of 5% to 7%. Exposure to heavy amounts of smog and smoke can also increase the HbCO levels.

MetHb is produced when the ferrous iron in Hb is oxidized to the ferric state, usually secondary to chemical ingestion. Such Hb cannot combine with oxygen. An increase in the normally very low levels of metHb results in a functional anemia with a decreased oxygen-carrying capacity.

Plasma

Total blood volume

Packed cells

50% of total blood volume

Sulfhemoglobin is another abnormal form of Hb formed by a combination of oxidative and denatured damage. The denatured Hb can precipitate in the red cell and be detected as Heinz bodies (detected by special stain performed on a peripheral smear).

Polycythemia is an increase in the RBC count, Hb, and hematocrit and may be primary, secondary, or spurious. Primary polycythemia is uncommon and is caused by an uncontrolled proliferation of hematopoietic cells within the bone marrow and is known as polycythemia vera (one of the myeloproliferative disorders).

Secondary polycythemia is more common and is seen in patients who have chronic stimulation of the bone marrow to produce more RBCs secondary to some other disorder. This is most commonly seen in patients with chronic hypoxemia as a result of pulmonary disorders such as chronic obstructive pulmonary disease, obstructive sleep apnea, or pulmonary fibrosis. It is also seen in people who live at high altitude and in some patients with chronic heart disease. Each of these disorders causes chronic hypoxemia that stimulates renal production of erythropoietin, which in turn causes the bone marrow to produce and release more RBCs to help compensate for the oxygen deficit.

Heavy smokers are also prone to develop secondary polycythemia. The carbon monoxide associated with cigarette smoke binds tightly with the Hb and reduces oxygen transport. This results in a functional anemia to which the bone marrow responds by increasing red cell production.

Both primary and secondary polycythemia involve a real or absolute increase in the total RBC mass. Sometimes relative polycythemia occurs because of a decrease in the plasma volume. This is seen in patients who are dehydrated for various reasons and is a condition known as spurious polycythemia. It often occurs in personality type "A" men who smoke, have hypertension, and are obese. Spurious or relative polycythemia does not represent a true increase in the number of circulating RBCs.

Although polycythemia is helpful in increasing the oxygen-carrying capabilities of the blood, it may be detrimental to the heart and circulation. Polycythemia increases the viscosity of the blood, causing an increased workload for the heart and increasing risk of clots.

SIMPLY STATED

Patients with an elevated red blood cell count and history of smoking may have secondary polycythemia caused by chronic hypoxemic lung disease.

Nucleated RBCs are referred to as reticulocytes. They represent immature RBCs and normally do not circulate in the peripheral blood. Their presence may indicate extreme stress being placed on the marrow to produce RBCs, thereby releasing cells at a younger stage. Nucleated RBCs also occur in the peripheral blood in some of the myeloproliferative disorders because of uncontrolled or malignant proliferation of bone mar-

row cells. Nucleated RBCs are also seen commonly in premature infants.

Reticulocyte Count

Reticulocytes are slightly larger and have an increased amount of ribonucleic acid (RNA) in the cytoplasm. Dyes, such as methylene blue or cresyl blue, stain the RNA material to identify these cells. A reticulocyte count is performed by obtaining the percentage of reticulocytes among the RBCs. The reticulocyte count is reported as a percentage of the RBC count. The average reticulocyte count is approximately 1.5%.

The reticulocyte count helps evaluate anemia. If the absolute reticulocyte count is high, it indicates that the marrow is producing increased numbers of RBCs, and the anemia probably is a result of peripheral blood loss or destruction. However, if the reticulocyte count is low, then the anemia probably is the result of decreased bone marrow production.

Sedimentation Rate

If blood is placed in a vertical tube, the RBCs tend to fall to the bottom. A measurement of the speed at which they fall (distance per unit of time) is known as the *sedimentation rate*. The most commonly used methods are known as the *Wintrobe* and *Westergren,* which differ mainly in the use of different tube sizes. The sedimentation rate is a nonspecific test that is increased in a multitude of disorders, especially in inflammatory diseases. This is largely because of an increase in various plasma proteins. The proteins surround the RBCs and decrease the normal repelling effect between the cells caused by external negative charges on the cell surface. Anemia also increases the sedimentation rate as a result of the lower concentration of erythrocytes.

Platelet Count

Platelets are the smallest formed elements in the blood. They have an important function in blood coagulation through formation of blood clots. Platelets usually are counted electronically, with normal platelet counts in the range of 140,000 to 440,000/mm^3. Like the other blood cells, platelets may be decreased as a result of either increased destruction or decreased bone marrow production.

When the platelet count is decreased significantly (less than 20,000/mm^3), patients are more likely to have bleeding problems, especially with trauma such as surgery or arterial punctures. The bleeding that results from decreased platelets usually manifests as small skin hemorrhages (petechiae and ecchymoses) or oozing from mucosal surfaces. However, when the platelet count becomes extremely low (less than 5000/mm^3), the patient is at risk for serious spontaneous internal hemorrhage (e.g., brain hemorrhage). The disorders most likely to result in decreased platelets are side effects of drugs such as heparin, bone marrow diseases, and idiopathic thrombocytopenia purpura, an autoimmune disorder in which antibodies are produced that destroy the person's own platelets.

An increase in platelets may be simply a nonspecific reaction to stress placed on the body or may be caused by bone marrow disease (usually one of the myeloproliferative disorders). If the platelet count is extremely high, there may be an increased tendency to form blood clots (thromboses).

Coagulation Studies

The evaluation of hemostasis (ability to prevent hemorrhage, form a blood clot) can be complex, and many tests are available. However, four basic screening tests are generally used: the bleeding time, platelet count (already discussed), APTT, and PT/INR (INR allows comparison of PT between laboratories).

The bleeding time measures the ability of the small skin vessels to constrict and evaluates the function of platelets. It is performed by making standardized puncture wounds in the skin and timing how long it takes for the bleeding to stop. Various methods are used, but normal values usually are up to 6 minutes. The bleeding time and platelet count measure the first two steps in the body's defense for preventing hemorrhage: vascular integrity (ability of vessels to constrict) and formation of a platelet plug (requiring adequate numbers of platelets and their normal function). The bleeding time is a somewhat crude test that can be difficult to reproduce and interpret. It is now used infrequently.

Clotting depends on an interaction between platelets and multiple proteins in the plasma. These proteins are labeled with Roman numerals, factors I to XIII. There is an intrinsic pathway activated by damaged vascular endothelium and an extrinsic pathway activated whenever tissue gains access to circulating blood. The APTT assesses predominantly the intrinsic system by measuring the length of time required for plasma to form a fibrin clot once the intrinsic pathway is activated. Normal values range from 24 to 32 seconds. The PT/INR is performed similarly, using activation of the extrinsic system as a beginning point. Normal values generally range from 12 to 15 seconds or INR less than 1.2. These tests are abnormal if one or more of the involved clotting factors are decreased significantly. Usually, further studies are required to delineate the specific factors implicated. Factor deficiencies may be either congenital (e.g., hemophilia, which is a congenital absence of factor VIII) or acquired (e.g., liver disease with a decrease in factors II, VII, IX, and X). The APTT is used for monitoring heparin therapy, whereas PT/INR is used for monitoring warfarin (Coumadin) therapy.

SIMPLY STATED

The respiratory therapist who is about to perform an arterial puncture should review the patient's chart for clinical laboratory results that document the patient's blood-clotting ability. The platelet count, PT, and APTT are important test results to review in such cases.

CHEMISTRY

Electrolyte Concentrations

Electrolytes are the free ions in body fluids. The normal functioning of all cells depends on proper concentrations of these elements, so the body must maintain close control of these substances. Monitoring of electrolyte concentrations of the plasma is extremely important in patients whose body fluids are being endogenously or exogenously manipulated (e.g., intravenous therapy, renal disease, diarrhea).

The four electrolyte concentrations commonly measured are sodium (Na^+), potassium (K^+), chloride (Cl^-), and total CO_2. Ninety percent of the total CO_2 is made up of HCO_3^-. Normal values for the electrolyte concentrations and other common chemistry tests are listed in Table 6-4.

Sodium is the major cation (an ion having a positive charge) of extracellular fluid. The kidney, influenced by hormones secreted by the adrenal gland (aldosterone) and hypothalamus (antidiuretic hormone [ADH]), regulates the concentration of sodium in the serum very closely. Normal values are 137 to 147 mEq/L.

Sodium is mainly responsible for the osmotic pressure of the extracellular fluid. Increased serum Na^+ (hypernatremia) is seen when the body loses water without salt (e.g., profuse sweating, diarrhea, renal diseases, prolonged hyperpnea), if there is lack of sufficient water intake, or when there are hormonal abnormalities such as diabetes insipidus. Patients with hypernatremia typically complain of excessive thirst and a dry, sticky mouth.

Decreased sodium concentration (hyponatremia) is caused by either excess free water intake/retention or excess sodium loss. Theoretically, healthy people could become hyponatremic by drinking too much water, but water retention is most commonly associated with syndrome of inappropriate secretion of ADH (SIADH). SIADH can be associated with many illnesses, but most commonly they are neurologic, pulmonary, or malignant. These people may become severely hyponatremic despite normal total body salt stores. Hyponatremia caused by sodium

Table 6-4	Normal Values in Chemistry
Test	**Normal Value**
Sodium	137-147 mEq/L
Potassium	3.5-4.8 mEq/L
Chloride	98-105 mEq/L
Carbon dioxide	25-33 mEq/L
Blood urea nitrogen	7-20 mg/dL
Creatinine	0.7-1.3 mg/dL
Total protein	6.3-7.9 g/dL
Albumin	3.5-5.0 g/dL
Cholesterol	150-220 mg/dL
Glucose	70-105 mg/dL

loss is most often associated with use of diuretics but can also be caused by diarrhea, severe sweating, or Addison's disease (in which destruction of the adrenal glands impairs production of aldosterone, which promotes sodium reabsorption in the kidneys). Patients with severe hyponatremia (less than 115 mEq/L) may show confusion, abnormal sensorium, muscle twitching, and sometimes, even seizures.

Potassium is the major cation occurring within cells. Extracellular concentration is normally low, with the usual serum concentration in the range of 3.5 to 4.8 mEq/L. Hypokalemia, or decreased serum K^+, occurs when there is increased loss of potassium, decreased intake, or when K^+ ions shift from extracellular to intracellular water space.

Increased loss of potassium occurs when K^+-containing fluid is lost (e.g., with vomiting, nasogastric suctioning, and diarrhea) with some kidney diseases and with the use of some diuretics. Decreased intake of potassium is often a dietary problem (Box 6-3). Total body potassium depletion is present in such cases.

Metabolic alkalosis causes a shift of K^+ ions from the extracellular to the intracellular space in exchange for hydrogen ions in an attempt to maintain a more neutral extracellular pH (see Chapter 7). Hypokalemia is not associated with true depletion of potassium in such cases, and in fact the level of total body potassium may be elevated.

Hypokalemia is important to detect, because it can be associated with cardiac, skeletal muscle, and gastrointestinal dysfunction. Weaning from mechanical ventilation may be difficult if hypokalemia is present. Patients with hypokalemia often have nausea, vomiting, abdominal distention, muscle cramps, lethargy, confusion, and arrhythmias.

Hyperkalemia, an elevated K^+ concentration, can occur with increased intake, with decreased output, or when K^+ ions shift from intracellular to extracellular water space. Actual body levels of potassium are not elevated in the latter example. Pseudohyperkalemia may occur when K^+ ions leak out of RBCs or WBCs with hemolysis of the blood sample or significant leukocytosis (Box 6-4).

Hyperkalemia caused by increased intake is often the result of dietary supplementation. Decreased output of potassium is seen in kidney disease (where potassium is no longer discarded) and with the use of certain diuretics. Metabolic acidosis causes an increased level of H^+ in the extracellular fluid. In an effort to buffer this acidosis, intracellular K^+ ions exchange with extracellular H^+. This helps maintain a more neutral extracellular pH but leads to increased extracellular levels of K^+. Correcting the acidosis usually corrects the hyperkalemia.

Hyperkalemia is important to identify, because it can lead to significant cardiac arrhythmias. The electrocardiographic changes associated with hyperkalemia include tall peaked T waves, loss of P waves, wide QRS complexes, and sine waves.

Chloride is the chief anion (an ion having a negative charge) in the extracellular fluid. Normal concentration is 98 to 105 mEq/L. Decreased serum Cl^- (hypochloremia) occurs when there is prolonged vomiting (loss of HCl), chronic respiratory acidosis (which causes elevated HCO_3^- levels), Addisonian crisis, and certain kidney diseases. Increased serum Cl^- (hyperchloremia) is seen with prolonged diarrhea (loss of HCO_3^-), certain kidney diseases, and sometimes, hyperparathyroidism.

HCO_3^- is the second most plentiful anion in the serum and is part of the carbonic acid buffer system that plays a major role in acid-base balance within the body. An increase in serum HCO_3^- (total CO_2) occurs with metabolic alkalosis or as compensation for respiratory acidosis, whereas a decrease occurs with metabolic acidosis or as compensation for respiratory alkalosis.

Other electrolyte concentrations that are often measured include calcium (Ca^{2+}), phosphorus (PO_4^-), and magnesium (Mg^{2+}). The Ca^{2+} level is controlled by parathyroid hormone (PTH). Patients with increased PTH have increased calcium (hypercalcemia). Because bone contains a large amount of calcium, certain bone diseases or metastatic cancer to bone may result in hypercalcemia. Hypocalcemia occurs in vitamin D deficiency (rickets) and in various other hormonal aberrations. PO_4^-

BOX 6-3 Causes of Hypokalemia

Decreased Potassium Intake

Low-potassium diet
Alcoholism

Increased Loss of Potassium

Gastrointestinal loss
Renal disease
Diuretics

Extracellular to Intracellular Shift of Potassium

Alkalosis
Increased plasma insulin
Diuretic use

BOX 6-4 Causes of Hyperkalemia

Increased Potassium Intake

High-potassium diet
Oral potassium supplement
Transfusion of old blood

Decreased Potassium Excretion

Renal failure
Hypoaldosteronism

Intracellular to Extracellular Shift of Potassium

Acidosis
Crush injuries
Tissue hypoxia

Pseudohyperkalemia

Hemolysis
Leukocytosis

metabolism is closely linked to that of Ca^{2+}. Abnormalities of Mg^{2+} concentrations are common in the intensive care unit. Hypomagnesemia and hypocalcemia have been associated with respiratory muscle weakness, which makes weaning from the ventilator difficult.

SIMPLY STATED

Healthy electrolyte concentrations are essential for proper physiologic function of the body. The respiratory therapist is interested in the patient's electrolyte panel, because the results may be responsible for irregular heart rhythms or weak muscles of breathing.

Anion Gap

Cations and anions are present in the body in exactly equal amounts. However, not all anions are measured, and these missing anions are called the *anion gap*. Calculating the anion gap helps define the cause of a metabolic acidosis. High anion gap metabolic acidosis is usually caused by lactic acid (as in sepsis), ketoacids (diabetic ketoacidosis), sulfates (renal failure), and poisons (e.g., aspirin overdose). The normal anion gap is 8 to 16 mEq/L. The anion gap is calculated by subtracting the total of the total CO_2 (HCO_3^-) and chloride from the sodium: $Na^+ - (HCO_3^- + Cl^-)$.

Electrolyte Concentration of Sweat

The electrolyte concentration of the patient's sweat may be analyzed to assist in the diagnosis of cystic fibrosis. The sweat glands of patients with cystic fibrosis have a diminished ability to reabsorb Na^+ and Cl^-. As a result, a high concentration of Na^+ and Cl^- (more than 60 mEq/L) is present in the sweat.

Blood Urea Nitrogen and Creatinine

The most common screening tests in assessing renal function are the blood urea nitrogen (BUN) and creatinine (Cr). Urea is a waste product synthesized in the liver from ammonia, which is the end product of protein (amino acid) breakdown. Therefore urea is constantly being formed and is excreted by the kidneys. Normally, the serum level is maintained in the range of 7 to 20 mg/dL. Many kidney diseases result in decreased filtration and thereby increased retention of urea, leading to an elevated BUN level. Other conditions such as shock and heart failure, in which there is decreased renal perfusion and thereby decreased filtration, also cause an elevated urea level. Diet (protein intake), the state of hydration, and various hormones that affect protein metabolism also influence BUN.

Creatinine is another waste product constantly formed within muscle tissue and filtered out by the kidneys. The serum concentration of creatinine (0.7 to 1.3 mg/dL) is usually constant and reflects the balance between production of creatinine (proportional to the body's muscle mass) and its fil-

tration by the renal glomerulus. The creatinine level rises in kidney diseases in which 50% or more of the renal nephrons are destroyed. Creatinine is also elevated in muscle diseases. Neither the BUN nor the creatinine level is sensitive to early renal disease.

When the BUN and creatinine are elevated as a result of renal failure, metabolic acidosis may be present, because the renal function for acid-base balance is impaired (see Chapter 7). Metabolic acidosis stimulates the respiratory system to increase ventilation and reduce the arterial CO_2 tension ($PaCO_2$) as a compensatory mechanism. Therefore patients with renal failure often have increased respiratory rates and may appear to be short of breath. If the patient with renal failure also has respiratory disease, the onset of metabolic acidosis can add intolerable stress and result in respiratory failure.

Enzymes

Enzymes are found in all of the body's cells. These substances are responsible for most chemical reactions. When there is destruction of tissue cells, enzymes are released into the blood. Many enzymes occur widely throughout the body, but certain enzymes are associated with specific organs. Therefore elevation of a particular enzyme sometimes may be a clue to a diseased organ. Most enzymes are measured by assessing their activity in catalyzing chemical reactions. The results usually are expressed in units that reflect the rate of the reaction. Because many enzymes occur in multiple organs, *isoenzymes* (slightly different chemical forms of the same enzyme) that may be more specific for a particular site or disease have been identified for some enzymes. Most isoenzymes are identified by electrophoresis.

New terminology has recently been adopted for naming many of the enzymes. Most enzymes are commonly referred to by a series of capital letters that are abbreviations for the chemical names. In the following discussion, commonly tested enzymes are discussed. When applicable, both the old and new names are given, with the newer name listed first. In some cases, the older name is still used and understood more widely.

Aspartate aminotransferase (AST), formerly known as *serum glutamic-oxaloacetic transaminase* (SGOT), occurs in many tissues throughout the body. The highest concentrations are in heart and liver tissue, and the highest serum concentrations are seen in diseases involving those two types of tissue. The highest levels occur with acute hepatitis. Elevated AST levels occur on the second day following myocardial infarction. Although elevated AST levels occur in many diseases, the enzyme is used primarily in assessing liver disease and possible myocardial infarction.

Alanine aminotransferase (ALT), formerly known as *serum glutamic-pyruvic transaminase* (SGPT), is a liver enzyme that is elevated in hepatic disease similarly to AST. However, ALT is elevated minimally or not at all in myocardial infarction or other heart diseases, unless there is secondary severe liver congestion with destruction of some liver tissue. Therefore ALT is helpful in determining whether an AST elevation is the result of disease in the liver or in some other organ, especially the heart, because AST occurs in many organs, whereas ALT occurs in high concentrations mainly in the liver.

Alkaline phosphatase (ALP) is useful in evaluating liver disease and bone disease. Liver ALP is most elevated by extrahepatic obstruction of the bile duct. ALP also occurs in bone, placenta, spleen, kidney, and intestine, and isoenzyme evaluation can often distinguish the source. Elevated ALP from bone suggests increased new bone formation.

Acid phosphatase (ACP) occurs in high concentrations in the prostate gland. Lesser levels of a chemically different ACP occur in RBCs and platelets. Significantly elevated levels of ACP are seen almost exclusively in prostatic carcinoma. Prostate-specific antigen (PSA) is another substance specific for prostate origin that can be identified and quantified in the blood. It is being used increasingly to screen for prostate cancer.

Lactate dehydrogenase (LDH) is an enzyme that occurs in high concentrations in heart, liver, skeletal muscle, brain, kidney, and RBCs. Therefore elevated LDH levels occur in a variety of diseases. It is possible, using electrophoresis, to separate LDH into five isoenzymes. However, there is considerable overlap in the patterns from different organs. LDH elevations occur in patients with megaloblastic anemia, widespread carcinoma, and severe shock. Moderate elevations occur with many diseases including acute myocardial infarction, muscular diseases, leukemia, hemolytic anemia, infectious mononucleosis, liver disease, renal disease, and hypothyroidism.

Creatine kinase (CK), also known as *creatine phosphokinase* (CPK), is primarily contained in skeletal muscle, myocardium, and brain tissue. Isoenzyme patterns characteristic for the source of the enzyme can be determined by electrophoresis. CK values are most commonly elevated in myocardial infarction and various skeletal muscle diseases, because CK originating in the brain does not cross the blood-brain barrier and therefore does not appear in serum. In acute myocardial infarction, the CK elevation can be detected within the first 8 hours after infarction and persists for several days. The CK enzyme is made up of two subunits, which may be either identical or different. The CK isoenzyme that occurs in the brain is made up of two similar subunits and is called *CK-BB*. The isoenzyme that occurs in skeletal muscle is also made up of two identical subunits and is called *CK-MM*. The CK present in the myocardium has one component similar to that found in brain and one similar to that found in muscle and is known as *CK-MB*. The CK normally present in the blood is all from the skeletal muscle or CK-MM type. The presence of a CK-MB band on electrophoresis is characteristic of myocardial infarction.

Recently, two additional analytes have been found to be useful in the diagnosis of acute myocardial infarction. Myoglobin is present in cardiac, skeletal, and smooth muscle. Whenever there is significant muscle damage, myoglobin is elevated and can be measured. Myoglobin is released from damaged myocardium within 2 hours. This test is not very specific, because the myoglobin may be from noncardiac sources, but the test may be useful in early screening for myocardial infarction.

Troponin is a complex of three proteins that help regulate the contractile process in muscle tissue. It can be identified immunochemically and is a commonly used test for the diagnosis of myocardial infarction. It is both sensitive and specific for myocardial infarction. The elevation of troponin occurs more rapidly and to a higher level than that of CK-MB in myocardial infarction.

Amylase and lipase are enzymes used primarily in assessing pancreatitis. Amylase in the blood and urine is predominantly from the pancreas and salivary glands. Elevated serum levels occur within a few hours after the onset of pancreatitis. There is also significantly increased excretion of amylase in the urine, and determination of urinary amylase is more sensitive than serum amylase. Serum amylase may also be elevated in pancreatic carcinoma (usually late in the disease); diabetic ketoacidosis; and diseases of the gallbladder, stomach, and small intestine. Serum lipase levels are also elevated in acute pancreatitis, but those elevated levels appear later, rising more slowly. Their presence may help confirm the diagnosis of pancreatitis.

> **SIMPLY STATED**
> Disease affecting a certain organ causes a release of excessive amounts of the enzymes stored in that organ into the circulating blood. Evaluation of the enzyme levels in the blood may give the attending physician insight into what body system is causing the patient's symptoms.

Glucose

Glucose is the major substance produced from the digestion of dietary carbohydrates. Glucose is absorbed into the blood and carried throughout the body, where it is metabolized for energy production. Insulin is produced by the pancreas and is necessary for cells to be able to use glucose circulating in the blood. Patients with diabetes have decreased insulin levels (type 1) or a slow release of insulin in response to high blood sugar (type 2), both of which result in a decreased use of blood glucose and increased levels of glucose, a condition known as hyperglycemia. Steroids blunt the insulin response to glucose and can cause hyperglycemia. Hyperglycemia associated with acidosis caused by accumulation of ketoacids is called *ketoacidosis* and is a medical emergency.

Hypoglycemia (low blood glucose) causes sweating, shaking, weakness, headaches, lethargy, and coma in severe cases and is most often caused by insulin injection or oral diabetes medications. Blood sugar levels of patients requiring insulin or oral agents are checked regularly to prevent either high or low levels.

Fasting plasma glucose level (blood drawn after an overnight fast) normally is in the range of 70 to 105 mg/dL. After ingestion of carbohydrates, the glucose level normally rises in the first 60 to 90 minutes and then returns to the normal fasting level within 2 hours. Blood glucose levels present a snapshot of blood sugar control. In contrast, the glycosylated Hb (HbA$_{1c}$) shows the average level of control over a 4- to 6-week period.

The classical test for diagnosing diabetes mellitus (infrequently used) is the 3-hour glucose tolerance test. In this test, a standard glucose load is given and plasma levels of glucose are determined at 30 minutes, 1 hour, 2 hours, and 3 hours after the glucose is ingested. The normal pattern and two typical diabetic patterns are shown in Figure 6-4.

Significant hypoglycemia is thought to be present if the plasma glucose falls below 45 mg/dL, especially if clinical symptoms are present concurrently. Hypoglycemia occurring after a meal is known as *reactive hypoglycemia*. An extended glucose tolerance test, carried on for 5 hours with plasma levels tested every 30 minutes, is sometimes useful in evaluating patients with possible hypoglycemia.

Proteins

The plasma contains a variety of proteins that are essential not only for normal metabolic functioning but also as the body's chief building substance. The enzymes and coagulation factors discussed earlier are proteins. Immunoglobulins and hormones are also proteins. Albumin is a protein that functions as a transport and storage substance for many hormones, drugs, and electrolytes. Albumin is also important in maintaining the oncotic pressure of blood. It is maintenance of the oncotic pressure that keeps the water component of plasma within vascular spaces. Albumin also plays a primary role in lipid metabolism. The two most commonly ordered tests assessing protein are the total protein and albumin.

Total protein analysis is a rough screening test used to detect gross abnormalities in overall protein synthesis. A decreased total protein is seen in severe liver disease (many proteins are produced by the liver), in nephrotic syndrome (albumin lost through kidneys), and in severe malnutrition. The total protein level has many limitations and does not reveal which of the many serum proteins may be missing or abnormal. Serum protein electrophoresis (SPEP) separates the proteins using an electrical current and may show low protein subgroup levels in some diseases or very high protein subgroup levels in other diseases. A single protein subgroup overproduction is called a

monoclonal gammopathy and results in a spike in SPEP. Plasma cells (immunoglobulin-secreting cells) normally secrete a variety of different immunoglobulins, which form a broad band with electrophoresis. However, in multiple myeloma (malignant proliferation of plasma cells), each plasma cell secretes the same immunoglobulin, resulting in a high concentration of one immunoglobulin and forming a narrow band or spike pattern on electrophoresis.

Albumin is secreted by liver cells and makes up a large percentage of the total serum protein. Decreased albumin levels (hypoalbuminemia) are seen in various forms of protein malnutrition and in severe liver disease. Significant hypoalbuminemia leads to loss of fluid from vascular spaces and causes edema throughout the body (e.g., pulmonary edema).

Lipids

Lipids include a variety of complex substances used throughout the body as fuel storage and as building blocks for substances as divergent as hormones and cell walls. Two lipids most commonly measured in routine screening tests are triglycerides and cholesterol. Triglycerides are the main storage lipid in humans, and fatty tissue is made up chiefly of these substances. Cholesterol is produced in the body and is contained in eggs and other dietary animal proteins. Most of the attention focused on the serum levels of various lipids results from the correlation of increased lipid levels with a greater incidence of atherosclerotic disease. Lipids should usually be assessed in fasting patients, because dietary intake affects the serum level, especially of triglycerides. The cholesterol level normally increases with age, with average values for adults being approximately 160 mg/dL at 20 years, 200 mg/dL at 40 years, and 215 mg/dL at 60 years. There is probably a difference between the average value and the ideal value. The ideal value (or the value that is desirable for optimal health) is considerably lower than the average level. The triglyceride level in adults after 35 years of age averages approximately 140 to 150 mg/dL.

More recently, the emphasis has been on assessment of the lipoproteins. They can be separated into three categories by ultracentrifugation or electrophoresis: very low-density lipoproteins (VLDL), low-density lipoproteins (LDL), and high-density lipoproteins (HDL). The amount of cholesterol occurring within these separate categories gives more useful information than a simple total cholesterol level, especially when the cholesterol level is elevated. Increased LDL and VLDL levels result in higher cardiac risk, whereas increased HDL levels result in lower cardiac risk. Therefore if the elevated cholesterol is primarily HDL, there may not be an increased risk of cardiovascular disease.

Tumor Markers

Because of the prevalence of cancer in our society, there has been tremendous interest in identifying substances in the blood that can be detected easily and that indicate the presence of cancer in the body. Several hormones, enzymes, proteins, and oncofetal

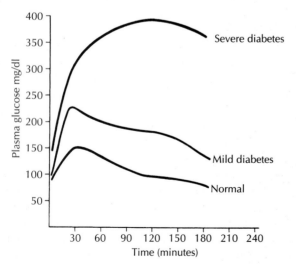

Figure 6-4 Typical blood glucose response to glucose tolerance test in healthy persons and in those with diabetes.

antigens have been found to be associated with various types of tumors. Unfortunately, none of these is specific enough to be used for general screening.

An oncofetal antigen is an antigen that is normally expressed by the cell only in fetal life. However, with the aberrations that take place in the development of cancer, the cancer cells may again express these fetal antigens. The most commonly tested oncofetal antigen is carcinoembryonic antigen (CEA). CEA is present in abundance in fetal life in the developing intestine and lung. Adult patients with gastrointestinal cancer may have elevated levels of CEA in their blood. However, CEA is not specific for any type of malignancy and can be elevated in many benign conditions, including hypothyroidism and inflammation, and in cigarette smokers. CEA is most useful in following patients with known colorectal cancer. An elevated CEA level occurring more than 6 weeks after resection of a colon cancer suggests recurrent disease. Alpha-fetoprotein is an oncofetal antigen used in the assessment of liver cell carcinoma (hepatoma) and testicular tumors. CA 125 is an oncofetal antigen sometimes associated with ovarian cancer. CA 15-3 is a breast cancer–associated antigen. PSA is associated with prostatic carcinoma, but its use as a general screening tool is controversial. Lung cancers often secrete ectopic hormones, but these are not useful for either diagnosis of tumor or evaluation of response to treatment.

Drug Monitoring

Some drugs have a narrow therapeutic window and are not helpful at slightly low blood levels and are harmful at slightly elevated blood levels. There is often individual variation in the rate of absorption, metabolism, and excretion of drugs, so there can be large variances in the blood levels of different patients taking the same drugs on the same dosage schedule. Drugs that are often tested include cardiac drugs (digoxin), anticonvulsants (phenytoin), bronchodilators (theophylline), and various antibiotics (gentamicin). Most of these substances are identified and quantified by chromatography (gas chromatography or high-performance liquid chromatography) or immunoassay. Immunoassay involves identifying a substance by an antibody specific for that substance and is used for quantitative analysis of many hormones. Radioimmunoassay is done by labeling an antibody with a radioactive material. The radioactive-antibody complex is then allowed to attach to the antibody's target. All unattached complexes are then washed away, and the amount of radioactivity left is directly proportional to the amount of initial target substance. A similar method known as *enzyme immunoassay* uses an enzyme to mark and quantify the substance being identified by the antibody. This method has the advantage of avoiding radioactive materials.

Theophylline has been used in treating bronchospasm. It usually is measured by chromatographic methods, and the normal therapeutic range is 5 to 15 mg/mL. The blood level should be measured after there has been time for the drug to reach the plateau or maximal level and just before the next dose. Side effects such as nausea, vomiting, loss of appetite, and abdominal pain usually occur when the level is greater than 15 mg/mL, but some patients begin to experience these side effects at levels

Table 6-5	Factors Affecting Theophylline Clearance	
Increased Clearance	**Decreased Clearance**
Young children	Liver disease
Smokers	Congestive heart failure
Use of rifampin	Cimetidine
Use of barbiturates	Erythromycin
	Propranolol
	Severe exacerbation of chronic obstructive pulmonary disease

above 10 mg/mL. More severe symptoms such as cardiac arrhythmias, seizures, and cardiac and respiratory arrest occur in the range of 20 to 60 mg/mL. Serum theophylline levels are determined by the dosage given and the ability of the liver to metabolize the drug. Factors that affect theophylline metabolism by the liver are listed in Table 6-5.

MICROBIOLOGY

Medical microbiology, sometimes called *bacteriology,* involves the isolation and identification of microorganisms from body tissues and fluids. The microbiology laboratory receives a variety of specimens. The handling of each specimen is determined by the site of origin of the sample and the specific organisms suspected by the patient's physician. The best information is gained from the specimen when the laboratory is provided with the proper clinical background. Many body sites are normally sterile, and the isolation of any organisms from these sites may be significant. Blood, pleural fluid, ascitic fluid, and tissue samples do not contain microorganisms in a state of health and, if collected in a sterile manner, will not grow any type of organisms when cultured. Other samples such as stool, urine, and sputum regularly contain or are routinely contaminated with large numbers of microorganisms known as *normal flora.* With these specimens, the number and type of organisms isolated must be evaluated to determine whether they represent pathogenic organisms or normal flora. Although bacteria are the most common organisms isolated, laboratories also may identify fungi, protozoa, helminths (worms), rickettsiae, and viruses. These different types of organisms require different procedures for proper identification. Viruses often are identified only in referral laboratories.

The initial step involved in the examination of most specimens is the immediate preparation and examination of a direct smear of the specimen. The smear may be stained by various methods, depending on the type of organism suspected. A Gram stain is used most commonly for bacterial organisms. Bacteria present may be classified as gram positive or gram negative, depending on their staining reactions. In addition, the shape of the organism can be determined, allowing further classification of bacteria as cocci (spherical) or rods (elongated).

Another bacterial stain often used for sputum and other specimens is the acid-fast stain (e.g., the Ziehl-Neelsen stain), which allows presumptive identification of the tuberculous and related organisms. The information derived from the Gram stain in combination with clinical information often allows the physician to suspect the proper diagnosis. Treatment may then be initiated based on the preliminary diagnosis.

A definitive identification of the microorganisms is made by culturing them on various types of media promoting the growth of organisms. Culture results usually are available anywhere from 24 hours to 6 weeks later. Most bacteria grow in 24 to 48 hours, but some bacteria (e.g., the tubercle bacillus) and fungi may require 6 weeks to grow. After an organism grows, additional time may be required for tests to permit full identification. Many laboratories are using procedures that allow more rapid culture and identification of organisms. Polymerase chain reaction (PCR) is especially useful in rapidly identifying tuberculosis bacilli and distinguishing them from other related organisms that stain positive for acid-fast bacilli (e.g., leprosy, other nontuberculous mycobacteria).

Along with the culture, a sensitivity test is often performed. The bacteria are cultured in the presence of various antibiotics, thereby permitting the determination of whether an organism is sensitive to a particular antibiotic (i.e., whether the antibiotic in appropriate concentration prevents the growth of organisms). This kind of information is of clinical importance in selecting the proper antibiotic therapy.

> ### SIMPLY STATED
> Sputum Gram stain and culture can be useful in determining the organism responsible for the patient's lung infection and the antibiotic most useful in treating the infection. Prior use of antibiotics by the patient can influence results of the Gram stain and culture.

Examination of Pulmonary Secretions

Sputum Collection

The goal of sputum collection is to obtain fresh, uncontaminated secretions from the tracheobronchial tree. This goal is achieved more readily when the alert patient is carefully instructed on the importance of the procedure and how the sample must come from the "windpipe." The patient should be instructed to rinse his/her mouth out with water and even brush his/her teeth before expectorating a specimen. This helps reduce contamination of the specimen with oral microbes. Most patients with respiratory infections have little problem producing an effective cough to produce secretions for analysis. However, occasionally the respiratory secretions may be minimal and sputum induction is necessary to obtain an acceptable sample. Sputum induction is accomplished by providing a slightly irritating mist (e.g., hypertonic saline) for the patient to breathe. The mist increases flow of bronchial secretions (bronchorrhea) and stimulates a cough. The resulting mild

bronchorrhea and cough usually results in an adequate mucous specimen.

If a culture is imperative and the patient has an unproductive cough and sputum induction is unsuccessful, sputum may be sampled with a bronchoscopic lavage. Transtracheal aspiration is not commonly performed but may be helpful in obtaining a specimen from the patient in a coma with a respiratory infection.

Sputum Examination

At the bedside, the sample should be grossly examined to determine its origin. Legitimate sputum samples from the tracheobronchial tree typically are more viscous and purulent than saliva. The specimen obviously containing mostly saliva should be discarded. Macroscopic examination of the sputum also identifies such characteristics as color, presence of blood, general viscosity, and odor. Yellow or green sputum often occurs when secretions are retained and may be seen in response to an allergic or infectious process. Stringy, mucoid sputum may be a sign of bronchial asthma. Certain respiratory infections may produce "classic" sputum samples. For example, respiratory infections with *Pseudomonas aeruginosa* typically produce thick, green sputum with a unique musty odor. Bronchiectasis typically produces a three-layered sputum sample that is foul smelling. Thick secretions may indicate the patient's need for hydration and aerosol treatment.

The first step in the microscopic examination of sputum is to determine whether the sputum is a reliable sample. Greater than 25 epithelial cells/high-power field (HPF) suggest oral contamination to the point that the specimen is useless. Oral secretions contain 100 times as many organisms per milliliter than do infected lower airway secretions, and as a result, a small amount of spit contaminates a large amount of sputum. A large number of leukocytes/HPF suggests that the sputum is from the lower airway and is a representative sample. The second step in microscopic examination of sputum is to determine whether the sputum is more likely related to allergy (asthma) or infection. If the leukocytes are predominantly eosinophils, then the cause of the sputum production is most likely allergy. If they are predominantly polymorphonuclear leukocytes (PMNs), the cause of the sputum production is more likely infection.

After a sputum specimen is determined to be reliable and most likely related to infection, it can be evaluated for the number of organisms, type of organisms (rods versus cocci) stain characteristics (gram positive versus gram negative), location (extracellular or within PMN), and whether the organism has a capsule. This information allows a presumptive organism diagnosis. The definitive organism diagnosis is provided later by culture characteristics.

Streptococcus pneumoniae is the most common cause of bacterial pneumonia. On Gram stain, these organisms have a distinctive appearance as encapsulated, lancet-shaped, gram-positive diplococci. Other agents that have a characteristic appearance on Gram stain and may cause pneumonia include *Staphylococcus aureus*, *Klebsiella pneumoniae*, and *Haemophilus influenzae*. *S. aureus* appears on Gram stain as intensely staining gram-positive cocci in clusters resembling clusters of concord grapes. *K. pneumoniae* appears on Gram stain as short, fat, encapsulated gram-negative rods. *H. influenzae* stains as very short gram-negative rods often described as coccobacilli.

Results of the sputum Gram stain and culture may be influenced by use of antibiotics by the patient. If the antibiotic is effective against the pathogen causing the infection, the Gram stain and culture do not demonstrate the offending organism but may show the presence of other bacteria not related to the infection. The patient usually appears to be clinically improving in such cases. If the antibiotic is not effective against the pathogen responsible for the patient's lung infection, the Gram stain and culture will not be influenced and will often demonstrate the offending pathogen. The specific infecting organism is never identified as often as 50% of the time, even in research studies using all available means for organism identification.

Bronchoalveolar Lavage

Bronchoalveolar lavage (BAL) is performed during bronchoscopy by injecting a large volume of sterile fluid into the patient's lung. This fluid mixes with the respiratory secretions within the airways and alveoli and is subsequently withdrawn for analysis in the laboratory. BAL has two main functions: (1) to evaluate the need for therapy in patients with interstitial lung disease (diseases that often cause pulmonary fibrosis) by analysis of the cells obtained in the lavage solution and (2) to collect organisms for evaluation to determine the cause of pneumonia. BAL is contraindicated in patients with severely reduced pulmonary function, reduced blood oxygen levels (hypoxemia), severe cardiovascular disease, or serious electrolyte disturbances.

Once the lavage solution is recovered from the patient, the sample is sent to the laboratory for microscopic analysis. Lavage solution obtained from healthy nonsmokers is 91% to 95% macrophages, 6% to 8% lymphocytes, and 1% granulocytes (neutrophils and eosinophils). The cellular composition of this fluid shows characteristic alterations in diseases such as pulmonary sarcoidosis or hypersensitivity pneumonitis.

Pleural Fluid Examination

Normal pleural fluid is clear and pale yellow. Usually, only small amounts of fluid (less than 20 mL) are present in the pleura. The fluid represents a balance between chest wall parietal pleural fluid production and lung (visceral) pleura absorption. Blood vessels feeding the parietal pleura come from the left side of the heart, which generates systolic pressures generally greater than 90 mm Hg, and these high pressures force 1 L of fluid/day out of the blood vessels into the pleural space. The visceral pleural is fed by blood vessels coming from the right side of the heart, which usually produces pressures of approximately 20 mm Hg, which allows the visceral pleura to rapidly absorb fluid. This normally leaves only a small amount of fluid in the pleura. This balance can be upset either by increased pleural vascular pressure so that the visceral pleura absorbs less

of the fluid produced by the parietal pleura or by any process that irritates the pleura, making it leak fluid more easily. Increased pleural pressures do no affect protein flow through the pleural vessel wall, so the resulting pleural effusion contains little protein. Irritation of the pleura makes the vascular walls more porous so that protein molecules escape from the vessels and the pleural fluid contains much more protein. This helps a physician determine the cause of a pleural effusion.

The most common cause of a low-protein effusion is congestive heart failure (because of increased visceral pleural vascular pressure). Common causes of high protein pleural effusions include cancer of the pleura, infection within the pleural space, pulmonary embolism with infarct of lung adjacent to the pleura, and chest wall trauma with bleeding into the pleural space. Opaque or turbid fluid is characteristic of infections or tumor metastasis in which there are large numbers of WBCs in the fluid. Cell counts may be performed on the fluid. The type of WBC present may be useful in determining the cause of the pleural effusion. The thoracic duct runs through the chest in its course from the abdomen to the subclavian vein. Disruption of the thoracic duct causes its fatty fluid to spill into the pleural space and results in a milky white pleural effusion. Hemorrhagic or bloody fluid most often results from malignancy but can occur with trauma, infections, pulmonary infarct, and various other disorders.

A low-protein pleural effusion is called a *transudate* and a high-protein pleural fluid is called an *exudate*. The classic dividing line between transudates and exudates is 3 g/dL. A protein level of less than 3 g/dL is characteristic of a transudate, whereas a level of greater than 3 g/dL is characteristic of an exudate. Culture of the fluid for microbiologic organisms and cytologic examination for malignant cells are other tests commonly performed on pleural fluid and are described elsewhere in this chapter.

URINALYSIS

Urinalysis is one of the most commonly performed tests in the clinical laboratory. It is helpful as a crude screening test for kidney disease and reflects the metabolic status of the patient. The examination of urine may also indicate the likelihood of urinary tract infection before culture results. The following features usually are noted in routine urinalysis: appearance, specific gravity, pH, protein, glucose, ketones, blood, bilirubin, urobilinogen, nitrite, and microscopic examination of urinary sediment.

The appearance simply denotes the color and whether the urine appears clear or cloudy. The specific gravity indicates the concentration of the urine. More concentrated urine is normally seen in dehydration, whereas more dilute urine is present with high fluid intake and in some kidney diseases in which the kidney is unable to concentrate urine normally. The pH of the urine reflects the acid-base status of the patient. The presence of protein in the urine, known as *proteinuria,* usually is indicative of renal disease. Glucose in the urine (glucosuria) appears most commonly in diabetes but sometimes is caused by renal disease.

Ketones occur with starvation and in diabetes mellitus. *Hematuria,* or blood in the urine, may originate in either the kidney or the bladder. Bilirubin occurs in the urine in the conjugated form and is seen when there is an obstruction to the outflow of bile from the liver. Urobilinogen appears in some liver diseases and hemolytic states. Nitrates may indicate that significant numbers of bacteria are present. Testing for most of the substances just mentioned is done by reagent strips that identify the presence of the substance but only roughly approximate the quantity. The degree of quantification is typically on a scale of 1^+ to 4^+.

The urine may then be centrifuged and the sediment examined microscopically. The presence and numbers of any blood cells (RBCs, WBCs), casts, and crystals are noted. Large numbers of WBCs suggest the presence of infection. Various types of casts may occur and may indicate renal disease.

HISTOLOGY AND CYTOLOGY

A small biopsy of lung tissue may be obtained either through a bronchoscope (bronchoscopic biopsy), or a large biopsy of lung tissue may be obtained at the time of thoracotomy or thoracoscopy (open lung biopsy). The tissue samples obtained are sent to the histology or surgical pathology laboratory. The tissue is processed over a period of time so that it can be cut very thin, placed on a slide, and stained so that the cells are visible when examined by a pathologist with a microscope. This can yield valuable information about infectious processes, chronic lung diseases, and benign and malignant tumors. An acid-fast (Ziehl-Neelsen) stain can be done on tissue to identify mycobacteria (TB or TB-like organisms). Gomori's methenamine silver (GMS) and periodic acid–Schiff (PAS) stains may be done to identify fungal organisms. GMS stains also identify *Pneumocystis* organisms (a parasite that causes pneumonia in AIDS patients and other immunocompromised patients). Tissue Gram stains also may be done.

Surgical removal of lung cancer requires close cooperation between the surgeon and surgical pathologist. The surgical pathologist must provide immediate reports to the surgeon regarding the presence of cancer in the resected lung, the type of cancer present, whether the surgical margins are clear, and whether there are metastases in local or regional lymph nodes. Because there is not time during surgery to process specimens in the usual way, the tissue is frozen so that it can be immediately sectioned and reviewed under the microscope. The frozen sections are thicker and more difficult to evaluate than standard sections but are usually adequate for surgical guidance. Final histology reports are issued after surgery, when standard stains have been completed.

Tumors of the lung may be either benign or malignant. A classification of malignant lung tumors is shown in Box 6-5. Benign lung tumors are less common than malignant tumors, with hamartoma (a benign proliferation of elements normally occurring in the lung) being seen most often. The first four tumors listed in Box 6-5 (squamous cell carcinoma, small cell carcinoma, adenocarcinoma, and large cell carcinoma) represent

---

> **BOX 6-5   Modified World Health Organization Histologic Typing of Malignant Tumors***
>
> 1. Squamous cell carcinoma
> 2. Small cell carcinoma
>   Oat cell carcinoma
>   Intermediate cell type
> 3. Adenocarcinoma
>   Bronchioloalveolar carcinoma
> 4. Large cell carcinoma
>   Giant cell carcinoma
> 5. Carcinoid tumor
> 6. Bronchial gland carcinoma
>   Adenoid cystic carcinoma
>   Mucoepidermoid carcinoma

*Indented categories represent common subtypes.

---

most primary lung tumors and often are called *bronchogenic carcinoma.* These tumors are usually related to smoking (with the possible exception of adenocarcinoma) and are highly malignant. Secondary or metastatic tumors to the lung are also common. Carcinoid tumors and bronchial gland carcinomas are much less common and usually are less aggressive. They are sometimes called *low-grade carcinomas* (they were previously called *bronchial adenomas*). Tumors consisting of a mixture of cell types and other rare types of tumors may occur.

Cytology is the study of fluids, secretions, or other body samples that contain cellular material but not actual fragments of intact tissue. The cells are smeared on a glass slide (Papanicolaou smear), stained, and examined by a pathologist. Often, the presence of malignancy and even the type of malignancy can be determined in this manner. Pulmonary samples that can be examined cytologically include sputum, bronchial washings, bronchial brushings, pleural fluid, and fine-needle aspiration (FNA) of lung tissue or lung masses. In FNA, a small needle (usually 22 gauge) is inserted into a mass, and some of the cellular material is aspirated into the needle and then expressed and smeared onto a slide. The slide is then stained and examined, often yielding accurate information about the nature of the mass. FNA of lung masses is performed under radiologic guidance. For many years, this procedure has been widely used to evaluate lung masses and has proved to be a safe, simple, and effective way to diagnose malignant tumors and other processes without requiring major surgery.

SKIN TESTING

Over the years, skin testing has proved to be a useful means of diagnosing disease entities that involve the entire body, as well as the lungs. The diseases include TB, coccidioidomycosis, histoplasmosis, sarcoidosis, blastomycosis, and allergic disorders.

The procedure requires a small amount of the protein essence of the organism or substance involved in causing the disease to be injected under the skin. The accuracy of the test depends on the material being placed precisely in the subcutaneous layer of the skin.

Patients may develop a condition, called anergy, in which the immune system does not react to skin testing. Unfortunately, some of the diseases diagnosed by skin testing render the patient anergic. Conditions that may cause a person to become anergic include aging, cancer, starvation or debilitation, and sarcoidosis. To evaluate the patient's reactions, the physician uses a marker skin test of a protein that would cause a reaction in most people, along with the material being used to test for a specific disease. If the marker test does not produce a reaction, the absence of a reaction to the skin test for disease is meaningless. The examiner should not accept this negative skin reaction as evidence that the patient does not have the suspected disease. The markers used are extracts of material that almost everyone has encountered and has developed immunity against but that do not cause disease. Some of the more common markers are protein derivatives of mumps, the fungus *Trichophyton*, and streptokinase-streptodornase.

The most commonly used skin test is the test for TB. The test requires that 0.1 mL of a material called *purified protein derivative (PPD)* be injected into the subcutaneous layer of skin. The test is evaluated 48 to 72 hours later. An intradermal or subdermal nodule present at 24 to 72 hours after injection of PPD shows a cellular reaction and demonstrates that the patient has been infected by a TB-like organism. TB causes the strongest reaction, but other nontuberculous mycobacteria can also produce weakly positive reactions. Because of this cross-reactivity, there is an elaborate set of criteria for interpreting a positive PPD. A normal healthy person without risk for exposure to TB is classified as PPD skin test positive only if the skin reaction produced a 15-mm diameter welt, whereas an HIV-positive or other immunocompromised patient is classified as positive with a 5-mm diameter skin nodule. It is important to note that the size of the nodule is the only diagnostic measurement; redness or erythema around the site of injection is not taken into account during test interpretation.

Older patients may have had a positive skin test in the past that eventually reverts to negative. A two-step skin test with the second test performed 3 weeks after the first test often shows a true positive when the first test produced a negative result. Multiple skin tests performed on a patient who has never been exposed to TB do not cause a positive result. Bacille Calmette-Guérin (BCG) vaccinations, which are common in countries with a high prevalence of TB, cause a positive PPD skin test until approximately 10 years after the vaccination; therefore positive PPD skin tests more than 10 years after BCG vaccination usually mean true TB infection.

SIMPLY STATED

The purified protein derivative skin test for tuberculosis must be interpreted in light of the patient's medical history.

CASE STUDY 1

B.K. is a 22-year-old white woman who was brought to the emergency department by her mother with chief complaints of cough, fever, and chills for the past 3 days. B.K. has a history of Down syndrome and lives at home with her parents. Initial examination reveals tachycardia, tachypnea, fever, and normal blood pressure. Chest auscultation identifies bronchial breath sounds and inspiratory and expiratory coarse crackles over the right lower lobe. The admitting physician orders a sputum Gram stain and culture, CBC, and chest film. The initial laboratory results are as follows:

CBC	Results	Normals
WBC ($\times 10^9$/L)	19.5	4.5-11.5
RBC ($\times 10^{12}$/L)	4.2	4.2-5.4
Hb (g/dL)	10.6	11.5-15.5
Hematocrit	34.9%	38%-47%
MCV	77.0	80.0-96.0
MCHC	30.4%	32%-36%

White blood cell differential		
Segmented neutrophils	82%	40%-75%
Lymphocytes	8%	20%-45%
Monocytes	4%	0%-6%
Eosinophils	1%	0%-6%
Basophils	0%	0%-1%
Bands	6%	0%-6%

Gram stain: 2+ gram-positive cocci; 1+ pus cells with many epithelial cells

Interpretation: Leukocytosis is present and appears to be the result of an increase in the neutrophils consistent with a bacterial infection (probably pneumonia). The slight increase in immature neutrophils (bands) represents a left shift indicating stress on the bone marrow to release more neutrophils to fight the infection. The relative decrease in the percentage of lymphocytes is caused by the absolute increase in the number of neutrophils and is not an abnormality.

The RBC count is within normal limits; however, the decreases in Hb, hematocrit, MCV, and MCHC are consistent with a microcytic, hypochromic anemia. Further investigation is needed to identify the cause, but iron-deficiency anemia is a likely reason.

The Gram stain of the sputum sample indicates that it was heavily contaminated with secretions from the mouth, because many epithelial cells were present. The sample should be discarded and another sputum sample obtained.

CASE STUDY 2

C.J. is a 65-year-old woman who was brought to the emergency department by her husband. C.J. is complaining of severe shortness of breath, weakness, and cough. C.J. has a long history of chronic obstructive pulmonary disease (COPD) and a 90-pack/year smoking history. She currently admits to smoking 1 pack/day. In the emergency department, C.J. appears acutely and chronically ill and is found to be using her accessory muscles to breathe. She is cyanotic and has decreased breath sounds bilaterally. C.J. is started on oxygen by nasal cannula, and the attending physician orders a CBC, electrolyte determination, and other tests. The results are as follows:

Test	Results	Normals
WBC ($\times 10^9$/L)	19.9	4.5-11.5
RBC ($\times 10^{12}$/L)	5.1	4.2-5.4
Hb (g/dL)	15.8	11.5-15.5
Hematocrit	48.5%	38%-47%
MCV	98.2	80.0-96.0
MCHC	31.6%	32%-36%

White blood cell differential

Segmented neutrophils	76%	40%-75%
Lymphocytes	12%	20%-45%
Monocytes	5%	0%-6%
Eosinophils	4%	0%-6%
Basophils	2%	0%-1%
Bands	1%	0%-6%

Electrolytes (mEq/L)

Na^+	137	137-147
K^+	4.8	3.5-4.8
Cl^-	87	98-105
Total CO_2	41	23-33

Interpretation: The increase in WBCs suggests leukocytosis and appears to be the result of an increase in the number of circulating neutrophils. This may be in response to a bacterial infection or acute stress. The RBC count, Hb, and hematocrit are slightly increased, consistent with polycythemia. These RBC differential findings are consistent with secondary polycythemia typical for patients with a chronic lung disease in which the arterial blood oxygen levels are persistently low.

The electrolyte values reveal a decreased serum Cl^- and an increased serum CO_2. This probably is related to the patient's long-term history of COPD. Some patients with COPD chronically retain CO_2 because of poor pulmonary function. To compensate for the elevated CO_2, the kidneys retain increased levels of serum HCO_3^- in an effort to maintain a near-normal serum pH. The resulting metabolic buildup of serum HCO_3^- is reflected as an increased total CO_2 in the venous blood sample. The increase in serum CO_2 (HCO_3^-) causes the kidneys to excrete more than the usual amount of Cl^- in an effort to maintain electrical neutrality. As a result, serum Cl^- levels typically are reduced in patients with chronically elevated serum CO_2.

CASE STUDY 3

B.T. is a 27-year-old man with a CD4 count of 120. He is concerned about his chronic cough and sputum production. The sputum is been negative for white cells and bacteria. A PPD skin test was placed on his right forearm 2 days ago, and there is now a 3-cm reddened area and a 5-mm nodule at the skin test site. Initial laboratory data results are as follows:

CBC	Results	Normals
WBC ($\times 10^9$/L)	5.0	4.5-11.5
Segmented neutrophils	70%	40%-75%
Lymphocytes	20%	20%-45%
Bands	5%	0%-6%
Monocytes	1%	2%-10%
Eosinophils	4%	0%-6%
Basophils	0%	0%-1%

Hb (g/dL)	14	13.5-16.5
Hematocrit	42%	40%-50%

Normal red cell indices

Sedimentation rate	40 (elevated)

Interpretation: The low CD4 count suggests moderate immunocompromise most likely caused by HIV. The elevated sedimentation rate suggests inflammation, which could be caused by TB or other infection. The large area of redness around the skin test site is not significant. The 5-mm nodule in this immunocompromised patient indicates TB infection. We anticipate that sputum cultures will be positive in 6 weeks. A PCR test for TB bacilli in the patient's sputum is likely to be positive. This patient's normal CBC is expected despite his chronic infection, because TB does not usually cause an elevated WBC count.

CASE STUDY 4

T.W. is a 20-year-old man who was brought to the emergency department by ambulance following a motor vehicle accident. T.W. was driving in a local canyon when a deer ran out in front of his car and caused him to lose control. The vehicle left the road and rolled over in the canyon. He complains of a stiff neck and left leg pain. Although T.W. was very upset and scared, he is conscious and able to move all extremities. Vital signs are normal except for a heart rate of 110/min. His initial CBC reveals the following:

Test	Results	Normals
WBC ($\times 10^9$/L)	14.9	4.5-11.5
RBC ($\times 10^{12}$/L)	5.1	4.2-5.4
Hb (g/dL)	15.0	11.5-15.5
Hematocrit	45.5%	38%-47%
MCV	95.2	80.0-96.0
MCHC	33.6%	32%-36%

White blood cell differential

Segmented neutrophils	76%	40%-75%
Lymphocytes	12%	20%-45%
Monocytes	5%	0%-6%
Eosinophils	4%	0%-6%
Basophils	2%	0%-1%
Bands	1%	0%-6%

Interpretation: The RBC count and indices are all normal. The elevated WBC count suggests possible infection; however, the lack of fever and minimal presence of bands on the white cell differential suggests otherwise. This is most likely a case of pseudoneutrophilia, where marginated neutrophils are released into circulation as a result of sudden stress (the accident). This type of neutrophilia is usually transient and resolves spontaneously in a matter of hours.

REVIEW QUESTIONS

1. Which of the following is *not* a component of the formed elements of the blood?
   a. RBCs
   b. Lipids
   c. WBCs
   d. Platelets

2. T F Blood serum is plasma from which the clotting factors have been removed by liquid chromatography.

3. T F In the presence of a significantly reduced RBC count, a normal oxygen-carrying capacity of the blood can be maintained.

4. Which of the following statements is (are) true regarding Hb?
   a. It functions in oxygen transport.
   b. It is the main component of RBCs.
   c. It functions in CO_2 transport.
   d. All of the above.

5. What is normal range for WBCs?
   a. 1000-3000/mm^3
   b. 3000-5000/mm^3
   c. 4500-10,000/mm^3
   d. 600-14,000/mm^3

6. Which of the following white cell types normally represents the largest percent in the differential?
   a. Neutrophils
   b. Eosinophils
   c. Basophils
   d. Lymphocytes

7. T F A tissue monocyte is called a *macrophage*.

8. Which of the following is the most common cause of anemia?
   a. Drug-induced RBC lysis
   b. Acute blood loss
   c. Iron deficiency
   d. None of the above

9. Which of the following is *not* true regarding polycythemia?
   a. It can be caused by chronic hypoxemia.
   b. It is defined as an increase in RBC, Hb, and hematocrit.
   c. It increases the oxygen-carrying capacity of the blood.
   d. It decreases the workload on the heart.

10. A left-shifted white cell differential is evidenced by which of the following findings?
    a. An increase in the number of eosinophils
    b. A decrease in the number of segmented neutrophils
    c. An increase in the number of bands (immature neutrophils)
    d. A decrease in the number of lymphocytes

11. Which of the following is a common finding in patients with bacterial pneumonia?
    a. Neutrophilia
    b. Leukopenia
    c. Lymphocytopenia
    d. Eosinophilia

12. Which of the following is a common finding in a patient with an allergic reaction?
    a. Neutropenia
    b. Leukopenia
    c. Eosinophilia
    d. Monocytosis

13. Viral infections typically produce which of the following abnormalities?
    a. Lymphocytosis
    b. Eosinophilia
    c. Basophilia
    d. Monocytosis

14. T F AIDS increases the ratio of T-helper to T-suppressor cells.

15. T F Leukemia is defined as an uncontrolled increase in the number of WBCs.

16. T F The sedimentation rate is a nonspecific test used to determine the general presence of disease.

17. Which of the following tests is used to assess the patient's blood-clotting ability?
    a. RBC count
    b. Hemoglobin
    c. Hematocrit
    d. Prothrombin time

18. Which of the following electrolytes closely affects muscle function?
    a. Sodium
    b. Potassium
    c. Chloride
    d. Phosphorus

19. Which of the following electrolytes is mainly responsible for extracellular water balance?
    a. Calcium
    b. Sodium
    c. Magnesium
    d. Potassium

20. What is the normal range for the anion gap?
    a. 2-5 mEq/L
    b. 6-10 mEq/L
    c. 8-16 mEq/L
    d. 22-29 mEq/L

21. Anion gap is useful in assessing which of the following situations?
    a. Cause of metabolic alkalosis
    b. Cause of metabolic acidosis
    c. Cause of respiratory acidosis
    d. Cause of respiratory alkalosis

22. An increase in the sweat electrolyte concentration is typical of which of the following diseases?
    a. Cystic fibrosis
    b. Patent ductus arteriosus
    c. Bronchiectasis
    d. Epiglottitis

23. Which of the following tests is (are) a measure of kidney function?
    a. BUN
    b. Creatine kinase
    c. Creatinine
    d. a and c

24. Which of the following enzymes is elevated in a patient who has had a myocardial infarction?
    a. AST
    b. LDH
    c. CPK
    d. All of the above

25. Which of the following is the therapeutic level for theophylline?
    a. 2-5 mg/mL
    b. 5-15 mg/mL
    c. 10-20 mg/mL
    d. 20-30 mg/mL

26. Which of the following decreases the clearance of theophylline?
    a. Cigarette smoking
    b. Congestive heart failure
    c. Youthful age
    d. All of the above

27. Which of the following bacteriologic tests is used to determine the effectiveness of antibiotics on a particular organism?
    a. Gram stain
    b. Culture
    c. Sensitivity
    d. Acid-fast stain

28. T F Bacteria that usually are present in a healthy person are called *normal flora*.

29. A Ziehl-Neelsen stain is used to identify which of the following organisms?
    a. *Staphylococcus aureus*
    b. *Pseudomonas aeruginosa*
    c. *Streptococcus pneumoniae*
    d. *Mycobacterium tuberculosis*

30. Which of the following items are evaluated during a macroscopic (gross) sputum examination?
    a. Color
    b. Consistency

c. Volume
d. All of the above

31. T   F   A sputum sample with many epithelial cells present is considered a reliable sample.

32. Which of the following is the most common cause of bacterial pneumonia?
   a. *Streptococcus pneumoniae*
   b. *Pseudomonas aeruginosa*
   c. *Haemophilus influenzae*
   d. *Klebsiella pneumoniae*

33. Which of the following findings is consistent with pleural infection?
   a. Bloody pleural fluid
   b. Low pleural fluid protein levels
   c. Opaque or turbid pleural fluid
   d. All of the above

34. T   F   Pleural fluid with a high protein content is called a *transudate*.

35. Which of the following tests performed during urinalysis could be helpful in diagnosing diabetes mellitus?
   a. Glucose
   b. pH
   c. Ketones
   d. All of the above

36. Proteinuria usually is indicative of which of the following?
   a. COPD
   b. Kidney disease
   c. Cardiovascular disease
   d. Spinal meningitis

37. T   F   Adenocarcinoma is responsible for producing primary lung carcinoma.

38. T   F   Cytologic studies are used to examine tissue samples by freezing and sectioning.

39. Which of the following may cause a patient to have a negative reaction to a skin test?
   a. He/she does not have the disease.
   b. He/she is anergic.
   c. The disease has progressed to a point beyond treatment.
   d. a and b

40. Which of the following is true regarding a PPD?
   a. It is positive with coccidioidomycosis infection.
   b. It is positive if the patient has previously had a BCG vaccination.
   c. It is negative if the induration produced is 12 mm in diameter.
   d. None of the above.

BIBLIOGRAPHY

Donahoe M, Rogers RM: Laboratory evaluation of the patient with chronic obstructive pulmonary disease. In Cherniack NS: *Chronic obstructive pulmonary disease,* Philadelphia, 1991, WB Saunders.

Henry J: *Clinical diagnosis and management by laboratory methods,* ed 19, Philadelphia, 1996, WB Saunders.

Kaplan JA, Pesce AJ, Kaxmierczak SC, editors: *Clinical chemistry,* ed 4, St Louis, 2003, Mosby.

McClatchey KD, editor: *Clinical laboratory medicine,* Baltimore, 1994, Williams & Wilkins.

Stiene-Martin EA, Lotspeich-Steininger CA, Koepke JA: *Clinical hematology,* ed 2, Philadelphia, 1998, Lippincott.

Wintrobe MM: *Clinical hematology,* ed 9, Philadelphia, 1993, Lea & Febiger.

7

Robert L. Wilkins

Interpretation of Blood Gases

LEARNING OBJECTIVES

Upon completion of this chapter, the reader should be able to accomplish the following:

1. Recognize why arterial blood rather than venous blood is useful in determining respiratory status.
2. Identify the importance of reviewing the laboratory data that reflect clotting ability before performing an arterial puncture.
3. Identify the common sites for arterial puncture.
4. Identify the test used to determine collateral circulation of the radial artery, how to perform this procedure, and how to interpret its results.
5. Recognize how the following factors generally affect blood gas analysis:
   a. Air bubbles in the syringe
   b. Failing to put the sample on ice
6. Identify the normal duration of arterial puncture site compression.
7. Identify the normal values for the following blood gas parameters at sea level and in room air:
   a. pH
   b. PaO_2
   c. $PaCO_2$
   d. HCO_3^-
   e. SaO_2
   f. $P(A - a)O_2$
   g. CaO_2
   h. Base excess
   i. $P\bar{v}O_2$
8. Recognize the clinical value of measuring the following indices of oxygenation:
   a. PaO_2
   b. $P(A - a)O_2$
   c. SaO_2
   d. CaO_2
   e. $P\bar{v}O_2$
   f. $C(a - \bar{v})O_2$
   g. HbCO
9. Define hypoxia and hypoxemia.
10. Identify the general classifications of hypoxemia.

11. Identify the physiologic causes, mechanisms, and most common physiologic cause of hypoxemia.
12. Describe how increases and decreases in $PaCO_2$, body temperature, and blood pH affect the oxyhemoglobin-dissociation curve and related SaO_2 measurements and oxyhemoglobin affinity.
13. Recognize how shifts in the oxyhemoglobin dissociation curve affect oxygen transport at the tissues and lungs.
14. Recognize a definition of, the significance of, and the factors that affect the following acid-base parameters:
    a. pH
    b. $PaCO_2$
    c. Plasma HCO_3^-
    d. Standard HCO_3^-
    e. Base excess
15. Identify the Henderson-Hasselbalch equation and the ratio of HCO_3^- to $PaCO_2$ needed to maintain a pH of 7.40.
16. Define simple and mixed acid-base abnormalities.
17. For the following simple acid-base disorders, identify the basic mechanism of impairment, how the body compensates for the disorder, common causes, and the expected values of compensating components:
    a. Respiratory acidosis
    b. Respiratory alkalosis
    c. Metabolic acidosis
    d. Metabolic alkalosis
18. For the simple acid-base disorders, identify the degree of compensation present given pH, $PaCO_2$, HCO_3^-, and base excess values.
19. Define mixed acid-base disorders and their common causes; given pH, $PaCO_2$, HCO_3^-, and base excess values, interpret the following mixed acid-base disorders:
    a. Metabolic and respiratory alkalosis
    b. Metabolic and respiratory acidosis
20. Recognize the significance of the 95% confidence limit bands as used to assess acid-base status.
21. Given the results of an arterial blood gas, interpret the acid-base and oxygenation status of the patient.

KEY TERMS

acidemia
acidosis
alkalemia
alkalosis
dead space
hypercapnia
hypercarbia
hypoxemia
hypoxia
respiratory acidosis
respiratory alkalosis

Table 7-1	Normal Arterial and Venous Blood Gas Measurements	
	Arterial*	Venous*
pH	7.35-7.45	7.34-7.37
P_{O_2}	80-100 mm Hg	38-42 mm Hg
P_{CO_2}	35-45 mm Hg	44-46 mm Hg
HCO_3^-	22-26 mEq/L	24-30 mEq/L

*Assumes normal respiratory and cardiac function in a patient breathing room air at sea level.

CHAPTER OVERVIEW

Analysis of the arterial blood sample provides precise measurement of acid-base balance and of the lungs' ability to oxygenate the blood and remove excess carbon dioxide (CO_2). For these reasons, assessment of the patient with respiratory dysfunction is more accurate and complete if arterial blood gas (ABG) measurements are reported. However, accurate interpretation of the measurements requires knowledge of the patient's total clinical picture, including any treatment the patient is receiving. This chapter provides insight into interpretation of ABG measurements in the clinical setting.

Arterial blood is used to assess respiratory function, because it contains oxygen and carbon dioxide levels determined primarily by the lungs. Venous blood does not reflect respiratory function, because it has been exposed to peripheral vascular beds, where gas exchange with the tissues alters the oxygen and carbon dioxide concentrations of the blood (Table 7-1). Mixed venous blood samples from the right atrium or pulmonary artery are useful to evaluate overall tissue oxygenation and are discussed later in this chapter. Peripheral venous blood, instead of arterial blood, may be obtained accidentally during the sampling procedure, especially in the patient with hypotension. Analysis of venous blood reflects local metabolic rates and is of little value. An inaccurate assessment results if the venous sample is analyzed and interpreted as arterial.

Because of the cost and risk to the patient, ABG analysis must be performed only when clinically indicated. If ABG measurements are not obtained when needed, improper assessment and treatment of the patient may result. ABG analysis is indicated if the patient's symptoms, medical history, physical examination, or laboratory data suggest significant abnormalities in respiratory or acid-base status (Box 7-1). The analysis is helpful in evaluating the effects of treatment and should also be obtained when significant changes in mechanical ventilation settings are initiated.

ARTERIAL BLOOD SAMPLING

Before arterial puncture, the clinician may find it helpful to review the patient's chart for clinical laboratory studies that reflect the patient's blood clotting ability (see Chapter 6). Abnormalities such as low platelet counts or increased bleeding time may indicate that postpuncture bleeding will pose a problem. In such cases, the puncture site should be pressurized longer than usual to prevent hemorrhage.

The arterial blood sample is obtained by inserting a needle into a major artery (*arteriotomy*). The arterial blood sample may be obtained from the radial, dorsalis pedis, brachial, or femoral arteries in the adult. The radial artery is the preferred puncture site, because it is accessible and easy to stabilize after the puncture. Adequate collateral circulation can be evaluated and is usually available if the radial artery becomes obstructed during the puncture procedure.

The degree of collateral circulation to the hand is evaluated by a modified *Allen's test* before puncture of the radial artery. To perform this test, the clinician should instruct the patient to make a tight fist. Then compress both the radial and ulnar arteries (Figure 7-1). Now instruct the patient to open his/her fist gently to a relaxed position, revealing a blanched palm and fingers. Then release the pressure over the ulnar artery while observing the patient's palm for changes in color. If collateral flow is adequate, the patient's hand will "pink up" within 10 to 15 seconds; this constitutes a positive Allen's test. A positive result documents that collateral blood flow is adequate and that the radial artery is an acceptable puncture site. If the test is negative (the palm does not pink up rapidly), the radial artery is not an acceptable site for puncture. In such cases, the other wrist is evaluated or the brachial artery used for the puncture site.

Because arteriotomy causes trauma to the puncture site, an indwelling arterial catheter should be used when a need for frequent sampling is anticipated. The catheter must be inserted by well-trained personnel, and its use must be reserved for patients in an intensive care unit under close observation.

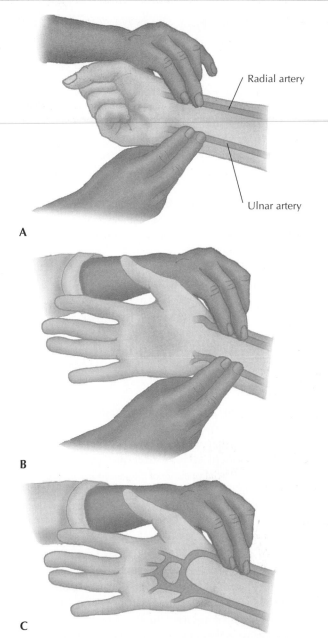

BOX 7-1	Clinical Findings That May Indicate the Need to Obtain an Arterial Blood Gas Sample

Symptoms

Acute dyspnea
Chest pain
Hemoptysis
Cough, fever, and sputum production consistent with
    pneumonia
Symptoms of headache and blurred vision consistent with CO
    poisoning

Past Medical History

History of chronic obstructive pulmonary disease (chronic
    bronchitis and emphysema), especially with cor pulmonale
History of cystic fibrosis
History of pulmonary fibrosis
History of exposure to environmental dusts known to harm the
    lung
History of diabetes with ketoacidosis
Significant smoking history (more than 20 pack/years)

Physical Examination

Cyanosis
Diffuse crackles and wheezing on auscultation
Severe tachypnea or abnormal breathing pattern
Heavy use of accessory muscles
Unexplained confusion
Evidence of chest trauma

Laboratory Data

Unexplained polycythemia
Severe electrolyte abnormalities (e.g., abnormal total CO_2)

Chest Radiograph

Diffuse infiltrates
Hyperinflation
Significant atelectasis
Pneumothorax
Large pleural effusion
Enlarged heart
Lobar consolidation

Radial artery

Ulnar artery

A

B

C

Figure 7-1 Assessment of collateral circulation before radial artery sampling. **A,** Patient clenches fist while examiner obstructs radial and ulnar arteries. **B,** Patient gently opens hand while pressure is maintained over both arteries. **C,** Pressure over ulnar artery is released, and changes in color of patient's palm are noted. (From Wilkins RL, Stoller JK, Scanlan CL: *Egan's fundamentals of respiratory care*, ed 8, St Louis, 2003, Mosby.)

Regardless of which artery is chosen, the process of arterial puncture must be well planned and carefully executed by a skilled technician. The sample must be obtained without being exposed to the environment. Exposure can occur when large air bubbles are trapped within the syringe. The oxygen and carbon dioxide gas tensions of the bubbles may equilibrate with the blood and result in erroneous measurements. Once the sample is obtained, air bubbles should be removed and the sample stored in an ice water bath to inhibit continued metabolism within the sample. Samples held at room temperature must be analyzed within 10 to 15 minutes of drawing, and those placed in an ice water bath should be analyzed within 1 hour.[1] Immediate placement of the sample in ice water is important when the patient's white blood cell or platelet count is ele-

vated.[2] Attention to the blood sample must not prevent proper care of the puncture site. After the needle is withdrawn, the wound should be pressurized for a period of at least 3 to 5 minutes, or longer if clotting problems exist.

Once the arterial sample is obtained and the puncture site is stabilized, the sample is taken to the laboratory for analysis. The iced sample should be analyzed within 1 hour for the most accurate results to be obtained. For the results to be reliable, analysis of the blood sample must be performed with properly maintained and calibrated equipment.

INTERPRETATION OF BLOOD GAS MEASUREMENTS

The measurements obtained from analysis of arterial and mixed venous blood samples are useful in evaluating the following:

- Acid-base balance (pH, $PaCO_2$, HCO_3^-, base excess [BE])
- Oxygenation status (PaO_2, SaO_2, CaO_2, $P\bar{v}O_2$)
- Adequacy of ventilation ($PaCO_2$)

Abbreviations associated with blood gas interpretation are as follows:

Acid-base

pH   Hydrogen ion concentration in blood
HCO_3^- Plasma bicarbonate concentration
$PaCO_2$ Partial pressure of carbon dioxide in arterial blood
BE   Base excess

Oxygenation

PaO_2 Partial pressure of oxygen in arterial blood
PAO_2 Partial pressure of oxygen in the alveoli
SaO_2 Percent of hemoglobin (Hb) saturated with oxygen in arterial blood
CaO_2 Content of oxygen in arterial blood (mL/dL)
$P\bar{v}O_2$ Partial pressure of oxygen in mixed venous blood
FIO_2 Fraction of oxygen in inspired gas (often expressed as a percentage)
$P(A-a)O_2$ Difference in pressure between alveolar and arterial blood oxygen
PIO_2 Partial pressure of oxygen in inspired gas

The following discussion describes the use of blood gases to assess oxygenation and acid-base balance in the clinical setting.

Assessment of Oxygenation

The important process of evaluating the oxygenation status of the patient involves two basic steps. First, the measurements provided by blood gas analysis must be evaluated to identify the quantity of oxygen transported in the blood. Second, the patient's tissue oxygenation status must be determined. The following discussion describes the evaluation of measurements available from blood gas analysis that reflect oxygenation. This is followed by a brief description of the basic techniques used in clinical assessment of the patient's overall oxygenation condition.

Oxygen in the blood is primarily transported bound to hemoglobin. A smaller portion is transported as dissolved gas in the blood plasma. Assessment of the basic blood gas measurements reflecting oxygenation involves interpreting data that identify the partial pressure of oxygen in the plasma (PaO_2), the amount of oxygen bound to hemoglobin (SaO_2), and the total content of oxygen in the arterial blood (CaO_2).

Partial Pressure of Oxygen in Arterial Blood (PaO_2)

NORMAL VALUE: approximately 75 to 95 mm Hg in room air

PaO_2 is a measurement of the pressure or tension of oxygen in the plasma of the arterial blood. PaO_2 reflects the ability of

the lungs to allow the transfer of oxygen from the environment to the circulating blood.

The normal predicted PaO_2 depends on the barometric pressure, the patient's age, and the concentration or fraction of inspired oxygen (FIO_2). Healthy lungs allow oxygen to move from the alveoli to the blood in direct proportion to the alveolar partial pressure of oxygen (PAO_2). At sea level, where the barometric pressure is 760 mm Hg, the PAO_2 and predicted PaO_2 are higher than at an elevated altitude, where the barometric pressure may be significantly lower than 760 mm Hg. The predicted normal PaO_2 of a person living in Denver, Colorado (elevation of 5280 ft), is significantly lower than that of a person of the same age living at sea level.

As age increases, the efficiency of the lungs to oxygenate the blood is reduced; the predicted normal PaO_2 is also reduced (Table 7-2).

PAO_2 and therefore PaO_2 are influenced by the FIO_2 according to the following alveolar-air equation:

$$PAO_2 = FIO_2 (PB - PH_2O) - (PaCO_2 \times 1.25)$$

where

FIO_2 = fraction of inhaled oxygen
PB = barometric pressure
PH_2O = water vapor pressure in alveoli, assumed to be 47 mm Hg
$PaCO_2$ = partial pressure of carbon dioxide in arterial blood, assumed to be equal to the partial pressure of carbon dioxide in the alveoli
1.25 = mathematic factor that takes into account the ratio of carbon dioxide production to oxygen consumption

For example, a patient breathing room air at 760 mm Hg with a $PaCO_2$ of 40 mm Hg has a predicted PAO_2 of approximately 100 mm Hg.

$$PAO_2 = 0.21 (760 \text{ mm Hg} - 47 \text{ mm Hg}) - (40 \times 1.25)$$
$$= (0.21 \times 713 \text{ mm Hg}) - 50 \text{ mm Hg}$$
$$= \sim 150 \text{ mm Hg} - 50 \text{ mm Hg}$$
$$= \sim 100 \text{ mm Hg}$$

Table 7-2	Relationship Between Age and Normal Predicted PaO_2
Age (yr)	Predicted (mm Hg)
≤ 10	95-103
20	91-99
30	87-95
40	83-91
50	78-86
60	74-82
70	70-78
80	66-74
90	62-70

Predicted PaO_2 (supine position) = $103.5 - (0.42 \times \text{age}) \pm 4$

Adapted from Burton G, Hodgkin JE: *Respiratory care, a guide to clinical practice,* ed 3, Philadelphia, 1990, Lippincott Williams and Wilkins.

When the measured Pa_{O_2} is below the predicted range for a patient breathing room air, regardless of the actual F_{IO_2}, it is called hypoxemia. As long as the Pa_{O_2} remains above the minimally acceptable limit, hypoxemia does not exist, regardless of the actual F_{IO_2}. Hypoxia is a term often associated with hypoxemia and indicates a condition in which tissue oxygenation is inadequate. Hypoxemia may result in hypoxia in patients with limited cardiac performance, but the two terms are not synonymous. Hypoxemia may be classified as mild, moderate, or severe according to the measured Pa_{O_2}. For patients breathing 21% oxygen (room air) and who are younger than the age of 60 years, a Pa_{O_2} of 60 to 79 mm Hg is considered mild hypoxemia; a Pa_{O_2} of 40 to 59 mm Hg is considered moderate hypoxemia; and a Pa_{O_2} of less than 40 mm Hg is considered severe hypoxemia. At any age, a Pa_{O_2} of less than 65 mm Hg is considered hypoxemia and a Pa_{O_2} of less than 40 mm Hg is considered severe hypoxemia.

Hypoxemia occurs in most patients when the inhaled gas does not match up with the pulmonary capillary blood flow. For example, mucus plugging or bronchospasm diminishes ventilation of specific parts of the lung. Blood that flows into those underventilated regions of the lung does not pick up normal amounts of oxygen and results in arterial blood that is not optimally oxygenated. This is an example of ventilation/perfusion ($\dot{V}/\dot{Q}$) mismatching and it is the most common cause of hypoxemia in patients with lung disease. Hypoxemia can also occur with diffusion defect and hypoventilation. Each is discussed briefly in the following section.

Abnormalities in the lung structure that slow the diffusion of oxygen from the inhaled gas through the alveolar-capillary membrane result in hypoxemia from diffusion defect. True examples of diffusion defect are not common. Hypoxemia occurring from diffusion defect typically is responsive to oxygen therapy.

Elevation of Pa_{CO_2} from hypoventilation reduces the Pa_{O_2}. As Pa_{O_2} falls, Pa_{O_2} decreases also. If the hypoventilation is occurring in a patient with lung disease, the hypoxemia usually is a result of a combination of $\dot{V}/\dot{Q}$ mismatching and hypoventilation. When hypoventilation occurs in patients without lung disease (e.g., drug overdose), the hypoxemia is strictly the result of an elevated Pa_{CO_2}.

Hypoxemia may also occur with low P_{IO_2}. Pa_{O_2} is determined directly by the partial pressure of oxygen in the inhaled gas (P_{IO_2}). At high altitudes, the P_{IO_2} is significantly lower than that at sea level, and hypoxemia occurs even if respiratory function is optimal. Patients with a marginal Pa_{O_2} at sea level should avoid traveling to high altitudes without supplemental oxygen.

One other situation in which a reduction in P_{IO_2} may occur is when the patient is attached to breathing circuits. If equipment fails, the patient may not receive proper F_{IO_2} and hypoxemia will occur. This can take place while the patient is receiving general anesthesia or mechanical ventilation. For this reason, the F_{IO_2} should be monitored closely during mechanical ventilation.

> ### SIMPLY STATED
> Hypoxemia is a measured Pa_{O_2} below the predicted range. It most often results from $\dot{V}/\dot{Q}$ mismatching.

Oxygen Saturation (Sa_{O_2})

NORMAL VALUE: greater than 95%

The Sa_{O_2} is an index of the actual amount of oxygen bound to hemoglobin expressed as a percentage of the total capacity. Some laboratories report only a calculated Sa_{O_2} when equipment is not available for actual measurements. True Sa_{O_2} can be determined only from a co-oximeter and is more reliable. Calculated Sa_{O_2} may be erroneously high, especially with carbon monoxide poisoning. (See discussion of carboxyhemoglobin later in this chapter.)

The relationship between Pa_{O_2} and Sa_{O_2} is demonstrated by the *oxyhemoglobin dissociation curve* (Figure 7-2). This curve demonstrates that Pa_{O_2} and Sa_{O_2} do not have a linear relationship.

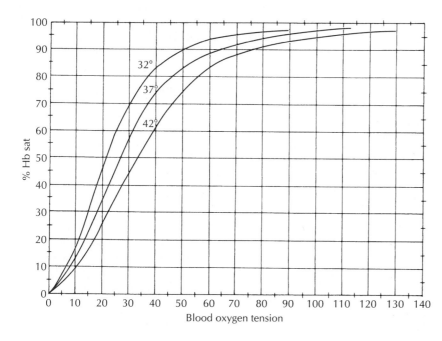

Figure 7-2 Oxygen dissociation curve of blood at a pH of 7.40, showing variations at three temperatures. For a given oxygen tension, the lower the blood temperature, the more the hemoglobin holds onto its oxygen, maintaining higher saturation. (From Scanlan CL, Wilkins RL, Stoller JK: *Egan's fundamentals of respiratory care*, ed 7, St Louis, 1999, Mosby.)

As PaO_2 increases above 80 mm Hg in the flat part of the curve, SaO_2 increases very little, whereas PaO_2 changes below 80 mm Hg in the steep portion of the curve cause significant changes in SaO_2 and thus in oxygen content.

The SaO_2 measurement is affected by body temperature, arterial blood pH, $PaCO_2$, and other factors (Box 7-2). Alkalosis, hypocapnia, hypothermia, fetal hemoglobin, and carboxyhemoglobin shift the curve to the left, resulting in higher SaO_2 values at the same PaO_2. Conversely, acidosis, hypercapnia, and fever shift the curve to the right and result in lower SaO_2 values for the same PaO_2. In other words, shifts to the left cause tighter or easier binding of oxygen with hemoglobin and make unloading of oxygen at the tissues more difficult, whereas shifts to the right have the opposite effect, resulting in decreased oxygen affinity for hemoglobin, allowing easier unloading of oxygen at the tissues.

Arterial Oxygen Content (CaO₂)

NORMAL VALUE: 16 to 20 mL/dL blood

The CaO_2 is a function of the amount of oxygen bound to hemoglobin and dissolved in the plasma. It is one of the most important blood gas measurements, because it significantly influences tissue oxygenation. Because most oxygen (99%) is carried in the blood bound to hemoglobin, CaO_2 cannot be normal without adequate circulating red blood cells containing hemoglobin (Table 7-3).

CaO_2 is calculated from the following:

$$\begin{array}{r} 1.39 \text{ mL} \times Hb \times SaO_2 = O_2 \text{ combined with Hb} \\ + 0.003 \text{ mL} \times PaO_2 = O_2 \text{ dissolved in plasma} \\ \hline \text{Total} = CaO_2 (\text{vol \%}) \end{array}$$

Anemic patients without lung disease may have normal PaO_2 and SaO_2, but CaO_2 is reduced because of the inadequate amount of hemoglobin, and tissue hypoxia may occur without adequate circulatory compensation. Conversely, patients with polycythemia may have mild reductions in PaO_2 and SaO_2 while maintaining CaO_2 values within or near normal limits (see Table 7-3). As with SaO_2, true measurements of CaO_2 can be achieved only from a co-oximeter. CaO_2 measurements from laboratories without a co-oximeter are only calculated values.

Table 7-3   Relationship Between Hemoglobin Concentration, PaO₂, Saturation, and Oxygen Content*

Hemoglobin (g/dL)	PaO₂ (mm Hg)	SaO₂ (%)	CaO₂ (vol%)
5.0	50	86	5.9
5.0	100	96	6.7
7.5	50	86	8.8
7.5	100	96	9.9
10.0	50	86	11.7
10.0	100	96	13.2
12.5	50	86	14.6
12.5	100	96	16.4
15.0	50	86	17.4
15.0	100	96	19.6

*Using factor of 1.39 mL of oxygen per gram of hemoglobin.

A reduced measured CaO_2 can also occur when the hemoglobin is bound to other gases. In such cases a normal level of hemoglobin in the circulating blood is of little value, because most of it is not available for transporting oxygen. For example, carbon monoxide poisoning probably is present in the patient who has inhaled a significant amount of smoke from a fire. Carbon monoxide has an increased affinity for hemoglobin and binds tightly with any hemoglobin it contacts. Measured CaO_2 is very low although adequate hemoglobin and dissolved oxygen are present in the circulating blood. (See discussion of carboxyhemoglobin later in this chapter.)

SIMPLY STATED

The single most important parameter that reflects the quantity of oxygen carried in the arterial blood is the CaO_2. An adequate hemoglobin concentration must be present for this parameter to be normal.

Alveolar-Arterial Oxygen Difference [P(a – a)o₂]

NORMAL VALUE: 10 to 15 mm Hg on room air

The $P(A - a)O_2$ is a measurement of the pressure difference between the alveoli and the arterial blood of oxygen. In normal lungs, oxygen is transferred readily from the alveoli to the blood, and only a small PO_2 difference is present. When the lungs become diseased, oxygen gas exchange is often hindered and a larger $P(A - a)O_2$ develops.

The predicted normal $P(A - a)O_2$ depends on the FIO_2 and the age of the patient. When the patient is breathing room air, the normal $P(A - a)O_2$ can be estimated by multiplying 0.4 by the patient's age in years. The higher the FIO_2 and the older the patient, the larger the predicted normal $P(A - a)O_2$. The $P(A - a)O_2$ is determined by subtracting the PaO_2 (obtained from ABG measurements) from the calculated PAO_2 (obtained

BOX 7-2   Factors Influencing the Oxygen Dissociation Curve

Shift to left (increase in hemoglobin-oxygen affinity)

Alkalosis
Hypocapnia
Hypothermia
Fetal hemoglobin
Carboxyhemoglobin

Shift to right (decrease in hemoglobin-oxygen affinity)

Acidosis
Hypercapnia
Fever

from use of the alveolar air equation described earlier in this chapter). Calculation of the PAO_2 requires a known FIO_2 and $PaCO_2$. The $P(A-a)O_2$ cannot be determined in patients breathing supplemental oxygen with low-flow devices (nasal cannula) for which the FIO_2 is not known.

An increase in $P(A-a)O_2$ is strictly an indication of respiratory defects in oxygenation ability. Most respiratory dysfunctions that produce hypoxemia are accompanied by an elevated $P(A-a)O_2$.

There are two situations in which hypoxemia may occur with a normal $P(A-a)O_2$: primary hypoventilation and high altitudes. Primary hypoventilation elevates the alveolar and arterial PCO_2 and reduces PAO_2. In this situation, hypoxemia may occur, but $P(A-a)O_2$ remains within normal limits. At high altitudes, PIO_2 is significantly reduced and hypoxemia occurs. The hypoxemia is the result of a decrease in PAO_2, and $P(A-a)O_2$ remains within normal limits. In summary, hypoxemia occurring with a normal $P(A-a)O_2$ is caused by either a decreased PIO_2 or primary hypoventilation.

Partial Pressure of Oxygen in Mixed Venous Blood ($P\bar{v}O_2$)

NORMAL VALUE: 38 to 42 mm Hg

The heart and lungs must work together to provide adequate tissue oxygenation, because oxygen delivery is a function of cardiac output and the CaO_2. PaO_2, SaO_2, and CaO_2 provide only evaluation of the respiratory component, leaving the assessment of tissue oxygenation incomplete.

One dimension capable of indicating the tissue oxygenation status in most cases is the $P\bar{v}O_2$. A true mixed venous sample can be achieved only by sampling the pulmonary artery blood through a pulmonary artery catheter. For this reason, analysis of $P\bar{v}O_2$ usually is reserved for the patient in an intensive care unit, where pulmonary artery catheters can be maintained adequately.

Normally, only approximately 25% of the oxygen in the arterial blood is given up at the tissue vascular beds. If oxygen extraction (consumption) remains constant as cardiac output decreases, the venous oxygen level is reduced below normal. The venous oxygen level is also reduced in patients with limited cardiac performance when oxygen consumption increases, as with fever. Therefore $P\bar{v}O_2$ is a reflection of the relationship between oxygen delivery to the tissues and the rate at which oxygen is consumed.

A $P\bar{v}O_2$ lower than 35 mm Hg is strong evidence that tissue oxygenation is less than optimal, and further evaluation is warranted. A sudden decrease in $P\bar{v}O_2$ most often occurs when circulation is impaired and oxygen delivery to the tissues is reduced. This may happen with hypovolemia, the addition of positive pressure ventilation, or left-sided heart failure. Rapid assessment of the cause of the decrease in $P\bar{v}O_2$ must be done so that appropriate treatment can be implemented.

A normal $P\bar{v}O_2$ may indicate that tissue oxygenation is adequate, but it is not always reliable. In some very sick patients, the $P\bar{v}O_2$ reads normal or elevated despite significant tissue hypoxia. The exact mechanism for this faulty reading is not known; however, the inability of the tissues to utilize oxygen is one theory.

SIMPLY STATED

$P\bar{v}O_2$ is an excellent parameter to assess overall tissue oxygenation. Values lower than 35 mm Hg suggest reduced cardiac output or severe hypoxemia in the patient with limited cardiac function.

Arteriovenous Oxygen Content Difference $C(a-\bar{v})O_2$

NORMAL VALUE: 3.5 to 5.0 vol%

Measurement of $C(a-\bar{v})O_2$ (commonly called the *arteriovenous oxygen difference*) requires simultaneous sampling of arterial and mixed venous blood. The mixed venous sample must be acquired from a pulmonary artery catheter to be most reliable. The two blood samples are taken to the laboratory for determination of the CaO_2 and $C\bar{v}O_2$. The difference between the oxygen content of the two samples provides an estimation of the tissue perfusion and oxygenation according to the following equation:

$$\dot{Q}T = \frac{\dot{V}O_2}{C(a-\bar{v})O_2}$$

The equation demonstrates that in a patient with a steady oxygen consumption ($\dot{V}O_2$), the cardiac output ($\dot{Q}T$) and $C(a-\bar{v})O_2$ are inversely proportional. As $\dot{Q}T$ decreases, $C(a-\bar{v})O_2$ increases; as $\dot{Q}T$ increases, $C(a-\bar{v})O_2$ decreases. $\dot{V}O_2$ usually can be assumed to be stable in most patients unless the patient is restless or having significant variations in body temperature.

Increases in $C(a-\bar{v})O_2$ in a patient with a stable $\dot{V}O_2$ indicate that the perfusion of the body organs is decreasing. Without adequate perfusion, the tissues do not receive adequate oxygenation and tissue hypoxia occurs. When the $C(a-\bar{v})O_2$ exceeds 6.0 vol%, cardiovascular decompensation is occurring and tissue oxygenation is inadequate.

A reduction in $C(a-\bar{v})O_2$ occurs when perfusion exceeds the normal level with a steady $\dot{V}O_2$ or when $\dot{V}O_2$ is reduced significantly (as with hypothermia) with a normal $\dot{Q}T$. A $C(a-\bar{v})O_2$ lower than 3.5 vol% may also occur when the tissue utilization of oxygen is impaired.

Carboxyhemoglobin (HbCO)

NORMAL VALUE: approximately 0.5%

The HbCO is a reflection of the quantity of carbon monoxide (CO) bound to the hemoglobin molecules and can be obtained only from the co-oximeter. Carbon monoxide is a highly diffusible, odorless, and colorless gas that has an affinity for hemoglobin 200 to 250 times that of oxygen. Inhalation of gas containing carbon monoxide results in a tight bond between the carbon monoxide and the hemoglobin and shifts the oxyhemoglobin dissociation curve to the left. Hemoglobin bonded with carbon monoxide is less capable of carrying oxygen, and CaO_2 decreases accordingly. The resulting shift to the left of the oxyhemoglobin dissociation curve further promotes tissue hypoxia by inhibiting the unloading of oxygen from the hemoglobin to the tissues.

A mild elevation of HbCO (5% to 10%) occurs with tobacco or cigarette smoking and exposure to polluted environments. A more significant elevation of HbCO (greater than 10%) occurs from inhalation of large amounts of smoke, automobile exhaust, or exhaust from other gas-powered engines in an enclosed space.[3] In such cases, CaO_2 (but not necessarily PaO_2) is reduced significantly, and tissue oxygenation may be in jeopardy. The patient generally complains of headache, dyspnea, and nausea and appears hypoxic (tachycardia, tachypnea), but cyanosis does not occur. At HbCO levels of 40% to 60%, visual disturbance, myocardial toxicity, loss of consciousness, and eventually, death occur. Laboratories without a co-oximeter do not easily detect the abnormality, because measured PaO_2 and calculated SaO_2 are often normal when carbon monoxide poisoning is present.

SIMPLY STATED

Carbon monoxide poisoning represents double trouble for tissue oxygenation. It reduces the oxygen-carrying capacity of the hemoglobin and inhibits unloading of oxygen at the tissues.

Clinical Assessment of Oxygenation

The ultimate goal of respiratory and cardiovascular function is to provide adequate oxygenation of the body tissues. Therefore assessment of oxygenation should evaluate the ability of the lungs to oxygenate the blood and the ability of the cardiovascular system to distribute the blood. Respiratory function can be evaluated by interpreting the ABG measurements previously reviewed and summarized in the following discussion. However, ABG analysis cannot assess the adequacy of tissue oxygenation. Tissue perfusion and oxygenation are evaluated better in the non–intensive care unit setting by using the findings of a physical examination as described in Chapter 5.

Hypoxemia occurs when the respiratory system fails to oxygenate arterial blood adequately. The PaO_2, SaO_2, and usually, CaO_2 are reduced. The degree of abnormality can be assessed by looking at the relationship between FIO_2 and PaO_2 or at $P(A-a)O_2$. Large $P(A-a)O_2$ values indicate severe respiratory abnormality. Hypoxemia occurring with a normal $P(A-a)O_2$ may be the result of low PIO_2 at high altitude or hypoventilation. The $P(A-a)O_2$ cannot be calculated when the FIO_2 is not known.

If hypoxemia exists at an FIO_2 of 0.21 and the sum of the PaO_2 and $PaCO_2$ is 110 to 130 mm Hg, the cause of the hypoxemia is hypoventilation. If the sum is less than 110 mm Hg, the cause of the hypoxemia is related to defects in the lungs' ability to oxygenate the blood. If the sum of the PaO_2 and the $PaCO_2$ is greater than 130 mm Hg, the patient probably is breathing supplemental oxygen, or an error has occurred.

The most important factor indicating the oxygenation status of the arterial blood is the CaO_2. Assessment of the hemoglobin concentration from either the complete blood cell count (CBC) or co-oximeter measurement is crucial in identifying the potential for CaO_2. A reduction in hemoglobin (anemia) dis-allows the possibility of a normal CaO_2, regardless of the PaO_2 and SaO_2, because 99% of the CaO_2 is bound to hemoglobin.

Other than hypoxemia and anemia, a reduction in CaO_2 can occur with carbon monoxide poisoning. Carbon monoxide poisoning usually is suggested by the initial history (exposure to smoke or automobile exhaust) and confirmed by co-oximeter measurements. SaO_2 and CaO_2 are reduced significantly, and the PaO_2 is higher than the predicted value for the SaO_2. Without co-oximeter measurements, carbon monoxide poisoning is difficult to identify, especially if the patient is comatose and the history of present illness is not provided.

The clinical recognition of hypoxemia often is first suggested by the patient complaining of shortness of breath, especially with exertion. Common clinical manifestations of hypoxemia include tachycardia, tachypnea, hypertension, cyanosis, and confusion. Cyanosis is identified when the level of hemoglobin is at or near normal and its saturation with oxygen drops below 90%. Cyanosis is not recognized in the patient with anemia even if the hypoxemia is severe. As hypoxemia worsens to the extent of tissue hypoxia, metabolic acidosis, bradycardia, and hypotension occur and the patient often becomes comatose. In the intensive care unit, $P\bar{v}O_2$ less than 35 mm Hg and increases in $C(a-\bar{v})O_2$ above 5 vol% may indicate tissue hypoxia.

Tissue hypoxia also may occur with normal arterial oxygenation when inadequate perfusion exists. Clinical signs of an inadequate cardiac output include hypotension, cool extremities, weak or absent pulses, reduced urine output, and coma.

Assessment of Acid-Base Balance

Normal metabolism produces approximately 12,000 mEq of acid each day in the average adult. It is the responsibility of the lungs and kidneys to excrete the metabolic acids, maintaining an appropriate acid-base balance in the body. Numerous blood buffers are also available to prevent a buildup of acid. The lungs remove most metabolic acids by removing carbon dioxide from the blood through the process of ventilation. The respiratory system serves as an important regulator of acid-base balance through the control of PCO_2. The kidneys remove a smaller quantity of acid but help restore the buffer capacity of the body fluids by replenishing the HCO_3^- concentration. Respiratory or renal dysfunction may cause a breakdown in the process of maintaining acid-base balance and result in acid-base disorders.

Accurate assessment of the patient's acid-base balance requires interpretation of the measurements provided by blood gas analysis. The measurements that reflect acid-base status are described in the following paragraphs. This is followed by a discussion of the common acid-base disorders and the clinical situations in which they occur.

Hydrogen Ion Concentration (pH)

NORMAL VALUE: 7.40 with a range of 7.35 to 7.45

The arterial blood pH is a measurement of the hydrogen ion (H^+) concentration in the plasma. Because *acids* are defined as solutions capable of *donating* H^+ and *bases* as solutions capable of *accepting* H$^+$, the pH is a reflection of the acid-base status of the arterial blood.

The actual concentration of H$^+$ in the arterial blood serum is low (0.00004 mEq/L) and is a cumbersome number with which to work. To solve this problem, the proposal has been made to convert the H$^+$ term to pH by taking the negative logarithm (base 10) of the hydrogen ion, resulting in more manageable numbers. Because pH is a logarithmic expression of the H$^+$, changes in pH of 1 unit (e.g., changes from 7.40 to 6.40) represent a 10-fold alteration in the H$^+$ of the blood.

The relationship between pH and H$^+$ is expressed as follows and demonstrates an important concept: H$^+$ and pH are inversely related.

As H$^+$ increases from the addition of acids, pH decreases. Therefore pH values below 7.35 represent increases in the H$^+$ concentration, and the blood is *acidotic* or *acidemic*. When the pH increases above 7.45, the H$^+$ has decreased, and the blood is *alkalotic* or *alkalemic*. It is more exact to refer to deviations in plasma pH with the terms acidemia and alkalemia rather than with acidosis and alkalosis, because the reported pH is that of the blood plasma and the latter terms do not indicate the compartment that is sampled.

The pH of the arterial blood is important to monitor, because the majority of body functions occur optimally at or near a pH of 7.40. Significant alterations in pH have a profound effect on many systems of the body, especially the central nervous system (CNS). Acidosis results in depression of the CNS. The patient with acidosis initially appears lethargic and disoriented. As the acidosis worsens, the patient eventually becomes comatose. The major effect of alkalosis is overexcitability of the CNS and peripheral nerves. The nerves become so responsive that they automatically and repetitively depolarize, resulting in tetany. Extreme alkalosis may result in muscular spasms of the extremities, face, and body. Respiratory failure may occur if the nerves and muscles of ventilation are involved. Significant alterations in arterial blood pH also may reduce the ability of the heart muscle (myocardium) to contract and effectively pump blood throughout the body.

Partial Pressure of Arterial Carbon Dioxide (Paco$_2$)

NORMAL VALUE: 35 to 45 mm Hg

Paco$_2$ is a reflection of the respiratory component of acid-base status. It identifies the degree of ventilation in relation to the metabolic rate. Carbon dioxide is a waste product of normal metabolism and must be removed, at least in part, by the lungs exchanging air with the blood. In healthy persons, as the metabolic rate increases (as with fever or exercise), ventilation also increases to maintain a normal Paco$_2$. A normal or increased metabolism without adequate ventilation results in an elevated Paco$_2$ and represents a failure of the respiratory system to remove carbon dioxide at an acceptable rate. An elevated Paco$_2$ (higher than 45 mm Hg), called hypercapnia or hypercarbia, most often results from less than adequate alveolar ventilation (*hypoventilation*). A Paco$_2$ value of less than 35 mm Hg, called hypocapnia or hypocarbia, occurs when alveolar ventilation exceeds normal levels (*hyperventilation*).

Paco$_2$ alters pH according to the following equation:

$$CO_2 + H_2O \rightleftharpoons H_2CO_3 \rightleftharpoons HCO_3^- + H^+$$

An increase in Paco$_2$ shifts the equilibrium equation to the right, resulting in an increase in H$^+$; this is called respiratory acidosis. A decrease in Paco$_2$ shifts the equation to the left and lowers H$^+$; this is called respiratory alkalosis. Appropriate adjustments in the plasma HCO$_3^-$ concentration by the kidneys compensate for respiratory acid-base disorders, which are discussed later in this chapter.

Paco$_2$ is the most reliable measurement for evaluating the effectiveness of ventilation and should be interpreted in light of the patient's minute volume ($\dot{V}E$). A normal Paco$_2$ should be accompanied by a normal $\dot{V}E$. An increased $\dot{V}E$ should result in hypocapnia unless metabolism is increased or dead space ventilation is increased. Dead space ventilation occurs when the portion of the tidal volume ($\dot{V}T$) that does not come into contact with blood flow is increased. An increase in dead space ventilation occurs most often when the perfusion of the lungs is reduced.

A reduction in $\dot{V}E$ below normal usually produces hypercapnia unless metabolism is reduced significantly. If the $\dot{V}E$ is reduced and Paco$_2$ is elevated, the effectiveness of ventilation may be normal but the quantity insufficient. In this case, the cause of hypoventilation usually lies outside the lungs and often is the result of neuromuscular disease or response to certain medications, such as morphine, that depress the drive to breathe.

SIMPLY STATED

The best parameter for evaluating the adequacy of ventilation is the Paco$_2$.

Arterial Blood Bicarbonate (HCO$_3^-$)

NORMAL VALUE: 22 to 26 mEq/L

The plasma HCO$_3^-$ is primarily a reflection of the metabolic component of acid-base balance and is regulated by the renal system. When plasma HCO$_3^-$ levels decrease below normal, the pH also decreases because HCO$_3^-$ is a base; metabolic acidosis results. Metabolic alkalosis occurs when the plasma HCO$_3^-$ increases, resulting in an elevated pH. The HCO$_3^-$ level may also change as a compensatory response to primary changes in Paco$_2$ levels; this usually requires 12 to 24 hours to occur.

The plasma HCO$_3^-$ is affected slightly by acute changes in Paco$_2$ according to the following equation:

$$CO_2 + H_2O \rightleftharpoons H_2CO_3 \rightleftharpoons H^+ + HCO_3^-$$

Increases in Paco$_2$ shift the reaction to the right and result in immediate but small increases in plasma HCO$_3^-$. Decreases in Paco$_2$ shift the equation to the left and result in a reduced HCO$_3^-$ level. For every 10- to 15–mm Hg increase in Paco$_2$ above 40 mm Hg, the HCO$_3^-$ increases 1 mEq/L. For every 5–mm Hg decrease in Paco$_2$ below normal, the serum HCO$_3^-$ decreases by 1 mEq/L.

Standard bicarbonate

Because plasma HCO_3^- levels are influenced by acute alterations in $PaCO_2$, some laboratories report a standard HCO_3^-. *Standard bicarbonate* is defined as the plasma HCO_3^- concentration that would be present if the $PaCO_2$ were 40 mm Hg. This theoretically eliminates the respiratory influence on plasma HCO_3^- and allows evaluation of the pure metabolic component. The normal standard HCO_3^- is 22 to 26 mEq/L.

Base Excess and Base Deficit

NORMAL VALUE: ±2 mEq/L

Base excess is a measurement reflecting the nonrespiratory portion of acid-base balance. It is a standard deviation of the standard HCO_3^- that takes the buffering capabilities of the red blood cells into account. The calculation of base excess is made from the measurements of pH, $PaCO_2$, and hematocrit concentration. The hematocrit is considered in the calculation because red blood cells contain significant blood buffers. The total quantity of buffer anions in the blood is 45 to 50 mEq/L, or approximately twice that of HCO_3^-. Thus HCO_3^- accounts for only approximately half of the total buffering capacity of the blood. Therefore the base excess provides a more complete analysis of the metabolic buffering capabilities.

Base excess is reported as a positive or negative value depending on the direction in which the buffer base has deviated from normal. The larger the value, the more severe the deviation in the metabolic component. A positive value indicates that either base has been added or acid has been removed, whereas a negative value (*base deficit*) indicates that acid has been added or base has been removed.

Measurement of base excess allows analysis of the pure metabolic components of acid-base balance. Changes in plasma HCO_3^- from metabolic components alter base excess, whereas acute changes in plasma HCO_3^- from the respiratory component (PCO_2) do not.

Respiratory and Metabolic Acid-Base Disorders

The previous discussion demonstrates that there are two basic types of acid-base disorders: metabolic and respiratory. Metabolic disorders are recognized by abnormalities in plasma HCO_3^-, whereas respiratory disorders alter $PaCO_2$. The effects of $PaCO_2$ and plasma HCO_3^- on acid-base balance are defined in the following Henderson-Hasselbalch equation:

$$pH = pK + \log \frac{HCO_3^- \text{ (renal)}}{PaCO_2 \times 0.03 \text{ (lungs)}}$$

where

pK = 6.1 ionization constant
0.03 = solubility factor to convert mm Hg to mEq
Normal example:

$$pH = 6.1 + \log \frac{24}{40 \times 0.03}$$

$$pH = 6.1 + \log 20$$
$$pH = 6.1 + 1.30$$
$$pH = 7.40$$

The equation demonstrates that arterial blood pH is determined by the ratio of HCO_3^- to $PaCO_2$. This ratio normally is 20:1. Changes in one component disrupt the 20:1 ratio, resulting in an abnormal pH. Abnormalities in one component can be compensated for by changes in the other component to return the ratio to 20:1. Therefore pH is not determined by absolute values of $PaCO_2$ and plasma HCO_3^- but by the ratio of one to the other.

For example, an increase in $PaCO_2$ from 40 to 60 mm Hg changes the ratio from 20:1 to 20:1.8, or 13.3:1. This results in a pH of 7.23 according to the Henderson-Hasselbach equation:

$$pH = 6.1 + \log \frac{24}{60 \times 0.03}$$

$$pH = 6.1 + \log (24/1.8)$$
$$pH = 6.1 + \log 13.33$$
$$pH = 6.1 + 1.13$$
$$pH = 7.23$$

Most acid-base abnormalities occur as simple disorders. Simple disorders involve a primary abnormality in one component (either $PaCO_2$ or HCO_3^-) that may be compensated for by changes in the other component. Therefore a near-normal pH does not rule out the possibility of an acid-base disorder but may indicate that compensation has occurred. When a combination of simple disorders occurs, a mixed acid-base disorder exists. The recognition of simple and mixed acid-base disorders in the clinical setting is described in the following section.

CLINICAL RECOGNITION OF SIMPLE AND MIXED ACID-BASE DISORDERS

In many situations, the most meaningful and accurate interpretation of ABG measurements is obtained by considering the results in relation to other clinical findings. This is especially true in interpreting mixed acid-base disorders. The following discussion focuses first on interpreting simple acid-base disorders. These are important and must be understood before mixed disturbances can be interpreted. The discussion then proceeds to mixed acid-base disorders and the clinical situations in which they may occur.

Simple Acid-Base Disorders

Simple Respiratory Acidosis

Simple respiratory acidosis is an abnormal condition in which there is a primary reduction in alveolar ventilation relative to the rate of carbon dioxide production. It indicates that ventilation is inadequate. Respiratory acidosis is present when the $PaCO_2$ is elevated above normal or when it is higher than the expected level of compensation. Respiratory acidosis may result from a variety of respiratory and nonrespiratory abnormalities. They are as follows:

Respiratory
  Acute upper airway obstruction
  Severe diffuse airway obstruction (acute or chronic)
  Massive pulmonary edema
Nonrespiratory
  Drug overdose
  Spinal cord trauma
  Neuromuscular disease
  Head trauma
  Trauma to thoracic cage

Respiratory acidosis is compensated for as the kidneys increase the reabsorption of HCO_3^-. Acute respiratory acidosis usually is uncompensated, because renal changes of plasma HCO_3^- are slow to occur. Uncompensated respiratory acidosis is identified by an elevated $Paco_2$, a decreased pH, and a normal plasma HCO_3^- and base excess. Partial compensation occurs when the plasma HCO_3^- is elevated above the normal range but the pH is not yet within normal limits. If the plasma HCO_3^- is elevated enough to return the pH to within normal range, it is called *completely compensated respiratory acidosis*. The plasma HCO_3^- does not rise enough to overcorrect the pH above 7.39, because the impetus of the body to compensate diminishes as the pH gets closer to normal.

When respiratory acidosis occurs, identifying the expected change in plasma HCO_3^- is useful in determining whether the degree of compensation is appropriate. For acute respiratory acidosis, the plasma HCO_3^- increases 1 mEq/L for each 10 to 15 mm Hg that the $Paco_2$ increases. In chronic respiratory acidosis, the plasma HCO_3^- is expected to increase 4 mEq/L for each 10 mm Hg that $Paco_2$ increases. If the expected compensation is not occurring, a complicating metabolic disorder may be present.

If the respiratory acidosis is caused by a neuromuscular disease or airway obstruction disorder, the patient will be short of breath and breathing rapidly. In contrast, if the respiratory center is impaired (e.g., with narcotics), the respiratory rate will be reduced.

The combination of an acutely elevated $Paco_2$ and acidosis usually has a significant effect on the clinical findings and produces an anesthetic effect on the CNS. The patient with hypercapnia often is confused, semiconscious, and eventually, comatose. Coma may be observed at CO_2 tensions above 70 mm Hg if the onset of hypercapnia is acute. Even higher levels of Pco_2 may be well tolerated in patients with chronic respiratory acidosis. As the $Paco_2$ acutely increases, the patient may complain of a headache and appear sleepy and lethargic. Because hypercapnia often is associated with hypoxemia in patient's breathing room air, the clinical manifestations of hypoxemia are also identified commonly.

Because elevations in $Paco_2$ cause systemic vasodilation, cardiovascular manifestations may be seen with hypercapnia. Peripheral vasodilation and an increased cardiac output promote warm flushed skin and a bounding pulse. Arrhythmias are occasionally observed. Cerebral vasodilation also occurs, resulting in elevated intracranial pressures, retinal venous distention, papilledema, and headache. Increases in serum HCO_3^- levels as a

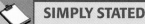

SIMPLY STATED

Respiratory acidosis is present when the $Paco_2$ is higher than the expected level. It is not limited to a $Paco_2$ above 45 mm Hg.

result of renal compensation are accompanied by decreased chloride levels.

Simple Respiratory Alkalosis

Simple respiratory alkalosis is an abnormal condition in which there is a primary increase in alveolar ventilation relative to the rate of carbon dioxide production. Respiratory alkalosis is identified by a $Paco_2$ below the expected level and indicates that ventilation is exceeding the normal level. Hyperventilation usually is the result of an increased stimulus or drive to breathe. This occurs with pain, hypoxemia (Pao_2, 55 to 60 mm Hg), acidosis, and anxiety.

The kidneys compensate for respiratory alkalosis by excreting plasma HCO_3^-. A normal plasma HCO_3^- with a low $Paco_2$ and increased pH is called *uncompensated respiratory alkalosis*. Partial compensation occurs when the plasma HCO_3^- falls below normal but the pH is still above 7.45. Full compensation occurs when the plasma HCO_3^- decreases enough to return the pH to within normal range.

The expected compensatory change in plasma HCO_3^- with respiratory alkalosis depends on the severity and duration of the hyperventilation. Acute respiratory alkalosis should result in a decrease in plasma HCO_3^- of 1 mEq/L for every 5 mm Hg the $Paco_2$ decreases. For chronic respiratory alkalosis, the plasma HCO_3^- should decrease 5 mEq/L for every 10 mm Hg the $Paco_2$ decreases. If the expected compensation is not present, a complicating metabolic disorder may be present.

One advantage of a reduction in $Paco_2$ is the increase in Pao_2. According to Dalton's law, a reduction in $Paco_2$ allows an increase in Pao_2 and potentially in Pao_2. Therefore when hypoxemia and respiratory alkalosis occur together, it is safe to say that the Pao_2 would probably be even lower if the $Paco_2$ increased to normal. If Pao_2 is barely adequate and respiratory alkalosis is present, it is likely that hypoxemia would occur if $Paco_2$ returned to normal range.

Clinical signs and symptoms associated with respiratory alkalosis include tachypnea, dizziness, sweating, tingling in the fingers and toes, and muscle weakness and spasm. Respiratory alkalosis may be induced accidentally in patients receiving intermittent positive-pressure breathing treatments when the treatments are administered improperly or with mechanical ventilation when not properly monitored.

Simple Metabolic Acidosis

Metabolic acidosis is identified when the plasma HCO_3^- or base excess falls below normal. This occurs whenever buffers are not produced in sufficient quantities or when they are lost excessively. In addition, metabolic acidosis can occur when an increased load of H^+ ions is present or when a decreased ability to excrete acids exists. Following is an outline of the causes of metabolic acidosis:

Loss of HCO_3^-
  Diarrhea
  Renal disease
Increase in metabolic acid production
  Ketoacidosis
  Lactic acidosis
  Ingestion of certain toxins (e.g., methanol)
  Posthypocapnia disorder

When metabolic acidosis occurs as a result of the buildup of organic or inorganic acids in the body, the anion gap is elevated above 16 mEq/L (see Chapter 6 for a discussion of the anion gap).

Normal metabolism requires both oxygen and glucose. When either element is not present in sufficient quantity, an increased amount of nonvolatile acids is produced and accumulates in the blood. A lack of cellular oxygen results in the formation of lactic acid; this is called *lactic acidosis*. Lactic acidosis is accompanied by signs of tissue hypoxia. The oxygen deficits must be corrected rapidly, usually by improving arterial blood oxygenation and perfusion.

A lack of cellular glucose occurs with diabetes and starvation. Metabolism without sufficient glucose produces ketone bodies from the breakdown of proteins and is called *ketoacidosis*.

Metabolic acidosis may also be the result of renal failure. The kidneys are responsible for excreting excess H^+ ions and reabsorbing HCO_3^- ions. Renal disease may disrupt either function and result in metabolic acidosis. In such cases, other signs of renal failure usually are present, including increases in blood urea nitrogen and creatinine and decreases in urine output.

A reduction in $PaCO_2$ through hyperventilation compensates for metabolic acidosis. Uncompensated metabolic acidosis rarely occurs, because $PaCO_2$ is rapidly altered by changes in ventilation. A normal or elevated $PaCO_2$ in the presence of metabolic acidosis indicates that a ventilatory defect is also occurring. The predicted compensatory alteration in $PaCO_2$ for metabolic acidosis can be estimated by the following equation:

$$PaCO_2 = (1.5 \times HCO_3^-) + 8 \pm 2$$

If the $PaCO_2$ is not at the expected level, a respiratory abnormality may also be present.

In most cases, metabolic acidosis causes a rapid and significant response by the respiratory system. Rapid and deep ventilation, called *Kussmaul's respiration*, is the most common and obvious sign of metabolic acidosis. This change in the pattern of breathing may not be clinically obvious, especially if the acidosis is not severe. With more severe cases, the patient may complain of dyspnea, headache, nausea, and vomiting. Confusion and stupor may follow. Constriction of the venous blood vessels often occurs with acidosis and may shift the blood flow to the pulmonary system.

SIMPLY STATED

Metabolic acidosis puts extra stress on the respiratory system to reduce $PaCO_2$ as a compensatory response. This may precipitate respiratory failure in the patient with lung disease.

Pulmonary edema may result. Arrhythmias can occur with severe acidosis when pH or PaO_2 decreases significantly.

Simple Metabolic Alkalosis

Metabolic alkalosis is identified by an above-normal elevation of the plasma HCO_3^-. This occurs whenever HCO_3^- ions accumulate in the blood or when an abnormal number of H^+ ions are lost from the plasma. Following is a listing of the most common causes of metabolic alkalosis:

- Hypokalemia or hypochloremia
- Nasogastric suction (loss of stomach acid)
- Persistent vomiting (loss of stomach acid)
- Posthypercapnia disorder
- Diuretic therapy
- Steroid therapy
- Excessive administration of sodium bicarbonate

Certain electrolyte imbalances can reduce the number of H^+ ions in the plasma or increase the number of HCO_3^- ions. Hypokalemia (reduced plasma potassium) promotes movement of H^+ ions into the intracellular fluids in exchange for K^+ ions. Hypokalemia also increases the renal excretion of H^+ ions, further increasing the blood base.

Hypochloremia (reduced plasma chloride) results in the loss of anions from the blood plasma, and these must be replaced by another anion, usually HCO_3^-, to maintain electrical balance. Therefore hypochloremia may lead to increases in the plasma HCO_3^- concentration and metabolic alkalosis.

Gastric suction often results in excessive loss of the hydrochloric acid (HCl) of the stomach. Loss of the combination of H^+ ions and Cl^- ions leads to a proportionate increase in the blood base.

Excessive administration of bicarbonate can lead to metabolic alkalosis and occurs most often during cardiopulmonary resuscitation. Cardiac arrest and tissue hypoxia result in metabolic acidosis, which is treated by the rapid administration of bicarbonate. If bicarbonate administration is not monitored carefully with ABG measurements, an excessive amount may be administered, resulting in metabolic alkalosis.

Hypoventilation and an elevation of $PaCO_2$ compensate for metabolic alkalosis. Hypoventilation does not occur to a significant degree in the awake, alert patient; metabolic alkalosis tends to remain uncompensated. In the comatose patient, metabolic alkalosis may result in significant hypoventilation and hypercapnia. In such cases, the hypercapnia tends to promote hypoxemia unless the FIO_2 is increased above room air levels.

Uncompensated metabolic alkalosis is identified by an elevated plasma HCO_3^-, an increase in pH, and a normal $PaCO_2$. Partial compensation occurs when the $PaCO_2$ is elevated above 45 mm Hg but the pH is not yet within normal range. Complete compensation is identified when the $PaCO_2$ rises enough to return the pH to normal. Predicting the expected compensation for metabolic alkalosis is difficult for the reasons mentioned previously. When the $PaCO_2$ is elevated significantly in the presence of metabolic alkalosis, the hypercarbia may actually represent respiratory acidosis.

Limitations of Compensation for Acid-Base Disorders

When severe deviations from the normal range occur with one acid-base component, it is not always possible for the other component to compensate completely. In a patient with a primary metabolic acid-base disorder and a normal respiratory system, compensation by elevated or decreased $PaCO_2$ can occur only within the limitations of the respiratory system. Changes in plasma HCO_3^- (only within the limitations of the renal system) can compensate for primary respiratory acid-base disorders.

The likelihood of compensation returning the pH to a normal range is inversely proportional to the degree of the primary disturbance. For example, in chronic respiratory acidosis, at a $PaCO_2$ of 50 mm Hg, 75% of patients may have a pH within a normal range. At a $PaCO_2$ of 60 mm Hg, the likelihood decreases to 15%.

The extent of compensation that is possible for any respiratory or metabolic disorder has been determined by human and animal studies. The data accumulated from these studies have been developed into 95% confidence limit bands.[4] The confidence limit bands describe the compensation limits the majority of patients (95%) are able to achieve and aid in the proper interpretation of acid-base disorders. For example, a pH of 7.38 and $PaCO_2$ of 85 mm Hg with an elevated plasma HCO_3^- traditionally would be interpreted as completely compensated respiratory acidosis. However, the 95% confidence limit bands demonstrate that most patients' HCO_3^- cannot elevate enough to fully compensate for a $PaCO_2$ of 85 mm Hg. In this example, the correct interpretation is probably chronic respiratory acidosis with a superimposed metabolic alkalosis. Serial ABG measurements and consideration of other clinical data usually are helpful in the interpretation of ABG measurements, because the exact limitations of compensation cannot be determined for any one patient.

Mixed Acid-Base Disorders*

When two of the simple acid-base abnormalities previously reviewed occur simultaneously, a mixed acid-base disorder results. Mixed disorders are less common than simple disorders

*Portions of this section are adapted from Narins RG, Emmett M: Simple and mixed acid-base disorders: A practical approach, *Medicine (Baltimore)* 59:161-187, 1980.

and can be more difficult to identify. When both components of acid-base balance (HCO_3^- and $PaCO_2$) simultaneously deviate from the normal range toward either acidosis or alkalosis, the mixed acid-base disorder can be identified more readily. However, if one component alters toward acidosis or alkalosis and the other component alters toward the opposite acid-base imbalance, the mixed disorder is more difficult to recognize.

Accurate interpretation of mixed disorders requires a complete understanding of the simple disorders and the clinical situations in which they occur. In most situations, the first clue to a mixed acid-base disorder comes from the clinical findings of the patient's history, physical examination, and other laboratory tests. In addition, each simple disorder alters acid-base balance and electrolyte concentration in a predictable manner. Identification of mixed disorders requires a thorough understanding of the extent of metabolic and respiratory compensation that should occur for each simple disorder. When the degree of compensation for what is thought to be the primary simple disorder is not appropriate, a mixed disorder usually is present (Table 7-4). A brief review of the criteria and clinical situations associated with the more common mixed acid-base disorders follows.

Respiratory and Metabolic Acidosis

Mixed acid-base disorders such as respiratory and metabolic acidosis are identified easily by an elevated $PaCO_2$ and a reduction in plasma HCO_3^-. Hypercapnia and low plasma HCO_3^- act synergistically to reduce pH significantly. Even mild hypercapnia ($PaCO_2$ = 50 mm Hg) occurring with a moderate reduction in plasma HCO_3^- (15 to 17 mEq/L) results in profound acidosis

Table 7-4	Summary of Expected Compensation for Acute and Chronic Acid-Base Disorders
Primary Disorder	**Expected Compensation**
Acute respiratory acidosis	For a 15 mm Hg increase in $PaCO_2$ the HCO_3^- increases 1 mEq/L; significant compensation takes 24-48 hr
Chronic respiratory acidosis	For every 10 mm Hg the $PaCO_2$ increases, the HCO_3^- increases 4 mEq/L
Acute respiratory alkalosis	For every 5 mm Hg decrease in $PaCO_2$, HCO_3^- decreases 1 mEq; significant compensation requires 24-48 hr
Chronic respiratory alkalosis	HCO_3^- falls 5 mEq/L for every 10 mm Hg fall in $PaCO_2$
Metabolic acidosis	$PaCO_2$ = last two digits of pH $PaCO_2 = (1.5 \times HCO_3^-) + 8 \pm 2$
Metabolic alkalosis	$PaCO_2$ change is variable; $PaCO_2$ usually does not elevate above 50-55 mm Hg. For each 1 mEq/L increase in HCO_3^-, $PaCO_2$ increases 0.6 mm Hg

(pH less than 7.15). This mixed disorder occurs in a variety of situations, including the following.

Cardiopulmonary resuscitation

Sudden failure of the heart to pump blood results in apnea and diffuse tissue hypoxia. The combination of tissue hypoxia and hypoventilation, often seen during resuscitation, is manifested as lactic (metabolic) and respiratory acidosis. Adequate ventilation, oxygenation, and perfusion must be reestablished if resuscitation is to be successful.

Chronic obstructive pulmonary disease and hypoxia

Many patients with chronic obstructive pulmonary disease (COPD) have chronic elevation of $PaCO_2$. Even if hypoxemia is also present, most patients with COPD maintain adequate tissue oxygenation by increasing hematocrit and cardiac output. However, metabolic acidosis may occur with significant electrolyte disturbances, sudden hypotension, renal failure, or anemia. Sudden hypotension and anemia result in tissue hypoxia and lactic acidosis. In these situations, plasma HCO_3^- may be reduced and $PaCO_2$ may remain elevated, resulting in the mixed acid-base disorder.

Poisoning and drug overdose

Many cases of poison and drug overdose result in depression of the respiratory center and respiratory acidosis. The poisons and drugs may also be metabolized to strong acids and produce metabolic acidosis. The hypoventilation usually is recognized as a result of shallow and slow breathing. The history of drug overdose or poisoning and the clinical signs of hypoventilation should be enough to prompt initiation of intubation and mechanical ventilation without waiting for ABG results. Metabolic acidosis is identified only by ABG measurements and is treated with infusion of bicarbonate in some cases.

Metabolic and Respiratory Alkalosis

This is a mixed acid-base disorder that is recognized by an elevated plasma HCO_3^- and a $PaCO_2$ below normal. The additive effects of simultaneous respiratory and metabolic alkalosis may result in severe alkalosis. The superimposition of one disorder on the other does not allow any compensation for either primary disorder. The resulting degree of alkalosis depends on the severity of the two primary disorders but usually is significant. Two clinical situations that can result in these mixed disorders are reviewed briefly.

Critical care unit

Respiratory alkalosis in the critical care unit may be induced by hypoxemia, hypotension, neurologic damage, excessive mechanical ventilation, anxiety, pain, or any combination of these and other problems. Metabolic alkalosis often results from

nasogastric suctioning, vomiting, blood transfusions, or antacid therapy. The resulting alkalosis can be severe and can result in a number of complications (e.g., cardiac arrhythmias).

Ventilator-induced alkalosis

Ventilator-induced alkalosis often occurs when patients with COPD are intubated and mechanically ventilated. These patients often have chronic hypercapnia with compensatory elevated plasma HCO_3^- levels. Acute respiratory failure may occur, requiring the temporary institution of mechanical ventilation. If the mechanical ventilation is excessive and reduces $PaCO_2$ to a normal range (35 to 45 mm Hg) or below, respiratory alkalosis results. The plasma HCO_3^- remains elevated, yielding the mixed alkalosis. This problem can be avoided if initial ventilator settings are set to maintain $PaCO_2$ at normal values for that patient or if the ventilator is adjusted to lower $PaCO_2$ slowly.

Metabolic Acidosis and Respiratory Alkalosis

Mixed disorders such as metabolic acidosis and respiratory alkalosis may be more difficult to recognize, because either abnormality usually compensates for the other. Most often, metabolic acidosis occurs as the primary disorder, and a predictable degree of hypocapnia compensates for the acidosis. Whenever metabolic acidosis is accompanied by a $PaCO_2$ that is lower than the predicted level for the degree of acidosis, a respiratory alkalosis is occurring simultaneously. In this situation, the pH may be elevated slightly above 7.40 and give the appearance of a compensated respiratory alkalosis. Conversely, this mixed disorder may be diagnosed in a patient with primary respiratory alkalosis when the degree of reduction in plasma HCO_3^- exceeds the predicted amount. Serial ABG measurements and clinical evaluation of the patient make the assessment of this mixed disorder accurate.

The situations that cause metabolic acidosis or respiratory alkalosis have already been reviewed. Critically ill patients are most likely to have mixed acid-base disorders and have been shown to have a poor prognosis when this mixed acid-base disorder occurs.

Metabolic Alkalosis and Respiratory Acidosis

When a patient with respiratory acidosis has an inappropriate elevation of plasma HCO_3^- concentration, the mixed disorder of metabolic alkalosis and respiratory acidosis may be diagnosed. Conversely, when a patient with a known metabolic alkalosis has an inappropriately elevated $PaCO_2$, a complicating respiratory acidosis is occurring. The pH in such situations is determined by the severity of each simple disorder and may be lower than, higher than, or within normal range. A pH of 7.40 occurring simultaneously with significant abnormalities in $PaCO_2$ and plasma HCO_3^- indicates that a mixed disorder is present, because normal compensation of a single disorder never returns pH to 7.40.

A typical clinical situation in which mixed metabolic alkalosis and respiratory acidosis may occur is treatment of the patient with COPD who has chronic respiratory acidosis. This type of patient often is treated with diuretics and steroid therapy, which can induce metabolic alkalosis. The complicating metabolic alkalosis may promote further hypoventilation and worsen the clinical picture. Metabolic alkalosis can make weaning of the patient from mechanical ventilation difficult because it decreases the patient's drive to breathe. Recognition and treatment of the metabolic alkalosis is vital to optimizing the patient's respiratory function and often results in a significant reduction in $PaCO_2$.

SUMMARY OF INTERPRETING BLOOD GAS MEASUREMENTS

Acid-Base Assessment

Step 1

Identify the pH measurement. If pH is within normal range, a normal acid-base status, a completely compensated acid-base disorder, or a mixed acid-base disorder is present. A normal acid-base status is obvious by a normal $PaCO_2$ (35 to 45 mm Hg) and plasma HCO_3^- (22 to 26 mm Hg). If plasma HCO_3^- and $PaCO_2$ are both abnormal with a pH within the normal range, either a fully compensated or mixed acid-base disorder is present.

If pH is lower than 7.35, an acidosis is occurring. Look at plasma HCO_3^- and $PaCO_2$ to identify which is contributing to the acidosis. An elevated $PaCO_2$ (greater than 45 mm Hg) indicates respiratory acidosis, whereas a decrease in plasma HCO_3^- (less than 22 mEq/L) indicates metabolic acidosis.

If pH is greater than 7.45, alkalosis is present. An increase in plasma HCO_3^- (more than 26 mEq/L) indicates metabolic alkalosis, whereas a decrease in $PaCO_2$ (less than 35 mm Hg) indicates respiratory alkalosis.

Step 2

Once the acid-base disorder is identified as respiratory or metabolic, look for the degree of compensation occurring. An elevation in plasma HCO_3^- compensates for respiratory acidosis, and a decrease in plasma HCO_3^- compensates for respiratory alkalosis. A decrease in $PaCO_2$ compensates for metabolic acidosis, and an elevation in $PaCO_2$ compensates for metabolic alkalosis.

In general, the degree of compensation is classified as *uncompensated* when the compensatory component is within normal range, *partially compensated* when the compensatory component is appropriately abnormal but pH is not yet within normal range, and *fully compensated* when the compensatory component alters enough to return the pH to normal range. Full compensation is not likely if the primary disorder is severe. When fully compensated acid-base disorders are present, the original abnormality can be identified by comparing the pH to the $PaCO_2$ and plasma HCO_3^-. If the pH is on the acid side of 7.40 (7.35 to 7.39), the acid-base component that lends itself to acidosis (either increased $PaCO_2$ or decreased plasma HCO_3^-) is the

component for which compensation is taking place. If the pH is on the alkaline side of 7.40 (7.41 to 7.45), the acid-base component that lends itself to alkalosis (either decreased $PaCO_2$ or increased plasma HCO_3^-) is the component for which compensation is taking place (Table 7-5).

Compensation for a primary acid-base disturbance often occurs in a predictable manner. This is particularly true for metabolic acidosis, respiratory alkalosis, and respiratory acidosis. A mixed acid-base problem probably is present when the predicted compensation is not present.

Oxygenation Assessment

Step 1

Identify the PaO_2 and determine whether it is below or within normal range. The normal predicted PaO_2 is dependent on the patient's age, FIO_2, and barometric pressure. In general, a PaO_2 lower than 80 mm Hg in a patient younger than 60 years of age is abnormal, and hypoxemia is occurring. A PaO_2 of 60 to 79 mm Hg is considered mild hypoxemia, 40 to 59 mm Hg is considered moderate hypoxemia, and less than 40 mm Hg is considered severe hypoxemia. A significant difference between PaO_2 and PaO_2 [$P(A - a)O_2$] indicates shunt, $\dot{V}/\dot{Q}$ mismatching, or diffusion defect. Hypoxemia with a normal $P(A - a)O_2$ may occur with an elevated $PaCO_2$ and when breathing at high altitude.

Step 2

Identify the level of oxygen saturation on the hemoglobin (SaO_2). SaO_2 should be maintained above 90% in the upper flat portion of the oxyhemoglobin dissociation curve in most cases.

Table 7-5	Summary of Simple Acid-Base Disorders		
	pH	$PaCO_2$	HCO_3^-
Respiratory alkalosis			
Uncompensated	↑	↓	N
Partially compensated	↑	↓	↓
Fully compensated	N	↓	↓
Respiratory acidosis			
Uncompensated	↓	↑	N
Partially compensated	↓	↑	↑
Fully compensated	N	↑	↑
Metabolic acidosis			
Uncompensated	↓	N	↓
Partially compensated	↓	↓	↓
Fully compensated	N	↓	↓
Metabolic alkalosis			
Uncompensated	↑	N	↑
Partially compensated	↑	↑	↑
Fully compensated	N	↑	↑

N, Within normal range; ↑, above normal range; ↓, below normal range.

In the upper portion of the curve, moderate decreases in the PaO_2 do not cause significant reductions in SaO_2 and oxygen content of the hemoglobin. If the SaO_2 is below 90% in the steep part of the oxyhemoglobin dissociation curve, small changes in PaO_2 will produce significant changes in SaO_2. SaO_2 may be abnormally decreased with hypoxemia and carbon monoxide poisoning. Actual measurement of SaO_2 with a co-oximeter is crucial when carbon monoxide poisoning is suspected.

Step 3

Identify the hemoglobin concentration and CaO_2, if available. Hemoglobin and CaO_2 measurements from co-oximeters are reliable. CaO_2 measurements from laboratories without co-

oximeters are calculated and may not be accurate. A recent hemoglobin measurement from the CBC can provide an estimation of the oxygen-carrying capacity of the blood when a co-oximeter is not available. A normal PaO_2 and SaO_2 are of little value without an adequate hemoglobin concentration.

Step 4

Assess the adequacy of tissue oxygenation using available data. Tissue oxygenation depends on adequate oxygenation and circulation of the arterial blood. Evaluation of circulation and tissue oxygenation can be achieved by assessment of the sensorium, blood pressure, extremity temperature and pulses, and mixed venous oxygen ($P\bar{v}O_2$).

CASE STUDY 1

J.B. is a 52-year-old white man admitted to the hospital following a sudden onset of severe chest pain and shortness of breath. Thirty minutes after admission to the intensive care unit, J.B. suffered a cardiopulmonary arrest. Cardiopulmonary resuscitation was initiated and was successful after approximately 10 minutes.

The initial examination after cardiopulmonary resuscitation revealed that J.B. had hypotension with a spontaneous respiratory rate of 40 breaths/min and a heart rate of 120 beats/min. He was comatose, with central cyanosis, cool extremities, inspiratory and expiratory course crackles, and weak pulses. The initial blood gas measurements after resuscitation were as follows:

	Results	Normal Range
pH	7.16	7.35-7.45
$PaCO_2$	40 mm Hg	35-45 mm Hg
PaO_2	60 mm Hg	74-82 mm Hg
SaO_2	85%	>92%
CaO_2	11 vol%	16-20 vol%
HCO_3^-	14 mEq/L	22-26 mEq/L
Base excess	(−14)	±2
FIO_2	1.0	—
$P(A-a)O_2$	665 mm Hg	50-70 mm Hg

Interpretation: The pH is well below normal, indicating that acidosis is present. The plasma HCO_3^- is reduced and

the $PaCO_2$ is normal, indicating metabolic acidosis as the primary problem.

When primary metabolic acidosis is occurring, the expected compensatory change in $PaCO_2$ can be calculated by using the following formula:

$$PaCO_2 = (1.5 \times HCO_3^-) + 8 \pm 2$$

$$\text{Expected } PaCO_2 = (1.5 \times 14) + 8 = 29 \pm 2$$

Because the measured $PaCO_2$ is higher than this value, a ventilatory disorder also must be occurring. A lack of adequate pulmonary perfusion probably is resulting in an increase in wasted or dead space ventilation. Metabolic and respiratory acidosis are present in this case.

The PaO_2 of 60 mm Hg is considered mild hypoxemia; however, considering that J.B. is breathing 100% oxygen, the PaO_2 is significantly below the predicted value. The $P(A-a)O_2$ is elevated significantly because of shunt, $\dot{V}/\dot{Q}$ mismatching, diffusion defect, or a combination of these. The SaO_2 and CaO_2 are significantly lower than normal. Because CaO_2 is reduced proportionally more than SaO_2, the patient must be anemic.

The clinical signs of tissue hypoxia and metabolic acidosis probably are related. The lack of adequate oxygenation and circulation of the arterial blood is resulting in anaerobic metabolism and lactic acidosis. Whenever hypoxemia and the clinical signs of inadequate perfusion occur simultaneously, metabolic acidosis from the production of lactic acid is a possibility.

CASE STUDY 2

K.M. is a 12-year-old boy brought to the emergency department with chief complaints of shortness of breath and cough. His past medical history was positive for allergies and atopic disorders (eczema). His family history was also positive for allergies and asthma. Physical examination revealed the following:

Pulse	124 beats/min
Respiratory rate	35 breaths/min
Blood pressure	120/76 mm Hg
Temperature	98.9° F

K.M. was restless and used his accessory muscles to breathe. Bilateral expiratory wheezes were heard on auscultation. His chest was clear to percussion but appeared hyperexpanded. His expiratory phase was prolonged. The CBC demonstrated a slight increase in white blood cells as a result of eosinophilia. The hemoglobin and hematocrit levels were within normal limits. ABG measurements were as follows:

	Results	Normal Range
pH	7.49	7.35-7.45
$PaCO_2$	32 mm Hg	35-45 mm Hg
PaO_2	68 mm Hg	95-103 mm Hg
SaO_2	91.5%	>95%
CaO_2	16 vol%	16-20 vol%
HCO_3^-	22 mEq/L	22-26 mEq/L
Base excess	(−1)	±2
FIO_2	0.21	—
$P(A − a)O_2$	40 mm Hg	<10 mm Hg

Interpretation: The pH is alkalotic and corresponds to the decrease in $PaCO_2$. Because plasma HCO_3^- is within normal range, the acid-base status is classified as simple uncompensated respiratory alkalosis.

PaO_2 and SaO_2 are reduced mildly and indicate mild hypoxemia. However, the CaO_2 is within the lower limits of normal. Therefore anemia must not be present. The increase in $P(A − a)O_2$ indicates that the respiratory disturbance is causing shunt, $\dot{V}/\dot{Q}$ mismatching, or diffusion defect. The clinical signs of hypoxemia are evident by the tachycardia and tachypnea. The hypoxemia probably would be worse if the patient were not hyperventilating.

The respiratory alkalosis is a result of the tachypnea and air hunger. The patient has an increase in the work of breathing because of diffuse airway obstruction, as evidenced by the expiratory wheezing. It is important to note that, although the ABG measurements do not identify any severe abnormalities, the patient's cardiopulmonary system is working hard to maintain these borderline measurements. Without proper treatment, the patient's condition could deteriorate rapidly.

CASE STUDY 3

C.B. is a 57-year-old white man with a history of chronic cough and sputum production. He was admitted to the hospital for abdominal surgery. On admission, C.B. was noted to be using his accessory muscles to breathe, and he appeared mildly short of breath at rest. He had diminished breath sounds bilaterally, increased anteroposterior diameter, and increased resonance to percussion. He has an 80-pack/year smoking history. As part of the preoperative evaluation, blood gases were drawn and revealed the following:

	Results	Normal Range
pH	7.41	7.35-7.45
$PaCO_2$	61 mm Hg	35-45 mm Hg
PaO_2	66 mm Hg	76-84 mm Hg
SaO_2	91.4%	>93%
CaO_2	12.2 vol%	16-20 vol%
HCO_3^-	37 mEq/L	22-26 mEq/L
Base excess	+11	±2
FIO_2	2 L/min via cannula	—

Interpretation: The pH is within normal range; however, the $PaCO_2$ and plasma HCO_3^- are elevated above normal. The initial temptation is to interpret the acid-base status as completely compensated metabolic alkalosis, because the pH is on the alkaline side of 7.40. However, in light of the patient's history and physical examination findings and because patients with normal respiratory systems usually do not hypoventilate significantly to compensate for metabolic alkalosis, the correct interpretation probably is respiratory acidosis and metabolic alkalosis. A mixed acid-base disorder is occurring. A cause for metabolic alkalosis must be sought to optimize respiratory function before surgery.

Mild hypoxemia is present even though the patient is breathing supplemental oxygen through a nasal cannula. The hypoxemia probably is a result of hypoventilation and $\dot{V}/\dot{Q}$ mismatching. The CaO_2 is reduced because of the hypoxemia and anemia.

CASE STUDY 4

V.S. is a 25-year-old woman with no previous history of cardiopulmonary disease. She was admitted to the hospital with a history of frequent urination, excessive thirst, and nausea for the past 3 days. At the time of admission, her skin was warm and dry and her breathing was notably deep. She was drowsy but coherent. Blood gas and chemistry results were as follows:

	Results	Normal Range
pH	6.96	7.35-7.45
$PaCO_2$	17 mm Hg	35-45 mm Hg
PaO_2	110 mm Hg	90-99 mm Hg
SaO_2	99%	>95%
CaO_2	19 vol%	16-20 vol%
HCO_3^-	3.5 mEq/L	22-26 mEq/L
Base excess	(−24)	±2
FIO_2	0.21	—
Na^+	142	137-147 mEq/L
K^+	5.7	3.5-4.8 mEq/L
Cl^-	106	98-105 mEq/L

Interpretation: The pH is well below normal range (acidemia) and corresponds to the decrease in plasma HCO_3^-.

The PCO_2 is significantly reduced, indicating that the respiratory system is attempting to compensate for the severe metabolic acidosis.

The expected compensation for the metabolic acidosis can be calculated as follows:

$$PCO_2 = (1.5 \times 3.5) + 8 \pm 2$$
$$PCO_2 = (5.25) + 8 \pm 2$$
$$PCO_2 = 13.25 \pm 2$$

Because the measured PCO_2 is 17 mm Hg, a slight respiratory problem may be present. This slight increase in the PCO_2 above the expected level probably is explained by the fact that severe decreases in pH (less than 7.1) do not increase the patient's drive to breathe as much as when the pH is near 7.1.

The anion gap is 32 mEq/L. This result is well above the normal range of 8 to 16 and indicates that an anion gap metabolic acidosis is present, consistent with severe diabetic ketoacidosis.

The patient's oxygenation status is normal, with the PaO_2 actually higher than the predicted normal range. This has occurred because the profound hyperventilation has reduced the $PaCO_2$ and simultaneously raised the PAO_2 and PaO_2.

 CASE STUDY 5

M.P. is a 68-year-old man with a 10-year history of COPD. He produces sputum most days, especially in the morning hours. Although he smoked for more than 40 years, he currently is a nonsmoker. He came to the emergency department complaining of severe dyspnea and cough. His physical examination revealed increased anteroposterior diameter, cyanosis of the oral mucosa, expiratory wheezing, and heavy use of accessory muscles. His respiratory rate was 30 breaths/min and his heart rate was 110 beats/min. The emergency department physician ordered arterial blood gas studies, which revealed the following:

	Results	Normal Range
pH	7.28	7.35-7.45
$PaCO_2$	58 mm Hg	35-45 mm Hg
PaO_2	44 mm Hg	>80 mm Hg
SaO_2	84%	>94%
CaO_2	15.5 vol%	16-20 vol%
HCO_3^-	24 mEq/L	22-26 mEq/L
Base excess	(−4)	±2
FIO_2	2 L/min via cannula	—

Interpretation: The pH is well below normal range and indicates that an acidosis is present. The $PaCO_2$ is elevated, indicating the acidosis is at least partly respiratory in origin.

Given this patient's history, we can assume that a chronic respiratory acidosis is likely. The expected compensation for chronic respiratory acidosis is an elevation of the plasma bicarbonate approximately 4 mEq/L for each 10 mm Hg the $PaCO_2$ is elevated above 40 mm Hg. Because this patient's $PaCO_2$ is nearly 60 mm Hg (20 above 40), the plasma bicarbonate should be approximately 32 mEq/L (24 + 8) to compensate for the respiratory acidosis. Because the measured plasma bicarbonate is well below this number, a coinciding metabolic acidosis must also be present. Mixed respiratory and metabolic acidosis is occurring. The cause for the metabolic acidosis needs to be identified to allow prompt treatment. The acidosis is a potent stimulus to the patient's drive to breathe and is probably contributing to his sensation of dyspnea.

The PaO_2 of 44 mm Hg indicates that moderate hypoxemia is present despite the application of low-flow oxygen therapy. Given that the CaO_2 is reduced only minimally, the patient must not be anemic and probably has mild polycythemia. The hypoxemia is also a potent stimulus to the patient's drive to breathe and is contributing to his sensation of breathlessness. The FIO_2 should be increased, and further assessment of his respiratory system is needed (e.g., chest radiograph) to identify the causes of the hypoxemia.

REVIEW QUESTIONS

1. T F Arterial blood reflects lung function better than venous blood, because arterial blood is not affected by tissue metabolism.

2. Before an ABG is obtained, the patient's clotting parameters should be evaluated because:
   a. They may affect the patient's PaO_2.
   b. If reduced, they may hinder filling of the syringe with blood during the draw.
   c. Bleeding time may be prolonged if they are abnormal.
   d. All of the above.

3. Which of the following is a common site for arterial puncture?
   a. Radial artery
   b. Aorta
   c. Temporal artery
   d. Jugular artery

4. Which of the following tests is performed to check the collateral circulation of the radial artery before puncture?
   a. Wilson's test
   b. Perfusion scan
   c. Sack's test
   d. Allen's test

5. For the test in Question 4, "pinking up" of the hand is normal if it occurs within _____ seconds.
   a. 10-15
   b. 15-20
   c. 20-25
   d. 25-30

6. T F Air bubbles in the blood gas syringe after puncture do not affect the values obtained during the analysis of the blood gas.

7. An arterial puncture site normally should be compressed for a minimum of ___ minutes after the puncture.
   a. 1-2
   b. 3-5
   c. 5-7
   d. 8-10

8. What is the normal value for arterial pH?
   a. 7.20-7.30
   b. 7.35-7.45
   c. 7.45-7.50
   d. Greater than 7.50

9. What is the normal value for PaO_2?
   a. 50-60 mm Hg
   b. 60-70 mm Hg
   c. 70-80 mm Hg
   d. 80-100 mm Hg

10. What is the normal value for CaO_2?
    a. 16-20 vol%
    b. 12-16 vol%
    c. 8-12 vol%
    d. 4-8 vol%

11. What is the normal value for $P\bar{v}O_2$?
    a. 25-29 mm Hg
    b. 32-35 mm Hg
    c. 38-42 mm Hg
    d. 45-55 mm Hg

12. Which of the following factors affects the PaO_2?
    a. Patient age
    b. Altitude
    c. Inspired oxygen concentration
    d. All of the above

13. Which of the following is the best indicator of oxygen transport?
    a. PaO_2
    b. SaO_2
    c. CaO_2
    d. $P(A-a)O_2$

14. T F $P\bar{v}O_2$ can be used as an indicator of tissue oxygenation.

15. T F A decrease in tissue oxygenation is called *hypoxia*.

16. Which of the following is *not* a true statement regarding the term *hypoxemia*?
    a. It occurs when the patient's PaO_2 is lower than the predicted range when breathing room air.
    b. It indicates a condition in which the tissue oxygenation is inadequate.
    c. It is classified as mild, moderate, or severe.
    d. It occurs at different PaO_2 levels depending on the age of the patient.

17. Which of the following physiologic causes of hypoxemia is the most common?
    a. Hypoventilation
    b. $\dot{V}/\dot{Q}$ mismatch
    c. Shunt
    d. Diffusion defect

18. Which of the following shifts the oxyhemoglobin dissociation curve to the left?
    a. Increased $PaCO_2$
    b. Decreased pH
    c. Increased body temperature
    d. None of the above

19. T   F   A shift to the right in the oxyhemoglobin dissociation curve results in an increased affinity of hemoglobin for oxygen.

20. T   F   A shift to the left in the oxyhemoglobin dissociation curve is an advantage at the tissues.

21. The negative log of the hydrogen ion concentration is defined as which of the following?
    a. $Paco_2$
    b. Base excess
    c. Standard HCO_3^-
    d. pH

22. T   F   An arterial blood pH less than 7.35 is called *acidosis*.

23. T   F   Alkalosis results in depression of the CNS and may lead to coma.

24. Which of the following parameters is the respiratory component of acid-base status?
    a. $Paco_2$
    b. HCO_3^-
    c. Pao_2
    d. Base excess

25. T   F   Air increase in $Paco_2$ causes a direct increase in plasma HCO_3^-.

26. Which of the following is the best indicator of metabolic acid-base status?
    a. Plasma HCO_3^-
    b. Base excess
    c. Standard HCO_3^-
    d. T40 HCO_3^-

27. Which of the following ratios of $HCO_3^-/Paco_2$ result in a pH of 7.40?
    a. 20:1
    b. 10:0.5
    c. 7:0.35
    d. All of the above

28. Which of the following is a correct representation of the Henderson-Hasselbalch equation?
    a. $pK = pH - \log (Paco_2 \times 0.03)/HCO_3^-$
    b. $pK = pH - \log HCO_3^-/(Paco_2 \times 0.03)$
    c. $pH = pK + \log HCO_3^-/(Paco_2 \times 0.03)$
    d. $pH = pK - \log HCO_3^-/(Paco_2 \times 0.03)$

29. T   F   An example of a simple acid-base disorder is one in which both the respiratory and the metabolic components cause alkalosis.

30. A 32-year-old man comes to the emergency department after a traffic accident with the following data: pulse, 118 beats/min; respiratory rate, 27 breaths/min; blood pressure, 100/68 mm Hg; paradoxical chest movement on left side; breath sounds decreased on left; and ABG (21%) as follows: pH, 7.32; $Paco_2$, 70 mm Hg; Pao_2, 57 mm Hg; HCO_3^-, 23 mEq/L; base excess, 0; Sao_2, 86%, Cao_2, 15.2 vol%; Hb, 13.0 g/dL; $P(A - a)o_2$, 18 mm Hg. Based on this information, what is the primary cause of the patient's hypoxemia?
    a. Overall hypoventilation
    b. $\dot{V}/\dot{Q}$ mismatch
    c. Diffusion defect
    d. Shunt

31. Which of the following is true regarding respiratory alkalosis?
    a. The $Paco_2$ is less than 35 mm Hg.
    b. An increase in HCO_3^- compensates for respiratory alkalosis.
    c. It is called completely compensated if the pH is 7.52.
    d. It is called partially compensated if the pH is in the normal range.

32. A patient has the following ABG results:
    pH 7.25
    $Paco_2$ 32 mm Hg
    HCO_3^- 16 mEq/L
    Base excess −10 mEq/L
    Based on these findings, the patient has which of the following?
    a. Compensated metabolic acidosis
    b. Uncompensated respiratory acidosis
    c. Uncompensated metabolic acidosis
    d. Compensated respiratory acidosis

33. A 35-year-old, 54-kg woman with congestive heart failure enters the emergency department short of breath. An ABG shows the following results:
    pH 7.50
    $Paco_2$ 30 mm Hg
    HCO_3^- 23 mEq/L
    Base excess +2 mEq/L
    The patient's ABG results indicate which of the following?
    a. Uncompensated respiratory alkalosis
    b. Compensated respiratory acidosis
    c. Uncompensated metabolic alkalosis
    d. Uncompensated metabolic acidosis

34. Given the following ABG results, interpret the acid-base status:
    pH 7.44
    $Paco_2$ 25 mm Hg
    HCO_3^- 17 mEq/L
    Base excess −6 mEq/L
    a. Compensated metabolic acidosis
    b. Uncompensated respiratory alkalosis
    c. Uncompensated respiratory acidosis
    d. Compensated respiratory alkalosis

35. A 17-year-old man is brought into the emergency department. Vitals are as follows: pulse, 100 beats/min; respiratory rate, 4 breaths/min; and blood pressure, 100/65 mm Hg. The patient was at a party, where he was discovered by his friends to be slumped in a chair and unresponsive. ABG results are as follows:

    pH   7.29
    $PaCO_2$ 68 mm Hg
    HCO_3^- 31 mEq/L
    Base excess +1 mEq/L

    The patient's acid-base status is classified as which of the following?
    a. Uncompensated respiratory acidosis
    b. Partially compensated respiratory acidosis
    c. Compensated respiratory alkalosis
    d. Uncompensated metabolic acidosis

36. Given the following ABG parameters, how would the acid-base status be interpreted?

    pH   7.53
    $PaCO_2$ 31 mm Hg
    PaO_2 90 mm Hg
    HCO_3^- 25 mEq/L
    Base excess +5 mEq/L

    a. Uncompensated metabolic alkalosis
    b. Partially compensated respiratory alkalosis
    c. Metabolic and respiratory alkalosis
    d. Compensated respiratory alkalosis

37. T F An acute increase in $PaCO_2$ of 10 to 15 mm Hg causes an increase in plasma HCO_3^- of 1 mEq/L.

38. T F A chronic decrease in $PaCO_2$ of 5 mm Hg causes a decrease in plasma HCO_3^- of 1 mEq/L.

39. Which of the following could cause metabolic acidosis?
    a. Kidney disease
    b. Diabetic ketoacidosis
    c. Diarrhea
    d. All of the above

    Answer the following questions based on the following blood gas data:
    pH   7.21
    $PaCO_2$ 67 mm Hg
    PaO_2 49 mm Hg
    SaO_2 76%
    Hb   10.1 g/dL
    CaO_2 10.4 vol%
    Bicarbonate 26 mEq/L
    Base excess −2 mEq/L

40. The 95% confidence limit bands in ABG interpretation refers to which of the following statements?
    a. They are the percentage of research data supporting the idea of buffer compensation.
    b. They are the percentage of mixed acid-base disorders achieving complete compensation.

c. Complete compensation occurs when the pH returns to 95% of normal.
d. They are compensation limits that most patients are able to achieve.

41. Which of the following is true regarding the PaO_2?
    a. It is adequate.
    b. It shows mild hypoxemia.
    c. It shows moderate hypoxemia.
    d. It shows severe hypoxemia.

41. Which of the following is true regarding oxygen-carrying capacity?
    a. It is normal.
    b. It is increased.
    c. It is decreased.
    d. Unable to determine with the given data.

42. The acid-base status is classified as which of the following?
    a. Uncompensated metabolic alkalosis
    b. Partially compensated metabolic alkalosis
    c. Uncompensated respiratory acidosis
    d. Partially compensated respiratory acidosis

43. Which of the following could cause this patient's problem?
    a. Anxiety and fear
    b. Acute airway obstruction
    c. Lactic acid production
    d. All of the above

REFERENCES

1. AARC clinical practice guideline: Sampling for arterial blood gas analysis. American Association for Respiratory Care, *Respir Care* 37:913-917, 1992.
2. AARC Clinical practice guideline: Blood gas analysis and hemoximetry: 2001 revision and update, *Respir Care* 46:498-505, 2001.
3. Hawkes AP, McCammon JB, Hoffman RE: Indoor use of concrete saws and other gas-powered equipment. Analysis of reported carbon monoxide poisoning cases in Colorado, *J Occup Environ Med* 40:49-54, 1998.
4. McCurdy DK: Mixed metabolic and respiratory acid-base disturbances: Diagnosis and treatment, *Chest* 62 (Suppl):35S-44S, 1972.

BIBLIOGRAPHY

Kacmarek RM: Assessment of gas exchange and acid-base balance. In Pierson DJ, Kacmarek RM, editors: *Foundations of respiratory care*, New York, 1992, Churchill Livingstone.
Shapiro BA and others: *Clinical application of blood gases*, ed 4, St Louis, 1989, Mosby.
Wilkins RL, Stoller JK, Scanlon CL: *Egan's fundamentals of respiratory care*, ed 8, St Louis, 2003, Mosby.

C H A P T E R

8

Richard L. Sheldon

Pulmonary Function Testing

LEARNING OBJECTIVES

Upon completion of this chapter, the reader should be able to accomplish the following:

1. Recognize the general purpose of performing pulmonary function tests (PFTs).
2. Recognize the situations in which PFTs are indicated.
3. Identify a definition of the following terms:
   a. Spirometer
   b. Spirograph
   c. Spirogram
4. Identify how the following factors affect PFT measurements:
   a. Height and weight
   b. Gender
   c. Age
   d. Patient effort
5. Identify the standard equipment found in a PFT laboratory and its basic uses.
6. Recognize the primary abnormalities associated with obstructive and restrictive lung disease.
7. Given a specific site of airway obstruction, identify the part of the spirogram affected.
8. Identify the criteria for establishing a restrictive defect and the diseases that can cause restrictive patterns.
9. Identify two diseases that exhibit combined restrictive and obstructive defects.
10. Recognize a definition, approximate normal value, factors affecting, and significance of the following spirometric volumes and capacities:
    a. Tidal volume
    b. Minute volume
    c. Total lung capacity
    d. Vital capacity and slow vital capacity
    e. Residual volume (RV)
    f. Expiratory reserve volume
    g. Functional residual capacity (FRC)
    h. Inspiratory reserve volume
    i. Inspiratory capacity
    j. Maximal voluntary ventilation
11. Identify the theory and methods used to measure RV and FRC using the following techniques:

a. Body plethysmography
b. Open-circuit nitrogen washout
c. Closed-circuit helium dilution

12. Identify a definition, approximate normal value, factors affecting, and significance of the following spirometric flow measurements:
    a. Forced expiratory volume at 1 second (FEV_1) and FEV_1/forced vital capacity (FVC)
    b. Forced expiratory volume at 3 seconds (FEV_3) and FEV_3/FVC
    c. Forced expiratory flow 25% to 75%
    d. Peak expiratory flow
13. Given a description of a flow volume loop or a tracing of a flow volume loop, identify the respective patterns for obstructive and restrictive disease.
14. Identify the following regarding before and after PFT bronchodilator assessment:
    a. Purpose
    b. Criteria for improvement
    c. Validity in asthma versus other chronic obstructive pulmonary diseases
15. Identify the method of measurement, normal value, factors affecting, and significance of the following specialized pulmonary function studies:
    a. Diffusion capacity
    b. Airway resistance
    c. Compliance studies
    d. Nitrogen washout
    e. Closing volume (single breath nitrogen test)
    f. Volume of isoflow
    g. Respiratory quotient
    h. Bronchoprovocation testing
    i. Work of breathing
16. Recognize the general applications to respiratory care and pulmonary medicine of the following exercise tests:
    a. Stress electrocardiograph
    b. Ventilatory capacity
    c. Blood gases before and after exercise
    d. Exercise challenge
    e. Anaerobic threshold
    f. Maximal oxygen uptake

17. Identify the significance of the following applications of pulmonary function testing:
    a. Smoking cessation
    b. Intensive care
    c. Surgery
    d. Sleep apnea
    e. Environmental lung diseases
18. Given a PFT, interpret the results in terms of obstructive, restrictive, or normal lung function.

CHAPTER OUTLINE

Purpose of Pulmonary Function Testing
Normal Values
   Height and Weight
   Gender
   Age
   Other Considerations
Standard Pulmonary Function Laboratory Equipment
Classification: Obstructive and Restrictive Defects
   Obstructive Defects
   Restrictive Defects
   Combined Defects
Anatomy of a Normal Spirogram
   Tidal Volume
   Minute Volume
   Vital Capacity
   Total Lung Capacity
   Residual Volume
   Expiratory Reserve Volume
   Functional Residual Capacity
   Inspiratory Reserve Volume and Inspiratory Capacity
   Indices of Flows
   Maximal Voluntary Ventilation
   Flow Volume Curves (Flow Volume Loops)
   Pulmonary Function Testing Before and After Aerosol Bronchodilators
Specialized Pulmonary Function Studies
   Diffusion Capacity
   Airway Resistance
   Compliance Studies
   Nitrogen Washout
   Closing Volume
   Respiratory Quotient
   Exercise Testing
   Bronchoprovocation Testing
Other Applications of Pulmonary Function Testing
   Smoking Cessation
   Surgery
   Sleep Apnea
   Environmental Lung Diseases
Clinical Interpretation of Pulmonary Function Testing

KEY TERMS

airway resistance (Raw)
bronchoprovocation testing
capacity
closing volume (CV)
compliance
diffusion capacity (D_L)
expiratory reserve volume (ERV)
forced vital capacity (FVC)
functional residual capacity (FRC)
inspiratory capacity (IC)
inspiratory reserve volume (IRV)
maximal voluntary ventilation (MVV)
minute volume ($\dot{V}_E$)
nitrogen washout
obstructive disease
peak expiratory flow (PEF)
respiratory quotient (RQ)
restrictive disease
spirogram
spirograph
spirometer
vital capacity (VC)
volumes

CHAPTER OVERVIEW

Pulmonary function testing (PFT) is the process of having the patient perform specific inspiratory and expiratory maneuvers while breathing in and out of tubing attached to equipment that measures a variety of variables. The pulmonary function technician is responsible for explaining the testing procedure to the patient and coaching the patient in order to obtain the best possible results. The results are then documented and given to the attending physician for interpretation and follow-up treatment if needed. This chapter describes the tests respiratory therapists should be familiar with even if they do not work in a pulmonary function laboratory. It is not uncommon for a patient to be admitted to the hospital who has had previous PFT that is reported in the current chart. A quick review of these results may be instrumental in decision making about current treatment. In addition to defining the common pulmonary function tests performed, a brief discussion of what may cause abnormalities in the results is included.

PURPOSE OF PULMONARY FUNCTION TESTING

PFT is a way to determine the functional status of the lungs as it relates to how much gas (air) can be moved in and out of the lungs, how fast the gas can be moved, the stiffness of the lung and chest wall, the diffusion characteristics of the alveolar-capillary membrane through which the gas moves, and how well the lung responds to therapy. By using a combination of lung function tests, a nearly complete assessment of the pulmonary system can be made. The purpose of this chapter is to present the fundamentals of interpreting PFT results.

The patient is brought to a laboratory for testing where the necessary equipment is carefully maintained and calibrated by a skilled technician. In most cases, the patient should be stable and not in need of acute treatment before complete PFT is performed (Box 8-1). For example, the asthmatic patient in acute distress is not likely to tolerate much of the PFT that requires significant effort. Currently, PFT is used for the following:

- Screening for the presence of pulmonary disease (especially useful in determining which patients will be most harmed by smoking)[1]
- Evaluating the patient before surgery to determine the patient's ability to tolerate the surgical procedure
- Evaluating the effectiveness of therapy (e.g., determining if the patient responds to bronchodilators)
- Documenting the progression of pulmonary disease over time
- Studying the effects of exercise on the patient's lung function
- Measuring the degree of airway hyperresponsiveness ("bronchoprovocation testing")

NORMAL VALUES

The usefulness of PFT improves with the ability to predict normal ranges accurately. Then, as the measured values deviate from the normal predicted values, a judgment can be made regarding the severity of the disease process or the rate of recovery taking place within the lung. Nomograms are useful in rapidly determining predicted normals for spirometry (Figure 8-1).

The following basic variables may have an impact on lung function.

Height and Weight

Height is the most important factor influencing lung size and predicted values. Generally, the taller the person, the larger the lung size and predicted lung volumes.

As a person gains weight, lung size does not necessarily change unless the lower range of weight gain is considered separately from the higher range of weight gain. If a person gains weight by putting on muscle, a muscularity effect is seen by an increase in lung size. As the weight gain continues because of an increase in body fat, there is a reduction in lung size, which, if

---

BOX 8-1   Contraindications for Pulmonary Function Testing (PFT)*

Recent abdominal, thoracic, or eye surgery
Hemodynamic instability
Symptoms indicating acute severe illness (e.g., chest pain typical of angina, nausea and vomiting, high fever, severe dyspnea)
Recent hemoptysis
Pneumothorax
Recent history of abdominal, thoracic or cerebral aneurysm

*These conditions may interfere with obtaining reliable results, or the PFT may worsen the problem
Modified from American Association for Respiratory Care Clinical Practice Guideline: Spirometry, *Respir Care* 41:629, 1996.

---

allowed to continue, results in the obesity effect and reduced lung volumes. This two-phased weight effect makes it difficult to predict normal values in PFT. To account for this change in body habitus, the concept of surface area may be a better scale for predicting normal lung volumes than height and weight.

Gender

Some measurements in lung function vary with the sex of the individual. When individuals are matched for height and weight, male patients normally have larger lungs than female patients.

Age

The vital capacity (VC)—maximal amount of air that can be exhaled after a maximal inspiratory effort—increases in a person until the mid-20s. Lung size begins to decrease as the person ages past the 20s. An average 20-year-old has a predicted VC slightly over 5 L. By age 70, the same person's predicted VC will have fallen to approximately 4 L.

Other Considerations

Other poorly defined predictors of pulmonary function may include race, environmental factors, and altitude. The exact effects of these variables on lung function are not known.

In considering patient performance, it should be noted that many PFTs require maneuvers that are effort dependent, so variability occurs in each person on a day-by-day basis. This should be taken into consideration when interpreting and reviewing test results with a patient, especially when comparing current and previous studies. The technician coaching the patient during the PFT procedures should note the apparent level of effort by the patient and communicate this to the attending physician for consideration during interpretation of the results.

The quality of pulmonary function data can be compromised by various issues that can lead to errors in measurement and interpretation. Routine procedures that can reduce errors include accurate calibration of all testing equipment, selecting reference equations and lower limits of normal appropriate for both the patients studied and the equipment being used to study them (pediatric versus adult patients), avoiding the use of too many measurements to generate an interpretation, and taking into consideration the patient's clinical state when doing the interpretation (e.g., for the patient who has undergone a thoracotomy [surgical removal of one lung], interpretation is unique).

SIMPLY STATED
Height is the most important factor influencing predicted pulmonary function results. The taller the patient, the larger the predicted lung volumes.

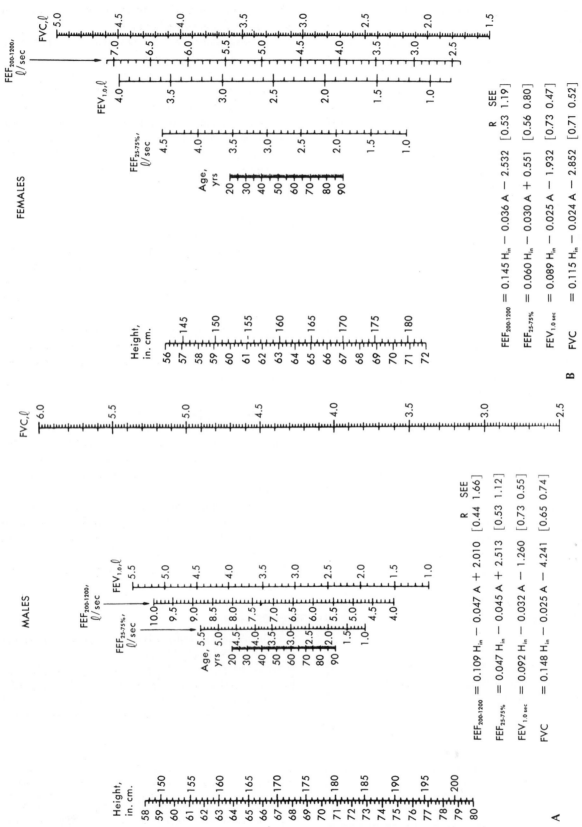

Figure 8-1 Spirometric standards for (**A**) males and (**B**) females (BTPS). (From Morris JF, Koski WA, Johnson LC: *Am Rev Resp Dis* 103:57, 1971.)

STANDARD PULMONARY FUNCTION LABORATORY EQUIPMENT

The primary instrument used in PFT has been the spirometer. It is designed to measure lung volumes and can measure only the lung volume compartments that exchange gas with the atmosphere. Spirometers with electronic signal outputs also measure flow (volume per unit of time). A device may be attached to the spirometer that graphically records the movement of gas in and out of the chest. This attachment is called a spirograph and the resulting tracing is a spirogram.

The American Thoracic Society has published a monograph that is useful in selecting and calibrating equipment.[2] Standardization of the methods for performing tests and reporting the results is necessary because of the numerous laboratories and variety of testing equipment available. It is recommended that PFT technicians make sure the equipment meets ATS standards before purchase and use.[3] Once purchased, the equipment must be calibrated on a daily basis to ensure accurate results.

State or Federal regulation of pulmonary function laboratories is currently unsettled. Clinical Laboratory Improvement Amendments (CLIA) regulations cover only the blood gas determinations. Of great concern is the lack of certification of competency of the individuals performing PFTs. Many State Licensing Boards are currently addressing the issue of how to regulate the technicians who perform PFTs.

Most equipment includes microprocessors to handle computerized evaluation and reporting. The modern pulmonary function laboratory has the following equipment (blood gas equipment is not included here):

- Spirometer with spirograph (for routine flows and volume)
- Body plethysmograph (for total lung capacity and airway resistance studies)
- Diffusion system (for measuring lung diffusion)
- Gas analysis (carbon dioxide, carbon monoxide, helium, nitrogen, and oxygen)

CLASSIFICATION: OBSTRUCTIVE AND RESTRICTIVE DEFECTS

Pulmonary function abnormalities can be grouped into two main categories: obstructive and restrictive defects. This grouping is based on the fact that the routine spirogram, as the centerpiece of PFT, measures two basic components: flow and volume. Obstructive disease is present if expiratory flow is below normal. If lung volume is reduced, a restrictive disease probably is present.

Obstructive Defects

Obstruction can occur in the upper and larger airways (larynx, trachea, right or left mainstream bronchi, bronchi) or in small airways (less than 2 mm). The anatomic site of obstruction to flow may be suggested by the part of the spirogram that is abnormally altered. Upper airway obstruction will reduce flow rates in the initial 25% of a forced expiratory VC maneuver. Obstruction in the smaller airways will reduce flow rates in the later portion of the exhaled volume.

It is important to recognize that the initial portion of the flow/volume curve generated by the patient's forced exhalation is to a large degree effort dependant. The harder he pushes, the more flow results. The later two thirds of the curve is the opposite—it is effort independent. This indicates that no matter how hard the patient tries to increase his flow rate, he can only reach a certain maximum speed. However, in order to reach this flow rate limitation at any given lung volume, the patient must generate sufficient intrathoracic pressure by exhaling very forcefully.

Restrictive Defects

A restrictive defect is present when lung volumes are reduced to less than 80% of predicted levels as measured by the routine spirogram or body plethysmograph. This category of disease includes chest wall dysfunction, neurologic diseases resulting in paralysis of the muscles of inspiration, dysfunction of the diaphragm, absent lung tissue, and scarring of the lungs as with interstitial lung disease. Atelectasis and obesity are two of the more common causes of a restrictive lung defect.

Combined Defects

Certain diseases can result in both obstructive and restrictive defects. Two examples are sarcoidosis* and emphysema. Sarcoidosis in its final stages severely reduces volume and limits airflow.

A better example of combined defects is severe emphysema, which results in obstruction to airflow out of the lungs. Thus the residual volume gas in the lung slowly increases and eventually restricts the volume of air that can be inspired. The net result is a combined obstructive and restrictive defect.

> **SIMPLY STATED**
> Obstructive lung diseases cause reduced expiratory flows, and restrictive lung diseases cause reduced lung volumes.

---

*Sarcoidosis is a disease of unknown cause characterized by the deposition of micronodules, called noncaseating granulomas, throughout the body. The granulomas have a predilection for the lungs. They also invade the brain, eyes, heart, liver, skin, and lymph nodes. Sarcoidosis has profound immunologic consequences. Treatment is usually inadequate. Some cases are self-limiting, with an occasional patient showing spontaneous remission of the entire disease process. The usual course is a slow progression of lung fibrosis.

ANATOMY OF A NORMAL SPIROGRAM

Before defining each part of the spirogram, it is worthwhile to note that lung volumes are single compartments in the lung. Adding two or more volumes together results in a lung capacity.

Volumes and capacities routinely identified are as follows (Figure 8-2):

- Tidal volume (V_T)
- Minute volume ($\dot{V}_E$)
- Vital capacity (VC)
- Total lung capacity (TLC)
- Residual volume (RV)
- Expiratory reserve volume (ERV)
- Functional residual capacity (FRC)
- Inspiratory reserve volume (IRV)
- Inspiratory capacity (IC)
- Maximal voluntary ventilation (MVV)

Tidal Volume

Tidal volume is the volume of air exhaled or inhaled during quiet breathing. The average values for healthy adults show considerable variation but usually fall between 350 and 600 mL. A decreased V_T can occur with both restrictive and obstructive disease. A fall in V_T without an increase in rate may result in hypoventilation and retention of arterial carbon dioxide tension (Pa_{CO_2}). Restrictive lung disease usually causes the patient to breathe with a smaller V_T. The breathing rate of the patient with restrictive lung disease increases in proportion to the loss in lung volume.

Minute Volume

The minute volume is the volume of gas expired over 1 minute. $\dot{V}_E$ is determined by adding each measured V_T in 1 minute or, if the patient's V_T is consistently the same size, by multiplying the rate by the average V_T. Normal $\dot{V}_E$ ranges

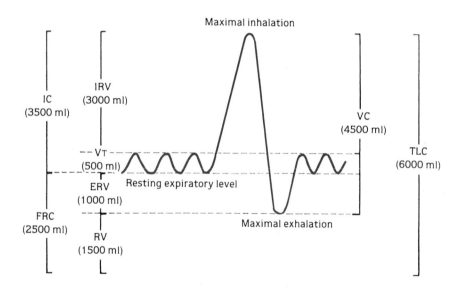

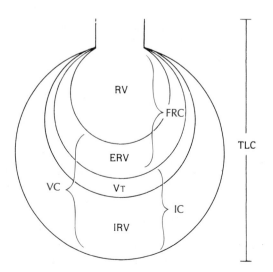

Figure 8-2 Lung volumes and capacities. Representation of a normal spirogram and divisions of lung volumes and capacities. Numbers are for average-sized young adults. See text for abbreviations. (From Scanlan CL, Spearman CB, Sheldon RL: *Egan's fundamentals of respiratory care*, ed 5, St Louis, 1990, Mosby.)

from 4 to 12 L/min at rest, depending on the size of the patient. The $\dot{V}E$ is the best index of ventilation when used in conjunction with arterial blood gas measurements. The $\dot{V}E$ should increase in response to exercise, fever, pain, hypoxia, and acidosis, regardless of whether the acidosis is caused by carbon dioxide retention (respiratory acidosis) or lactic acid or ketone body retention (metabolic acidosis).

Vital Capacity

Vital capacity is measured after the person has taken the deepest breath possible. The following exhaled volume should be the maximal amount the patient can exhale and is measured as the VC. If the patient forcefully exhales the volume, it is called the forced vital capacity (FVC) and is the most frequent way the VC is reported (Figure 8-3).

Proper coaching of the patient during the FVC maneuver is extremely important because the most common cause of erroneous results is suboptimal coaching.[4] The technician should use exaggerated body language to demonstrate the three phases of the FVC maneuver: (1) the maximal inspiratory effort, (2) the initial expiratory blast, and (3) the forceful emptying of the lungs. During the third phase, yelling at the patient to keep blowing is not recommended because it may lead to more air trapping in the obstructed patient.[4,5] Instead, the patient should pay attention to the motion of the bell of the volume spirometer or the computer incentive display to encourage complete emptying of the lungs. The PFT technician should also grade the patient effort during the PFT to communicate to the physician the level of confidence to be placed on the results.[4]

VC is not thought of as abnormally increased, only as abnormally decreased. Both restrictive and obstructive diseases can decrease VC. Restrictive lung disorders reduce FVC by shrinking the lung. Obstructive lung dysfunction causes a decrease in the FVC by causing a slow rise in the RV. Because the lung is contained in the thoracic cage, which is a rigid structure, room must be made for this expanding RV. The only space readily available is that used by VC. Therefore, as the RV increases, VC decreases.

VC is also reported as slow vital capacity (SVC). The SVC test is performed by having the patient completely exhale, slowly, following a maximal inspiration. A slow exhalation may allow more air to be exhaled from the lung because a slow

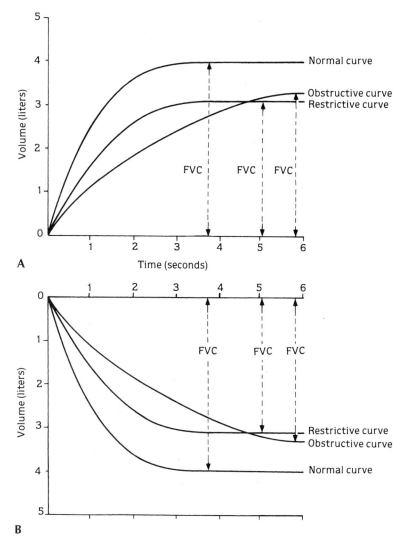

Figure 8-3 Forced vital capacity (FVC) curves comparing normal, obstructive, and restrictive disorders. **A,** Curves as they appear on commonly available spirometers with tracings beginning at bottom left corner. **B,** Same curves as they appear on some spirometers that begin tracings at upper left corner. (From Scanlan CL, Wilkins RL, Stoller JK: *Egan's fundamentals of respiratory care,* ed 7, St Louis, 1999, Mosby.)

exhalation helps reduce air trapping. In some patients forceful exhalation causes airways to close prematurely because of the high intrathoracic pressures produced. This early closure may spuriously decrease the measured VC volume as gas is trapped distal to the airway closure and cannot be exhaled. The SVC is intended to reduce the likelihood of this happening and allows for all of the VC volume to be exhaled and measured. If measured FVC is significantly smaller than SVC, air trapping is occurring.

VC is an important preoperative assessment factor. Significant reduction in VC (less than 20 mL/kg of ideal body weight) indicates that the patient is at a high risk for postoperative respiratory complications. This is because VC reflects the patient's ability to take a deep breath, cough, and clear the airways of excess secretions. VC is also useful in evaluating the patient's need for mechanical ventilation. A VC of less than 15 mL/kg indicates that the adult patient's ventilatory reserve is decreased significantly.

SIMPLY STATED

VC is an important indicator of the patient's ventilatory reserve. A significant reduction in VC indicates that the patient is at higher risk for respiratory failure, especially after surgery.

Total Lung Capacity

Total lung capacity is the sum of VC and RV. TLC is a function of the person's size, age, and gender. It is increased with most obstructive lung diseases and decreased with restrictive disorders. To measure TLC, the RV must be determined. The RV or FRC is obtained in one of three ways: body plethysmograph (body box), open-circuit nitrogen washout, or closed-circuit helium dilution. After the RV is obtained, it is added to the VC to determine TLC. More is said about VC and RV and how the FRC relates to the RV later in this chapter. The following sections briefly describe the body plethysmograph, open-circuit nitrogen washout method, and closed-circuit helium dilution method.

Body Plethysmography (Body Box)

The body plethysmograph (Figure 8-4) takes advantage of Boyle's law, which says that the pressure and volume of a gas vary inversely if temperature is constant. The body plethysmograph measures all of the gas within the chest. When the patient is placed in the body box, two volumes are considered: the volume of the gas in the lung (the unknown) and the volume of the box itself (known). The formula for identifying the unknown volume is derived from the following:

$$\frac{\text{Unknown lung gas volume } (V_1)}{\text{Known body box gas volume } (V_2)} = \frac{\text{Gas pressure of the box } (P_2)}{\text{Gas pressure of the lung } (P_1)}$$

Thus

$$V_1 = \frac{V_2 \times P_2}{P_1}$$

Because the cost of a body box is high, this method of determining lung volumes is performed only in hospitals and research facilities. The body box determination is more accurate than the gas dilution methods described next, because it measures the communicating and noncommunicating or poorly communicating spaces (volumes) of the lung. Examples of noncommunicating lung volumes are seen with COPD, where "air-trapping" occurs and with pneumothorax. When body box methods of determining lung volumes are compared with gas dilution methods, body box results show slightly larger volumes. Because patients with a known pneumothorax should never be placed in a body box, and air trapping accounts for a small amount of the increase in lung volumes seen with COPD, the simpler and less costly gas dilution methods (open-circuit nitrogen washout and closed helium dilution methods) are more commonly used.

Open-Circuit Nitrogen Washout Method

The nitrogen washout method is shown in Figure 8-5. This method requires that the patient breathe 100% oxygen and measures the nitrogen washout from the lungs down to a low concentration. This test is based on the principle that the gas within the lung is approximately 79% nitrogen. If the amount of nitrogen washed out of the lungs is measured, this measurement represents 79% of the unknown lung volume.

There are several problems with this method: The actual amount of nitrogen "resident" in the lung before washout starts cannot be measured precisely, so an estimate is required; a significant amount of nitrogen is washed out of the tissue with the nitrogen washed out of the lung; and if a patient's lungs have significant areas of poor communication with outside air, as in emphysema, this test along with the helium dilution method will underestimate total lung volume.

The test assumes that the nitrogen concentration in the lungs is in equilibrium with the nitrogen in the atmosphere. The patient breathes 100% oxygen for approximately 7 minutes. As the nitrogen washes out of the lungs, the volume and nitrogen percentages of the exhaled gas are measured. The test is stopped when the nitrogen concentration plateaus. The following formula is then applied:

$$FRC \times N_2\% \text{ at start of test} = \text{Expired volume} \times N_2\% \text{ at end of test}$$
$$\text{or } V_1 \times N_1 = V_2 \times N_2$$

Closed-System Helium Dilution Method

The closed-system helium dilution method is illustrated in Figure 8-6. It is another way to measure FRC and RV. As with the nitrogen washout method, the RV is added to the VC to determine TLC.

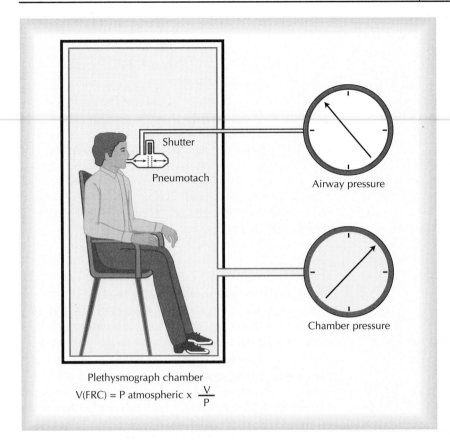

Plethysmograph chamber

$$V(FRC) = P \text{ atmospheric} \times \frac{V}{P}$$

Figure 8-4 Body plethysmography method for measuring lung volumes. P_1, initial alveolar volume; P_2, test of alveolar pressure (shutter closed); V_1, initial thoracic gas volume (unknown); V_2, test of thoracic gas volume (shutter closed). (From Wilkins RL, Stoller JK, Scanlan CL: *Egan's fundamentals of respiratory care,* ed 8, St Louis, 2003, Mosby.)

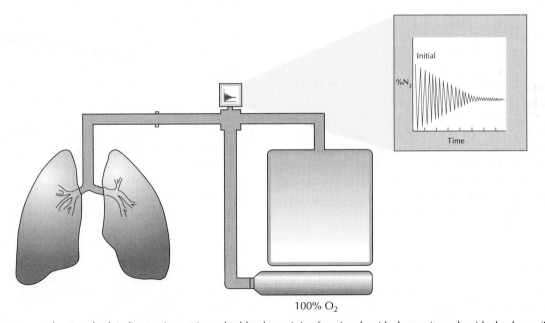

100% O_2

Figure 8-5 Nitrogen washout method. Indirect spirometric method for determining functional residual capacity and residual volume. (From Wilkins RL, Stoller JK, Scanlan CL: *Egan's fundamentals of respiratory care,* ed 8, St Louis, 2003, Mosby.)

Helium is used because it is an inert gas and is not significantly absorbed from the lungs by the blood. This test is based on the principle that if a known volume and concentration of helium is added to the patient's respiratory system, the helium will be diluted in proportion to the size of the lung volume to which it is added.

Helium is breathed at VT while oxygen is added to replace the oxygen that is consumed by the patient during the test. Because the patient adds carbon dioxide to the closed system, the carbon dioxide must be absorbed out of the closed system to prevent an increase in the dilutional effect on the helium and a falsely enlarged FRC measurement.

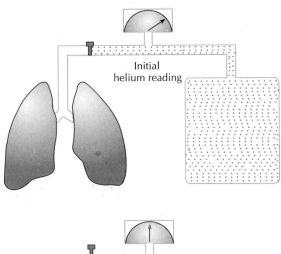

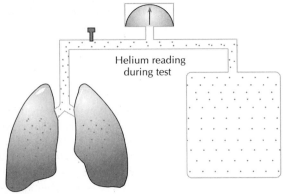

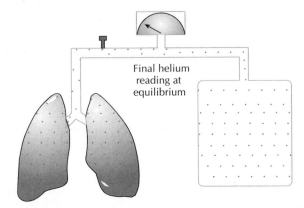

Figure 8-6 Helium dilution method. Indirect spirometric method for measuring functional residual capacity and residual volume. (From Wilkins RL, Stoller JK, Scanlan CL: *Egan's fundamentals of respiratory care*, ed 8, St Louis, 2003, Mosby.)

If leaks occur with this method, the measured volumes will be overestimated. Other factors influencing the quality of the test include the blower speed of the device, how soon the technician stops the test after equilibration is achieved, and the ventilatory pattern of the patient being tested. As just mentioned, if parts of the lung communicate poorly with the atmosphere, the results will be inaccurate.

The patient breathes in a closed system of a known volume containing a known concentration of helium. The test usually takes about 7 minutes. When the helium meter shows that equilibrium has been reached, the following formula can be used:

$$\text{Volume in spirometer} = \frac{\text{Helium added (in milliliters)}}{\% \text{ Helium at first reading}}$$

The FRC can now be calculated using V for the volume in the spirometer with the following formula:

$$\text{Volume in spirometer} = \frac{\text{Helium added (in millimeters)}}{\% \text{ Helium at first reading}}$$

$$\text{FRC} = \frac{(\text{Initial helium} - \text{Final helium}) \times V \times \text{BTPS}}{\text{Final helium}}$$

where BTPS = values at body temperature and pressure standardized.

Residual Volume

Residual volume measurement cannot be obtained from the routine spirogram. It is obtained from the studies already described in the TLC section. RV can be determined by subtracting the VC from the TLC or by subtracting the ERV from the FRC (described later). RV is the amount of gas left in the lung after the patient exhales all that is physically possible. RV is reduced in restrictive dysfunction and increased in moderate to severe obstructive dysfunction. RV increases with obstructive disease as air trapping occurs.

Expressed as a ratio to TLC and VC, RV is normally 25% of TLC and 33% of VC. This ratio is a dependable and clinically useful measurement. If RV is greater than 33% of VC, COPD is probably present. In restrictive dysfunction the ratio is usually normal. There are no clinical states in which RV/TLC or RV/VC is reduced.

Expiratory Reserve Volume

The expiratory reserve volume is the volume that can be maximally exhaled following a passive exhalation. It can be calculated by subtracting the RV from the functional residual capacity (see below). This volume is of limited clinical usefulness. It is reduced in obese persons, those making a poor effort to perform the test, and those with restrictive disease.

Functional Residual Capacity

When the values representing RV and ERV are added together, the result is the functional residual capacity (FRC). This is the resting volume in the lungs following exhalation of a VT breath. It represents a balance between the expanding chest wall forces and the contractile rebound forces of lung tissue.

Any dysfunction that causes a loss of lung tissue (e.g., emphysema) increases FRC because the forces that expand the chest wall have a decreasing amount of opposition. Respiratory disorders that cause partial or more complete collapse of the lung (e.g., pneumothorax) reduce FRC.

Inspiratory Reserve Volume and Inspiratory Capacity

Inspiratory reserve volume and inspiratory capacity are measured by the routine spirogram but are not used widely in evaluating pulmonary dysfunction. Both of these measurements can be normal in restrictive and obstructive diseases (see Figure 8-2).

Indices of Flows

The expiratory side of the FVC curve provides data regarding the contractile state of the airways. This part of the curve evaluates the amount of obstruction present in the patient's airways. To better study this curve, the recording device is sped up at the instant the patient starts to exhale. This spreads the recording out and allows for more detailed study of its shape. One of the features that separates an expensive PFT device from a less costly one is the timing device gears and mechanisms that recognize the instant expiration starts and automatically speed up the recorder. Flows routinely identified are the following:

- Forced expiratory volume at 1 second (FEV_1)
- Forced expiratory volume at 3 seconds (FEV_3)
- Forced expiratory flow, mid-expiratory phase ($FEV_{25\%-75\%}$)
- Peak expiratory flow (peak flow, PEF)

Forced Expiratory Volume at 1 Second

The FEV_1 measures the maximal volume of air exhaled during the first second of expiration. It is a forced maneuver, is highly significant, and is the best indicator of obstructive diseases. It reflects the flow characteristics in the larger airways.

The FEV_1 is reported as a raw number, but it is best expressed as a percentage of the observed FVC (FEV_1/FVC). The normal value varies with age, sex, and height, although most patients should be able to exhale approximately 75% of their VC in 1 second. The FEV_1/FVC is decreased in acute and chronic obstructive pulmonary disease and usually is normal in purely restrictive disorders.

SIMPLY STATED
The normal FEV_1/FVC is about 0.75. It is reduced with obstructive disease and normal with restrictive disease.

Forced Expiratory Volume at 3 Seconds

The FEV_3 looks at the 3-second point of the expired curve and gives an indication of the flow in the smaller airways. It is not as reproducible and sensitive as the FEV_1 but is helpful.

The FEV_3 can also be reported as a percentage of the FVC and tends to decrease normally with age, as does the FEV_1. Normal FEV_3/FVC is approximately 95%.

Forced Expiratory Flow, Midexpiratory Phase

The $FEF_{25\%-75\%}$ is a different way of looking at expiratory flows and is a sensitive test. It is expressed in liters per second and is therefore a real indicator of flow (speed). The first 25% of the exhaled curve is disregarded because of the lungs' initial inertia. The last 25% is also disregarded because of effort dependency. This leaves the middle 50% of the curve's slope to reflect the degree of airway patency. This measurement is sensitive enough to be an early indicator of obstructive dysfunction. $FEF_{25\%-75\%}$ can also be reduced in restrictive dysfunction, but its primary usefulness is in evaluating obstructive disorders. There are other points along the expired curve that are also observed, including the $FEF_{50\%}$ and the $FEF_{75\%}$. These measurements show the 50% and 75% points, respectively, on the expired slope. They are not as useful as the $FEF_{25\%-75\%}$.

Peak Expiratory Flow

The peak expiratory flow (PEF) is the maximum flow rate achieved by the patient during the FVC maneuver. It may be recorded in liters per second or liters per minute. PEF may be determined by identifying the steepest part of an FVC spirogram or by use of a handheld portable flowmeter. Use of a portable device allows rapid and repeatable assessment of PEF in a variety of clinical settings such as the emergency room or the outpatient setting.[6,7]

In asthmatics, the PEF correlates well with the FEV_1 and can be used to identify the severity of the airways obstruction.[7] If the PEF is less than 100 L/min, severe obstruction is present; 100 to 200 L/min indicates moderate obstruction; and PEF over 200 L/min suggests mild disease. Once therapy is started, PEF is useful in guiding treatment management of the asthmatic patient, providing objective data regarding the patient's response to therapy. Because inexpensive portable devices are available, PEF measurements can be used by the asthmatic patient to self-monitor home care.

SIMPLY STATED
PEF is a popular measurement in pulmonary function testing of patients with obstructive lung disease. Asthmatic patients can use it to monitor their condition at home.

Maximal Voluntary Ventilation

Maximal voluntary ventilation (MVV) measurement requires the patient to breathe as rapidly and fully as possible for 12 to 15 seconds. The total volume exhaled is measured to obtain total volume. This volume is then multiplied by the appropriate number (5 if tested for 12 seconds, 4 if tested for 15 seconds) and reported as the volume moved by the lungs in 1 minute. This number is probably larger than if the patient actually performed the maneuver for 1 full minute. Because of rapid fatigue of the respiratory muscles or possible syncope from hyperventilation, it is unreasonable to have the patient inhale and exhale rapidly for a full minute. Healthy young adults have a predicted MVV of about 170 L/min.

The MVV reflects the status of the respiratory muscles, compliance of the thorax-lung complex, and airway resistance (Raw). Normal values vary widely. Only large decreases in MVV are clinically significant. The test is popular with surgeons as a quick assessment of the state of the patient's lungs before surgery. A poor performance on this test suggests that the patient may have significant respiratory problems postoperatively. Because this test is very effort dependent, it is generally not useful.

Flow Volume Curves (Flow Volume Loops)

Flow volume loops are generated by integrating flow with volume on graph paper. Volume is plotted on the horizontal axis and flow on the vertical axis. The inspiratory loop is shown below the horizontal line and the expiratory loop is shown above the line (Figure 8-7). Recall that the initial one third of the expiratory part of the curve is effort dependent and that the later two thirds is effort independent. The shape of the flow volume loop changes when gases differing from the density of air are inhaled (low-density mixture of 80% helium and 20% oxygen or heliox).

The flow volume loop usually reveals a pattern that is distinctive for certain diseases. These diseases include restrictive pulmonary disease, upper airway (tracheal) obstruction, and obstructive pulmonary disease (Figure 8-8). This test can be particularly useful in looking for upper airway obstruction and small airway obstruction. Restrictive disease is shown as a shortened loop in the horizontal volume line (see Figure 8-8).

A common way to report PFTs in today's practice of pulmonary medicine is to show two flow volume curves superimposed on one another. The first curve is done without the patient having inhaled a standard bronchodilator. After the patient inhales the bronchodilator, the flow volume maneuver is repeated. If there has been a good response to the medication, a graphic visualization of the improvement is easily seen on the upper or expiratory half of the loop (see discussion below).

Pulmonary Function Testing Before and After Aerosol Bronchodilators

In most pulmonary function laboratories, if airway obstruction is identified, bronchodilators are administered to the patient after the routine flow and volume study (spirogram). This is done to assess the reversibility of the airway obstruction seen on the initial spirogram. The type of drug used is a β_2 sympathomimetic, but the specific drug is not standardized from one laboratory to another. The bronchodilator is delivered to the patient as an aerosol via a metered dose inhaler (MDI), preferably with a "spacer device" used to improve delivery. It is recommended that two out of three of the measurements—FVC, FEV_1, and $FEF_{25\%-75\%}$—improve before response to the inhaled bronchodilator is considered present. The amount of improvement needed is as follows:

- FVC: increase greater than 10%
- FEV_1: increase of 200 mL or 15% over baseline FEV_1
- $FEF_{25\%-75\%}$: 20% to 30% increase

A positive response to a bronchodilator is thought to be most often predictive of subsequent usefulness in asthmatic patients, but it can be misleading in other patients with COPD. This is due to the day-by-day variability seen in the natural course of the disease coincidentally occurring when the PFT is performed.

Many practitioners ask a common question: If there is no response to bronchodilators, should they be used in treatment? Bronchodilators are given a trial even when no positive response is documented by the laboratory. Prolonged exposure to these drugs or a combination of steroids and sympathomimetics may be required before a response is seen clinically. The response to bronchodilators in the laboratory setting is often a predictor of ease of control in the clinical setting. If there is no response to the bronchodilator in the laboratory, clinical control may be difficult.

SPECIALIZED PULMONARY FUNCTION STUDIES

Specialized PFTs go beyond the routine spirogram and are usually available only at larger medical centers. The special tests described here are often used to clarify or quantify the lung abnormalities detected by the simple spirogram. Some of these tests can also be used to detect abnormalities that are present but not detectable by spirograms. These studies include the following:

- Diffusion capacity (DL_{CO})
- Airway resistance (Raw)
- Compliance studies (static, dynamic, static-effective, and frequency-dependent) (C_L)
- Nitrogen washout
- Closing volume (CV)
- Respiratory quotient (RQ)
- Exercise testing
- Bronchoprovocation testing (i.e., methacholine [Provocholine] challenge)

Diffusion Capacity

The ability of gas to diffuse across the alveolar-capillary membrane can be measured and is known as the diffusion capacity (D_L). The determinants of gas exchange across the membrane include the following:

- Diffusion coefficient of the gas used in testing
- Surface area of the membrane
- Thickness (diffusion characteristics) of the membrane
- Blood volume and flow in the pulmonary capillary tree
- Distribution of the inspired gas (matching of ventilation to perfusion)
- Hematocrit

Diseases that reduce surface area of the membrane, such as emphysema, can reduce D_L. Emphysema also has a negative effect on the distribution of the inhaled gas. Interstitial diseases

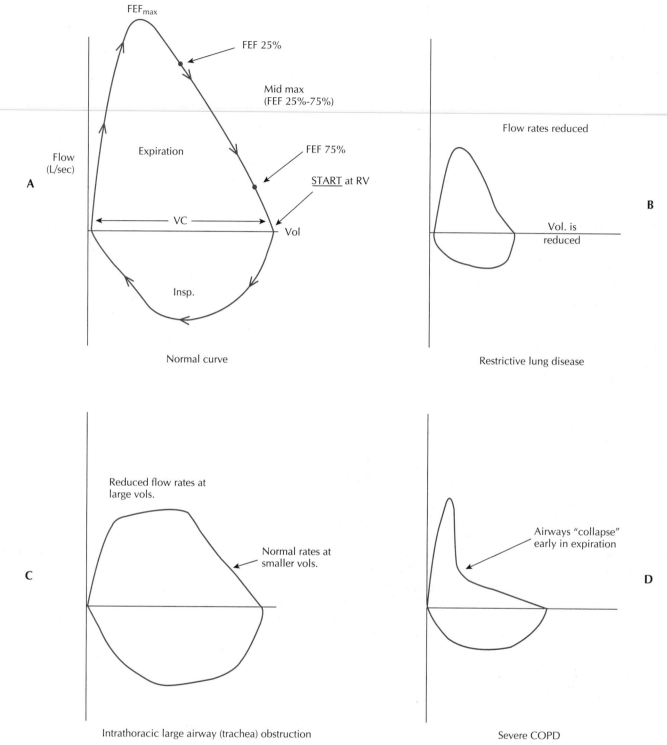

Figure 8-7 Flow volume loop. These flow volume loops are typical patterns seen with **(A)** normal, **(B)** restrictive lung diseases, **(C)** upper airway obstruction, and **(D)** severe chronic obstructive lung disease.

such as pulmonary fibrosis, asbestosis, and sarcoidosis alter the integrity of the membrane and cause a reduction in diffusion. The perfusion status of the pulmonary capillaries determines the ability of oxygen in the lung to be absorbed across the alveolar-capillary membrane. Minimal diffusion will occur if the blood volume of the pulmonary capillaries is significantly

reduced. The patient's hematocrit also affects D_L for the same reason. The hemoglobin level of the blood influences the carrying capacity of the blood because oxygen is carried primarily by the red blood cells.

Diffusion is most commonly measured by using a single breath of carbon monoxide (CO) at minute levels (0.4%). The

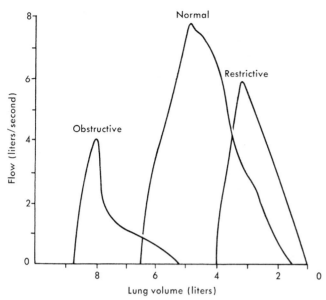

Figure 8-8 Maximum expiratory flow volume curve comparing normal with obstructive and restrictive disorders. Displayed as flows at actual lung volumes. (From Scanlan CL, Wilkins RL, Stoller JK: *Egan's fundamentals of respiratory care,* ed 7, St Louis, 1999, Mosby.)

designation of the test is then DL_{CO-SB}, where D_L = diffusion-lung, CO = carbon monoxide, and SB = single-breath.

Because of CO's intensive affinity for hemoglobin (over 200 times greater binding power to hemoglobin than oxygen), the ability of CO to diffuse is limited by the membrane and not by capillary blood flow. It is therefore a diffusion-limited gas rather than a perfusion-limited gas.

Using CO mixed with an insoluble tracer gas (usually helium) in a closed system, the patient inhales and holds his/her breath for 10 seconds. CO's rate of removal from this closed system is an indication of the biologic state of the alveolar-capillary membrane.

DL_{CO} is measured in milliliters per minute per millimeter of mercury and is reported as both the raw number and percentage of predicted value. Normal DL_{CO} is approximately 25 mL/min/mm Hg. The equation used to determine diffusion is as follows:

$$DL_{CO} = [V_A \times 60 \div (Pbar - 47) \times t] \times [ln \times (PACOi \div PACOt)]$$

where V_A = original lung volume, Pbar = barometric pressure, t = breath holding time, and PACOi and PACOt = initial and final partial alveolar pressures of carbon monoxide.

In interpreting diffusion abnormalities, the practitioner should consider the fact that patients with small lungs will have apparent diffusion abnormalities that must be differentiated from patients with true diseases of the alveolar capillary membrane. By establishing a ratio between diffusion (D_L) and alveolar ventilation (V_A), it can be noted that patients with normal but small lungs will have a decreased D_L but normal D_L/V_A. Patients with true diffusion problems will have both a decreased D_L and D_L/V_A.

Other methods of determining D_L are the "steady state" and "rebreathing" methods. Both methods are more complex and time consuming but can be used during exercise. They are less affected by ventilation/perfusion abnormalities when compared

with the single-breath method described above. The single-breath technique is most widely used, however, because normal values for this technique are well established, making interpretation easier.[8]

Other important considerations in measuring and interpreting diffusion studies include:
1. Severe anemia reduces the number of red blood cells that remove CO from the closed system and thereby reduces DL_{CO}.
2. If pulmonary capillary blood flow to an area is reduced, the diffusion of CO will not occur, thus reducing DL_{CO}.
3. The size of the individual will influence results. Large individuals will have larger diffusion capacities.

> **SIMPLY STATED**
> The DL_{CO} is useful in determining the ability of the lung to transfer gas with the blood. The most common causes of reduced DL_{CO} values are emphysema and pulmonary fibrosis.

Airway Resistance

Narrowing of the airways in acute and chronic obstructive pulmonary disease causes airflow resistance to increase. It is sometimes useful to document the precise airway resistance (Raw) level as a means of indicating the severity of the disease and effect of therapy. The equipment used to determine Raw is shown in Figure 8-9. This study uses the same closed, tightly sealed body box (plethysmograph) described earlier for the determination of TLC.

Normally Raw is greater on expiration than on inspiration. It increases with any pathologic process that narrows the airways or causes inflammation, edema, or bronchoconstriction (e.g. asthma, COPD). Because the elastic rebound of the lung tends to hold open the airways, loss of elasticity causes the airway to collapse on exhalation and thus increases resistance. This process is seen in emphysema.

The normal resistance is 0.5 to 3.0 cm $H_2O/L/sec$ at a flow rate of 0.5 L/sec. Sometimes resistance is reported as conductance, which is the reciprocal of resistance. Resistance is usually reported as a percentage of normal. A report of 100% ± 20% is considered within normal limits.

Compliance Studies

Compliance is defined as volume change per unit of pressure change. Compliance measurements are useful in identifying the relative stiffness of the lung. Lungs with low compliance require greater pressure changes to expand with a specific volume as compared with more compliant lungs. Esophageal pressure closely approximates intrapleural pressure and can be used to identify changes in thoracic pressures that occur with changes in lung volume. Lung compliance can be determined by having the patient swallow a balloon catheter approxi-

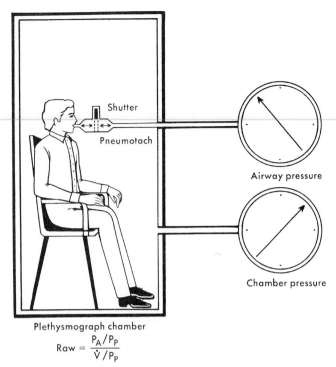

$$Raw = \frac{P_A/P_P}{\dot{V}/P_P}$$

Figure 8-9 Measurement of airway resistance (Raw) by body plethysmograph. P_A, Airway pressure; P_P, chamber pressure; $\dot{V}$, ventilation. (From Scanlan CL, Wilkins RL, Stoller JK: *Egan's fundamentals of respiratory care*, ed 7, St Louis, 1999, Mosby.)

mately 10 cm into the esophagus. The proximal end of the catheter is connected to a pressure transducer, and serial pressure measurements are recorded at various lung volumes. For the patient who is intubated, intrathoracic pressure can be determined by using a pressure manometer in line with the breathing circuit, avoiding the need for an esophageal balloon.

Compliance may be measured either at a point of no flow (*static compliance*) or when gas is flowing into the lung (*dynamic compliance*). Healthy persons exhibit values for dynamic compliance that are slightly less than values for static compliance. When Raw is elevated, however, dynamic compliance decreases well below static compliance. Both static and dynamic compliance values decrease when the lung becomes stiffer, as with atelectasis, pneumonia, and pulmonary fibrosis.

The total compliance of the respiratory system is made up of two distinct compliance units: lung tissue and chest wall. These two compliance units are parallel and not in series; therefore the effect of the sum of the two units would be expressed as follows:

$$\frac{1}{\text{Total CL}} = \frac{1}{\text{CL of the thorax}} + \frac{1}{\text{CL of the lung}}$$

The compliance curve is derived from the following formula:

$$\text{CL} = \frac{\text{Change in volume}}{\text{Change in pressure}}$$

The typical compliance curves for various diseases are shown in Figure 8-10. The flat curve reflects a stiff lung, whereas the curve for emphysema demonstrates a highly compliant lung that has lost its recoil ability.

Nitrogen Washout

Nitrogen washout is used to determine whether there is gross maldistribution of ventilation. As the patient breathes 100% oxygen, the nitrogen analyzer measures a continuously diminishing concentration of nitrogen from the lungs. *Fast ventilatory spaces* may occur and, if so, will empty first. *Slower ventilating spaces* empty slowly and erratically, making the downward slope uneven. This pattern confirms the presence of uneven ventilation, as is commonly seen in obstructive lung diseases such as emphysema (Figure 8-11).

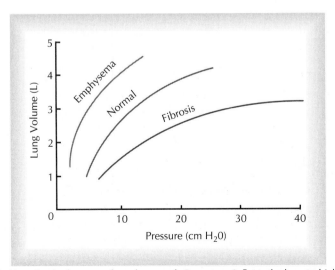

Figure 8-10 Pressure-volume curves. Note that in the case of emphysema, less pressure inflates the lung to higher volumes, indicating that the lung has become less elastic. With patients who have pulmonary fibrosis, their lung is stiffer because of the development of scarring (fibrosis). Thus their lung requires a lot of pressure in order to inflate it to the lowest of volumes. (Modified from Martin L: *Pulmonary physiology in clinical practice: the essentials for patient care and evaluation*, St Louis, 1987, Mosby.)

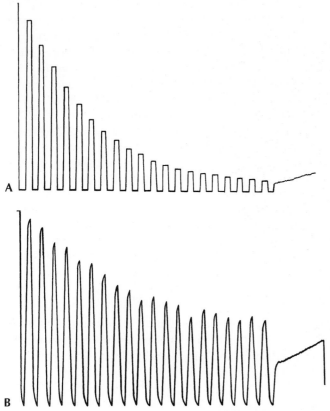

Figure 8-11 Nitrogen washout tracing showing **(A)** normal and **(B)** abnormal washout curves.

Closing Volume

Closing volume (CV) is a special form of nitrogen washout used for early diagnosis of obstruction in the small airways. In the standard nitrogen washout test, the patient "washes out" the lung nitrogen by breathing in 100% oxygen for 7 to 10 minutes. In contrast, the CV is determined by having the patient inhale a single breath of 100% oxygen and then slowly exhale while the levels of nitrogen in the exhaled breath are monitored. Normally, four phases are seen on the test curve (Figure 8-12). Phase I is the extreme upper airway (dead space) gas consisting of 100% oxygen, phase II is a mixture of dead space and alveolar gas, phase III is a plateau produced by the exhalation of alveolar gas, and phase IV is identified by an abrupt increase in the concentration of nitrogen, which continues until the patient reaches RV. Phase IV occurs when the small airways in the dependent lung zones close, which stops gas flow out of the bases. Gas flow out of the apices now dominates exhalation, and it has a higher concentration of nitrogen than gas from the lower lung zones. This occurs because the lower lung regions receive more of the 100% oxygen inhaled than the upper regions, because there is proportionately more of the RV gas in the apices after maximum exhalation than in the bases.

There are some significant technical problems in getting an accurate and useful curve. As a consequence, some laboratories have stopped offering CV as a diagnostic aid. Nevertheless, four varied but valuable test results are available from the CV curve:

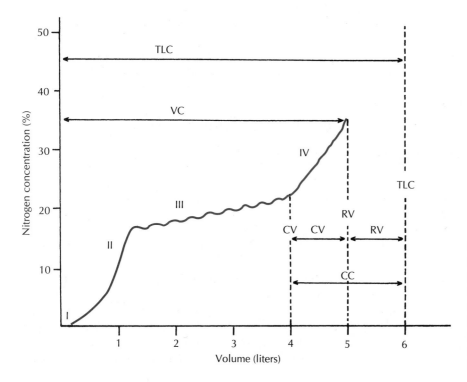

Figure 8-12 Single-breath nitrogen test curve for measuring closing volumes and capacity. Phase I: expired dead space gas. Phase II: mixed dead space and alveolar gas. Phase III: alveolar plateau. Phase IV: airway closure. See text for abbreviations. (From Scanlan CL, Spearman CB, Sheldon RL: *Egan's fundamentals of respiratory care,* ed 5, St Louis, 1990, Mosby.)

- Closing volume: representation of the state of the small airways; early airway narrowing can be detected in this test
- Delta nitrogen (ΔN_2): index of distribution of ventilation
- TLC and RV: done by integrating the area under the expired nitrogen curve
- Fowler method: determination of anatomic airway dead space

Phase IV of the curve is where the CV occurs. CV is often reported as a percentage of the VC, and in this situation the term *closing capacity* may be used. Closing capacity is determined by adding the CV to the RV. CV is reported as a percentage of VC, and closing capacity is reported as a percentage of TLC; plus or minus 20% of the predicted value is considered normal. The normal predicted value increases with age. The value increases abnormally in early obstruction of the small airways.

Respiratory Quotient

The ratio of carbon dioxide produced to oxygen consumed is called the respiratory quotient (RQ). By using appropriate collectors to accurately measure the volume of expired gas and then analyzing the amount of carbon dioxide and oxygen in the expired gas, one can determine carbon dioxide produced and oxygen consumed.

Many metabolic activities affect the RQ. One of the most frequent uses of the RQ is to assess which food group (fats, carbohydrates, or protein) is being metabolized for energy. If the RQ is 0.7, fats are the sole energy source. If the RQ is 1.0, carbohydrates are the main source of energy. Depending on the activity level and nature of the food being ingested, the RQ can shift. Normally, it is 0.8 to 0.85, showing a mixed metabolism pattern.

There are many clinical applications for this information. One important use is in assessing the patient who is being weaned from a ventilator. Because a patient who is being fed a diet made up exclusively of glucose (carbohydrate) produces more carbon dioxide than usual, the work of breathing increases to blow off this excess carbon dioxide load. Carbon dioxide is a direct byproduct of carbohydrate metabolism, and the more of this foodstuff eaten, the more carbon dioxide produced. Knowledge of the patient's RQ allows intelligent adjustment of the patient's diet and may speed up the process of weaning the patient from the ventilator (see Chapter 17).

> **SIMPLY STATED**
> Normal RQ is 0.8 to 0.85. This figure represents the ratio of CO_2 produced to oxygen consumed each minute.

Exercise Testing

A complete review of exercise testing is not feasible here. The information has become so vast that entire books are written on the subject. The following list of possible exercise tests and their uses should serve as an introduction to this fascinating field in pulmonary medicine.

- Stress electrocardiography (ECG): Used for the noninvasive detection of coronary artery disease.
- Ventilatory capacity: Assesses the patient's ability to respond to exercise with the appropriate increase in rate and depth of ventilation.
- Blood gases (arterial oxygen [PaO_2] and carbon dioxide tension [$PaCO_2$]), alveolar-arterial oxygen tension difference [$P(A-a)O_2$], pH, base excess, before and after exercise: Detects the presence of oxygenation, ventilation, and oxygen usage problems not apparent at rest.
- Exercise challenge: The patient exercises hard and then the spirogram is used to see whether this challenge has incited the development of bronchospasm. Exercise-induced bronchospasm is a variant of asthma and usually responds to specific treatment when correctly identified.
- Anaerobic threshold: When the body is stressed enough during exercise, there is a point at which oxygen need exceeds availability, and a backup mode of metabolism called *anaerobic* (without oxygen) *metabolism* is brought into action. Exercise testing is useful to identify this point in persons such as athletes in training and patients with heart disease who may need an individualized exercise program that is safe for them. With proper exercise, the anaerobic threshold can be increased.
- Maximal oxygen uptake ($\dot{V}O_2$max): Designed to show the level of exercise that causes the patient to reach maximum oxygen consumption. Obtaining this information requires a well-ordered and well-staffed laboratory with calibrated equipment.

Recently the American Thoracic Society (ATS) has issued guidelines for the 6-minute walk test (6MWT). In this test the patient walks alone, with no assistance in pulling his/her supplemental oxygen source. No equipment like a treadmill is used. The test is intended to imitate the patient's true activities of daily living. Much information is taken from this test, including oxygen saturation and the perception of dyspnea. The test measures functional capacity in patients with moderate to severe impairment. The test is inexpensive to perform and is useful in measuring the response to therapeutic interventions in patients with both pulmonary and cardiac disease.[9]

Bronchoprovocation Testing

The most common cause of undiagnosed cough is "occult" asthma. Often the routine spirogram is normal in patients suspected of having nonspecific bronchial hyperresponsiveness (i.e., asthma or reactive airways disease [RADS]). This hyperresponsiveness is a constant feature of asthma even though airflow obstruction is often absent at the time of routine testing. Other causes of wheezing exist. Methods of uncovering this hyperresponsive state in a safe, controlled setting are necessary to determine which episodes of wheezing are caused by asthma and which ones are not.

In these settings, bronchoprovocation testing is useful. Several easy and safe techniques are used to document bronchial hyperresponsiveness. Challenging the patient with inhaled histamine or methacholine is most commonly used.

These medications have parasympathomimetic properties and therefore may induce bronchospasm. Spirogram studies are done, following the administration of the provoking agent, to determine the response of the airways. Healthy subjects without hyperactive airways tolerate the challenge without significant reduction in pulmonary function values. A 20% decrease in FEV_1 or other reliable measure of expiratory flow suggests that the patient has hyperactive airways.

The technique may be used safely in an outpatient setting if protocol is followed carefully. Other challenge techniques include cold air and exercise.

OTHER APPLICATIONS OF PULMONARY FUNCTION TESTING

PFT is useful in a variety of clinical settings. The following discussion presents some of the additional ways PFT can be valuable.

Smoking Cessation

There has been a significant drop in the consumption of cigarettes in the United States since the Surgeon General's report in the mid-1960s. This report, and many since, detailed the dangers of smoking cigarettes.

PFT can be performed on smokers to reinforce the need for smoking cessation, especially if considerable loss of lung function is documented. Smokers may be more motivated to stop smoking if evidence is presented to them that clearly demonstrates the damage cigarettes have imposed on their airways and lung function.

More important, PFT has proved to be the most useful single predictor of who will have cardiopulmonary disease as a result of smoking. Smoking is the main risk factor in the development of coronary artery disease (ahead of hypertension and abnormal cholesterol levels). Early changes in FEV_1 and FVC better predict future problems with cardiovascular disease than does a resting ECG.[1]

Surgery

In patients anticipating surgery who have known pulmonary disease, a significant smoking history, or symptoms of dyspnea or cough, PFT is crucial, especially if the surgery is involving the abdomen or chest. Surgeons want their patients to have quick and complication-free postoperative courses. One of the most dreaded postoperative complications is pneumonia and respiratory insufficiency or failure. With this in mind, PFT is frequently performed on high-risk patients to determine their current lung function status. Those patients who demonstrate significant impairment prior to surgery often benefit from preoperative and postoperative measures that optimize lung function.

Regardless of history or symptoms, patients who are to have all or part of a lung removed must have PFT performed before surgery. If the FEV_1 is less than 2 L, high-resolution computerized tomography (CT) or differential perfusion lung scans are recommended to assess the effect on oxygenation and ventilation resulting from the proposed lung resection. It is widely accepted than a postoperative FEV_1 less than 800 mL places a patient at high risk after surgery and may condemn them to a life of dyspnea.[10]

> ### SIMPLY STATED
> Preoperative pulmonary function screening is essential in patients with a history of lung disease, especially if the surgery involves thoracic or upper abdominal surgery.

Sleep Apnea

Approximately a third of our life is spent asleep, a state of profound physiologic change compared to when we are awake. Only recently have we begun to understand this remarkable phenomenon called sleep (see Chapter 18).

Sleep apnea can occur as a result of central nervous system problems (central sleep apnea [CSA]) or airway obstructive problems (obstructive sleep apnea [OSA]). OSA makes up approximately 90% of sleep apnea patients. Of this group, 20% have COPD. PFT can be performed in this group to better direct daytime treatment of chronic lung disease along with the nighttime treatment of sleep apnea. PFT can be helpful in assessing the patient with CSA.[11] In such patients a mixed obstructive and central apnea is often present and PFT may prove useful in evaluating the degree and severity of upper airway obstruction.

Environmental Lung Diseases

Twenty percent of the general population has some form of lung disease: a restrictive defect, COPD, or lung cancer. The workplace is a place where lung disease can start or can be made worse. Teams made up of PFT technicians, physicians, and statisticians have worked to identify and lessen the effect of the work environment on lung disease.[12] Studies have been performed on employees in a wide variety of work settings, including those places where exposure to asbestos and other harmful dusts may be present. Such studies are instrumental in determining if harmful exposure has occurred and what effect it has had on the lung. PFT is an important part of this process and often determines who gets disability payments as a result of their work environment.

CLINICAL INTERPRETATION OF PULMONARY FUNCTION TESTING

PFT is used to identify and evaluate obstructive and restrictive respiratory disorders (Table 8-1). Obstructive defects cause a reduction in the measurements of flow, including FEV_1/FVC, $FEF_{25\%-75\%}$, and PEF. VC is normal in mild obstructive disease but decreases as the obstruction becomes more severe. FRC and

Table 8-1	Summary of Pulmonary Function Tests			
Measurement	**How Determined**	**Units**	**Disease Process**	**Usefulness**
TLC	Body box	Liters and % predicted	↑ Obstructive, ↓ restrictive	+++
VC	Spirogram	Liters and % predicted	↓ Obstructive, ↓ restrictive	+++++
ERV	Spirogram	Liters and % predicted	↓ Restrictive	+
FRC	Derived: spirogram and body box or nitrogen washout/helium dilution	Liters and % predicted	↑ Obstructive, ↓ restrictive	+++
RV	Derived: spirogram and body box or nitrogen washout/helium dilution	Liters and % predicted	↑ Obstructive, ↓ restrictive	+++
V_T	Spirogram	Liters and % predicted	↑/N Obstructive, ↓ restrictive	++
IRV	Spirogram	Liters and % predicted	N Obstructive, ↓/N restrictive	+
IC	Spirogram	Liters and % predicted	N Obstructive, ↓/N restrictive	+
MVV	Spirogram	L min	↓ Obstructive, ↓ restrictive	+++
Frequency	Clock	No./min	↑ Obstructive and restrictive	+++
$\dot{V}_E$	Derived: $f \times V_T$	L min	↑ Obstructive, N restrictive	+++
FEV_1	Spirogram	% Predicted	↓ Obstructive and restrictive	++++
FEV_3	Spirogram	% Predicted	↓ Obstructive and restrictive	+++
$FEF_{25\%-75\%}$	Spirogram	% Predicted	↓ Obstructive	+++
PEF	Spirogram	% Predicted	↓ Obstructive	++
FEV_1/FVC	Spirogram	% Predicted	↓ Obstructive, N restrictive	++++
DL_{CO}	Carbon monoxide uptake	mL/min/mmHg	↓ Emphysema and restrictive	+++
CV	Nitrogen washout	% Predicted	↑ Obstructive	++
Raw	Body box	% Predicted	↑ Obstructive	+++
Compliance	Esophageal balloon	L/cm H_2O pressure	↑ Obstructive, ↓ restrictive	+++

N, Normal; +, least useful; +++, most useful.

TLC are initially normal to mildly increased with acute airway obstruction, but they are increased significantly with chronic defects such as emphysema. MVV is reduced in more severe cases.

Acute decreases in flow rate measurements are clinically associated with dyspnea, hypoxemia, hypocapnia, tachypnea, use of accessory breathing muscles, expiratory wheezing, and paradoxic pulse. Chronic airflow impairments are associated with an increased anteroposterior diameter of the chest, reduced voice and breath sounds, use of accessory muscles, increased resonance to percussion, and low, flat diaphragms (see Chapter 5).

Restrictive lung disorders are recognized by identifying a reduction in VC, RV, FRC, and TLC. The measurements of flow may be normal or mildly reduced. The FEV_1/FVC is normal in pure restrictive disorders.

Clinically, the patient who has restrictive lung disease may show signs of dyspnea on exertion, cyanosis, rapid shallow breathing, digital clubbing, reduced breath sounds, and late inspiratory crackles. In chronic advanced cases, the signs of chronic right heart failure (cor pulmonale) occur (see Chapter 5).

FINAL THOUGHTS

The scope of this single chapter limits inclusion of many important issues currently being investigated related to PFT. For example, the techniques and interpretations of data from children and the elderly continue to be researched.[13,14] Although such research on PFT is useful, the most important aspect of how PFT is accepted by the patient and how accurately the test reflects the state of the patient's lungs depends foremost on the quality of the coaching given by the technicians at the time of testing. As is so frequently the case in the application of health care, the human element is the most important issue in whether or not health care is perceived to be high quality.

CASE STUDY 1

M.W. is a 70-year-old man with a chief complaint of dyspnea on exertion. The dyspnea has increased gradually over the last several years. M.W. denies a history of cough, sputum production, smoking, working in a polluted environment, or respiratory disease. Physical examination reveals tachypnea, tachycardia, jugular venous distention, decreased breath sounds, digital clubbing, and kyphoscoliosis.

Personal data

Age: 70 years
Height: 66 in.
Weight: 155 lb
Sex: male

Spirometry

Report	Predicted	Observed	Predicted %
FVC (L)	3.78	1.46	39
SVC (L)	3.78	1.42	38
ERV (L)	0.67	0.34	51
IC (L)	3.10	1.07	35
FEV_1 (L)	2.57	1.40	54
FEV_3 (L)	3.59	1.46	41
FEV_1/FVC	70%	96%	—
FEV_3/FVC	95%	100%	—
MVV (L/min)	114	76	67
$FEF_{25\%-75\%}$ (L/sec)	2.46	2.01	82
PEF (L/sec)	5–8	6.20	—

Lung Volume Studies

(body box)	Predicted	Observed	Predicted %
VC (L)	3.78	1.79	47.4
ERV (L)	0.67	0.15	22.0
IC (L)	3.10	1.64	52.9
FRC (L)	2.42	2.01	83.0
RV (L)	1.75	1.86	106
TLC (L)	5.78	3.65	63.2
RV/TLC	30%	51%	—

Interpretation: Spirometry reveals a significant reduction in FVC, IC, FEV_1, and FEV_3. However, the measurements of flow are within normal limits. The lung volume studies identify a reduction in VC, IC, and TLC. The findings are consistent with restrictive lung disease. Arterial blood studies are indicated to further evaluate the degree of respiratory impairment.

The lung function studies are typical for a patient with kyphoscoliosis. Kyphoscoliosis causes a reduction in the size of the thoracic cage and severely compromises lung expansion.

CASE STUDY 2

J.D. is a 38-year-old man with a chronic complaint of dyspnea on exertion. His dyspnea has increased significantly over the past year and now occurs with minimal exertion. J.D. denies cough, chest pain, or sputum production. He has a 40-pack/year smoking history. His family history is positive for COPD. There is no history of exposure to environmental pollutants. Clinical examination is positive for chronic airflow obstruction (see Chapter 5).

Personal data

Age: 38
Height: 76 in.
Weight: 188 lb
Sex: male

Spirometry

Report	Predicted	Observed	Predicted %
FVC (L)	6.06	3.39	56
SVC (L)	6.06	4.49	74
ERV (L)	1.38	1.99	145
IC (L)	4.69	2.49	53
FEV_1 (L)	4.52	0.95	21
FEV_3 (L)	5.76	1.84	32
FEV_1/FVC	75%	28%	—
FEV_3/FVC	95%	54%	—
MVV (L/min)	189	48	25
$FEF_{25\%-75\%}$ (L/sec)	4.39	0.34	8
PEF (L/sec)	5–8	1.40	—

Lung Volume Studies

(body box)	Predicted	Observed	Predicted %
VC (L)	6.06	4.88	80.5
ERV (L)	1.38	1.83	133.0
IC (L)	4.69	3.05	65.1
FRC (L)	3.24	9.75	301.2
RV (L)	1.86	7.92	425.7
TLC (L)	7.75	12.80	165.1
RV/TLC	24%	61.90%	257.8

Interpretation and Discussion: Spirometry results demonstrate a reduction in FVC, SVC, IC, FEV_1, and FEV_3. The measurements of flow, FEV_1/FVC, and $FEF_{25\%-75\%}$ are also reduced markedly. At first glance this appears to be a combined restrictive and obstructive lung defect. However, the lung volume studies clearly reveal that the reduction in FVC is the result of air trapping, and only an obstructive defect is present. The significant difference in FVC and SVC measurements suggests that air trapping is occurring, especially during forced expiratory maneuvers.

Studies done after the use of bronchodilators and arterial blood gases and DL_{CO} measurements would be helpful to further evaluate J.D.'s respiratory status. There should be a high index of suspicion for the presence of α_1-antitrypsin deficiency in this patient, given the severity of his lung disease at such a young age. The DL_{CO} is expected to be markedly reduced if emphysema is the cause of this patient's dyspnea.

CASE STUDY 3

A 72-year-old female was admitted to the medical service complaining of weakness and shortness of breath. She had been recently diagnosed with asthma but previously was in good health.

The physical examination of the chest was remarkable in that little air entry was heard. There was no wheezing, but crackles were noted at both bases. The admitting chest radiograph revealed the presence of bi-basilar atelectasis but was otherwise clear. Her admitting lab work was normal. Her blood gases indicated that her pH was normal but her $PaCO_2$ was 54 mm Hg with a PaO_2 of 58 mm Hg while breathing room air.

After 3 days of standard therapy for asthma, to include inhaled bronchodilators and steroids, her respiratory symptoms were no better. Her $PaCO_2$ had increased to 62 mm Hg and her chest x-ray was unchanged. Her weakness was a little better. Pulmonary consultation was requested.

The consultant requested bedside spirometry and, finding little evidence of airflow obstruction as expected in an asthmatic, ordered full PFT. More blood testing was also ordered to include a sed-rate, ANA screen, and antiacetylcholine receptor antibody (anti-acetylcholine receptor [AChR] antibody). A more complete pulmonary function test indicated the following:

Personal data

Age: 72
Height: 63.5 in.
Weight: 166 lb
Sex: female

Spirometry

Report	Predicted	Observed	Predicted %
FVC (L)	2.80	1.45	52
SVC (L)	2.80	1.51	54
ERV (L)	0.61	0.30	49
FEV_1 (L)	2.13	1.19	56
FEV_3 (L)	2.56	1.38	54
FEV_1/FVC	75%	82%	—
FEV_3/FVC	95%	95%	—
MVV (L/min)	82.38	23.14	28
$FEF_{25\%-75\%}$ (L/sec)	1.90	0.34	18

Interpretation and Discussion: The second round of blood work revealed a normal sedimentation rate and normal ANA screen. The anti-AChR antibody titer was elevated, suggesting the diagnosis of myasthenia gravis. Now, a more focused history and physical examination were performed, which strengthened the belief that this patient had myasthenia gravis instead of asthma. The final confirmation of this belief occurred with a positive Tensilon test.

Myasthenia gravis afflicts 1 in 7500 patients of any age and occurs more frequently in women. The disease is an acquired autoimmune disorder associated with an AChR deficiency at the motor end-plate. The motor end-plate is where the nerve ends and stimulates the muscle to contract. (Please consult a standard medical textbook for a more detailed discussion of this complex disease.) The weakness caused by myasthenia gravis is peculiar in that it worsens as muscle groups are used. The standard physical examination performed by physicians does not fully evaluate muscle strength, so this physical finding can be easily missed. As the disease worsens, respiratory muscles weaken and the patient goes into hypercapnic respiratory failure ("myasthenia crisis"). This is the reason for the patient's rising $PaCO_2$. The patient's chest x-ray findings of small volumes and bi-basilar atelectasis are also explained by weakening respiratory muscles. Further misleading information in this case is that high-dose steroids can constitute partial treatment for myasthenia gravis, which explains why the patient felt better.

The PFTs show marked reduction in all the volumes. Note the flow determinations when expressed as percentages of FVC are normal. Since little air was brought into the lungs because of muscle weakness, little air was exhaled; thus the percentages appear to be normal. These findings are compatible with myasthenia gravis. There is no evidence of bronchoconstriction needed to support a diagnosis of asthma causing this level of disease.

REVIEW QUESTIONS

1. T F PFTs measure the ability of the lungs to exchange respiratory gases.

2. In which of the following situations is a PFT least useful?
   a. Documenting the progression of pulmonary disease
   b. Evaluating the probability of getting a pulmonary disease
   c. Exercise evaluation
   d. Weaning from mechanical ventilation

3. The tracing obtained from a PFT is called a:
   a. spirograph
   b. spiroagnew
   c. spirogram
   d. spirometer

4. Which of the following factors is the most important in predicting PFT measurements?
   a. Weight
   b. Age
   c. Gender
   d. Height

5. T   F   Male patients generally have larger lung volumes and flows than female patients of similar height and weight.

6. T   F   Most PFTs are independent of patient effort.

7. Which of the following pieces of standard PFT equipment is (are) used to determine total lung capacity and resistance of the airways?
   a. Body plethysmography
   b. Spirometry
   c. Diffusion systems
   d. All of the above

8. Which of the following are consistent with obstructive lung disease?
   a. Increased expiratory flows
   b. Decreased expiratory flows
   c. Decreased lung volumes and flows
   d. Increased lung volumes and flows

9. An anatomic obstruction located in the upper airway will affect which part of the spirometric tracing?
   a. Initial portion
   b. Middle portion
   c. End portion
   d. All of the above

10. Which of the following is true regarding restrictive lung disease?
    a. It is characterized by reduced lung volumes on the PFT.
    b. It can be caused by obesity.
    c. Expiratory flows generally are normal.
    d. All of the above.

11. T   F   Emphysema can produce both obstructive and restrictive defects in lung function.

12. Which of the following is true regarding tidal volume (V_T)?
    a. It is normally 4 to 5 L.
    b. It is normally 50% of TLC.
    c. It is defined as the volume inhaled and exhaled during quiet breathing.
    d. It is increased in restrictive lung disease.

13. Total lung capacity is the sum of which of the following?
    a. Tidal volume and vital capacity
    b. Inspiratory reserve volume and expiratory reserve volume
    c. Residual volume and expiratory reserve volume
    d. Vital capacity and residual volume

14. Which of the following tests is useful in determining the need for mechanical ventilation?
    a. FEV_1
    b. FVC
    c. $FEF_{25\%-75\%}$
    d. TLC

15. T   F   A vital capacity of 12 mL/kg would suggest a high risk of postoperative pulmonary complications.

16. T   F   TLC is increased in most obstructive lung diseases.

17. Residual volume is normally which of the following values?
    a. 25% of VC
    b. 25% of V_T
    c. 33% of VC
    d. 33% of TLC

18. Which of the following is true regarding FRC?
    a. It is the sum of the RV and ERV.
    b. It is increased in obstructive disease.
    c. It is reduced in restrictive disease.
    d. All of the above.

19. Body plethysmography is based on which of the following gas laws?
    a. Boyle's law
    b. Charles's law
    c. Dalton's law
    d. Universal gas law

20. Open-circuit nitrogen washout can be helpful in measuring which of the following?
    a. RV
    b. TLC
    c. FRC
    d. All of the above

21. Which of the following tests is the best indicator of obstructive lung disease?
    a. FEV_3
    b. $FEF_{25\%-75\%}$
    c. FEV_1
    d. VC

22. Which of the following is the normal value for FEV_1?
    a. 25% of VC
    b. 50% of VC
    c. 60% of VC
    d. 75% of VC

23. T F The FEV_1/FVC is usually normal in purely restrictive disorders.

24. T F A PEF of 120 L/min indicates severe airway obstruction.

25. T F A shortened flow volume loop on the horizontal axis indicates obstructive lung disease.

26. Which of the following is true regarding prebronchodilator and postbronchodilator PFTs?
    a. It is used to assess the reversibility of airway obstruction.
    b. A 5% increase in FVC is considered proof of improvement.
    c. It is useful in all forms of obstructive lung diseases.
    d. All of the above.

27. Which of the following is true regarding a DL_{CO}?
    a. It is increased in emphysema.
    b. It uses 0.4% CO_2 as a test gas.
    c. It decreases with decreasing lung surface area.
    d. It is normally 35 mL/min/mm Hg.

28. T F A lung with an increased compliance requires less pressure to expand than a lung with reduced compliance.

29. Which of the following is true regarding bronchoprovocation testing?
    a. It is used to test for occult asthma.
    b. Methacholine is commonly used as a bronchoprovocation agent.
    c. Histamine is commonly used as a bronchoprovocation agent.
    d. All of the above.

30. Which of the following exercise tests is useful in determining coronary artery disease?
    a. Ventilatory capacity
    b. Exercise challenge
    c. Stress electrocardiograph
    d. Anaerobic threshold

31. The results of a PFT are as follows:
    Patient data
    Age: 68
    Height: 63 in.
    Weight: 135 lb
    Sex: male

Spirometry	Observed	Predicted	% Predicted
FVC	1.33 L	3.38 L	39
SVC	1.35 L	3.38 L	40
ERV	0.48 L	1.03 L	47
IC	1.01 L	2.35 L	43
FEV_1	1.21 L	2.36 L	51
FEV_3	1.29 L	3.21 L	40
FEV_1/FVC	91%	70%	—
FEV_3/FVC	97%	95%	—
MVV	77 L/min	97.5 L/min	79
$FEF_{25\%-75\%}$	2.0 L/sec	2.41 L/sec	83
PEF	6.1 L/sec	7.66 L/sec	80

Lung Volume Studies

Studies	Observed	Predicted	% Predicted
VC	1.44 L	3.38 L	43
ERV	0.27 L	1.03 L	26
IC	1.17 L	2.35 L	50
FRC	2.51 L	3.03 L	83
RV	2.24 L	2.00 L	112
TLC	3.68 L	5.38 L	68
RV/TLC	61%	37%	165

Which of the following is the correct interpretation of this PFT?
a. Restrictive disease
b. Obstructive disease
c. Combined obstructive and restrictive disease
d. Normal PFT

REFERENCES

1. Petty TL: Spirometry in smoking related diseases, *Intern Med* 12:35, 1991.
2. Official statement of the American Thoracic Society. Standardization of spirometry – 1994 update. *Am J Resp Crit Care Med* 152:1107-1136, 1995.
3. Crapo RO, Jensen RJ: Standards and Interpretive Issues in Lung Function Testing, *Respir Care* 48:764-772, 2003.
4. Enright PL: How to make sure your spirometry tests are of good quality, *Respir Care* 48:773-776, 2003.
5. Stoller JK, et al: Trial of standard versus modified expiration to achieve end-of-test spirometry criteria. *Am Rev Respir Dis* 148:275-280, 1993.
6. Mueller GA and others: Pediatric pulmonary function testing in asthma, *Pediatr Clin North Am* 39:1243, 1992.
7. Boggs PB, Wheeler D, Washburne WF, Hayati F: Peak expiratory flow rate control chart in asthma care, *Ann Allergy Asthma Immunol* 81:552, 1998.
8. Jensen RJ and Crapo RO: Diffusion capacity: how to get it right. *Respir Care* 48:777-780, 2003.
9. ATS statement: guidelines for the six-minute walk test. ATS committee on Proficiency Standards for Clinical Pulmonary Function Laboratories, *Am J Resp Crit Care Med* 166: 111, 2002.
10. Cottrell JJ and others: Preoperative assessment of the thoracic surgery patient. *Clin Chest Med* 13:47-52, 1992.
11. Hanly PJ: Mechanisms and management of central sleep apnea, *Lung* 170:1, 1992.

12. Enright PL: Surveillance for lung disease. Quality assurance using computers and a team approach, *Occup Med* 7:209, 1992.
13. Davis DD: Neonatal and pediatric respiratory diagnostics, *Respir Care* 48:367, 2003.
14. Malmstrom K and others: Quality assurance of asthma clinical trials. *Control Clin Trials* 23:143-156, 2002.

BIBLIOGRAPHY

American Association for Respiratory Care Clinical Practice Guideline: Spirometry, *Respir Care* 41:629, 1996.

Official statement of the American Thoracic Society. Standardization of spirometry – 1994 update. *Am J Resp Crit Care Med* 1995;152:1107-1136.

Ruppel G: *Manual of pulmonary function testing,* ed 7, St Louis, 1998, Mosby.

Wanger J. Editor-in Chief, Pulmonary function laboratory management and procedure manual 1998. Available at http://www.thoracic.org/education/lab-manual.asp.

Wilkins RL, Stoller JK, Scanlon, C, editors: *Egan's fundamentals of respiratory therapy,* ed 8, St Louis, 2003, Mosby.

Clinical Application of the Chest Radiograph

LEARNING OBJECTIVES

Upon completion of this chapter, the reader should be able to accomplish the following:

1. Identify the general method of how x-rays are produced.
2. Recognize the following regarding the density of the object being x-rayed:
   a. Relative amount of penetration depending on object density
   b. Definition of *radiolucent* and *radiopaque*
   c. Four classifications of radiographic density
3. Recognize how the distances between the x-ray source, film, and patient affects the radiographic appearance of anatomic structures on the film.
4. Recognize the standard distance between the x-ray source and film for a posteroanterior chest film.
5. Identify the clinical indications for the use of a chest x-ray.
6. Recognize the technique, indications, and advantages and disadvantages of the following chest radiographic views:
   a. Posteroanterior
   b. Left lateral
   c. Anteroposterior
   d. Lateral decubitus
   e. Apical lordotic
   f. Oblique
   g. Expiratory
7. Identify the correct position for endotracheal tube placement on a chest x-ray.
8. Identify the value in assessing a chest radiograph in the following situations:
   a. Central venous pressure line insertion
   b. Pulmonary artery catheter placement
   c. Nasogastric tube placement
   d. Chest tube insertion
   e. Thoracentesis
   f. Pericardiocentesis
   g. Bronchoscopy
9. Identify the technique, indications, and advantages and disadvantages for tomography and computed tomography.
10. Identify the relative use and indications for magnetic resonance imaging in lung disease.
11. Recognize the technique and indications for performing lung scans.
12. Identify how the following problems affect lung scans:
    a. Thromboembolism
    b. Atelectasis
    c. Pneumonia
13. Recognize the technique and indications for the use of pulmonary angiography.
14. Recognize the proper technique for assessing the following during technical evaluation of the chest x-ray:
    a. Placement on view box
    b. Adequacy of exposure
    c. Patient rotation
    d. Depth of inspiration
15. Recognize the proper technique for performing a systematic descriptive evaluation (interpretation) of the chest x-ray.
16. Identify the significance of the following special radiographic evaluation signs:
    a. Silhouette sign
    b. Air bronchogram
17. Recognize the limitations of the chest radiograph.
18. Recognize the typical clinical and chest radiographic findings for the following lung diseases:
    a. Atelectasis
    b. Pneumothorax
    c. Hyperinflation
    d. Interstitial lung disease
    e. Congestive heart failure
    f. Pleural effusion
    g. Consolidation

CHAPTER OUTLINE

Production of the Radiograph
Indications for the Chest X-Ray Examination
Radiographic Views
   Standard and Special Views
   Portable Chest Film (Anteroposterior View)
   Postprocedural Chest X-Ray Evaluation
Tomography

Computed Tomography
  Lung Tumors
  Chronic Interstitial Lung Disease
  Acquired Immune Deficiency Syndrome (AIDS)
  Occupational Lung Disease
  Pneumonia
  Bronchiectasis
  Chronic Obstructive Pulmonary Disease
Magnetic Resonance Imaging
Lung Scanning
Pulmonary Angiography
Evaluation of the Chest Radiograph
  Review of Clinical Findings
  Placing the Chest Film on the View Box
  Interpretation
  Limitations
Clinical and Radiographic Findings in Lung Diseases
  Atelectasis
  Pneumothorax
  Hyperinflation
  Interstitial Lung Disease
  Congestive Heart Failure
  Pleural Effusion
  Consolidation

KEY TERMS

air bronchogram
apical lordotic view
atelectasis
bronchoscopy
computed tomography
  (CT scanning)
exudate
Kerley's B lines
lateral decubitus view
magnetic resonance (MR)
oblique views
pneumothorax

positron emission
  tomography (PET)
posteroanterior (PA)
  view
pulmonary angiography
radiolucent
radiopaque
silhouette sign
target
thoracentesis
transudate

CHAPTER OVERVIEW

The introduction of x-ray technology in the early part of the last century gave medical workers a chance to see inside the human body without cutting into it. The result of this advance was revolutionary. It ushered in the era of modern medicine. Finally, the ability to detect disease expanded beyond what the examiners could identify with the history and physical examination.

The ease, accuracy, and reliability of radiographic examination allowed its use to proliferate rapidly. Within a decade or two, radiology became an entire hospital-based department and soon a special discipline within the field of medicine.

This chapter begins with a short description of the physics related to radiographs. The use of standard and special views in assessment of the patient with pulmonary disease is presented next. This is followed by a discussion of techniques for interpreting the chest film. Finally, some of the more common pathologic abnormalities seen on chest x-ray films and their related clinical findings are presented.

PRODUCTION OF THE RADIOGRAPH

X-rays are electromagnetic waves that radiate from a tube through which an electric current has been passed. The tube is made of a cathode that is attached to a low-voltage electron source (transformer). The end of the cathode wire is inside the vacuum-sealed tube, and as electrons flow through the wire, they are "boiled off," accelerate across a short gap, and strike a positively charged tungsten plate called the *anode*. The electrons coming off the cathode wire are focused to hit a small area on the anode. This area is called the target.

On striking the target, the electrons undergo physical changes, which result in the emission of x-rays. These x-rays are emitted in all directions, but because of the construction of the tube, only the few that escape through the window are actually used; the rest are absorbed harmlessly into the wall of the x-ray machine (Figure 9-1).

X-rays are not reflected back like light rays but penetrate matter. Their ability to penetrate matter is dependent on the density of the matter. Dense objects such as bone absorb more x-rays (allow less penetration) than air-filled objects such as lung tissue. A sheet of film is placed next to the patient's thorax opposite to where the x-ray tube is located to generate a chest film. The x-ray machine emits x-rays, which pass through the patient and are absorbed proportional to the density of the tissue through which they are passing. X-rays that pass through low-density (air-filled) objects strike the film full force and turn it black (radiolucent). X-rays that strike bone are partially absorbed; therefore less darkening of the corresponding area on the x-ray film is seen (radiopaque). Radiopaque areas are seen as white shadows on the film. The four different densities seen on the chest film (also called a chest radiograph) are bone, water, fat, and air.

The distance between the source of the x-ray and the patient is an important consideration. The closer the patient is to the source, the greater the magnification and distortion of the objects seen on the chest film. This concept can be demonstrated easily by placing your hand below a lamp and observing the shadow created on the surface below. The shadow becomes smaller and sharper as your hand is moved away from the light source and closer to the surface.

The patient and the film are positioned approximately 6 feet from the x-ray source for the conventional chest x-ray examination. At this distance the images seen on the chest film are in good focus, and the magnification effect is minimized.

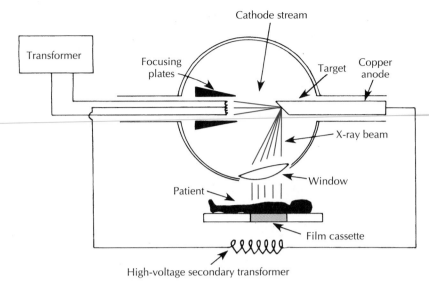

Cathode stream

Transformer

Focusing plates

Target   Copper anode

X-ray beam

Window

Patient

Film cassette

High-voltage secondary transformer

Figure 9-1 Electric current is generated by the transformer, passes through focusing plates, and arrives at the cathode. Electrons are "boiled off," making a cathode stream. The cathode stream then strikes the anode target and is transformed into x-rays. X-rays leave the sealed vacuum x-ray tube through a window and strike the patient, pass through the patient, and cast a shadow on the film cassette, making an image on the film. (From Scanlan CL, Spearman CB, Sheldon RL: *Egan's fundamentals of respiratory therapy*, ed 5, St Louis, 1996, Mosby.)

SIMPLY STATED

X-rays passing through low-density tissue (e.g., lung parenchyma) create a dark corresponding shadow on the film, and dense tissues (e.g., bone) create a white shadow on the film.

INDICATIONS FOR THE CHEST X-RAY EXAMINATION

The ability to "see inside" the body with the use of radiographs has proved to be of great benefit, especially when assessing the contents of the thorax. Production of the chest film has become one of the most popular and important procedures performed in the hospital. It can be used in the following ways:

• Detecting alterations of the lung caused by pathologic processes
• Determining the appropriate therapy
• Evaluating the effectiveness of treatment
• Determining the position of tubes and catheters
• Observing the progression of lung disease

Although the chest film provides important information about the status of the lungs, obtaining and interpreting the film must never delay fundamental treatment of the patient with obvious signs of hypoxia. In most situations, when the members of the healthcare team are well trained and work together, a chest film can be obtained without interrupting assessment and treatment.

Although only the physician can order a chest radiograph, the respiratory therapist (RT) may want to suggest to the attending physician that the chest film be obtained in certain circumstances. For example, an undiagnosed pneumothorax may suddenly cause deterioration of the mechanically ventilated patient. A stat portable chest film may be life saving if obtained early in the process. The RT is often at the bedside of

the mechanically ventilated patient and may be the first person to see the signs consistent with a potential pneumothorax and the need for a stat chest x-ray. For this reason, all RTs should be familiar with the clinical indications consistent with the need for a chest radiograph (Box 9-1).

RADIOGRAPHIC VIEWS

Standard and Special Views

The standard chest radiographs are taken in two directions. First, with the patient standing upright with his/her back to the x-ray tube, the anterior thorax is pressed against a metal cassette containing the film, and his/her arms are positioned out of the way. The patient is instructed to take a deep breath and hold it just before the x-ray is taken. The x-ray beam leaves the source, strikes the patient's posterior chest, moves through the chest, exits through the front (anterior), and then strikes the film. Because the beam moves from posterior to anterior, this is called a posteroanterior (PA) view. Because the heart is in the anterior half of the thorax, there is less cardiac magnification with a PA view. The patient is then turned sideways, and a lateral or side view is obtained. Generally, a left lateral view (left side against the cassette) is preferred. The left lateral view provides less cardiac magnification and a sharper view of the left lower lobe, which is partially obscured on the PA view by the cardiac shadow. However, if right-sided lesions are present, a right lateral view will provide a sharper view of the lesion.

Other views are sometimes obtained when special problems are identified. A lateral decubitus view is taken with the patient lying on the right or left side to see whether free fluid (pleural effusion or blood) is present in the chest. As little as 25 to 50 mL of pleural fluid can be detected with the lateral decubitus view. This view is also helpful in the identification of pneumothorax. Because air tends to rise and water tends to fall, patients with a suspected

BOX 9-1	Clinical Indications for the Chest Radiograph

Symptoms

Unexplained dyspnea
Cough, sputum, and fever
Persistent chest pain
Hemoptysis

Medical history

Recent history of chest trauma
History of aspiration of foreign body
History of tuberculosis
History of chronic obstructive pulmonary disease
Significant smoking history
History of pulmonary fibrosis
Employment history consistent with inhalation of certain dusts

Physical examination

Crackles or wheezes on auscultation
Sudden drop in blood pressure during mechanical ventilation
Unilateral decrease in breath sounds
Heavy use of accessory muscles
Respiratory rate >40/min
Loud P-2
Pedal edema
Cardiac murmurs
Signs of trauma

Arterial blood gas

Severe hypoxemia
Acute hypercarbia

Pulmonary function tests

Evidence of air trapping (e.g., increase in residual volume or functional residual capacity)
Marked reduction in expiratory flows or lung volumes
Reduced diffusing capacity of lung for carbon monoxide

Post procedure

Intubation
Central venous pressure or pulmonary artery catheter placement
Nasogastric tube placement
Chest tube placement
Thoracentesis
Pericardiocentesis
Bronchoscopy with transbronchial biopsy
Abdominal or thoracic surgery

Other

Sudden increase in peak airway pressure during mechanical ventilation
Following cardiopulmonary resuscitation
Routinely for mechanically ventilated patients
Routine screening for infectious disease

right-sided pneumothorax should be placed on their left side for radiologic examination and patients with suspected right-sided pleural fluid should be placed on their right side.

Projections made at approximately a 45-degree tube angulation from below, referred to as apical lordotic view, are sometimes required for a closer look at the right middle lobe or the top (apical region) of the lung. When the tube is angled upward, the shadows of the clavicles are projected above the thorax.

Oblique views are helpful in delineating a pulmonary or mediastinal lesion from structures that overlie it on the PA and lateral views. Oblique views are often obtained when bilateral lesions are present and to help localize the abnormality. In this view the patient is turned 45 degrees to either the right or left, with the anterolateral portion of the chest against the film.

Although chest radiographs are usually taken with the patient at full inspiration, an expiratory film can be helpful in certain situations. For example, a small pneumothorax can be difficult or impossible to detect in a routine inspiratory film. As the patient exhales, however, the lung volume is reduced, while the pleural air volume remains the same. The pneumothorax now occupies a greater percentage of the thoracic volume and therefore stands out more. In addition, the lung is denser in the expiratory position, and the contrast allows for the air density within the pleural space to be more easily visualized.

Portable Chest Film (Anteroposterior View)

Patients in intensive care units are too sick to be transported to the x-ray department for a standard PA chest film. In this instance, a portable x-ray machine is brought to the patient's bedside and positioned in front of the patient. The film cassette is placed carefully behind the patient's back. Thus the x-ray beam moves from front to back (anterior to posterior), generating an **anteroposterior (AP) film** instead of the usual PA film. The distance from the patient to the beam's origin must be consistent to prevent a magnification effect.

Interpreting an AP film requires advanced skills. The AP film is often not centered, is either overexposed or underexposed, or is not taken when the patient is in full inspiration. There may be many extrathoracic shadows superimposed on the film. These extra shadows include bedding, gowns, electrocardiogram leads, and tubing. The clinician has to be able to read the film accurately despite this artifact.

AP portable films are obtained to evaluate the lung status, to gain information on how well lines and tubing are positioned, and to see the results of invasive therapeutic maneuvers. Some of the lines and tubes needing evaluation are discussed in the following paragraphs.

> **SIMPLY STATED**
> The standard chest film is taken with the patient's chest pressed against the film cassette. The x-ray passes from back (posterior) to front (anterior), and the resulting chest film is called a PA film. The portable chest film is obtained with the x-ray passing from front (anterior) to back (posterior), producing an AP film.

Postprocedural Chest X-Ray Evaluation

Tracheal Intubation

The AP chest film often is used to evaluate the position of the endotracheal tube to be sure that the inferior tip comes to rest appropriately 3 to 5 cm above the carina after intubation (Figure 9-2). Accidental placement of the endotracheal tube in the right or left mainstem bronchus or esophagus must be recognized immediately to minimize potential harm to the patient. All manufacturers include a thin radiopaque strip in the wall of the entire length of the endotracheal tube to allow visualization of the tube's precise position in the chest on the radiograph.

Figure 9-3 shows a common incorrect endotracheal tube placement. Note that the tip of the endotracheal tube has come to rest in the right mainstem bronchus. The team doing the intubation probably did not have enough experience in assessing the size of the patient as it relates to the notation imprinted on the tube indicating its length from the tip. Thus the tube was inserted too deeply. Furthermore, the team did not auscultate the chest carefully after the tube was placed. In this case, there would have been prominent breath sounds on the right but absent breath sounds on the left. If this tube is not pulled back to the proper position, the entire tidal volume being delivered by the ventilator will go into the right lung and may cause barotrauma (pneumothorax), a potential cause of shock, hypoxia, and death.

After the tube is repositioned, the number of centimeters seen on the tube at the position of the patient's lips (teeth) should be noted, the tube carefully taped, and a repeat x-ray obtained for documentation that the tube's malposition has been corrected.

Central Venous Pressure Line

Evaluation of the central venous pressure (CVP) line is necessary to be sure that the catheter tip is in the proper position. The catheter is placed into the right or left subclavian or jugular vein and should come to rest in the confluence of the superior venae cavae and the right atrium of the heart. During placement of central catheters, it is possible to enter the lung accidentally by passing through the wall of the vein, entering the pleural space, and thus causing the lung to collapse. If fluids are being delivered (e.g., blood replacement, total parenteral nutrition), the fluid will end up in the chest cavity instead of the bloodstream. An AP portable chest film is required immediately after the line is thought to be in position and before it is sutured in place and fluid given.

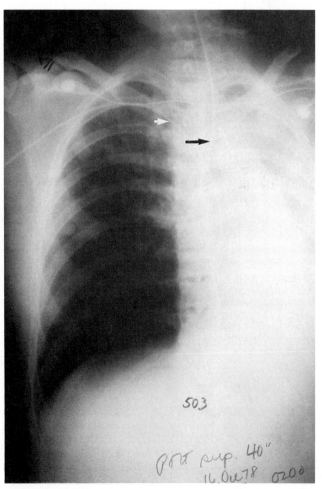

Figure 9-3 Anteroposterior chest film demonstrating placement of the endotracheal tube in the right mainstem bronchus (black arrow). The left lung has collapsed because of atelectasis. The central venous pressure line is in good position (white arrow).

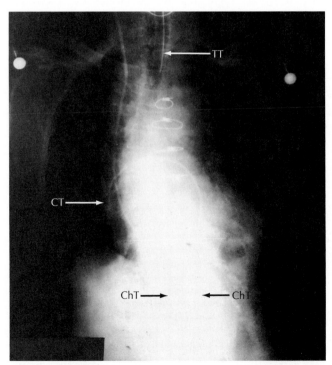

Figure 9-2 Pulmonary artery catheter (Swan-Ganz catheter) in its usual position in the right lower lung field. This view does not indicate whether the catheter is anterior or posterior within the chest. CT, Catheter tip; ChT, chest tube; TT, tracheal tube.

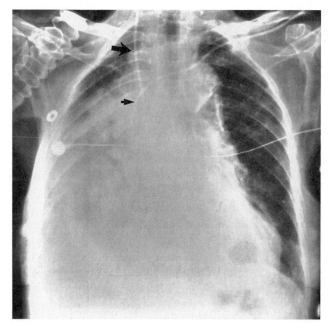

Figure 9-4 Anteroposterior chest film demonstrating a total parenteral nutrition line in the right jugular vein *(large arrow)*. The line has punctured the vein and entered the right lung. Nutritional substances have been infused into the right pleural space. Note that a left subclavian central venous pressure line is in good position *(small arrow)*.

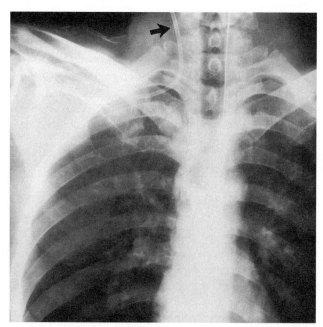

Figure 9-5 Anteroposterior chest film showing a central venous pressure line in the right subclavian vein. The tip of the line has moved retrograde up the internal jugular vein *(arrow)* and must be repositioned.

In Figure 9-3 the postplacement x-ray shows the tip of the CVP line to be in proper position, which is at the confluence of the superior venae cavae and the right atrium. Figure 9-4 shows the CVP catheter having missed the vein, entered the pleural space, nicked the lung, and caused a pneumothorax. To make matters worse, fluid delivery was started before the error was discovered. The fluid is seen contaminating the pleural space. A second invasive procedure is now required: the placement of a chest tube to relieve the pneumothorax and drain off the fluid, thereby preventing an empyema.

Figure 9-5 shows the most common malpositioning of a CVP line. It has gone up the neck on the right. If the catheter is withdrawn a short distance, manual pressure placed over the right jugular vein while the patient's head is turned will cause the catheter to flip around and pass down the superior venae cavae.

Figure 9-6 shows the venous anatomy in the area of the neck and upper thorax. Every vein shown has the potential for receiving a misdirected CVP line.

Pulmonary Artery Catheter Placement

After the pulmonary artery (Swan-Ganz catheter) is inserted, an AP portable chest film is obtained to identify the position of the catheter tip. Because these catheters usually stay in the patient for days or weeks, the chest film is used on a daily basis to monitor its position and effect on the pulmonary circulation. Figure 9-7 shows a pulmonary artery catheter in good position: the right midlung near the hilum.

The pulmonary artery catheter has a small inflatable balloon near the tip that is inflated with about 1 mL of air at the time of placement. The inflated balloon serves as a "sail" to allow the natural flow of blood to drag the rest of the catheter through the right atrium, tricuspid valve, right ventricle, and pulmonary valve and into the pulmonary artery. The catheter usually is swept into the right pulmonary artery, probably because the right lung is slightly larger than the left and has slightly more blood flow entering it. In addition, the right pulmonary artery is more directly in line with the trunk of the pulmonary artery in most people. Once the catheter wedges into a smaller pulmonary capillary (as noted on the pressure monitor), the balloon is deflated and a portable AP chest film is obtained. The catheter is sutured into place if the chest film demonstrates proper position of the catheter tip.

Most of the problems with these catheters are related to the inflatable balloon. It can rupture the artery whenever it is inflated to obtain the wedge pressure reading. Permanent damage to a portion of the lung can occur if the balloon is accidentally left inflated too long because the inflated balloon blocks blood flow to the lung tissue distal to the catheter tip. The portable chest film will demonstrate an area of pulmonary infarction in such cases.

Nasogastric Feeding Tubes

The AP chest film is useful to evaluate the position of the nasogastric (NG) feeding tube to ensure that it is located appropriately in the stomach or small bowel. Occasionally the NG tube can be inserted accidentally into the trachea. An AP chest film can reveal this complication.

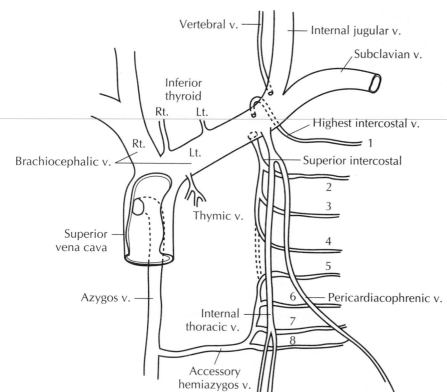

Figure 9-6 Venous anatomy of the neck. The central venous pressure line is intended to be located in the lower part of the superior vena cava. *Lt.,* Left; *Rt.,* right; *V.,* vein.

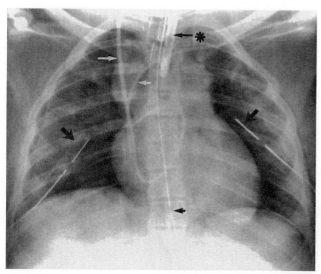

Figure 9-7 Portable chest film showing good position of the pulmonary artery catheter as it passes through the right side of the heart and into the right pulmonary artery *(long white arrow).* Note the position of the right and left chest tubes *(large black arrows),* endotracheal tube *(black arrow with asterisk),* and nasogastric tube *(small black arrow).* A short white arrow points to the left subclavian central venous pressure line in good position.

In the alert patient, the accidental placement of an NG tube into the trachea causes severe coughing and dyspnea. The patient complains bitterly. However, these tubes are often placed in the heavily sedated or comatose patient who cannot complain. NG tubes have been placed accidentally

into the trachea, down the mainstem bronchus, and deep into the lung. This can lead to numerous problems, such as pneumonia and pneumothorax, if not detected as soon as possible.

Chest Tubes

Chest tubes are large drainage tubes placed into the left or right thorax and attached to a set of three drainage bottles. These bottles are attached in series with the third bottle attached to wall suction of approximately 20 cm H_2O pressure. Their purpose is to drain excess air, blood, or pleural fluid from the pleural cavity.

Placing the chest tube is very painful for the patient and requires intravenous opiates and conscious sedation. Pain medication is usually needed as long as the tube remains in the chest. With proper precautions (monitoring the ECG and SaO_2), the tube can be placed at bedside and not in an operating room.

The attending physician will request a portable chest x-ray after the chest tube has been inserted. Figure 9-8 shows good placement of the tube. The tip of the tube should be posterior and near the apex of the lung so drainage can occur with the patient lying on his/her back. The tube is sutured in place and heavily bandaged to reduce pain if the patient inadvertently rolls onto the insertion wound. Periodic portable chest x-rays may be needed to ensure that the tube is draining and remaining in the correct position.

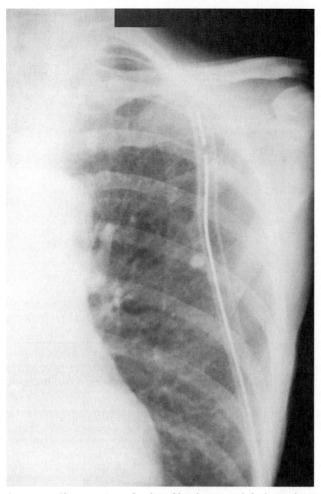

Figure 9-8 Close-up view of a chest film showing a left chest tube in good position. Note that three distinct lines are seen along the tube. The thicker line in the middle is a radiopaque stripe that allows visualization of the entire length of the tube. The other two lines are the edges of the tube itself; they would not be visible if the tube was accidentally placed in the soft tissues of the chest wall.

Procedures Requiring Evaluation with an AP Portable Film

- Thoracentesis: temporary placement of a needle into the pleural space to withdraw fluid for analysis (pleural effusion analysis).
- Pericardiocentesis: temporary placement of a needle into the sac surrounding the heart to draw off abnormally accumulated fluid for treatment and analysis.
- Bronchoscopy: a device used for direct viewing of the larynx, trachea, and large airways can be passed down an oral or nasal tracheal tube. This device, called a bronchoscope, allows visualization of the trachea and some bronchi. Tissue and secretions can be obtained for analysis, or, if a lobe or segment is blocked, the offending blockage can be removed. After this is done, an AP portable x-ray film is obtained to look for any positive or negative effects of the procedure.

SIMPLY STATED

The chest radiograph is used not only to diagnose lung disease, but also to confirm the correct placement of tubes and catheters and the effect of procedures on the lung.

TOMOGRAPHY

Tomograms are a special type of x-ray examination in which the x-ray tube is rotated throughout exposure on an armature above the patient, focusing the rays into a central point or "cut" (Figure 9-9). In the case of chest tomograms, the patient is placed in the supine position on the x-ray table, and the armature holding the x-ray tube is rotated above the patient. Starting at the patient's back as a reference point, consecutive

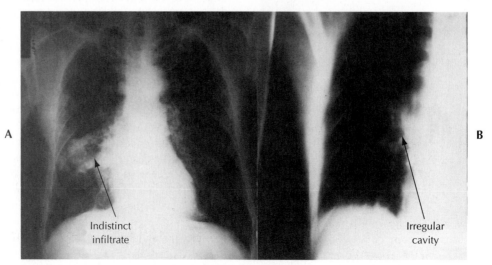

A — Indistinct infiltrate

B — Irregular cavity

Figure 9-9 A, Lesion in the right lung is indistinct. **B,** Single tomographic cut taken from a series of cuts done for a tomogram study of the lesion. Every other structure is blurred except for the lesion in question. Note the irregular cavity, which is highly suggestive of squamous cell carcinoma.

1-cm cuts are made, moving progressively anteriorly. Tomograms are useful for pinpointing chest lesions, thus detailing their shape and size.

This form of tomography has been replaced almost completely by computed tomography (CT). Other forms of imaging of the body inspired by the concept of tomography have also gained acceptance. Most noteworthy is magnetic resonance (MR). The clinical uses of CT and MR are presented in the following sections.

COMPUTED TOMOGRAPHY

Computed tomography (CT scanning) is a high technology approach to evaluating patients via x-ray examination. The technique involves computed enhancement of x-ray shadows. What results is an amazingly clear look at internal anatomy. CT scanning has revolutionized radiology and is especially useful in pulmonary medicine.

This technique is so widely used in U.S. hospitals that CT scanners are available to scan heads and chests in most hospitals and are used nearly around the clock. Big metropolitan hospitals have these scanners in emergency rooms for easy evaluation of trauma cases. The technique and equipment have advanced to allow high-resolution CT scanning. This advance has increased the sensitivity of CT scanning so that lesions can be detected even before the patient begins to complain of symptoms.

The clarity of the image produced has made CT scanning indispensable in the medical management of pulmonary disease. The only drawback to the use of this technique is its cost (about $800 per procedure). CT scanning is extremely useful in the following areas.

Lung Tumors

Currently the most important use for CT scanning in the patient with lung cancer is to determine whether a lesion originating outside the chest has metastasized to the lung. The need for mediastinoscopy has been reduced significantly by the use of CT scanners in this situation. In looking for spread of cancer from extrathoracic sites to the lung, CT scanning is superior to conventional radiography. High-resolution CT scanning detects peripheral nodules as small as 2 to 3 mm.

Once a peripheral carcinoma of the lung (coin lesion) has been identified, CT is helpful in placing a biopsy needle into the lesion. Pneumothorax is the main complication and has been reported in 10% to 60% of cases, with chest tube insertion being required in 5% to 15% of the cases.[1]

Chronic Interstitial Lung Disease

High-resolution CT scanning is superior to conventional films in the evaluation of diffuse interstitial lung disease (Figure 9-10). The CT scan will demonstrate considerable changes even when the conventional chest film is read as normal. More than 100 diseases involve the pulmonary interstitium, with 10 of these diseases constituting 80% to 90% of all cases.[2] CT scanning is used selectively because of its high cost. Current research in this area is aimed at identifying the radiographic appearance of each individual interstitial disease with CT scanning. Eventually this may reduce or eliminate the need for open- or closed-lung biopsy, which is more expensive and dangerous.

Acquired Immune Deficiency Syndrome (AIDS)

CT scanning can be useful in the early detection of pneumonias that occur as a result of AIDS. The technique is also useful in detecting abscesses and cavities. The mediastinum also can be evaluated for enlarged lymph nodes caused by infection or the lymphoma-like cancers seen in AIDS.[3]

Occupational Lung Disease

The lung diseases resulting from the inhalation of dusts, fumes, irritant gases, organisms, and smoke are called *pneumoconioses,* or *extrinsic alveolitis.* Inhaling dusts and fumes can cause numerous respiratory problems, such as asthma and pulmonary fibrosis. CT scanning is very helpful in identifying the changes seen in the pleura and the lung parenchyma associated with occupational lung disease. The initial nodules and subsequent fibrosis are seen clearly on CT scan. Pleural plaques seen with asbestosis are readily demonstrated with CT scan.[4]

Pneumonia

The cost of CT has restricted its use in the evaluation of most pneumonias. However, CT scans of the lung are superior to conventional chest films in the visualization of pneumonias and related pathologic changes in the hila and pleura. Opportunistic pneumonias are detected sooner and more precisely by CT than by plain films.[5]

Bronchiectasis

In the past, bronchiectasis was visualized best with the bronchogram. This dangerous and invasive method has been replaced by the CT scan. The frequency with which unsuspected bronchiectasis is present has surprised many investigators.[6]

Chronic Obstructive Pulmonary Disease

CT scans of the emphysematous chest are almost breathtaking in their clarity and detail. The diagnosis of emphysema via conventional radiography is 65% to 80% accurate. With CT scanning, emphysematous changes of even mild to moderate degree are seen with such ease as to make diagnosis consistently in the high 90% range[7] (see Figure 9-10).

MAGNETIC RESONANCE IMAGING

The role of MR imaging in the diagnosis of intrathoracic lung disease has been limited. It has been used in conjunction with CT

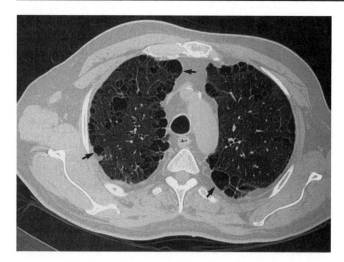

Figure 9-10 Computed tomographic slice through the upper lungs in a patient with pulmonary emphysema. Numerous cystic lucencies are present in both lungs. Note the absence of bronchovascular markings within the lucencies. Most of the emphysematous areas are located in a peripheral distribution (*arrows*) along the pleural surface (paraseptal). (From Wilkins RL, Stoller JK, Scanlan CL: *Egan's fundamentals of respiratory care,* ed 8, St. Louis, 2003, Mosby.)

scans, but so far MR imaging has added little or no new information to the understanding of lung disease. The one area in which MR imaging may be a little better than CT scanning is in the evaluation of hila. MRI is better able to differentiate hilar lymph node enlargement from enlarged hilar blood vessels than is CT.[8] This information is critical in determining to what extent lung cancer has spread. The patient is inoperable if a lung cancer has spread to the hilum and thus enlarged it (Figure 9-11).

Another area in which MRI may be superior to the CT scan is in the evaluation of chest wall invasion by lung cancer and the evaluation of the specific cancer called Pancoast's tumor or superior sulcus tumor. These tumors occur high in the lung and invade the nearby chest wall. The axillary nerves and superior mediastinal blood vessels may also be involved in the tumor spread.[9] MRI can determine the precise position of the tumors and the involvement with surrounding structures.

LUNG SCANNING

Lung scans are obtained by measuring gamma radiation emitted from the chest after radiopharmaceuticals are injected into the bloodstream or inhaled into the lung. This procedure, once thought of as a sophisticated research technique, is now widely available. Lung scanning is useful for studying the distribution of ventilation and perfusion and the effect disease may have on these two important functions. The major clinical application of lung scanning is in the evaluation of patients suspected of having a pulmonary embolism.

To perform perfusion lung scans, particulate radionuclides are injected into a peripheral vein. The venous blood flow carries the particles to the pulmonary circulation, where the radionuclides lodge in the pulmonary capillaries because the particles are larger than the capillaries. The particles remain

lodged for a considerable time and can be scanned to identify the distribution of perfusion in the lungs (Figure 9-12). A reduction in pulmonary blood flow to a part of the lung can be detected because the radioactivity over the affected area is decreased. This reduction in blood flow occurs with pulmonary embolism or any respiratory disease such as atelectasis or pneumonia that causes a localized area of vasoconstriction.

Ventilation lung scans are performed by having the patient breathe a radioactive gas or a nebulized aerosol of a radioactive material. Poorly ventilated regions can be detected easily because the radioactive material will not enter the affected lung regions. The ventilation scan is then compared with the perfusion scan to identify the matching of ventilation to perfusion (Figure 9-13). When a pulmonary embolism is present, the ventilation scan usually is normal and the perfusion scan shows a defect in the affected region. If the patient has pneumonia or atelectasis, both ventilation and perfusion scans are abnormal. In some cases of pulmonary embolism, the clot may cause atelectasis in the affected region and therefore lead to abnormal ventilation and perfusion. In such cases the lung scan results are not diagnostic for pulmonary thromboembolic disease.

The diagnosis of pulmonary embolism often is difficult. The current approach is to obtain a ventilation-perfusion ($\dot{V}/\dot{Q}$) scan as the first step. The current radiology wording for reporting the results of a $\dot{V}/\dot{Q}$ scan is "high probability," "indeterminant," or "low probability." "High probability" suggests that the scan is positive for pulmonary embolism but not 100% conclusive because lung scans are not diagnostic. "Indeterminant" indicates that the lung scan has an abnormality, but the defect may or may not be consistent with a pulmonary embolism. "Low probability" suggests that the lung scan is not demonstrating an abnormality typical of pulmonary embolism.

A recently reported large multicenter study has confirmed the concerns of clinicians having to diagnose pulmonary embolism using $\dot{V}/\dot{Q}$ scans and this reporting system. "High-probability" scans are falsely positive 12% to 14% of the time, and "low-probability" scans miss 16% to 40% of patients who have pulmonary embolism. This means that 12% to 14% of patients can undergo prolonged therapy with dangerous blood thinners (heparin and Coumadin for at least 2-4 months) or that 16% to 40% of patients may not be treated for a life-threatening condition.[10] The solution to the problems lies in the use of the more invasive pulmonary angiogram.

> ### SIMPLY STATED
> $\dot{V}/\dot{Q}$ scans are useful to evaluate the patient suspected of having a pulmonary embolism, but the results often are inconclusive.

POSITRON EMISSION TOMOGRAPHY (PET SCAN) (Figure 9-14)

A discussion of the physics involved in the production of photons by "annihilation of positrons" is well beyond the scope of

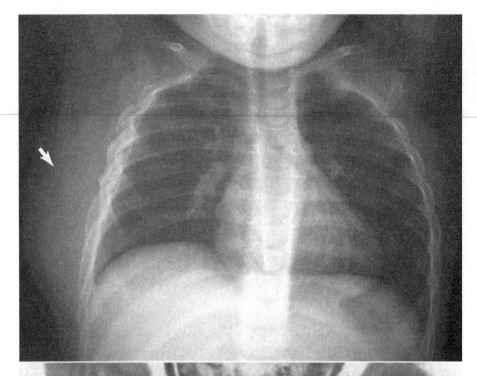

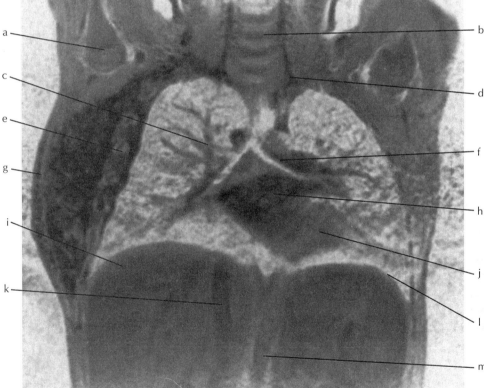

Figure 9-11 A, PA chest film demonstrating normal lung fields but severe soft tissue swelling along the right lateral chest wall *(arrow)* outside the thoracic cage (compare right to left side). This chest film is instructive because it demonstrates the importance of examining the entire chest, not just the lung fields. **B,** MRI view of posterior thorax in the same patient. *a,* humeral head; *b,* vertebral column; *c,* right lung and bronchi; *d,* left vertebral artery; *e,* rib; *f,* posterior wall of left main stem bronchus; *g,* soft tissue mass (lymphosarcoma); *h,* mediastinal metastasis of lymphosarcoma; *i,* hepatic view; *j,* posterior wall of heart; *k,* inferior vena cava; *l,* left hemi diaphragm; *m,* descending aorta.

this text. It is adequate to know that in order for this imaging to work, metabolically active radiopharmaceuticals labeled with positron emitters are required. A glucose analog fluorine-18 fluorodeoxyglucose is used in positron emission tomography (PET) scanning to diagnose and stage cancers.

When this compound is injected into a vein, malignant cells, having increased metabolic rates, selectively pick up the compound. Using the PET scanner, this area will "light up" and

produce a bright spot on the film. There are other disease states that may give false-positive results, but, in the proper settings, this scanning technique has greatly improved the ability to differentiate between tumors and nonmalignant tissues.

For instance, in the diagnosis of coin lesions 1 cm or greater, PET scans have shown sensitivities of 95% or higher and specificities of 78% or higher. This scan can also demonstrate spread to local and distant tissues such as lymph nodes in the hilar and mediastinal area, and distant spread to brain, bone, and adrenal glands.

PULMONARY ANGIOGRAPHY

Angiography of the pulmonary circulation is done most often to evaluate thromboembolic disease of the lungs. It is generally done only after lung scanning and when results of the $\dot{V}/\dot{Q}$ scan are uncertain. To perform pulmonary angiography, a contrast medium is injected into the pulmonary artery or one of its branches. Angiographic proof of pulmonary embolism is considered to be identification of one or more filling defects (Figure 9-15). The decision to use it must be made carefully because this procedure is invasive and costly.

EVALUATION OF THE CHEST RADIOGRAPH

This section is intended to introduce the basic principles of evaluation of the chest radiograph. It cannot teach the reader to interpret chest films any more than a book on surgery can teach the reader to operate. Interpreting chest films is a skill obtained only through hours of dedicated practice. The beginner is encouraged to view chest films initially with the help of qualified experts.

Familiarity with the anatomic landmarks seen on normal chest films is extremely helpful in learning to recognize abnormalities. Figure 9-16 identifies the more important landmarks on a normal PA chest radiograph.

Review of Clinical Findings

The clinician will benefit from reviewing the patient's history and physical examination findings before viewing the chest film. This information can provide insight into the abnormalities to be looked for on the chest film.

Placing the Chest Film on the View Box

The chest film must be placed on the view box as if the patient were facing the clinician (i.e., the right side of the patient's chest is on the clinician's left, and vice versa). The left side of the patient's chest is easily identified by looking at the cardiac shadow, which is most often prominent on the left side of the chest. Also, the letters *L* and *R* identifying the patient's left and right sides may be visible to assist in identifying the correct placement. Once the film is on the view box, the nameplate should be inspected to make sure the name on the film matches the name of the patient being evaluated.

The first step in evaluating the chest film is to determine the technical quality of the film. The adequacy of exposure can be judged by looking at the vertebral bodies. The clinician should just be able to visualize the vertebral bodies through the cardiac shadow. If the vertebral bodies are seen easily, the film is probably overexposed and the lungs will appear black.

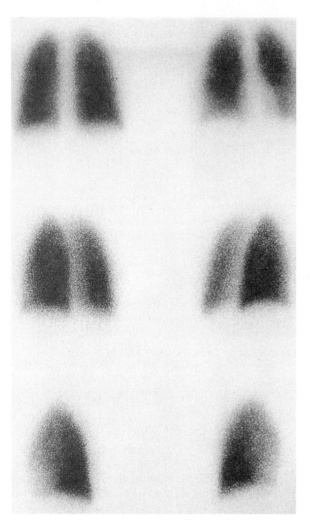

Figure 9-12 Normal lung perfusion scan. There is no evidence of perfusion defects in the anterior, posterior, oblique, or lateral views of the lungs.

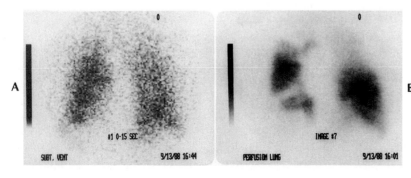

Figure 9-13 Abnormal ventilation-perfusion scan. The ventilation study **(A)** demonstrates bilateral lung filling without gross defects; however, the perfusion scan **(B)** shows multiple subsegmental perfusion defects of both lungs. These findings are highly suggestive of pulmonary emboli.

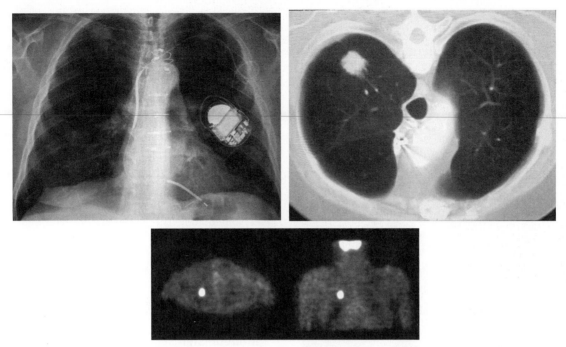

Figure 9-14 This series of images shows a coin lesion on routine chest x-ray, a CT scan of the lesion, and a PET scan. Only the PET scan is able to indicate, with a high sensitivity and specificity that this lesion is actually cancerous. The routine chest x-ray shows a faint density on the right, behind the right clavicle. The presence of the pacemaker overlying the left chest tends to direct the examiner's eye away from the right upper lobe lesion. The CT scan shows this lesion to be ominous. Is it a cancer or an old scar, and thus benign? Two views from the PET scan show this lesion "lights up." It is a cancer.

Underexposure makes identification of the vertebral bodies more difficult, and the lung fields appear whiter than on a properly exposed film. The pulmonary vascularity and some pulmonary abnormalities may be misinterpreted with overexposure or underexposure.

The film should be evaluated to make sure that the patient was not rotated when the chest film was obtained. If the patient is rotated, uniform exposure of both lungs will not be obtained, and one side of the film will be darker than the other. Patient rotation is assessed by identifying the relationship of the spinous processes of the vertebral column to the medial ends of the clavicles or to the tracheal air shadow (Figure 9-17). The spinous processes should be centered between the ends of the clavicles and directly behind the tracheal air shadow. If the medial end of one clavicle appears closer to the spine or if the spinous processes are to the side of the tracheal air shadow, the patient probably was rotated.

Finally, the degree of the patient's inspiratory effort is evaluated by counting the posterior ribs visible above the diaphragm. On a PA film, 10 ribs indicate a good inspiratory effort. A poor inspiratory effort may cause the heart to appear abnormally enlarged and increase the density of the lung fields so that they appear too white to allow detection of certain lung abnormalities.

SIMPLY STATED

A good inspiratory effort results in 10 posterior ribs visible above the diaphragm. The depth of the patient's inspiration is assessed to help determine the quality of the chest film.

Interpretation

Interpretation of the chest film requires a complete understanding of the x-ray principles introduced at the beginning of this chapter. The clinician must remember that x-ray penetration of structures is inversely proportional to the density of the structure. The greater the density, the less the penetration. X-rays that do not penetrate fully are absorbed, resulting in less exposure of the film and the casting of a white shadow on the film.

Normal lung tissue has a low density (air density), and normal lung fields appear as dark shadows on the chest film. If an area of the lung consolidates (increases in density) because of pneumonia, tumor, or collapse, that area will absorb more x-rays and appear as a white patch on the film. Abnormalities that decrease lung tissue density, such as cavities and blebs, absorb fewer x-rays and result in darker areas on the film.

The heart, diaphragm, and major blood vessels are considered to have the density of water. Because water is denser than air, water densities result in less exposure and therefore whitish-gray shadows on the film. The heart, diaphragm, and major blood vessels rarely alter in density, but may change in size, shape, and position. Evaluation of the shadows produced on the chest film by these structures allows a clear view of any deviation from normal in position or size.

The structures in the chest with the greatest density are the bones, including the ribs, clavicles, scapulae, and vertebrae. They are seen on the film as white shadows. Fractures and changes in position and density of bones may be evaluated with the chest film. A chest film should be obtained to evaluate the bony structures of the chest whenever the patient's history or physical examination suggests chest trauma. A recent history of

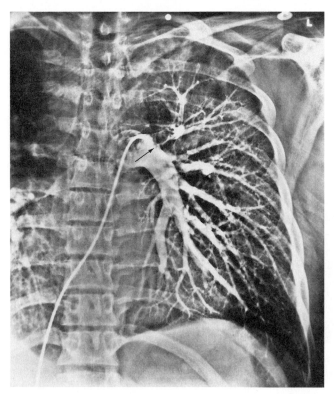

Figure 9-15 Abnormal pulmonary angiogram. The radiograph demonstrates a large clot in the pulmonary vascular tree. A small amount of dye was able to slip around the clot and outline the embolus *(arrow)*.

an automobile accident or blunt chest injury from any sudden impact indicates that a chest film is needed.

Identification of the abnormalities visible on the chest film requires a systematic review of all the structures shown on the film. The sequence in which the structures are evaluated is not important as long as all are included. Many experts encourage beginners to develop a habit of evaluating the bony structures and peripheral areas of the chest film first. This helps prevent overlooking subtle but important abnormalities in the less conspicuous areas of the film. Once the peripheral soft tissues and bony structures have been viewed, the lung, mediastinum, heart, and diaphragms are inspected carefully. A system using the alphabet—A to Z—has been recommended to remind the examiner which parts of the chest film to study. This system, starting with A for *airway*, B for *bones*, C for *cardiac shadow*, and so forth, may prove useful in organizing the approach to reading the chest radiograph.

The ability to localize abnormalities within the thorax is aided by special radiographic signs. Two of the most important and reliable methods are the silhouette sign and the air bronchogram.

Silhouette Sign

The silhouette sign is useful primarily in determining whether a pulmonary infiltrate is in anatomic contact with a heart border or the diaphragm. Normally, the significant difference in density between muscle tissue and lung tissue results in sharply delineating these borders. If the lung tissue in contact with either heart border or sections of diaphragm becomes consolidated, the contrast in densities is lost and the corresponding heart or diaphragm border is blurred (see Figure 9-17; Figure 9-18).

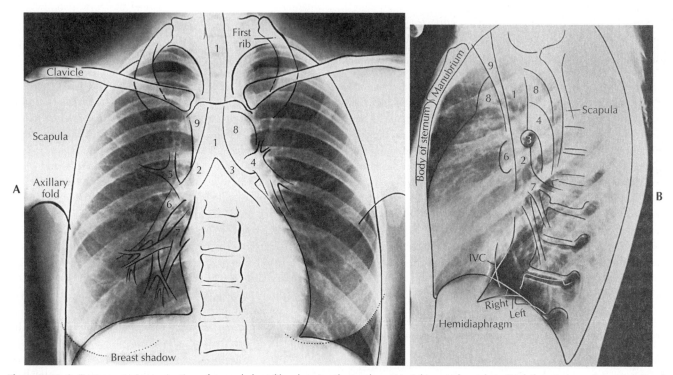

Figure 9-16 A, Posteroanterior projection of normal chest film showing the trachea *(1)*, right main bronchus *(2)*, left main bronchus *(3)*, left pulmonary artery *(4)*, right upper lobe pulmonary artery *(5)*, right interlobar artery *(6)*, right lower and middle lobe vein *(7)*, aortic knob *(8)*, and superior vena cava *(9)*. **B,** Lateral projection of normal chest film showing trachea *(1)*, right main bronchus *(2)*, left main bronchus *(3)*, left interlobar artery *(4; not visible this view [5])*, right main pulmonary artery *(6)*, confluence of pulmonary veins *(7)*, aortic arch *(8)*, and brachiocephalic vessels *(9)*. (From Fraser RS, Pare RD: *Diagnosis of diseases of the chest*, Philadelphia, 1970, WB Saunders.)

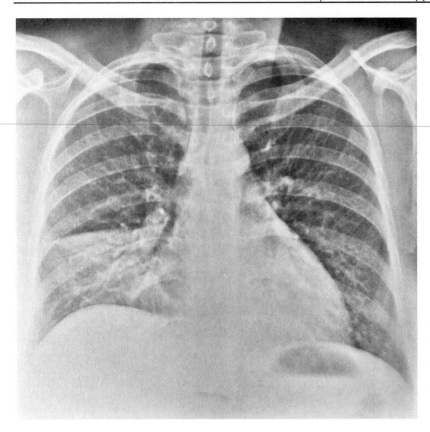

Figure 9-17 Note how the spinous processes of the vertebrae are centered within the tracheal air shadow, indicating that the patient was not rotated when the chest film was obtained. Also note the consolidation in the patient's right lung. The infiltrate must be in the right middle lobe because the right heart border is blurred (see description of silhouette sign in text).

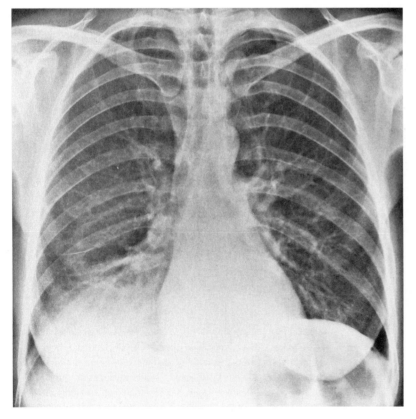

Figure 9-18 Right lower lobe pneumonia. Note how the right heart border is clearly seen, indicating that the infiltrate must be in the lower lobe, which is posterior to the heart. Also note that the right hemidiaphragm is obscured. This provides further evidence that the consolidation is in the right lower lobe.

Because the heart is located in the anterior thorax, any infiltrate that obliterates the heart border must also be located in the anterior segments of the lungs. Infiltrates that appear to overlap the heart border on the film but do not affect its sharpness are located in posterior segments and are not in anatomic contact with the heart. The same can be said of the diaphragm, except the diaphragms are under the lungs and span from the anterior to the posterior compartments of the lung. This allows for location of infiltrates that occur in the bases of the lungs.

> ### SIMPLY STATED
> Infiltrates in the lung will blur the edges of the heart or the diaphragm where the infiltrate touches them. This observation helps locate with better precision where the infiltrate is located in the lung.

Air Bronchogram

The air bronchogram is useful in determining whether an abnormality seen on the radiograph is located within the lung. Normally the intrapulmonary bronchi are not visible on the chest film because they contain air and are surrounded by air-filled alveoli. If the bronchi are surrounded by consolidated alveoli, they will be visible because the air within their lumina will stand out in contrast to the surrounding consolidation. In this situation the bronchi are seen as linear branching air shadows, signifying that the lesion is within the lungs and not located in the pleural space.

The air bronchogram is often seen in pneumonia and pulmonary edema. However, if the lesion fills the bronchi as well as the alveoli, air bronchograms will not be seen because no contrast is present. Therefore the absence of the air bronchogram is of little significance.

Limitations

Although the chest radiograph provides important information about the pathologic changes within the thorax, it does have certain limitations. Small lesions and those located in "blind" areas may not be seen. In addition, the chest film is often normal in patients experiencing significant respiratory symptoms. A typical example is the patient with asthma experiencing acute bronchospasm. Even though the patient may be experiencing cough and shortness of breath, the chest radiograph often appears normal.

CLINICAL AND RADIOGRAPHIC FINDINGS IN LUNG DISEASES

This section reviews the radiographic findings typical of the more common respiratory disorders. Familiarity with this information is helpful in the interpretation of chest films. In addition, this section presents the clinical findings typically associated with the different pathologic abnormalities described. In most cases, the most efficient and accurate assessment is achieved when clinical and radiographic findings are used together. The following categories of chest diseases are presented:

- Atelectasis
- Hyperinflation
- Interstitial lung disease
- Congestive heart failure (CHF)
- Pleural effusion
- Consolidation

Atelectasis

Loss of air in a portion of lung tissue results in a condition called atelectasis (Figure 9-19). Atelectasis is formed from the Greek *ateles* (incomplete) and *ektasis* (extension). Atelectasis may occur as a result of changes in the transpulmonary distending pressure and in such cases is called *compressive atelectasis*. It may also be caused by obstruction of one or more airways, which allows distal gas to be absorbed (see Figure 9-19). The latter type of atelectasis may be called *obstructive* or *absorption atelectasis*.

Compressive Atelectasis

Compressive atelectasis is seen in patients with pleural effusion, pneumothorax, hemothorax, and any space-occupying lesion. The degree of pulmonary compromise with compressive atelectasis depends on the size of the lesion. Small lesions may not disrupt pulmonary function significantly; however, larger

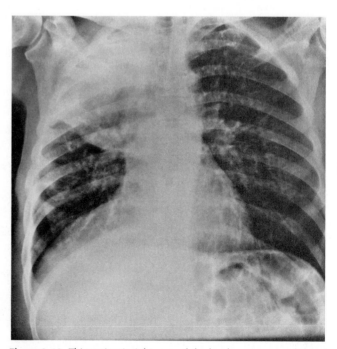

Figure 9-19 This patient's right upper lobe has become consolidated because of a tumor obstructing the right upper lobe bronchus. As a result, pneumonia has developed distal to the obstruction. Note the well-outlined horizontal fissure, slightly rotated up and delineating the inferior boundary of the right upper lobe. The upward displacement of the horizontal fissure suggests atelectasis in the right upper lobe.

lesions may compromise cardiac function as well as lung function if the mediastinum is shifted.

Obstructive Atelectasis

Obstructive atelectasis emphasizes the blockage of an airway so that ventilation of the affected region is absent. Many clinical situations can obstruct an airway, leading to collapse (atelectasis). When this happens, usually entire lobes or segments are involved rather than subsegments or smaller units (microatelectasis). Tumor, aspirated foreign substances, fibrosis, mucus plugging, mechanical obstruction, and scarring are some of the more common causes of obstructive atelectasis (see Figure 9-19).

As long as the airway obstruction remains incomplete, the distal lung will remain inflated. In fact, partial obstruction of a bronchus can lead to hyperinflation of the lung if the obstruction causes a one-way valve effect, allowing air to enter the lung but not escape. Complete obstruction of a larger airway usually leads to atelectasis of the distal lung; however, collateral ventilation may occur through alveoli ventilated by unobstructed airways and thus maintain partial alveolar patency.

A related form of atelectasis occurs in patients following surgery. It is not uncommon for atelectasis to develop in the postoperative period, especially if the patient has had upper abdominal or thoracic surgery or if the patient is obese or has a history of chronic lung disease. After surgery, lung secretions tend to be retained in the lung because of mucociliary stasis and suppression of coughing and deep breathing. Retained secretions can obstruct multiple distal airways, leading to underventilation and atelectasis of the affected region.

The physical examination findings of atelectasis vary with the amount of lung involved. With significant loss of lung volume, as occurs with lobar collapse, the findings are striking and usually include the following:
- Rapid shallow breathing
- Decreased to absent breath sounds
- Decreased to absent vocal fremitus
- Decreased resonance to percussion
- Cyanosis
- Shift of the mediastinum toward the affected side

The chest radiograph in most cases readily demonstrates the loss of lung volume caused by the atelectasis. With collapse of entire segments or lobes, characteristic densities are seen. Shift of the trachea, heart, and major thoracic vessels toward the affected side is often seen. The radiographic findings seen with postoperative atelectasis often are more subtle.

Abnormalities may not be detected during physical examination of the patient with atelectasis. If an entire lobe is collapsed (atelectatic), the surrounding healthy lung tissue may expand into the space previously occupied by the atelectatic region. Thus no abnormalities may be detected over the affected region. Careful examination of the chest film and other clinical findings are needed to detect this condition. The chest radiograph may not readily demonstrate the atelectasis when the degree of atelectasis is small. In these cases, more subtle signs of collapse must be looked for on the film. These signs include:

- Shift of the fissure lines toward the collapsed area (see Figure 9-19)
- Movement of the hilar structures toward the area of collapse
- Overall loss of volume in one lung
- Hemidiaphragm elevation

Pneumothorax

Pneumothorax is an extreme form of atelectasis (Figure 9-20). Pneumothorax is a condition in which air enters the pleural space either externally from a hole in the chest wall or internally from a hole in the lung. This leads to loss of the negative pressure normally found in the pleural space. As a result, the lung's normal elasticity, which causes it to contract, is unopposed, and the lung collapses.

This is serious enough, but the lung can develop a potentially more serious problem called a *tension pneumothorax* (Figure 9-21). With a tension pneumothorax, the hole formed has a flap on it that acts as a valve as the person breathes. The effect is to pump air into the pleural space, which now has positive pressure in it. This pressure eventually shifts the heart away from the involved lung and puts pressure on the good lung, altering blood and lymph flow. The good lung's ability to oxygenate is severely compromised, and the heart may not pump blood effectively. Not all pneumothoraces develop "tension." Clinical situations predisposing a person to pneumothorax are the following:
- Trauma, such as an automobile accident or stab wounds to the chest
- Fractured ribs poking through the pleural space

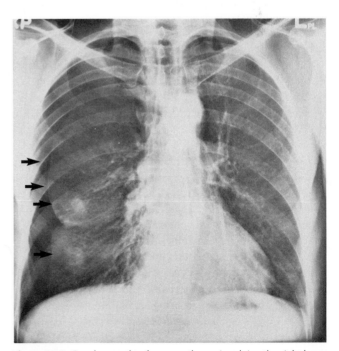

Figure 9-20 Good example of pneumothorax involving the right lung. Note the pleural line along the right lateral chest wall where the lung has pulled away from the chest wall as it collapsed toward the hilum.

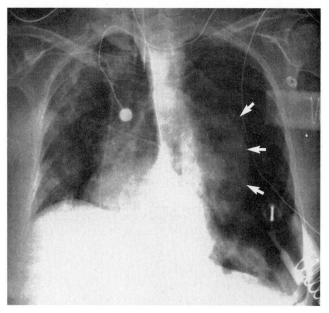

Figure 9-21 Portable chest film showing a left-sided tension pneumothorax. Note that the pressure in the left hemithorax has depressed the diaphragm on that side and forced the heart into the right side of the chest. A chest tube must be inserted immediately into the left chest.

- Hospital procedures such as chest surgery thoracentesis, or placement of a CVP line, hyperalimentation line, or pulmonary artery catheters
- Elevated mean airway pressures, as occur during positive-pressure ventilation with stiff lungs
- Spontaneous rupture of blebs along the lung margins
- Improper placement of an oral or nasal tracheal tube, resulting in the tip of the tube coming to rest in the right or left mainstem bronchi

Physical findings associated with pneumothorax without tension reveal the following:
- Chest wall: reduction in movement in the chest wall on the side where the pneumothorax has occurred
- Auscultation of the lung: loss of breath sounds or at least distant breath sounds on the affected side
- Percussion: increased resonance to percussion on the affected side
- Heart: usually a rapid heart rate (tachycardia) and tachypnea
- Other: cyanosis, an external wound, or bruising, with a sucking noise on the involved side, usually seen when a tension pneumothorax is present
- Absent whispered voice sounds and tactile fremitus

With a tension pneumothorax, shift of the mediastinal structures (the trachea, heart, and lung) away from the involved side results in deviation of the trachea from the affected side. In Figure 9-20 the chest film shows a pleural line that comes down the right side of the chest wall and even shows the invagination caused by the horizontal fissure. With the lung pulled away from the chest wall it is easy to see why there is a decrease in breath sounds and increased resonance with percussion during physical examination.

> **SIMPLY STATED**
> Tension pneumothorax is a life-threatening condition that is seen on the chest film as extreme hyperlucency on the affected side, with a shift of the mediastinal structures away from the air-filled pleural space.

Hyperinflation

The most common cause of hyperinflation is obstructive lung disease. The diagnosis of chronic obstructive pulmonary disease (COPD) does not depend solely on radiographic changes. The history, physical examination, and pulmonary function data are crucial. The chest film reveals dependable, consistent changes that help support the diagnosis of asthma, chronic bronchitis, and emphysema: the three diseases that constitute COPD. In some cases of COPD the chest film may be read as normal, especially when the disease process is mild.

The functional residual capacity (FRC), residual volume (RV), and total lung capacity (TLC) increase and are seen as hyperinflation on the chest radiograph with COPD. The specific findings of hyperinflation seen on the chest film (Figure 9-22) are as follows:
- Large lung volumes
- Increased anterior air space, as seen on the lateral film (see Figure 9-22, *B*)
- Depressed diaphragms
- Small narrow heart, especially with emphysema
- Enlarged intercostal spaces

The physical examination findings that correlate with the x-ray examination include the following:
- Large barrel chest, with increased AP dimension of the chest wall
- Increased resonance to percussion
- Decreased breath sounds
- Limited motion of low-set diaphragms
- Wheezing (may not be present with fatigue)
- Prolonged expiratory phase
- Rapid respiratory rate
- Use of accessory muscles to breathe

> **SIMPLY STATED**
> The severity of the emphysema in the patient with COPD is often predicted by the size of the retrosternal air space. The larger it is, the more severe the emphysema.

Interstitial Lung Disease

Many diseases can cause a pattern on the chest film called *interstitial lung disease* (Figures 9-23 to 9-25). Fortunately, it occurs in a small number of patients. A list of the diseases causing this

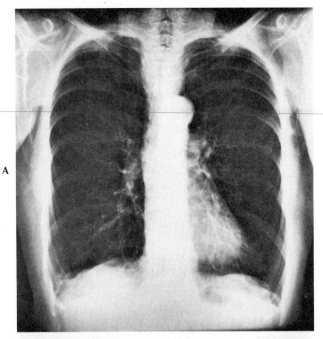

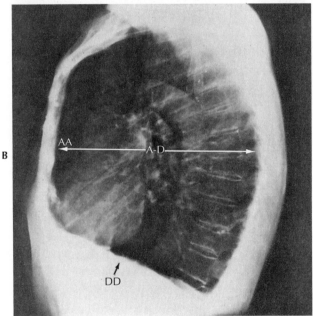

Figure 9-22 A, Posteroanterior chest film. Note marked hyperinflation with large lung volumes, low-set diaphragm, small, narrow heart, and enlarged intercostal spaces. **B,** Lateral view. Hyperinflation is manifested by increased anterior air space, depressed diaphragm, and increased anteroposterior chest dimensions (barrel chest). *AA,* Anterior air space; *DD,* depressed diaphragm; *A-D,* anteroposterior dimension.

type of infiltrate is included to acquaint the reader with the terms (Box 9-2).

The basic pathologic process associated with pulmonary fibrosis is shown in Figure 9-23. Some substance (etiologic agent) insults the lung's immune system, causing the lung to scar or become fibrotic. The fibrotic process usually is progressive, leading to more and more scarring of the lung with each

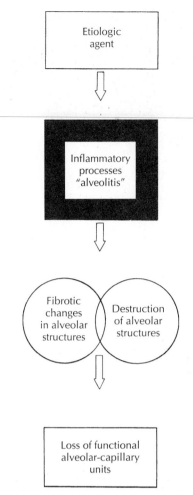

Figure 9-23 Theoretic explanation for development of pulmonary fibrosis. Patients who develop interstitial fibrosis are prone to develop other complications such as pneumothorax, cancer, and pneumonia. (Modified from Simmons DH: *Current pulmonology,* New York, 1981, Elsevier.)

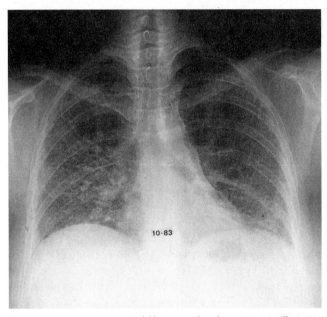

Figure 9-24 Severe interstitial fibrosis in the chest. (From Wilkins RL, Stoller JK, Scanlan CL: *Egan's fundamentals of respiratory care,* ed 8, St Louis, 2003, Mosby.)

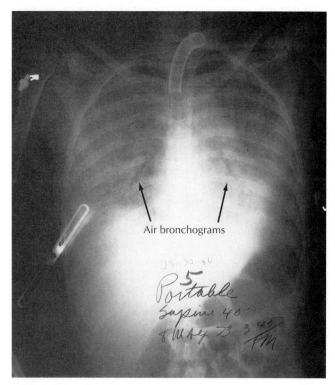

Figure 9-25 Typical alveolar filling pattern.

passing year. The end result for the majority of these patients is combined cardiac and respiratory failure after many years of a slow, progressively debilitating disease. In a few instances the disease is self-limiting, and spontaneous cures have been seen.

Initially, the patient afflicted with interstitial lung diseases may notice a dry, nonproductive cough and dyspnea on exertion (DOE). This usually brings the patient in for medical care. The history is probably the most important element in helping to determine what has incited the immune response, causing the lung damage. A history of industrial exposure to silica or asbestos is crucial. A history of systemic symptoms such as swallowing disorders or joint or muscle pain may suggest a collagen-vascular disease causing the fibrosis.

The pattern seen on the chest film may give a clue to the cause (see Figure 9-24). Upper lobe fibrosis is unusual. Most of the time the fibrotic infiltrates occur in the lower lobes; however, ankylosing spondylitis, tuberculosis, and silicosis all have a predilection for the upper lobes. If the pattern of fibrosis present is favoring the upper lung fields, the disorders just mentioned are suggested.

The term *alveolar pattern* is favored by some and disliked by others when referring to interstitial lung disease. The term has some usefulness in helping to identify the disease by looking at the pattern of the infiltrate. The alveolar pattern results when the alveoli begin to fill up with water, blood, pus, protein, or cells (see Figure 9-25). If the patient is coughing up any of these materials or has been known to have inhaled some of these substances (e.g., near-drowning victims), the pattern on the x-ray film is better understood (Table 9-1).

BOX 9-2 Interstitial Lung Diseases

Infections

Viruses: measles, chickenpox, influenza
Rickettsiae: Q fever, Rocky Mountain spotted fever
Bacteria: tuberculosis; mycoplasm, staphylococcal, and strepto coccal infection; *Klebsiella;* salmonellosis; others
Fungi: histoplasmosis, coccidioidomycosis, others
Parasites

Occupational Causes

Mineral dusts: asbestosis, silicosis, berylliosis, others
Chemical fumes: nitrogen dioxide, ammonia, chlorine, acetylene, many others

Neoplastic Causes

Bronchioalveolar carcinoma, hematogenous metastases, lym phangitis, leukemia, lymphoma

Congenital or Familial Causes

Cystic fibrosis, Niemann-Pick disease, Gaucher's disease, tuberous sclerosis, familial dysautonomia (Riley-Day syndrome), pulmonary alveolar microlithiasis, familial idiopathic pulmonary fibrosis

Metabolic Causes

Uremic pneumonitis

Physical Agents

Postirradiation fibrosis, thermal injury, oxygen toxicity, blast injury

Circulatory Causes

Thromboembolism
Hemodynamic, congestive heart failure

Immunologic Causes

Hypersensitivity pneumonia: inhaled antigens, drug reactions
Collagen diseases: scleroderma, rheumatoid arthritis, lupus erythematosus, Wegener's granulomatosis, dermatomyositis, Goodpasture's syndrome

Unknown

Sarcoidosis, histiocytosis X, idiopathic hemosiderosis, pulmonary alveolar proteinosis, desquamative interstitial pneumonia, idiopathic fibrosis

Adapted from Braunwald E and others, editors: *Harrison's principles of internal medicine,* ed 11, New York, 1987, McGraw-Hill.

The alveolar pattern of pulmonary fibrosis may lead to visualization of air bronchograms. This occurs as a result of the alveolar spaces becoming infiltrated and denser. The air-filled airway is seen as clear and as a dark, straight shadow with several attached branchings. Around the area is a whitened ground-glass–appearing area, representing affected alveolar spaces.

Physical examination of the patient with interstitial lung disease typically identifies a rapid and shallow breathing

Table 9-1   Alveolar Space Pathology

Alveolar Space

Fills with	Possible Causes
Water	Congestive heart failure
	Drowning or near drowning
Blood	Goodpasture's syndrome
	Idiopathic pulmonary hemosiderosis
Purulent exudate (pus)	Pneumonia
Protein	Pulmonary alveolar proteinosis
Cells	Desquamative interstitial pneumonitis
	Bronchioalveolar (alveolar cell) carcinoma

The alveolar pattern exists when the following is noted on the chest x-ray film in contrast to the interstitial pattern:

Interstitial Pattern	Alveolar Pattern
Peripheral distribution (especially in lower lobes)	Perihilar in distribution
Small volume with contracted lungs	Minimal volume loss
Linear stranding	Early in the process small mulberry-like infiltrates are seen; later, nodules are seen that coalesce into a ground-glass appearance
No air bronchogram	Air bronchogram is seen.

pattern. The interstitial fibrosis causes a decrease in lung compliance that results in the patient breathing with a smaller tidal volume. As the tidal volume decreases, the respiratory rate must increase to maintain adequate ventilation. Auscultation usually identifies fine inspiratory crackles that do not clear with deep breaths or changes in position. The crackles often are more noticeable over the lower lobes. If the interstitial lung disease is severe, significant hypoxemia and cyanosis may be present.

The final diagnosis of interstitial lung disease usually requires the physician to obtain a piece of lung by open lung biopsy or transbronchial biopsy using a flexible bronchoscope. Even after a lung biopsy, the final diagnosis and determination of the cause with this group of diseases often are difficult.

Congestive Heart Failure

Pulmonary edema can be diagnosed by many different routes, but perhaps the earliest indication is obtained with the chest film. Early CHF causes definite changes in the chest film (Figure 9-26). These changes include the following:

1. Redistribution of pulmonary vasculature to the upper lobes. Usually the normal chest film shows the pulmonary blood vessels prominent in the lower lobes. With CHF, fluid collects in the dependent portions of the lung. The ability to exchange oxygen in these lower lung fields is impeded. To compensate for this altered physiology, the blood flow is redirected to the upper lung fields, where the lung tissue is

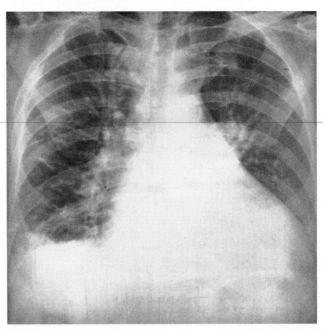

Figure 9-26 Congestive heart failure with upper lobe redistribution of vasculature markings, especially on the right, increased cardiothoracic, ratio, Kerley's B lines, and increased interstitial markings. Cardiac shadow should not be over half of the entire width of the thoracic cage; here it is well over half.

still free of edema fluid. With CHF, the chest film shows enlarged prominent blood vessels in the upper lobes, where they should be small and barely noticeable.

2. Increase in the ratio of the width of the heart at its greatest span to the width of the thorax: the cardiothoracic (C/T) ratio. Normally, this ratio does not exceed 0.5. In CHF the heart enlarges and its width exceeds one half of the width of the thoracic cage. This enlargement is abnormal and consistent with CHF (see Figure 9-26).

3. Development of Kerley's B lines. These lines, usually seen in the right base, are 1 mm thick and approximately 1 to 2 cm in length. They are horizontal and start at the periphery, extending into the lung approximately 1 to 2 cm. They are pleural lymphatic vessels filled with fluid (see Figure 9-26).

4. Miscellaneous signs.
   a. Increased interstitial markings
   b. Pleural effusion in the right hemithorax only
   c. Enlarged pulmonary artery segments

CHF in patients with severe hyperinflation (especially emphysema) may not result in some of the signs just mentioned. The development of an enlarged heart may be delayed in patients with emphysema because of the pathologic changes already present in the thoracic cage. With tissue destruction, common in emphysema, redistribution to the upper lobes already may have occurred before CHF develops. Also, redistribution in such cases may not occur when the vascular bed has been altered by bullae.

The physical examination findings that correlate with the x-ray findings center around crackles (rales) at the bases. The crackles may be heard in the apices in more severe cases. The patient has a rapid respiratory rate and is anxious, usually sitting upright to breathe and resisting lying down because of the dyspnea associated with reclining (orthopnea). Other important findings that relate to CHF are associated with cardiac abnormalities. The patient's neck veins are distended, and on auscultation of the heart, the following are noted:

- Rapid heart rate, either regular or irregular in rhythm. (The rhythm regularity is vital and must be noted.)
- Third heart sound (S_3), a consistent finding in CHF.
- Murmurs, usually not present if CHF is the only cardiac abnormality.
- Increased closure sound of the pulmonary component of the second heart sound.

Other findings outside the chest but related to CHF include the following:

- Enlarged liver (hepatomegaly).
- Pulsus alternans: On palpating the peripheral pulse, a strong pulsation alternates with a weak one. This is an indicator of severe heart failure.
- Ankle edema (swelling) that is pronounced during the day and improves after a night of sleep. This is usually accompanied by having to get up several times each night to urinate (nocturia).

Historically, the patient complains of nocturia, orthopnea, coughing (sometimes productive of a bloody and frothy sputum), and paroxysmal nocturnal dyspnea (attacks of severe shortness of breath that awaken the patient from sleep). Fatigue and weakness are common complaints.

> **SIMPLY STATED**
> The size of the heart on the chest film is an important parameter to evaluate. If the width of the heart exceeds 50% of the width of the thorax, an enlarged heart is present. Remember that a portable AP chest film causes the heart shadow to appear slightly larger because of the magnification effect of the heart being closer to the source of the x-ray.

Pleural Effusion

Free fluid may form in the intrapleural space (Figures 9-27 and 9-28). Usually 100 mL must be present before the fluid can be seen on the chest radiograph. The fluid can be a clear watery material; low in protein content (less than 3 g/L), called a transudate; or more commonly a fluid with a high protein content (over 3 g/dL), called an exudate.

The causes of transudative pleural effusion are limited and include CHF and atelectasis. The possible causes of exudative pleural effusions are more numerous and include bacterial pneumonia, pulmonary embolism, malignancy, viral disease, tuberculosis, and fungal infections.

Other free fluids can collect in the pleural space. These include blood (hemothorax), a fatty fluid called chyle (chylothorax), and pus (empyema or pyothorax). The chest x-ray findings of pleural effusion depend on the volume of fluid collected in the pleural space. Small volume findings (see Figure 9-27) are:

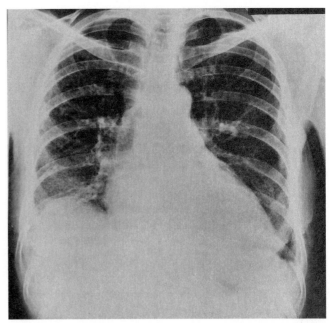

Figure 9-27 A small pleural effusion has developed in the right chest, resulting in a blunted right costophrenic angle and partially obscured right hemidiaphragm.

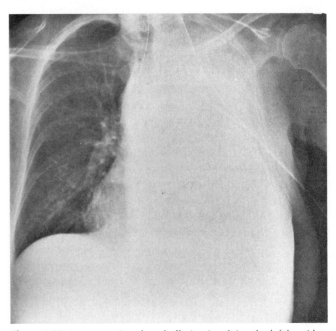

Figure 9-28 Large massive pleural effusion involving the left hemithorax. This has caused the x-ray film to appear as a whiteout of the involved side, completely obscuring all structures in the left chest.

- Blunting of the otherwise sharp angle between the chest wall and the point at which the diaphragm touches the chest wall laterally (the costophrenic [CP] angle).
- Small meniscus sign. The meniscus sign is seen whenever fluid starts to track up the side of the chest wall, much as water slides for a short distance up the side of a glass container, thus forming a meniscus.
- Partially obscured diaphragm with elevation of the diaphragm from its normal position.

Large (massive) volume findings (see Figure 9-28) are:

- Complete whiteout of the involved side
- Complete obscuring of the hemidiaphragm

If there is a question as to whether an effusion is present, or if the fluid is free to move about, a lateral decubitus film is obtained. This helpful study requires only that the patient lie on the side suspected of having the pleural effusion while the radiograph is taken. This is called the *lateral decubitus view* (Figure 9-29). The special positioning of the patient allows visualization of a fluid line on the chest film.

The physical findings with pleural effusion are related to the volume of free fluid in the chest. The patient may complain of pain on inspiration; a dull, heavy feeling in the involved area; coughing; or shortness of breath. Small volumes of fluid are symptom free and undetectable on physical examination. However, when the size of the pleural effusion is significant, the findings may include the following:

- Dullness to percussion in the involved area
- Egophony just above the area of dullness
- Decreased breath sounds on the affected side
- Tachypnea

Consolidation

A section of lung can become airless, fill up with fluid, and not collapse. In this instance the involved lung area is said to be consolidated. The usual cause of this state is bacterial pneumonia. Many times the bacterial pneumonia is a result of obstruction of the airways by aspirated foreign bodies (e.g., peanuts or very small toys) or tumorous growths. Figures 9-17 and 9-18 show good examples of consolidation. The radiographic signs of consolidation include the following:

- Minimal loss of volume
- Usually lobar distribution
- Homogeneous density late in the process
- Air bronchogram if the airway leading to the consolidated area is open

The physical findings associated with a consolidated lung include the following:

- Dullness to percussion over the involved area
- Bronchophony and bronchial breath sounds
- Crackles often heard over the involved area
- Whispered voice sounds increased, and egophony present (if airway is patent)
- Tachypnea and fever

The patient reports typical symptoms associated with pneumonia. These include a cough with sputum production, weakness, fever and chills, chest pain (pleural in nature), and shortness of breath. If the consolidation is chronic, the patient may have mild symptoms. Surprisingly, some patients with a consolidated lung may not request medical care for some time because the symptoms are minimal.

> **SIMPLY STATED**
> When lung tissue becomes consolidated, it is airless, with little loss of volume. It usually occurs to a lobe of the lung that is obstructed at its bronchus. The physical findings over the area are easily demonstrated.

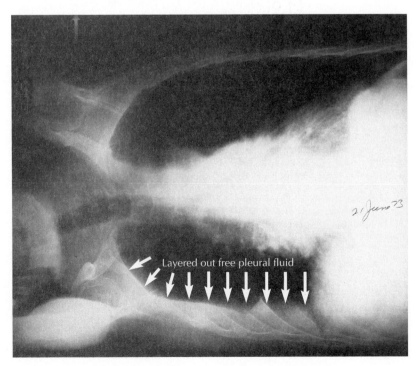

Layered out free pleural fluid

Figure 9-29 Patient lying on side so that pleural effusion fluid has moved to the dependent area of the chest cavity *(line indicated by arrows)*. This is called a lateral decubitus view. Important information is available from this view: confirmation of the effusion's presence and the fact that the effusion is free and not loculated, or trapped, by adhesions in one area of the chest cavity.

REVIEW QUESTIONS

1. T F X-rays are produced by positron emission.

2. T F Increasing object density increases the amount of x-ray penetration.

3. Which of the following is *not* a radiographic density?
   a. Water
   b. Air
   c. Mineral
   d. Fat

4. T F An item that is white on the radiograph would be called radiopaque.

5. Which of the following is true regarding the distance between the x-ray source, film, and patient when taking a chest x-ray?
   a. Distance has no effect on the image on the film
   b. As the distance between the source and the patient decreases, magnification increases
   c. As distance between the source and patient decreases, the image becomes sharply focused
   d. None of the above

6. Which of the following is the standard distance between the x-ray source and the film for a posteroanterior x-ray?
   a. 3 feet
   b. 4 feet
   c. 5 feet
   d. 6 feet

7. In which of the following situations would a chest x-ray *not* be indicated?
   a. During cardiopulmonary resuscitation
   b. After intubation to assess the position of the endotracheal tube
   c. To assess the progression of a patient's pneumonia
   d. To check the effectiveness of chest physical therapy

8. Which of the following is/are true regarding a posteroanterior chest x-ray?
   a. Patient rotation usually is present and makes interpretation difficult
   b. Heart size is subject to less magnification
   c. It is the standard for bedridden hospitalized patients
   d. All of the above

9. Which of the following views helps to evaluate for the presence of small amounts of free pleural fluid?
   a. Apical lordotic
   b. Expiratory
   c. Oblique
   d. Lateral decubitus

10. T F Chest x-rays normally are taken during a full inspiration.

11. Which of the following problems may be associated with a portable (anteroposterior) chest x-ray?
    a. Poor radiographic exposure
    b. Patient is not centered on the film
    c. Artifactual shadows may be present on the film
    d. All of the above

12. Which of the following films is especially helpful in identifying a pneumothorax?
    a. Lateral
    b. Oblique
    c. Expiratory
    d. Lateral decubitus

13. Correct positioning of an endotracheal tube is confirmed if the tip of the tube is approximately _____ cm above the carina on the chest x-ray.
    a. 0–1
    b. 2–3
    c. 3–5
    d. 7–9

14. Which of the following *cannot* be assessed via the use of a chest x-ray?
    a. CVP line position
    b. Chest tube position and effectiveness
    c. Nasogastric tube placement
    d. Cardiac pacemaker effectiveness

15. T F Tomography is especially useful in visualizing masses in the mediastinum and chest.

16. Which of the following is/are true regarding the use of MR imaging in lung disease?
    a. It is widely used.
    b. It is a useful diagnostic tool for detecting pulmonary problems.
    c. It is better than CT in evaluating the hilar areas for lymph node and vascular enlargement.
    d. All of the above.

17. Which of the following is/are true regarding lung scanning?
    a. It can be used to detect abnormalities in ventilation compared to perfusion.
    b. It uses radioactive tracers.
    c. It can be used to detect pulmonary thromboembolism.
    d. All of the above.

18. T F Pneumonia can cause a decrease in perfusion and ventilation on a lung scan.

19. Which of the following is the best method to evaluate for the presence of the thromboembolism?

a. Lung scan
b. Angiography
c. CT
d. MR imaging

20. T   F   An x-ray is considered properly exposed if the thoracic vertebrae are easily visible through the heart shadow on an AP or PA film.

21. The depth of inspiration on an x-ray is adequate if _____ posterior ribs are visible above the diaphragm on a PA or AP film.
a. 5
b. 7
c. 8
d. 10

22. T   F   Interpretation of the chest x-ray primarily involves identification of abnormal findings.

23. What is the significance of the silhouette sign?
a. It allows differentiation between alveolar and interstitial infiltrates.
b. It can aid in detecting pleural effusion.
c. It helps determine the anterior or posterior position of an infiltrate based on the appearance of the heart shadow.
d. All of the above.

24. T   F   A chest x-ray can be normal in the presence of significant pulmonary disease.

25. Which of the following clinical or chest x-ray findings are consistent with a tension pneumothorax?
a. Increased radiolucency on the affected side
b. Mediastinal shift toward the pneumothorax
c. Dullness to percussion on the affected side
d. Bronchial breath sounds on the affected side

26. Which of the following is/are radiographic sign(s) of atelectasis?
a. Increased radiopacity
b. Hemidiaphragm elevation
c. Hilar shift toward atelectasis
d. All of the above

27. Which of the following could be seen on a chest x-ray of a patient with congestive heart failure?
a. Low and flat diaphragms
b. Increased cardiothoracic ratio
c. Tracheal deviation
d. Increased retrosternal airspace on a lateral film

28. Which of the following clinical or chest x-ray findings might be found in a patient with consolidation due to pneumonia?

a. Lobar radiopaque pattern of the infiltrate
b. Increased resonance to percussion over the affected area
c. Stridorous breath sounds upon auscultation of the affected area
d. All of the above

29. Which of the following chest x-ray findings is/are consistent with hyperinflation?
a. Large lung volumes
b. Widened intercostal spaces bilaterally
c. Small and narrow heart
d. All of the above

30. Which of the following chest x-ray findings is *not* consistent with a small pleural effusion?
a. Air bronchograms on the affected side
b. Blunted costophrenic angle
c. Meniscus sign
d. Partially obscured and elevated hemidiaphragm

REFERENCES

1. Gardner D and others: CT-guided transthoracic needle biopsy, *Cardiovasc Int Radiol* 14:17, 1991.
2. Hansell DM: Computed tomographic diagnosis of diffuse lung disease, *Curr Opin Radiol* 69, 1992.
3. Naidich DP, McGuinness G: Pulmonary manifestations of AIDS: CT and radiographic correlations, *Radiol Clin North Am* 29:999, 1991.
4. Aberle DR, Balmes JR: Computed tomography of asbestos related pulmonary parenchymal and pleural diseases, *Clin Chest Med* 12:115, 1991.
5. Hommeyer SH, Godwin JD, Takasugi JE: Computed tomography of air-space disease, *Radiol Clin North Am* 29:1065, 1991.
6. Westcott JL: Bronchiectasis, *Radiol Clin North Am* 29:1031, 1991.
7. Sanders C: The radiographic diagnosis of emphysema, *Radiol Clin North Am* 29:1019, 1991.
8. Gualdi GF and others: Computed tomography and magnetic resonance in the TNM staging of pulmonary carcinoma [in Italian], *Clin Ter* 141:493, 1992.
9. Weinreb JC: Thoracic magnetic resonance imaging, *Clin Chest Med* 12:33, 1991.
10. *Medical knowledge self-assessment program IX, pulmonary medicine and critical care,* 1992, part C, book 3, p. 884.

BIBLIOGRAPHY

Fraser R, Pare J: *Diagnosis of diseases of the chest,* ed 4, Philadelphia, 1999, WB Saunders.
Murray JF, Nadel JA: *Textbook of respiratory medicine,* Philadelphia, 1988, WB Saunders.

Sheldon RL, Dunbar RD: Systematic analysis of the chest radiograph. In Scanlon CL, Sheldon RL, Spearman CB, editors: *Egan's fundamentals of respiratory therapy,* ed 6, St Louis, 1995, Mosby.

Scott WJ, Dewan NA: Use of the positron emission tomograph to diagnose end stage lung cancer. *Clinical Pulm Med,* 1999;6:198-204.

Smith JP, Pierson DJ: Diagnostic imaging. In Pierson DJ, Kacmarek RM, editors: *Foundations of respiratory care,* New York, 1992, Churchill Livingstone.

CHAPTER

10

Traci L. Marin
Robert L. Wilkins

Bedside Interpretation of Electrocardiogram Tracings

LEARNING OBJECTIVES

Upon completion of this chapter, the reader should be able to accomplish the following:

1. Discuss the clinical value of the electrocardiogram (ECG).
2. Identify the clinical findings that indicate the need for an ECG recording.
3. Identify the key components of the electrical conduction system of the heart and the role of each component.
4. Recognize definitions of depolarization and repolarization.
5. Identify the specific electrical activity of the heart associated with each wave and interval of the normal ECG.
6. Identify normal values for the PR interval and the QRS complex.
7. Given a 12-lead ECG recording, identify the ventricular rate and position of the mean QRS vector.
8. List the steps for ECG interpretation.
9. Identify the ECG criteria for each of the following abnormalities:
   a. Sinus bradycardia
   b. Sinus tachycardia
   c. Sinus dysrhythmia
   d. Premature atrial contraction
   e. Atrial flutter
   f. Atrial fibrillation
   g. Premature ventricular contractions
   h. Ventricular tachycardia
   i. Ventricular fibrillation
   j. Asystole
   k. First-, second-, and third-degree atrioventricular (AV) block
10. Identify the ECG abnormalities associated with chronic lung disease.
11. Discuss the identification of ischemia, injury, and infarction using the 12-lead ECG tracing.
12. Describe how to assess patients with chest pain.

CHAPTER OUTLINE

What Is an ECG?
What Is the Value of an ECG?
When Should an ECG Be Obtained?
Cardiac Anatomy and Physiology
Causes and Manifestations of Dysrhythmias
Important Abbreviations and Acronyms
Basic ECG Waves
    ECG Paper and Measurements
ECG Leads
    Limb Leads
    Chest Leads
    Evaluating the Mean QRS Axis
Steps of ECG Interpretation
Identification of Common Dysrhythmias
    Sinus Bradycardia
    Sinus Tachycardia
    Sinus Dysrhythmia
    Paroxysmal Atrial Tachycardia
    Atrial Flutter
    Atrial Fibrillation
    Premature Ventricular Contractions
    Ventricular Tachycardia
    Ventricular Fibrillation
    Asystole
    Pulseless Electrical Activity
    AV Heart Block
    Idioventricular Rhythm
    Junctional Rhythm
Evidence of Cardiac Ischemia, Injury, or Infarction
Assessing Chest Pain
ECG Patterns with Chronic Lung Disease

KEY TERMS

atrial kick	ectopic impulse
automaticity	escape beat
depolarization	focus
dysrhythmia	repolarization

Cindy Tait, RN, MPH, CCRN, contributed to this chapter in the previous edition.

CHAPTER OVERVIEW

Given the hands-on nature of respiratory care, the likelihood of a respiratory therapist (RT) observing a patient during the acute onset of an ischemic cardiac event or lethal dysrhythmia is significant. Thus, it is vital for RTs to have basic knowledge in electrocardiogram (ECG) interpretation because they may serve as the first link in the chain of survival for a patient experiencing such an event. Early recognition may potentially minimize cardiac damage or prevent death due to a myocardial infarction. In addition, understanding the significance of the subtle and often progressive aspects of ECG changes provides the RT with information that will enhance the assessment of a patient's cardiopulmonary health.

This chapter describes the electrophysiology of normal and abnormal ECG tracings. Ultimately, it is intended to explain how to recognize basic and life-threatening ECG patterns that may be observed while performing respiratory care. After a review of cardiac physiology related to the production of electrical activity within the heart, numerous abnormal rhythms (dysrhythmias) are described. Criteria for recognition and possible causes are reviewed for each abnormality presented.

WHAT IS AN ECG?

An ECG (also called an EKG) is an indirect measurement of the electrical activity within the heart. A recording of the electrical currents within the heart is obtained by placing electrodes containing a conductive media to each extremity and to numerous locations on the chest wall to create a 12-lead ECG. Each specific position of an electrode provides a tracing referred to as a *lead.* The purpose of using 12 leads is to obtain 12 different views of the electrical activity in the heart and therefore a more complete picture.

Current standard of practice in most hospitals calls for patients at risk for cardiac events or dysrhythmias to be placed on continuous ECG monitoring using the three-lead system or the five-lead system. These systems use only three or five leads, placed on the patient's chest, which is less cumbersome and allows for more patient mobility than the 10 leads placed on the chest and extremities for a 12-lead ECG. Although these modified systems do not provide the overview that a 12-lead ECG does, they do allow for the recognition of gross abnormalities in the electrical conduction of the heart. Identification of a rhythm abnormality on a three-lead or five-lead tracing often indicates the need to obtain a more detailed 12-lead view of the heart.

WHAT IS THE VALUE OF AN ECG?

The ECG provides valuable information about the cardiac status of a patient presenting with signs and symptoms suggestive of heart disease. For example, if a patient presents with dyspnea and chest discomfort, an ECG can aid in the diagnosis of an ischemic cardiac event. In addition, the ECG may indicate an increased workload on the myocardium as a compensatory response to the chronic dysfunction of another body system, such as the respiratory system. Both acute and chronic conditions may have adverse effects on the heart. The severity of such effects (e.g., myocardial infarction, ventricular hypertrophy, or abnormal heart rhythms known as dysrhythmias) may be assessed on interpretation of the ECG. The ECG may also be used to monitor the heart's response to treatment of an event that causes changes in the ECG. Therefore, several ECGs may be needed over the course of treatment.

It is important to note that the ECG tracing does not measure the pumping ability of the heart. It is not unusual for a patient with a low cardiac output to have a normal ECG tracing. This is because the ECG does not directly depict abnormalities in cardiac structure such as defects in the heart valves or interventricular septum. Another limitation worth noting is that the probability of any patient having an acute problem such as myocardial infarction cannot be predicted from a resting ECG tracing.

SIMPLY STATED

The resting ECG does not reflect the pumping ability of the heart or the likelihood of the patient having a myocardial infarction in the near future.

WHEN SHOULD AN ECG BE OBTAINED?

Because an ECG is noninvasive and does not present a risk to the patient, it is reasonable to obtain an ECG whenever the patient has signs and symptoms suggestive of an acute or chronic cardiac disorder such as myocardial infarction or congestive heart failure (Box 10-1). Of course, the process of obtaining the ECG should never delay the initiation of critically needed care such as oxygen therapy, airway placement, or cardiopulmonary resuscitation (CPR).

An ECG is often used as a screening tool to determine the patient's health status before major surgery. An ECG is especially helpful in this situation if the patient is older or has a history of heart disease. If an abnormality is identified, it may need to be treated before the operation is performed.

CARDIAC ANATOMY AND PHYSIOLOGY

Before discussing the interpretation of ECGs, it is important to review the cardiac anatomy and physiology related to electrical activity within the heart. The heart is made up of four chambers: two upper chambers called *atria* and two lower chambers called *ventricles* (Figure 10-1). The heart typically is described as having two sides, the right and the left. The right atrium receives deoxygenated blood from the venae cavae and directs the blood into the right ventricle. Right ventricular contraction ejects blood into the pulmonary artery, which carries blood to the lungs for oxygenation. The oxygenated blood returns to the

BOX 10-1 Clinical Findings Suggestive of the Need for an ECG

Medical History

Chief Complaints

Chest pain (centrally located and may radiate to the shoulder or back)
Dyspnea on exertion in a patient older than age 40 years
Orthopnea
Paroxysmal nocturnal dyspnea
Pedal edema
Fainting spells
Palpitations
Unexplained and persistent nausea and indigestion in a high-risk patient

Past Medical History

History of heart disease
History of cardiac surgery

Physical Examination

Unexplained tachycardia at rest
Hypotension
Decreased capillary refill
Abnormal heart sounds or murmurs
Pedal edema
Cool, cyanotic extremities
Abnormal heaves or lifts on the precordium
Diaphoresis
Jugular venous distention
Abnormal sensorium
Hepatojugular reflex
Bilateral inspiratory crackles in the dependent lung zones

left atrium of the heart via the pulmonary veins, where it is directed into the left ventricle. Left ventricular contraction ejects blood into the aorta, which branches off into the systemic circulation. Since the left side of the heart pumps blood throughout the entire body, it normally has a significantly larger muscle mass than the right side.

Cardiac muscle is referred to as the *myocardium.* Myocardial contraction occurs as a response to electrical stimulation. For the heart to move blood effectively, stimulation of the myocardium must be coordinated. Initiating and coordinating the electrical stimulation of the myocardium is the responsibility of the electrical conduction system, which is made up of special pacemaker and conducting cells (Table 10-1).

Normally, the electrical activity of the heart is initiated in the sinus or sinoatrial (SA) node located in the right atrium (Figure 10-2). The SA node is a collection of specialized cells capable of spontaneously generating electrical signals. Cells that have the ability to generate electrical activity spontaneously are said to have automaticity. Because the SA node normally has the greatest degree of automaticity of all the cardiac cells, it usually controls the rate at which the heart beats. In this way, the SA node serves as the primary pacemaker of the heart, discharging at about 60 to 100 beats/min at rest.

The SA node is strongly influenced by the autonomic nervous system. For this reason, the rate at which the SA node fires can vary significantly. Increased activity of the sympathetic system increases the heart rate. Stimulation of the sympathetic system occurs with stress, anxiety, exercise, and the administration of certain medications. On the other hand, slowing of the heart rate occurs due to vagal stimulation, which is a parasympathetic response.

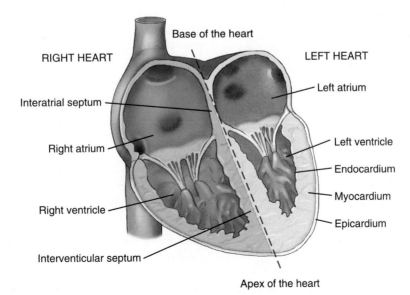

Figure 10-1 Anatomy of the heart. (Redrawn from Huszar RH: *Basic dysrhythmias: interpretation and management,* ed 2, St Louis, 1994, Mosby.)

Once the SA node initiates the electrical signal, the impulse spreads across the atria in a wavelike fashion. The electrical impulse travels through the atria by way of the internodal pathways, causing depolarization and then contraction. Contraction of the atria just before ventricular contraction (systole) aids in filling the ventricles with blood and accounts for about 10% to 30% of cardiac output. This atrial contraction is often referred to as the atrial kick.

After the electrical impulse passes through the atria, it reaches the atrioventricular (AV) junction. This junction acts as an electrical bridge between the atria and the ventricles. The AV junction contains the AV node and the bundle of His (see Figure 10-2). Once the electrical impulse reaches the AV node, it is delayed for approximately 0.1 second before passing on into the bundle of His. The delay is believed to serve the purpose of allowing more complete filling of the ventricles before ventricular contraction. In addition, the AV node can protect the ventricles from excessively rapid atrial rates that the ventricles could not tolerate.

The AV junction normally only guides the electrical impulse from the atria into the ventricles. Under certain circumstances, however, it can also serve as the backup pacemaker. The AV junction has automaticity qualities similar to those of the SA node. If the SA node fails to function properly and does not pace the heart, the AV junction can serve as the pacemaker for the ventricles. When this occurs, the ventricular rate is usually between 40 and 60 beats/min and the ECG reveals a distinct pattern, described later in this chapter (Figure 10-3).

After the electrical impulse leaves the AV node, it travels rapidly through the bundle of His and then into the left and right bundle branches (see Figure 10-2). The stimulus travels simultaneously through the bundle branches into the myocardium. At the end of the bundle branches are countless fingerlike projections called *Purkinje fibers*. The Purkinje fibers pass the electrical impulse rapidly throughout the myocardium to create a coordinated contraction of the left and right ventricles.

SIMPLY STATED

The SA node normally has the greatest degree of automaticity and therefore normally controls the pace of the heart rate. The AV junction acts as the backup pacemaker.

Because most of the cardiac cells have automaticity characteristics, the heartbeat may be paced by heart tissue other than the SA node. When this occurs, it often indicates that the SA node is not functioning normally or that myocardial tissue is irritated. Any impulse that originates outside the SA node is called an ectopic impulse, and the site from which the ectopic impulse originates is called the focus. Ectopic impulses can originate from foci in either the atria or the ventricles. When

Table 10-1	Types of Heart Cells
Pacemaker cells	Specialized cells that have a high degree of automaticity and provide the electrical power for the heart
Conducting cells	Cells that conduct the electrical impulse throughout the heart
Myocardial cells	Cells that contract in response to electrical stimuli and pump the blood

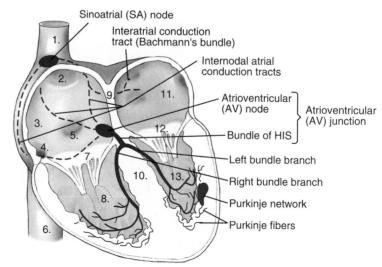

1. Superior vena cava
2. Inlet of the superior vena cava
3. Right atrium
4. Inlet of the inferior vena cava
5. Coronary sinus
6. Inferior vena cava
7. Tricuspid valve
8. Right ventricle
9. Interatrial septum
10. Interventricular septum
11. Left atrium
12. Mitral valve
13. Left ventricle

Sinoatrial (SA) node
Interatrial conduction tract (Bachmann's bundle)
Internodal atrial conduction tracts
Atrioventricular (AV) node
Atrioventricular (AV) junction
Bundle of HIS
Left bundle branch
Right bundle branch
Purkinje network
Purkinje fibers

Figure 10-2 Electrical conduction system of the heart. (Redrawn from Huszar RH: *Basic dysrhythmias: interpretation and management,* ed 2, St Louis, 1994, Mosby.)

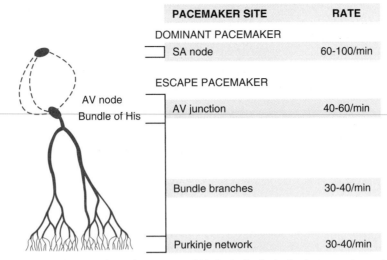

PACEMAKER SITE	RATE
DOMINANT PACEMAKER	
SA node	60-100/min
ESCAPE PACEMAKER	
AV junction	40-60/min
Bundle branches	30-40/min
Purkinje network	30-40/min

Figure 10-3 Dominant and escape pacemakers. (Redrawn from Huszar RH: *Basic dysrhythmias: interpretation and management,* ed 2, St Louis, 1994, Mosby.)

the ectopic impulse results from depression of the normal impulse origin, it is called an escape beat.

The myocardium must receive a constant supply of oxygen and nutrients to pump blood effectively. Oxygen and nutrients are supplied to the myocardium via the left and right coronary arteries and their branches. The main coronary arteries arise from the ascending aorta and direct arterial blood into branches that feed various regions of the heart. Blockage of one or more of the coronary vessels leads to regionalized ischemia and tissue death (infarction). The size and location of the region affected by the coronary vessel blockage determines the resulting physiologic and clinical impact. Infarction of a major portion of the left ventricle is likely to cause significant arterial hypotension, abnormal sensorium, and a backup of blood into the pulmonary circulation. Infarction of the tissues associated with pacing the heart (e.g., the SA or AV junction) can lead to significant dysrhythmias and diminished blood flow to all regions of the body.

SIMPLY STATED

Blockage of one of the coronary arteries leads to ischemia and infarction of a portion of the myocardium. This leads to dysrhythmias and reduced cardiac output in most cases.

CAUSES AND MANIFESTATIONS OF DYSRHYTHMIAS

Disturbances in cardiac conduction are called dysrhythmias. Dysrhythmias can occur even in healthy hearts. Often minor dysrhythmias produce no symptoms and resolve without any treatment. More serious dysrhythmias indicate significant acute or chronic heart disease. When serious dysrhythmias occur, medication or electrical therapy often is required to increase or decrease the ventricular rate or to suppress an irritable area within the myocardium. Occasionally, surgical intervention or thrombolytic therapy is needed to prevent the progression of injury or infarct, thereby salvaging viable tissue. The application and improved delivery of oxygen often is a key factor in reducing or eliminating cardiac irritability. Causes of dysrhythmias include the following:

- **Hypoxia:** This results from inadequate delivery of oxygen to the myocardium and may be referred to as *ischemia.* Inadequate delivery may be caused by reduced arterial oxygen levels, reduced hemoglobin levels, or reduced perfusion (blood flow).
- **Ischemia:** Ischemia can lead to myocardial injury and infarction. Myocardial cells deprived of oxygen do not conduct nor contract well.
- **Sympathetic stimulation:** Physical or emotional stress or conditions such as hyperthyroidism and congestive heart failure can elicit dysrhythmias. Sympathetic stimulation can also result in cardiac ischemia due to an increased workload on the myocardium without concurrent increase in blood flow, such as in the case of diseased coronary arteries.
- **Drugs:** Many medications taken in nontherapeutic ranges or in the presence of inadequate biotransformation or clearance may produce dysrhythmias. Illegal use of sympathomimetic agents such as cocaine or methylphenidate (Ritalin) may cause myocardial irritability and even infarction.
- **Electrolyte imbalances:** Potassium, magnesium, and calcium are the most common electrolytes that cause dysrhythmias when present in abnormal serum concentrations.
- **Rate:** Rhythms that are too slow or too fast result in inadequate cardiac output. Cardiac output is a product of stroke volume and cardiac rate. Stroke volume is the volume of blood pumped by one ventricle during one beat. Therefore, if the heart rate is too slow and the stroke volume is not increased proportionally, the cardiac output

will be reduced. On the other hand, if the heart rate is too fast, the ventricles do not have enough time to fill with blood and stroke volume may be significantly reduced, resulting in poor cardiac output.

- **Stretch:** Atrial or ventricular hypertrophy can produce dysrhythmias. Hypertrophy may be a result of a genetic disorder or a consequence of increased workload on the myocardium (e.g., chronic, uncontrolled high blood pressure).

IMPORTANT ABBREVIATIONS AND ACRONYMS

Before coming in contact with a patient, the RT will receive a verbal report regarding the patient or review the patient's chart. It is important to understand the meaning of descriptive terms, abbreviations, and acronyms related to cardiology and ECG interpretation that may be presented by report or in reviewing the chart. Box 10-2 provides a list of some of the most common

cardiology abbreviations and acronyms that may assist in the assessment of the patient's underlying disease process or cardiac conduction abnormalities.

BASIC ECG WAVES

The spread of electrical stimuli throughout the heart causes depolarization of the myocardial cells. Depolarization occurs when a polarized cell is stimulated. Polarized cells carry an electrical charge on their surface, the inside of the cell being more negatively charged than the outside of the cell. The sudden loss of the negative charge within the cell is called depolarization. This is a result of potassium moving out of the cell and sodium moving into the cell. The return of the negative electrical charge is called repolarization (Figure 10-4) and is a result of potassium moving back into the cells and sodium moving out of the cell. This process of depolarization and repolarization produces waves of electrical activity that travel back and forth across the heart. These waves of electrical activity are

BOX 10-2	Common Cardiology Abbreviations		
AIJR	Accelerated idiojunctional rhythm	MAT	Multiformed atrial tachycardia
AIVR	Accelerated idioventricular rhythm	MCL	Modified chest lead
ARP	Absolute refractory period	ms	Milliseconds
A-tach	Atrial tachycardia	mV	Millivolt
AV	Atrioventricular	NSR	Normal sinus rhythm (see RSR)
BBB	Bundle branch block	PAC	Premature atrial complex
bpm	Beats per minute	PEA	Pulseless electrical activity
BVH	Biventricular hypertrophy	PJC	Premature junctional complex
CABG	Coronary artery bypass graph	PJT	Paroxysmal junctional tachycardia
CAD	Coronary artery disease	PMI	Point of maximal impulse
CK-MB	Creatinine kinase-myocardial band	PSVT	Paroxysmal supraventricular tachycardia
CO	Cardiac output	PTCA	Percutaneous transluminal coronary angioplasty
CV	Cardiovascular	PVC	Premature ventricular complex
DC	Direct current	PVR	Pulmonary vascular resistance
ECG	Electrocardiogram	QTc	QT interval corrected for heart rate
EF	Ejection fraction	RAE	Right atrial enlargement
EKG	Electrocardiogram (German abbreviation)	RBBB	Right bundle branch block
EMD	Electromechanical dissociation (see PEA)	RSR	Regular sinus rhythm
EP	Electrophysiologic	RVH	Right ventricular hypertrophy
f-wave	Fibrillatory wave	SA	Sinoatrial
F-wave	Flutter wave	SVR	Systemic vascular resistance
HR	Heart rate	SVT	Supraventricular tachycardia
ICD	Implantable cardioverter/defibrillator	TdP	Torsade de pointes
IVR	Idioventricular rhythm	VF	Ventricular fibrillation
LA	Left atrial	VSD	Ventral septal defect
LAE	Left atrial enlargement	VT	Ventricular tachycardia
LAHB	Left anterior hemiblock	WAP	Wandering atrial pacemaker (also called multiformed atrial rhythm)
LAP	Left atrial pressure		
LBBB	Left bundle branch block	WPW	Wolff-Parkinson-White syndrome
LPHB	Left posterior hemiblock	1°AVBL	First-degree AV block
LVH	Left ventricular hypertrophy	2°AVBL	Second-degree AV block types I or II
mA	Milliamperes	3°AVBL	Third-degree AV block

represented by waves detected by the ECG electrodes. The magnitude or amplitude of the each wave is determined by voltage generated by depolarization of a particular portion of the heart.

Depolarization of the atria creates the initial wave of electrical activity detected on the ECG tracing, known as the *P wave* (Figure 10-5). Because the atria usually are small, the atria generate less voltage than the ventricles and the resulting P wave is small. Repolarization of the atria is not seen on the ECG because it usually is obscured by the simultaneous depolarization of the ventricles.

Depolarization of the ventricles is represented by the *QRS complex.* Because the ventricular muscle mass is larger than the atria and produces more voltage during depolarization, the QRS complex is normally taller than the P wave in most cases (see Figure 10-5). Ventricular repolarization is seen as the *T wave.* The T wave is normally upright and asymmetrically rounded.

Just after the T wave but before the next P wave, a small deflection known as the *U wave* is sometimes seen. The U wave is thought to represent the final phase of ventricular repolarization. In most cases the U wave is not seen. The clinical significance of its presence or absence is not known.

QRS complexes usually consist of several distinct waves, each of which has a letter assigned to it as a label. This labeling system is needed because the precise configuration of the QRS complex can vary from one lead to the next and from one patient to the next. To establish a standardized labeling system, several guidelines have been developed. If the first deflection of the QRS complex is downward (negative), it is labeled a *Q wave.* The initial upward (positive) deflection is called an *R wave.* The first negative deflection following an R wave is called an *S wave* (Figure 10-6). If the QRS complex has a second positive deflection, it is labeled *R′* (R prime), and if a second S wave is also present it is called *S′* (S prime). A negative deflection can be called a *Q wave* only if it is the first wave of the complex. In clinical practice, each ventricular depolarization complex is called a *QRS complex* whether it has all three waves or not.

> **SIMPLY STATED**
>
> The QRS complex is important to evaluate in the ECG because it reflects the electrical activity of the ventricles.

ECG Paper and Measurements

The electrical activity of the heart is recorded on paper that has gridlike boxes with light and dark lines running horizontally and vertically (Figure 10-7). The light lines circumscribe small boxes (1 × 1 mm) and the dark lines circumscribe larger boxes (5 × 5 mm).

Time is measured on the horizontal axis of the ECG paper. The ECG paper moves through the electrocardiograph at a speed of 25 mm/sec. Therefore, each small square (1 mm) represents 0.04 second and each larger square (5 mm) represents 0.2 second. Five large boxes represent 1.0 second.

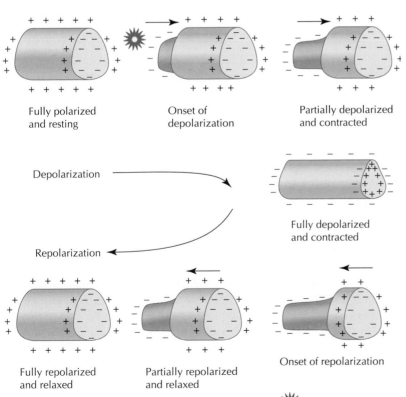

Fully polarized and resting

Onset of depolarization

Partially depolarized and contracted

Depolarization

Fully depolarized and contracted

Repolarization

Fully repolarized and relaxed

Partially repolarized and relaxed

Onset of repolarization

Electrical impulse

Figure 10-4 Depolarization and repolarization of a cardiac cell. (Modified from Huszar RH: *Basic dysrhythmias: interpretation and management,* ed 2, St Louis, 1994, Mosby.)

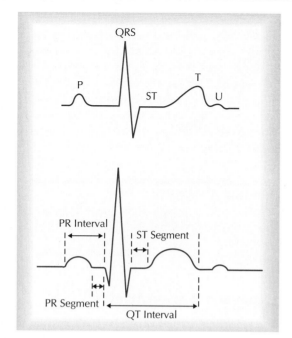

Figure 10-5 Normal configuration of ECG waves, segments, and intervals.

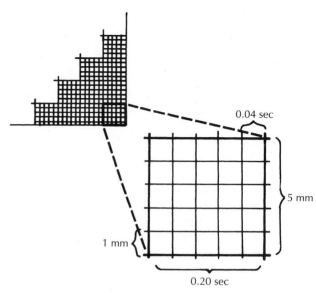

Figure 10-7 Gridlike boxes of ECG paper illustrating the 1-mm and 5-mm boxes.

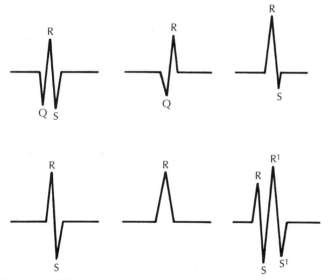

Figure 10-6 QRS nomenclature. See text for explanation.

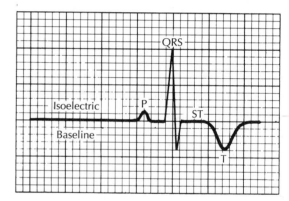

Figure 10-8 Isoelectric baseline used for measuring voltage of ECG waves. (From Goldberger AL, Goldberger E: *Clinical electrocardiography,* ed 4, St Louis, 1990, Mosby.)

On the vertical axis, voltage, or amplitude of the ECG waves, is measured. The exact voltage of any ECG wave can be measured because the electrocardiograph is standardized so that 1 mV produces a deflection 10 mm in amplitude. Therefore, the standard for most ECG recordings is 1 mV = 10 mm. Each small square represents 1 mm.

To measure the amplitude of a specific wave, the isoelectric baseline must be identified. This is the flat line seen just before the P wave or right after the T or U wave (Figure 10-8). Any movement of the ECG stylus above this line is considered positive; any downward movement is considered negative. To measure the degree of positive or negative amplitude of a specific wave, the isoelectric line is used as a reference point marking zero voltage.

R waves are measured from the isoelectric line to the top of the R wave. Q and S waves are measured from the isoelectric line to the bottom of the wave (see Figure 10-6). P waves can be either positive or negative and are also measured from the isoelectric line to the top (if positive) or bottom (if negative) of the wave.

In addition to the amplitude of any wave, the duration of waves, intervals, and segments can be measured. A *segment* is a straight line between two waves. An *interval* encompasses at least one wave plus the connecting straight line.

The normal P wave is less than 2.5 mm in height and not more than 0.10 second in length. The *PR interval* is an important measurement that provides information regarding conduction time. This interval is measured from the beginning of the P wave, where the P wave lifts off the isoelectric line, to the beginning of the QRS complex (see Figure 10-5). The PR interval represents the time it takes for the electrical stimulus to spread through the atria and to pass through the AV junction. The normal PR interval is between 0.12 and 0.2 second (three to five small boxes). If conduction of the impulse through the AV junction is abnormally delayed, the PR interval will exceed 0.2 second. A prolonged PR interval is called *first-degree block* and is discussed later in this chapter.

The duration of ventricular depolarization is determined by measuring the *QRS interval*. This interval is measured from the first wave of the QRS complex to the end of the last wave of the QRS complex. Normally the QRS interval does not exceed 0.12 second (three small boxes). The amplitude of the QRS complex may range from 2 to 15 mm, depending on the lead and the size of the ventricular mass.

A very important segment to evaluate is the *ST segment*. This segment is the portion of the ECG cycle from the end of the QRS complex (even if no S wave is present) to the beginning of the T wave (see Figure 10-5). It measures the time from the end of ventricular depolarization to the start of ventricular repolarization. The normal ST segment is isoelectric (no positive or negative voltage) or at least does not move more than 1 mm above or below baseline. Certain pathologic abnormalities such as myocardial ischemia or injury cause the ST segment to be elevated or depressed (Figure 10-9). The duration of the ST segment is not as important as its configuration.

Figure 10-9 ST segments. **A,** Normal. **B,** Abnormal elevation. **C,** Abnormal depression.

> **SIMPLY STATED**
>
> In patients suspected of having acute myocardial ischemia, the ST segment is important to evaluate. Significant elevation or depression of the ST segment must be recognized and responded to immediately.

The *RR interval* is useful in identifying the rate and regularity of ventricular contraction. The distance in millimeters is determined from one R wave to the next in successive QRS complexes. This is done for several different RR intervals. ECG calipers can be helpful in making this measurement. The average of the measurements is determined and converted to time. Remember that each large box is equal to 0.2 second and five large boxes equal 1.0 second. If the RR interval is 1.5 seconds, the heart rate is 40 beats/min. If the RR interval is 1.0 second, the heart rate is 60 beats/min. If the RR interval is 0.5 second, the heart rate is 120 beats/min. This method for determining the heart rate is easy to apply if the RR interval falls conveniently on one of the numbers just described. Unfortunately, this is not usually the case. Other methods for calculating the heart rate are described later. Marked variation in the RR interval from one interval to the next indicates that the heartbeat is irregular and may be a sign of sinus dysrhythmia, which is described in more detail in the section about dysrhythmia identification.

The *QT interval* is measured from the beginning of the QRS complex to the end of the T wave (see Figure 10-5). This interval represents the time from the beginning of ventricular depolarization to the end of ventricular repolarization. The normal values for the QT interval depend on the heart rate. As the heart rate increases, the QT interval normally shortens; as the heart rate decreases, the QT interval increases. As a general rule, the QT interval that exceeds one half of the RR interval is prolonged if the heart rate is 80 beats/min or less. Common causes of an abnormally prolonged QT interval include hypokalemia (low potassium), hypocalcemia (low calcium), and the side effects of certain medications such as quinidine.

Evaluating Heart Rate

If the heart rate is regular, one of the easiest ways of determining the heart rate is to count the number of large (0.2 second) boxes between two successive QRS complexes and divide this number into 300. For example, if there is one large box between successive R waves, then each R wave is separated by 0.2 second. Over the course of 1.0 second there will be five QRS complexes and 300 QRS complexes in 60 seconds. Therefore, the heart rate is 300 beats/min. Following this logic:

> 2 large boxes = rate of 150 beats/min (300/2 × 150)
> 3 large boxes = rate of 100 beats/min (300/3 × 100)
> 4 large boxes = rate of 75 beats/min (300/4 × 75)
> 5 large boxes = rate of 60 beats/min (300/5 × 60)
> 6 large boxes = rate of 50 beats/min (300/6 × 50)

If the heart rate is irregular, this method will not be accurate because the spacing between QRS complexes will vary from beat to beat. In such cases, the average rate can be determined by counting the number of QRS complexes in a 6-second interval (30 large boxes) and multiplying the number by 10. Because the top of the ECG paper is marked with small vertical dashes every 3 seconds, 6-second intervals are easy to identify.

An increase or decrease in heart rate by more than 20% of the baseline value is a significant change and should be evaluated further. An abnormally slow heart rate may reduce cardiac performance to the point of compromised perfusion. Recall that cardiac output is a product of stroke volume and heart rate. A heart rate below 60 beats/min is referred to as an *absolute bradycardia*. However, bradycardia that may require intervention is relative to the individual patient. For example, a well-conditioned runner may present with a heart rate of

50 beats/min with no signs of inadequate cardiac output. On the other hand, a person with poor myocardial contractility that presents with a heart rate of 50 beats/min is likely to show signs of compromised perfusion. An abnormally rapid heart rate (tachycardia) will increase myocardial oxygen demand, possibly to the point of inducing ischemia if the demand exceeds the supply. An increase in heart rate above 130 beats/min may compromise cardiac performance. Significant tachycardia reduces the ventricular filling time, and as a result, cardiac output will diminish. In addition, significant tachycardia may induce ischemia because it shortens the diastolic period, which is the period when most coronary perfusion occurs.

ECG LEADS

Because the heart is a three-dimensional organ, a more complete picture of the electrical activity in the heart will be obtained if it is viewed from several different angles. The standard ECG uses 12 different leads to provide 12 different views from different angles of the heart. Interpretation of the 12 leads is a little more difficult, but the information obtained is more complete and abnormalities are not likely to be missed.

The 12 leads can be subdivided into two groups: six extremity (limb) leads and six chest leads. To obtain the six limb leads, two electrodes are placed on the patient's wrists and two on the patient's ankles. The ECG machine can vary the orientation of these four electrodes to one another to create the six limb leads. The chest leads are created by attaching six electrodes across the patient's chest. The chest leads are discussed after the limb leads are reviewed.

Limb Leads

The six limb leads are called leads I, II, III, aV_R, aV_L, and aV_F. Leads I, II, and III are bipolar. Each lead is created by comparing the difference in electrical voltage between two electrodes. For lead I, the ECG machine temporarily designates the electrode on the left arm as a positive lead and the electrode on the right arm as negative. The measured difference in voltage between these two leads results in lead I. For lead II, the right arm electrode remains negative and the left leg electrode is positive. Lead III is created by making the left arm negative and the left leg positive.

The other three limb leads (aV_R, aV_L, and aV_F) are called *augmented leads* because the ECG machine must amplify the tracings to get an adequate recording. This is because the augmented leads are created by measuring the electrical voltage at one limb lead, with all other limb leads made negative. For the augmented leads, the ECG machine must augment the recorded voltages by about 50% to get an adequate recording. Lead aV_R is created by making the right arm positive and all the others negative. Lead aV_L calls for the left arm to be positive, and lead aV_F is created by making the left leg positive.

The six limb leads view the heart in a vertical plane called a *frontal plane.* Any electrical activity that is directed up, down, left, or right is recorded by the limb leads (Figure 10-10). The

frontal plane can be envisioned as a giant circle that surrounds the patient and lies in the same plane as the patient. This circle can be marked off in 360 degrees, as shown in Figure 10-10.

The angle of orientation for each of the bipolar limb leads can be determined by drawing a line from the designated negative lead to the designated positive lead. For lead I, the angle of orientation is 0 degrees; for lead II, +60 degrees; and for lead III, +120 degrees. For the augmented leads, the angle of orientation can be determined by drawing a line from the average of the other three limb leads to the one that is designated as the positive lead. The angle of orientation is −150 degrees for lead aV_R, −30 degrees for lead aV_L, and 90 degrees for lead aV_F.

In review, the limb leads consist of three bipolar leads and three unipolar leads. The three bipolar leads are called leads I, II, and III. The three unipolar leads are called aV_R, aV_L, and aV_F. The abbreviation *a* refers to augmented, *V* to voltage, and *R, L,* and *F* to right arm, left arm, and left leg, respectively. The limb leads measure the electrical activity in the heart that occurs in the frontal plane, and each lead has its own specific view or angle of orientation to the heart (Table 10-2).

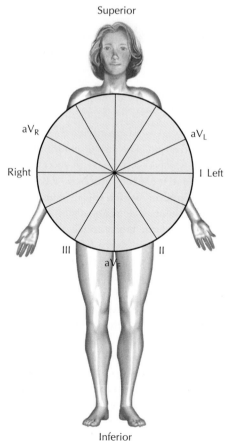

Frontal plane leads

Superior

aV_R

aV_L

Right

I Left

III

II

aV_F

Inferior

Figure 10-10 Frontal plane showing spatial relationships of six extremity leads. (Modified from Goldberger AL: *Clinical electrocardiography: a simplified approach,* ed 6, St Louis, 1999, Mosby.)

Table 10-2	The 12 Leads of an ECG and the Myocardial Wall That Each Set Views
Lead	View
I, aV_L, V_5, V_6	Lateral
II, III, aV_F	Inferior
V_1, V_2	Septal
V_3, V_4	Anterior

Chest Leads

The six chest leads, or precordial leads, are called leads V_1, V_2, V_3, V_4, V_5, and V_6. The chest leads are unipolar leads that are placed across the chest in a horizontal plane (Figure 10-11). The chest leads define a horizontal or transverse plane and view electrical voltages that move anteriorly and posteriorly. Like the limb leads, each chest lead has its own view or angle of orientation. Under normal conditions, leads V_1 and V_2 lie directly over the right ventricle, V_3 and V_4 lie over the interventricular septum, and V_5 and V_6 lie over the left ventricle. In addition, leads V_1 through V_4 often are called the *anterior* leads because they view the anterior portion of the heart. Leads V_5 and V_6 view the left lateral portion of the heart and are therefore called the *left lateral* leads (see Table 10-2).

> ### SIMPLY STATED
> The normal ECG has six limb leads that examine the heart in the vertical plane and six chest leads that look at the horizontal plane.

Evaluating the Mean QRS Axis

The QRS axis represents the general direction of current flow during ventricular depolarization. Although depolarization spreads through the ventricles in different directions, an average or mean direction can be determined. Normally, the mean QRS axis (vector) points leftward (patient's left) and downward, somewhere between 0 and +90 degrees in the frontal plane previously described (Figure 10-12).

The ECG records a positive (upward) QRS complex whenever the mean QRS axis is moving toward a positive electrode. When the mean QRS axis is moving toward a negative lead, the QRS complex is negative (downward). Because each of the six limb leads has its own angle of orientation as defined in the hexaxial reference system, a review of the recorded limb leads should identify the mean QRS axis in the frontal plane.

To identify the mean QRS axis, begin by sketching the hexaxial reference system, including labels for the points where the limb leads are located on the circle. Next, identify which limb lead has the QRS complex with the most voltage (positive or negative). This is accomplished by identifying the QRS complex with the largest deflection from baseline. If the largest

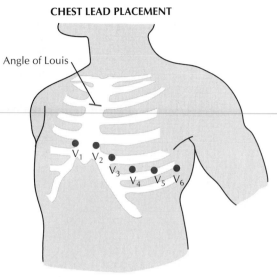

CHEST LEAD PLACEMENT

Figure 10-11 Position of the six chest leads. V_1 is located in the fourth intercostal space left of the sternum. V_2 is located in the fourth intercostal space right of the sternum. V_3 is placed between V_2 and V_4. V_4 is placed in the fifth intercostal space in the midclavicular line. V_5 is placed between V_4 and V_6. V_6 is placed in the fifth intercostal space in the midaxillary line. (Redrawn from Goldberger AL, Goldberger E: *Clinical electrocardiography,* ed 4, St Louis, 1990, Mosby.)

deflection is positive (R wave), the mean QRS axis points toward the lead with the tallest QRS. If the most voltage is negative (Q or S wave), the mean axis points away from that lead. For example, if the most voltage is found to be in lead II and it is positive, then the mean QRS axis must be about +60 degrees because this is where lead II is located on the hexaxial reference system (see Figure 10-12). This would be considered a normal axis because it falls between 0 and +90 degrees. If the most voltage is found in lead I and is negative, then the QRS axis is approximately 180 degrees because lead I is located at 0 degrees.

In some situations, the most voltage may be equally present in two leads. If two leads exhibit equal positive voltage, the mean axis must fall midway between the two leads. If the most voltage is equally negative in two leads, the mean axis is opposite the midpoint between the two leads.

As mentioned, a normal QRS axis is approximately 0 to +90 degrees. If the axis is found to be between +90 and 180 degrees, right axis deviation is present. Right axis deviation is common in patients with cor pulmonale (right ventricular enlargement due to chronic lung disease). In such cases, the QRS complex will be negative in lead I but positive in lead aV_F. Leads II and III are both positive in most cases of right axis deviation; however, lead III will be taller than lead II (Figure 10-13 and Table 10-3).

Left axis deviation is present when the mean axis is found to be between 0 and −90 degrees. Left axis deviation can occur in several different conditions, including left ventricular hypertrophy and blocks of the left bundle branch. In such cases, the QRS complex is positive in lead I and negative in lead aV_F. In addition, the QRS complex in lead III will demonstrate negative voltage with left axis deviation.

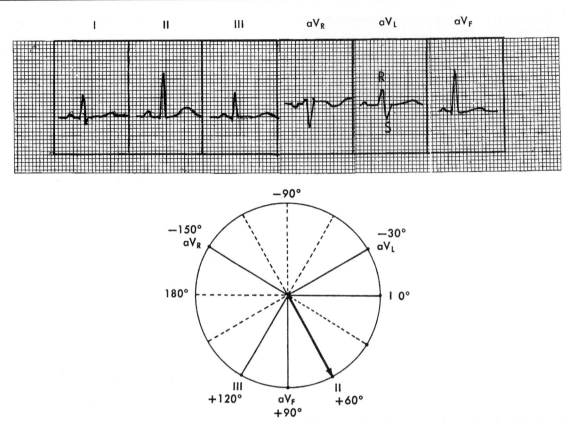

Figure 10-12 Normal mean QRS axis of 60 degrees. (From Goldberger AL, Goldberger E: *Clinical electrocardiography*, ed 4, St Louis, 1990, Mosby.)

RIGHT AXIS DEVIATION

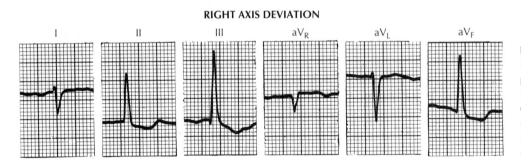

Figure 10-13 Sample ECG showing right axis deviation. Note the positive QRS complex (R wave) in leads II and III and the negative QRS complex (S wave) in lead I. (From Goldberger AL, Goldberger E: *Clinical electrocardiography*, ed 4, St Louis, 1990, Mosby.)

Table 10-3	Quick Axis Determination
Lead	**Axis**
I is Positive II is Positive	Normal
I is Positive II is Negative	Left Deviation
I is Negative II is Positive	Right Deviation
I is Negative II is Negative	Extreme Right Deviation

If the mean QRS axis is found to be between −90 and 180 degrees, extreme left or right axis deviation is present. This condition is not common. When the ECG recording indicates that it may be present, the extremity leads should be checked to make sure they are attached properly.

The same principles of axis evaluation can be applied to the P wave as to the QRS complex. When normal sinus rhythm is present and the atria are normal in size, the P wave is positive in lead II and negative in lead aV_R. Therefore, the normal P wave is directed toward lead II and away from lead aV_R, making the normal mean P wave axis about +60 degrees. In cor pulmonale, right atrial enlargement is common. The ECG will show tall, narrow P waves in leads II, III, and aV_F in such cases.

STEPS OF ECG INTERPRETATION

First and most importantly, the patient's condition must be evaluated. All dysrhythmias should be interpreted and evaluated in accordance with the patient's clinical presentation and medical history. Important signs and symptoms that may be associated with dysrhythmias may include:

- Chest pain
- Dyspnea
- Fine crackles
- Palpitations
- Pale, cool clammy skin
- Dizziness or syncope
- Sense of impending doom
- Low blood pressure (<90 systolic)
- Altered level of consciousness

Interpretation of dysrhythmias can be accomplished on three levels. The first level is simply identifying ventricular response. The contraction of the ventricles determines the majority of the cardiac output and perfusion of blood to the tissues. The ventricular response is determined by the QRS complexes and subsequent pulse strength. Abnormal conduction can be viewed as being:

- Too fast
- Too slow
- Too irritable
- Lethal or absent

Secondly, dysrhythmias can be placed into categories based on the origin of the impulse formation, which may include:

- Atrial
- Junctional
- Ventricular

Thirdly, dysrhythmias can be evaluated based on the electrophysiology (or pathway) of the conduction disturbance. These can be categorized as:

- Ectopic beats or rhythms
- Escape beats or rhythms
- AV blocks
- Bundle branch blocks

To make sure that all components of the ECG tracing are covered, use a systematic method. Read every strip from left to right and apply the stepwise process as described below. It is important to avoid assumptions as glancing at a strip may lead to misinterpretation. The steps are as follows:

1. *Identify the heart rate.* Most modern ECG monitors provide a display of the heart rate. Always take the patient's pulse to verify that the monitor is calculating the heart rate correctly. Note that the monitor may not provide an accurate rate if the rhythm is irregular. If this is the case,

a strip should be printed and calculation should be done as mentioned in the "Evaluating Heart Rate" section of this chapter. Rhythms are called bradycardic if the rate is below 60 beats/min and tachycardic if the heart rate is over 100 beats/min.

2. *Evaluate the rhythm.* Note whether the spacing between the QRS complexes is equal. Small variations of 0.04 second (40 msec) are considered normal. If the spaces are greater than 0.04 second, the rhythm is irregular. Irregularity may occur randomly or in patterns (e.g., occur every other beat or change with respirations). Irregular rhythms are present with the following dysrhythmias:

- Ectopic beats
- Escape beats
- Second-degree AV blocks
- Atrial fibrillation
- Sinus dysrhythmia

3. *Note the presence of P waves.* A normal P wave generally is positive, depending on the lead, and round in shape. Normal P waves are less than 0.11 second (110 msec) wide and less than 2.5 mm (2½ small boxes) tall. Oddly shaped P waves may indicate atrial enlargement. Normal rhythms will only have one P wave preceding each QRS complex, and each P wave should have the same configuration as the others. If there appears to be more than one P wave preceding a QRS complex, the rhythm may be:

- Atrial flutter
- Atrial fibrillation (each P wave will have a different configuration)
- Second-degree AV block
- Third-degree AV block

4. *Measure the PR interval.* The normal PR interval is 0.12 to 0.20 second (120 to 200 msec) wide. A PR interval that is wider than 0.20 second indicates a delay in conduction through the AV node, indicating the possibility of a block (Table 10-4).

5. *Measure the width of the QRS complex.* The normal QRS complex is less than 0.12 second (120 msec) wide. Wide QRS complexes can occur with:

Table 10-4	Summary of Normal Values for the ECG Interpretation	
Variable	Normal Range	Interpretation
Rate	60-100/min	Rates >100 = tachycardia Rates <60 = bradycardia
PR interval	0.12-0.20/sec	>0.20 = heart block
QRS interval	<0.12/sec	>0.12 = ectopic foci
ST segment	Isoelectric	Elevated or depressed = myocardial ischemia
T wave	Upright and round	Inverted with ischemia, tall and peaked with electrolyte imbalances

- Bundle branch blocks
- Ectopic beats originating in the ventricles (premature ventricular contractions)
- Ventricular dysrhythmias such as ventricular tachycardia, idioventricular rhythm, or premature ventricular complexes
- Third-degree AV block

6. *Inspect the ST segment in all leads.* ST segment elevation may indicate myocardial injury whereas ST segment depression may indicate myocardial ischemia. The portion or wall of the heart that is ischemic can be determined by identifying the leads looking at that portion of the heart (see Table 10-4). The ST segment is measured from the J point: the junction between the QRS complex and the ST segment (see Figure 10-8).

7. *Identify the mean QRS axis.* Most modern 12-lead ECG tracings indicate the QRS axis. Normal axis is 0 to +90 degrees. Left axis deviation is 0 to −90 degrees, and right axis deviation is +90 to 180 degrees (see Figure 10-12 and Table 10-3). Box 10-3 lists causes of axis deviation.

8. *Assess the waveform morphology.* Some QRS complexes may have additional deflections. If there is a second deflection, the second portion is called prime (see Figure 10-6). For example, a second R wave would be labeled R′.

9. *Evaluate the Q wave.* A Q wave is considered normal (or physiologic) if it is less than 0.04 second (40 msec) wide and less than one third the amplitude of the R wave. Q waves that exceed either of these values are considered pathologic and indicate a new or possibly old infarction.

10. *Look for signs of chamber enlargement.* High-voltage R waves in the precordial leads indicate ventricular hypertrophy. Large or abnormally shaped P waves indicate atrial enlargement (see review later in this chapter).

BOX 10-3   Causes of Axis Deviation

Right Axis

Left ventricular infarction
Right ventricular hypertrophy
Chronic obstructive lung disease
Acute pulmonary embolism
Infants up to 1 year old (normal)
Biventricular hypertrophy
Left posterior hemiblock

Left Axis

Right ventricular infarction
Left ventricular hypertrophy
Abdominal obesity
Ascites or large abdominal tumors
Third-trimester pregnancy
Left anterior hemiblock

SIMPLY STATED

A systematic step-by-step evaluation of the ECG is needed to find all abnormalities.

IDENTIFICATION OF COMMON DYSRHYTHMIAS

This section discusses the characteristics of some of the most commonly seen dysrhythmias. It is always important to treat a symptomatic dysrhythmia, but it is just as important to determine the underlying cause. Some of the most common causes of each dysrhythmia are also discussed.

Sinus Bradycardia

Sinus bradycardia meets all the criteria for a normal sinus rhythm except for the heart rate, which is below 60 beats/min (see Table 10-4). It is important at this point to understand the difference between an absolute bradycardia and a relative bradycardia. Absolute sinus bradycardia is simply a heart rate less than 60 beats/min and may be normal for a particular patient or tolerated well by the patient. For example, a conditioned runner may present with a heart rate of 55 beats/min with no negative cardiopulmonary signs and symptoms. By definition, this is an absolute bradycardia, but it is probably the patient's normal heart rate. A relative sinus bradycardia, on the other hand, is not tolerated well by the patient and will compromise cardiac performance. Marked sinus bradycardia may result in hypotension, syncope, diminished cardiac output, congestive heart failure, and shock.

Transient bradycardia may be caused by an increase in vagal tone as a result of direct carotid massage, manipulation of tracheostomy ties or tube, tracheal suctioning, or the Valsalva maneuver. Damage to the SA node, as may occur with a myocardial infarction, can cause a long-term bradycardia. Hypothyroidism, hypothermia, and hyperkalemia, and certain drugs may also result in bradycardia.

Systematic Evaluation (Figure 10-14):

Rate:	Less than 60 beats/min
Rhythm:	Regular
P Waves:	Normal configuration. Each P wave is followed by a QRS complex.
PR Interval:	Less than or equal to 0.2 second in length
QRS Complex:	Less than 0.12 second in width

Sinus Tachycardia

Sinus tachycardia is present when the heart rate is 100-150 beats/min, the SA node is the pacemaker, and all the normal conduction pathways in the heart are followed. Sinus tachycardia may be well tolerated by the patient; however, it increases myocardial oxygen demand and decreases the diastolic period, both of which can lead to myocardial ischemia. Sinus tachycardia results from sympathetic nervous system stimulation and

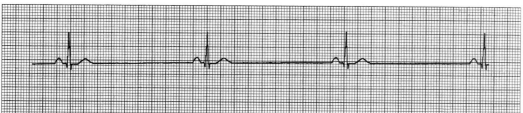

Figure 10-14 ECG tracing of sinus bradycardia.

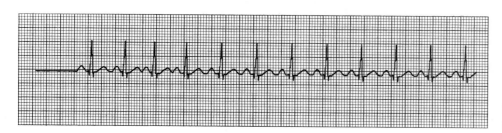

Figure 10-15 ECG tracing of sinus tachycardia.

almost always indicates a significant physiologic problem. Fever, pain, hypoxemia, hypovolemia, hypotension, sepsis, and heart failure are causes of sinus tachycardia. Tracheal suctioning, especially if it is performed without adequate oxygenation before, during, and after each catheter insertion, can cause sinus tachycardia. In addition, methylxanthines (or phosphodiesterase inhibitors) and the β-agonist bronchodilators often increase heart rate.

Systematic Evaluation (Figure 10-15):

Rate:	100 to 150 beats/min
Rhythm:	Regular
P Waves:	Normal configuration. Each P wave is followed by a QRS complex.
PR Interval:	Less than or equal to 0.2 second in length
QRS Complex:	Less than 0.12 second in width

Sinus Dysrhythmia

This is a benign dysrhythmia that meets all the criteria for normal sinus rhythm except that the rhythm is irregular. It usually does not produce symptoms in the patient and requires no treatment. In most cases of sinus dysrhythmia, no abnormality of the heart is present. Often the irregularities are related to the respiratory pattern, suggesting that changes in intrathoracic pressure are causing changes in the tone of the vagus nerve, which may produce the irregularity.

Systematic Evaluation:

Rate:	60 to 100 beats/min, may also present as a bradydysrhythmia (<60)
Rhythm:	Irregular
P Waves:	Normal configuration. Each P wave is followed by a QRS complex.
PR Interval:	Less than or equal to 0.2 second in length
QRS Complex:	Less than 0.12 second in width

Paroxysmal Atrial Tachycardia

Paroxysmal atrial tachycardia (PAT) occurs when an ectopic focus in the atrium usurps the pacemaking function of the SA node and paces the heart, usually at an abnormally rapid rate of 160 to 240 beats/min. It appears on the monitor as a series of normal-looking QRS complexes, each associated with a P wave. Because of the rapid rate, the P wave may be obscured by the preceding T wave.

Onset of this dysrhythmia is sudden and spontaneous; termination is similarly abrupt. PAT is seen in patients with normal hearts and in those with organic heart disease. The hazard of PAT is that it increases myocardial oxygen demand while decreasing pump effectiveness due to the diminished "filling time." PAT may precipitate hypotension, congestive heart failure, or an ischemic episode. PAT is especially dangerous for patients with compromised cardiovascular function, myocardial ischemia, preexisting heart failure, and recent myocardial infarction. Patients with PAT often complain of lightheadedness or palpitation. Occasionally PAT will cause the patient to faint. Some possible causes of PAT may include emotional stress, mitral valve disease, rheumatic heart disease, digitalis toxicity, or the use of alcohol, caffeine, or nicotine.

Systematic Evaluation (Figure 10-16):

Rate:	160 to 240 beats/min
Rhythm:	Regular
P Waves:	Abnormal configuration. May precede the QRS complex or may be hidden within the QRS complex. Usually appear pointed due to combined amplitude with the previous T wave. If observable, each P wave is followed by a QRS complex.
PR Interval:	Usually not measurable
QRS Complex:	Less than 0.12 second in width

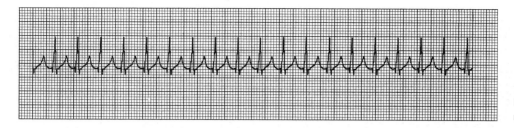

Figure 10-16 Short run of paroxysmal atrial tachycardia.

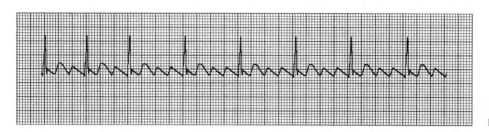

Figure 10-17 ECG tracing of atrial flutter.

Atrial Flutter

Atrial flutter is a dysrhythmia that produces a very distinctive ECG pattern, usually caused by a rapidly firing ectopic site in the atria that presents as a characteristic sawtooth pattern between normal-appearing QRS complexes. The sawtooth pattern of flutter waves (often referred to as *F waves*) represents the rapid flutter or contraction of the atria upon stimulation by a reentry circuit or accelerated automaticity. Atrial flutter results in diminished atrial "filling time," which results in minimal atrial assistance in filling the ventricles. Recall that the term *atrial kick* refers to the contraction of the atria forcing out blood at the latter part of systole and results in about 10% to 30% of cardiac output in a healthy person, but will be diminished in atrial flutter. A secondary problem with atrial flutter is that the pattern of blood flow in the atria causes areas of diminished blood movement near the atrial walls. This stagnation of blood promotes the formation of thrombi, often referred to as *mural thrombi,* along the wall of the atria. The patient is then at risk for embolization caused by the migration of a mural thrombus.

Atrial flutter usually is a short-lived dysrhythmia; it usually deteriorates to atrial fibrillation or the patient's previous rhythm returns spontaneously. Atrial flutter commonly is associated with pulmonary disease. Some possible causes of atrial flutter may include valvular heart disease, myocardial infarction, hypertensive heart disease, cardiomyopathy, myocarditis, and pericarditis.

Systematic Evaluation (Figure 10-17):

Atrial Rate:	180 to 400 beats/min
Ventricular Rate:	Varies but is always less than the atrial rate
Rhythm:	Regular
P Waves:	Sawtooth configuration and uniform. The relationship between the flutter waves and the QRS complexes may be regular (e.g., four flutter waves to each QRS complex) or variable

PR Interval:	Not measurable
QRS Complex:	Less than 0.12 second in width

Atrial Fibrillation

In atrial fibrillation, the electrical activity of the atria is completely chaotic and without coordination because it is arising from multiple ectopic sites within the atria. This results in a quivering of the atrial myocardium and complete loss of atrial pumping ability. Because the atria provide useful assistance in filling the ventricles from the *atrial kick,* there is a decrease in ventricular filling during atrial fibrillation. In most cases, the reduction in cardiac output is not serious enough to produce symptoms, although it reduces cardiac reserve and may limit the normal activities of daily living. Atrial fibrillation carries an even higher risk of mural thrombi formation and embolization than atrial flutter. Some possible causes of atrial fibrillation include all of those mentioned under atrial flutter but may also include hyperthyroidism, pulmonary disease, and congenital heart disease.

The ECG tracing shows a chaotic baseline between QRS complexes, with no regular pattern or organization. This irregular baseline is composed of what are called *fibrillatory* waves (f waves) that all have a different configuration due to their origin from different ectopic sites in the atria.

Systematic Evaluation (Figure 10-18):

Atrial Rate:	May be greater than 400 beats/min
Ventricular Rate:	Varies but is always less than the atrial rate
Rhythm:	Irregularly irregular
P Waves:	Fibrillatory waves (f waves) all having a different configuration. The relationship between the fibrillatory waves and the QRS complexes is irregular.
PR Interval:	Not measurable
QRS Complex:	Less than 0.12 second in width

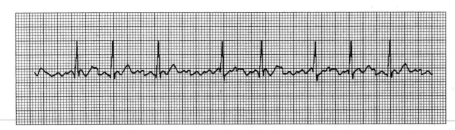

Figure 10-18 ECG tracing of atrial fibrillation.

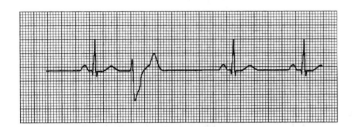

Figure 10-19 ECG tracing of a single premature ventricular contraction.

Premature Ventricular Contractions

Premature ventricular contractions (PVCs) represent ectopic beats originating in one of the ventricles due to enhanced automaticity. PVCs occur in both the normal heart and the diseased heart. PVCs commonly occur with anxiety or excessive use of caffeine, alcohol, or tobacco. Certain medications such as epinephrine and theophylline may also provoke PVCs in patients with normal hearts. Myocardial ischemia is a common cause of PVCs in patients with heart disease. Other causes may include acidosis, electrolyte imbalance, congestive heart failure, myocardial infarction, and hypoxia.

A single PVC poses no threat to the patient (Figure 10-19), but certain configurations of PVCs may signal a serious cardiac problem that may need immediate treatment. Although the idea that PVCs are "warning" dysrhythmias has not been proved by clinical research, the following conditions warrant further investigation and indicate the need for close monitoring of the patient:

- **Increased frequency:** Multiple PVCs occur in 1 minute (Figure 10-20)
- **Multifocal PVCs:** The QRS complexes of the PVCs have more than one configuration (Figure 10-21); this indicates that more than one area of the ventricles is irritated.
- **Couplets:** Two PVCs occur in a row.
- **Salvos:** Three or more PVCs occur in a row (sometimes called a *short run of ventricular tachycardia*).
- **R-on-T phenomenon:** The PVC occurs during the T wave of the preceding beat; this poses a real danger because it can precipitate ventricular tachycardia (Figure 10-22).

Systematic Evaluation (see Figure 10-19):
Rate: That of the underlying rhythm
Rhythm: Underlying rhythm is usually regular but irregular with a PVC

P Waves: None associated with the PVC
PR Interval: Not measurable
QRS Complex: More than 0.12 second in width, abnormal configuration, and premature. T wave following the PVC is deflected in a direction opposite to that of the QRS complex. There is a full compensatory pause following the PVC confirmed by measuring the interval between the normal QRS complex immediately before the PVC and the normal QRS complex immediately after the PVC; it will be double the normal RR interval for that patient.

Ventricular Tachycardia

Ventricular tachycardia appears on the monitor as a series of broad QRS complexes, occurring at a rapid rate, without identifiable P waves originating from an ectopic focus in the ventricles associated with enhanced automaticity or reentry. By definition, *ventricular tachycardia* is a run of three or more consecutive PVCs. It may occur as a single isolated burst or may persist for a long run. The rhythm is regular, and the rate is usually in the range of 140 to 300 beats/min. The majority of patients deteriorate rapidly with this dysrhythmia; therefore, it must be treated as an emergency. Without appropriate treatment, sustained ventricular tachycardia may lead to ventricular fibrillation (described later). When ventricular tachycardia occurs, the patient may become hypotensive and be slow to respond. If cardiac output deteriorates significantly, the patient usually becomes unresponsive. Ventricular tachycardia often is caused by problems similar to those that cause PVCs. When the heart is hypoxic, as occurs with severe myocardial ischemia, ventricular tachycardia is common and is a sign that the patient needs immediate care.

Systematic Evaluation (Figure 10-23):
Rate: 140 to 300 beats/min
Rhythm: Regular
P Waves: None associated with the QRS complex. They may occasionally occur because the SA node is still functioning.
PR Interval: Not measurable
QRS Complex: Abnormal and greater than 0.12 second in width

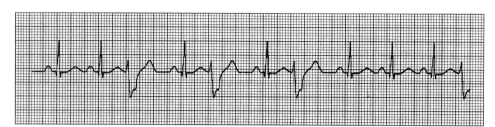

Figure 10-20 ECG tracing of frequent premature ventricular contractions.

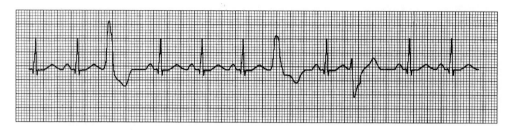

Figure 10-21 ECG tracing of multifocal premature ventricular contractions.

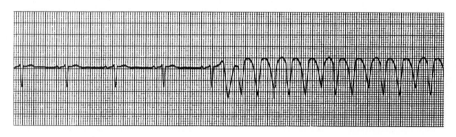

Figure 10-22 ECG tracing of R-on-T phenomenon.

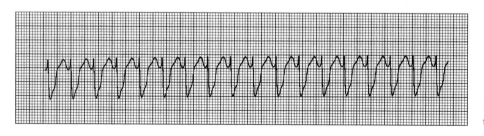

Figure 10-23 ECG tracing of ventricular tachycardia.

Ventricular Fibrillation

Ventricular fibrillation is the presence of chaotic, completely unorganized electrical activity in the ventricular myocardial fibers. It produces a characteristic wavy, irregular pattern on the ECG monitor. Depending on the amplitude of the electrical impulses, it can be mistaken for asystole or ventricular tachycardia. Because the heart cannot pump blood when fibrillation is occurring, the cardiac output drops to zero and the patient becomes unconscious immediately. This dysrhythmia is life threatening and must be treated immediately (defibrillation). Ventricular fibrillation often is caused by the same factors that precipitate ventricular tachycardia.

Systematic Evaluation (Figure 10-24):

Rate:	None
Rhythm:	Irregular, chaotic waves
P Waves:	None
PR Interval:	None
QRS Complex:	No waves appear with any regularity on the ECG tracing. There may be occasional low-amplitude waves that appear somewhat like ventricular-origin complexes, but they are sporadic in occurrence and totally irregular.

Asystole

Asystole is cardiac standstill and is invariably fatal unless an acceptable rhythm is restored. In fact, asystole is one of the criteria used for the determination of clinical death. Asystole is recognizable on the ECG monitor as a straight or almost straight line. The bedside clinician must take care to assess the patient with what appears to be asystole before initiating ther-

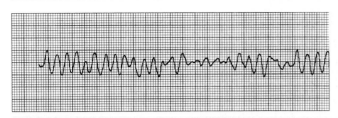

Figure 10-24 ECG tracing of ventricular fibrillation.

apy because a simple disconnection of the ECG leads can resemble asystole. Clinically, asystole is characterized by immediate pulselessness and loss of consciousness. The ECG tracing shows a line that is flat or almost flat, without discernible electrical activity (Figure 10-25).

Pulseless Electrical Activity

Pulseless electrical activity (PEA) is not a discrete dysrhythmia but rather an electromechanical condition that can be diagnosed clinically. As the name implies, there is a dissociation of the electrical and the mechanical activity of the heart. In other words, the pattern that appears on the ECG monitor does not generate a pulse. Fortunately, PEA is rare and does not occur without a precipitating event. Tension pneumothorax, cardiac trauma, and severe electrolyte or acid-base disturbances are among the most common causes of PEA. PEA sometimes is seen as a terminal event in an unsuccessful cardiac resuscitation effort.

There is no relationship between the electrical pattern appearing on the ECG monitor or tracing and the mechanical activity of the heart. PEA, therefore, is any rhythm that does not produce a pulse with the exception of ventricular tachycardia, ventricular fibrillation, and asystole.

AV Heart Block

AV heart block is a general term that refers to a disturbance in the conduction of impulses from the atria to the ventricles through the AV node. However, the block may be at the level of the AV node or the bundle of His or in the bundle branches. Classification of the AV blocks is based on the site of the block and the severity of the conduction disturbance.

Disturbances in AV conduction can occur as an adverse effect of medications such as digitalis, or when damage to the conduction system occurs with myocardial infarction. In some cases of complete heart block, the patient may develop symptoms associated with hypotension (fainting and weakness) if the ventricles are beating too slowly. In milder forms of heart block, the patient often is asymptomatic.

First-Degree AV Block

The mildest form of heart block is first-degree block, which is present when the PR interval is prolonged more than 0.2 second. In first-degree block, all the atrial impulses pass through to the ventricles but are delayed at the AV node. First-degree AV block may or may not compromise cardiac output. It is important to assess the patient as discussed earlier in the section on steps of ECG interpretation. Some potential causes of first-degree AV block include adverse effects of medications such as digitalis, increased vagal tone, hyperkalemia, myocarditis, and degenerative disease.

Systematic Evaluation (Figure 10-26):

Rate:	Underlying rhythm rate
Rhythm:	Regular
P Waves:	Normal sinus configuration, each preceding a QRS complex
PR Interval:	Greater than 0.20 second in length and constant
QRS Complex:	Less than 0.12 second in width

Second-Degree AV Block Type I (Mobitz I)

Second-degree AV block type is an intermediate form of heart block that presents with a PR interval that becomes progressively longer (changes in length) until the stimulus from the atria is blocked completely for a single cycle (dropped QRS complex). After the blocked beat, relative recovery of the AV junction occurs, and the progressive increasing of the PR interval starts all over again. The ventricular rhythm is almost always irregular. As with first-degree AV block, second-degree AV block type I may or may not compromise cardiac output; thus, it is important to assess the patient in conjunction with rhythm interpretation. Causes of second-degree AV block type one are similar to those of first-degree AV block.

Systematic Evaluation (Figure 10-27, *A*):

Rate:	Varies but ventricular rate is always less than the atrial rate
Atrial Rhythm:	Regular
Ventricular Rhythm:	Irregular
P Waves:	Normal sinus configuration, not always followed by QRS complex
PR Interval:	Varies, lengthening, and then dropping a QRS complex
QRS Complex:	Less than 0.12 second in width

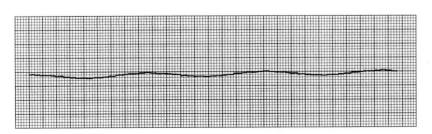

Figure 10-25 ECG tracing of asystole.

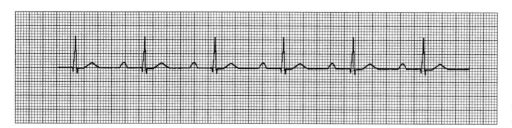

Figure 10-26 First-degree atrioventricular block with a PR interval of 0.30.

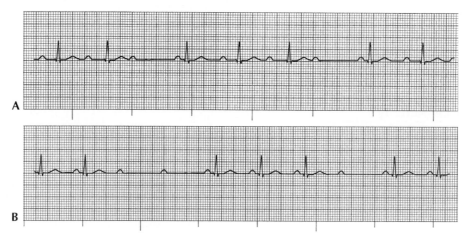

Figure 10-27 A, Second-degree atrioventricular block type I. **B,** Second-degree atrioventricular block type II.

Second-Degree AV Block Type II (Mobitz II)

Second-degree AV block type II is a rarer but more serious form of second-degree AV block and is characterized by a series of nonconducted P waves followed by a P wave that is conducted to the ventricles. It is important to note that each time the P wave is followed by a QRS complex, the PR interval is always fixed (not changing in length). This will help differentiate between the two types of second-degree AV block. Sometimes the ratio of nonconducted to conducted P waves is fixed (at 3:1 or 4:1, for example). This block should be considered serious and treated promptly. Common causes of second-degree AV block type II include extensive damage to the bundle branches after an acute anteroseptal myocardial infarction or degenerative disease.

Systematic Evaluation (see Figure 10-27, *B*):

Rate:	Varies, but ventricular rate is always less than the atrial rate
Atrial Rhythm:	Regular
Ventricular Rhythm:	May be regular if there is a constant conduction ration or irregular if conduction is not constant
P Waves:	Normal sinus configuration, not always followed by QRS complex
PR Interval:	Normal or prolonged but always constant
QRS Complex:	Less than 0.12 second in width

Third-Degree AV Block

The most extreme form of heart block is third-degree AV block, which is caused by conduction disturbances below the AV node in the bundle of His (producing a narrow QRS complex) or bundle branches (producing a wide QRS complex). This block does not allow any conduction of stimuli from the atrium to the ventricles. In this situation, the ventricles and atria beat independently of one another. Thus there is no distinguishable pattern between the atria and ventricles. Third-degree AV block may be transient or permanent but is always considered serious and should prompt immediate intervention. Possible causes of transient third-degree AV block may include inferior myocardial infarction, increased vagal tone, myocarditis, and digitalis toxicity. Permanent causes may include degenerative disease or acute anteroseptal myocardial infarction.

Systematic Evaluation (Figure 10-28):

Rate:	Usually less than 60 beats/min but may vary; ventricular rate is always less than the atrial rate
Rhythm:	Both atrial and ventricular rates are regular
P Waves:	Normal sinus configuration, not always followed by QRS complex
PR Interval:	Varies, no relationship
QRS Complex:	Usually greater than 0.12 second but may also be less than 0.12 second in width

Idioventricular Rhythm

Idioventricular rhythm occurs when the normal pacemaker does not set the pace for the ventricles. In this case, an ectopic focus in one of the ventricles becomes the pacemaker for the ventricles. The intrinsic rate of the ventricular tissue is usually less than 40 beats/min, so the ventricular rate is very slow (Figure 10-29). In idioventricular rhythm, the ECG pattern appears as a slow series of wide and bizarre QRS complexes. The slower ventricular rate and the loss of assistance in ventricular filling provided by the atria decrease cardiac output significantly and can lead rapidly to heart failure and more severe dysrhythmias.

There is a variation of idioventricular rhythm called *accelerated idioventricular rhythm*. In accelerated idioventricular rhythm, the rate is in the normal range (60 to 100 beats/min).

Systematic Evaluation (see Figure 10-29):

Rate:	30 to 40 beats/min or slower, unless accelerated — then it may be between 60-100 beats/min.
Rhythm:	Regular
P Waves:	Absent
PR Interval:	None
QRS Complex:	Greater than 0.12 second

Junctional Rhythm

In a junctional rhythm, an area in the AV junction assumes the pacemaking role and sends impulses down the normal conduction pathways in the ventricles. Because the normal conduction pathways in the ventricles are being used, the QRS complexes appear normal. The P wave may be present or absent. If present, it may appear immediately after the QRS, plainly demonstrating retrograde conduction. In this case, the P wave is almost invariably inverted, indicating that depolarization of the atria

followed a retrograde path. The P wave may appear before the QRS, but when it does, the PR interval is of less than normal duration (0.12 second). This indicates that there was not sufficient time for the P wave to be responsible for initiating the associated QRS complex. Some potential causes of a junctional rhythm may include AV node damage, electrolyte disturbances, digitalis toxicity, heart failure, valvular disease, rheumatic fever, and myocarditis.

Systematic Evaluation (Figure 10-30):

Rate:	Normal intrinsic junctional rate, 40 to 60 beats/min
	Accelerated junctional rate, 60 to 100 beats/min
	Junctional tachycardia, >100 beats/min
Rhythm:	Regular
P Waves:	Absent, inverted, or short
PR Interval:	Short if present
QRS Complex:	Less than 0.12 second

EVIDENCE OF CARDIAC ISCHEMIA, INJURY, OR INFARCTION

Normally the ST segment is isoelectric, meaning that it is in the same horizontal position as the baseline, isoelectric line. Significant deviations (1 mm) of the ST segment from baseline, either up or down, suggest an abnormality in myocardial perfusion and oxygenation.

Cardiac ischemia is seen on the ECG as depression of the ST segment (Figure 10-31) or inversion of the T waves. At this point, there is no permanent damage to the heart, and proper therapy usually reverses any ECG abnormalities. In many cases of myocardial infarction, however, this pattern of ischemia may not be seen because the event has already progressed to the injury phase.

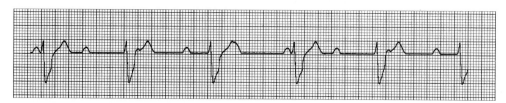

Figure 10-28 Third-degree heart block characterized by independent atrial (P wave) and ventricular activity. The atrial rate is always faster than the ventricular rate.

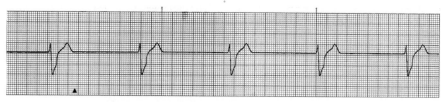

Figure 10-29 ECG tracing of idioventricular rhythm.

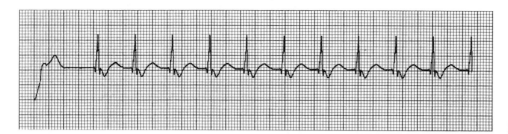

Figure 10-30 ECG tracing showing junctional tachycardia.

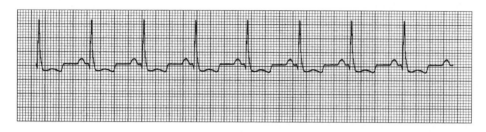

Figure 10-31 ECG tracing showing ST segment depression.

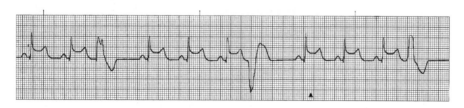

Figure 10-32 ECG tracing showing ST segment elevation with a PVC.

The typical pattern of acute myocardial injury is ST segment elevation in the leads that reflect electrical activity of the corresponding injured heart tissue (Figure 10-32). For example, an acute myocardial injury to the anteroseptal part of the heart will cause ST segment elevation in the leads that examine the anteroseptal portion of the heart (see Table 10-4; Figure 10-33). In general, the degree of damage to the heart caused by the ischemia determines the degree of ST segment elevation. The ST segment abnormality usually resolves when perfusion is restored. At some point after myocardial infarction, significant Q waves (0.04 second in length) will be seen on the ECG in the corresponding leads. Q waves may develop within hours of an infarction but may not evolve for several days in some patients. They persist for the remainder of the patient's life.

> **SIMPLY STATED**
>
> T-wave inversion and ST segment depression indicate myocardial ischemia. ST segment elevation indicates that an acute myocardial injury has occurred.

It can be helpful to identify ST segment abnormalities by drawing a straight line over the imaginary isoelectric line. This will reveal whether ST segment elevation or depression is present and to what degree. If the deviation from the isoelectric line is greater than 1 mm, significant changes have occurred and further investigation is appropriate. The patient should be monitored closely when this abnormality is identified.

ASSESSING CHEST PAIN

Pain and distress are subjective to the patient's perception of his/her condition and may be difficult to assess. However, it is essential that signs and symptoms associated with cardiac events be accurately reported both verbally and on the patient's chart. The following formula will provide you with a reference for assessing these signs and symptoms. Ask the patient:

O   When was the *o*nset of the symptoms?
P   What *p*rovoked the symptoms? (e.g., exercise, sleep, emotional upset)
Q   How would you describe the *q*uality of the pain? (e.g., sharp, dull)
R   Does the pain *r*adiate anywhere?
    Does anything provide *r*elief from the pain?
    In what *r*egion is the pain located?
    Does the pain change with deep *r*espiration?

S Placing severity on a *scale* of 0 to 10, how would you rate your pain?

T What is the *time* frame of your symptoms? Is this chronic or acute?

U What do *you* think is wrong? Is this different from any previous episodes?

The American Heart Association recommends that for chest pain or associated symptoms not relieved by nitroglycerin, a myocardial infarction should be suspected until proven otherwise. Remember that "time is muscle," and treatment interventions such as thrombolytic therapy or surgical intervention should be implemented quickly to salvage as much viable myocardium as possible.

The role of an RT in such cardiac events is to notify the patient's physician, evaluate and optimize oxygen delivery, obtain a 12-lead ECG, and stand by to participate as a member of the cardiac arrest team if needed.

ECG PATTERNS WITH CHRONIC LUNG DISEASE

The majority of patients with chronic obstructive pulmonary disease (COPD) have ECG abnormalities. Hyperinflation of the lungs and flattening of the diaphragm are associated with a more vertical position of the heart. This causes a clockwise rotation and contributes to the right axis deviation associated with COPD. (For quick axis determination, see Table 10-3.) Additionally, chronic pulmonary hypertension is common in patients with COPD and causes an enlargement of the right side of the heart. Enlargement of the right atrium causes the following:

- Rightward deviation of the P-wave axis
- Enlarged positive P waves greater than 2.5 mm in leads II, III, and aV_F
- A prominent and negative P wave in lead I

This syndrome is called *cor pulmonale.* Right ventricular enlargement may be associated with this syndrome and is recognized by the following characteristics:

- Right axis deviation of the QRS complex
- Increased R-wave voltage in leads V_1, V_2, and V_3

Reduced voltage in the limb leads (I, II, and III) is seen when severe pulmonary hyperinflation (emphysema) is present. This is seen as QRS complexes that are less than 5 mm tall in leads I, II, and III. Reduced voltage in precordial leads V_5 and V_6 may also be present. The reduced measured voltage appears to be caused by two factors:

- Reduced transmission of electrical activity through hyperinflated lungs
- A mean QRS axis directed posteriorly and perpendicular to the frontal plane of the limb leads, causing decreased voltage on the ECG

Dysrhythmias often are seen in patients with COPD and acute lung disease. Tachycardia, multifocal atrial tachycardia, and ventricular ectopic beats are some of the more common ECG abnormalities seen in COPD. Such dysrhythmias occur as the result of hypoxemia from lung disease and from adverse effects of medications (e.g., bronchodilators) used to treat the obstructed airways. Hypoxemia often worsens during sleep in patients with COPD and increases the prevalence of nighttime dysrhythmias.

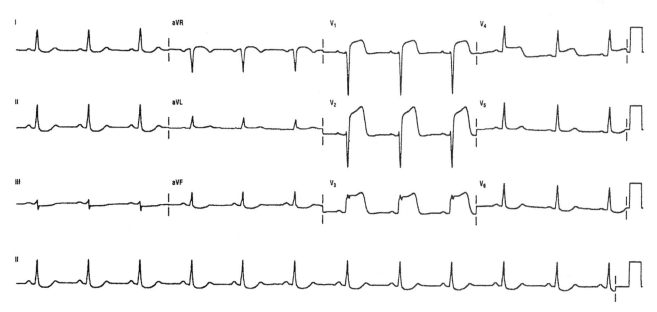

Figure 10-33 Twelve-lead ECG tracing showing ST segment elevation in leads V_1, V_2, V_3, and V_4. This pattern is indicative of acute anteroseptal myocardial injury.

REVIEW QUESTIONS

1. ECGs are useful to evaluate all but the:
   a. impact of lung disease on the heart.
   b. pumping ability of the heart.
   c. severity of the myocardial infarction.
   d. heart rhythm.

2. What clinical findings are suggestive of the need for an ECG?
   a. Headache and facial droop
   b. Orthopnea and syncope
   c. Fever and cough
   d. Joint pain and swelling

3. What is the normal intrinsic rate of the heart's primary pacemaker?
   a. 90 to 110 beats/min
   b. 60 to 100 beats/min
   c. 40 to 80 beats/min
   d. 40 to 60 beats/min

4. What is the normal intrinsic rate of the heart's secondary pacemaker?
   a. 80 to 100 beats/min
   b. 60 to 100 beats/min
   c. 40 to 60 beats/min
   d. 30 to 40 beats/min

5. What does the P wave on the ECG recording represent?
   a. Atrial depolarization
   b. Atrial repolarization
   c. Ventricular depolarization
   d. Ventricular repolarization

6. What does the QRS wave on the ECG recording represent?
   a. Atrial depolarization
   b. Atrial repolarization
   c. Ventricular depolarization
   d. Ventricular repolarization

7. What does the T wave on the ECG recording represent?
   a. Atrial depolarization
   b. Atrial repolarization
   c. Ventricular depolarization
   d. Ventricular repolarization

8. What is a normal PR interval?
   a. 0.10 second
   b. 0.20 second
   c. 0.30 second
   d. 0.40 second

9. What is the length of the normal QRS complex?
   a. 0.04 second
   b. 0.08 second
   c. 0.12 second
   d. 0.16 second

10. The QRS complexes are equally spaced with three large boxes between each complex. What is the heart rate?
    a. 150 beats/min
    b. 100 beats/min
    c. 75 beats/min
    d. 60 beats/min

11. A prolonged PR interval is indicative of:
    a. sinus dysrhythmia.
    b. sinus bradycardia.
    c. sinus block.
    d. AV block.

12. An early, widened QRS complex with an inverted T wave and no associated P wave is consistent with:
    a. PVC.
    b. ventricular tachycardia.
    c. ventricular fibrillation.
    d. ventricular asystole.

13. What ECG finding is suggestive of an acute myocardial infarction?
    a. Prolonged PR intervals
    b. Elevated ST segments
    c. Tall, peaked T waves
    d. Narrow QRS complexes

14. What ECG finding is suggestive of cor pulmonale?
    a. Inverted T waves
    b. Elevated ST segments
    c. Right axis deviation
    d. Small QRS complexes

15. Which of the following statements is/are true regarding sinus tachycardia?
    a. It is caused by sympathetic stimulation.
    b. It may be caused by a fever.
    c. It may be caused by hypotension.
    d. It may be caused by fear or pain.
    e. All of the above

Practice ECG Strips

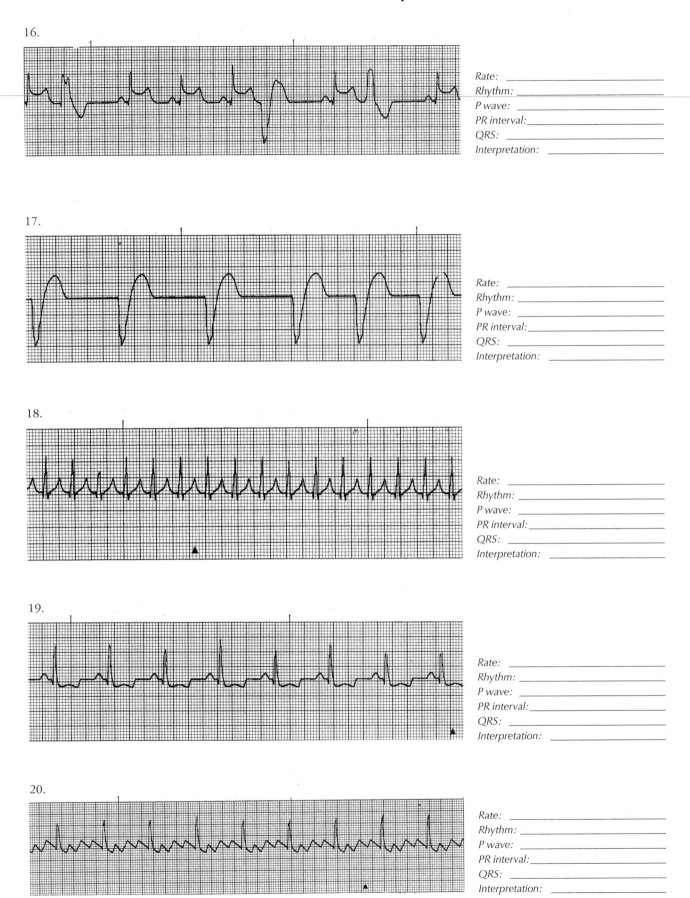

16.

Rate: _____

Rhythm: _____

P wave: _____

PR interval: _____

QRS: _____

Interpretation: _____

17.

Rate: _____

Rhythm: _____

P wave: _____

PR interval: _____

QRS: _____

Interpretation: _____

18.

Rate: _____

Rhythm: _____

P wave: _____

PR interval: _____

QRS: _____

Interpretation: _____

19.

Rate: _____

Rhythm: _____

P wave: _____

PR interval: _____

QRS: _____

Interpretation: _____

20.

Rate: _____

Rhythm: _____

P wave: _____

PR interval: _____

QRS: _____

Interpretation: _____

21.

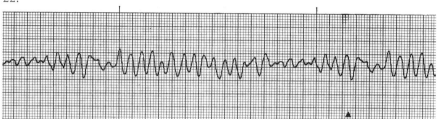

Rate: _____
Rhythm: _____
P wave: _____
PR interval: _____
QRS: _____
Interpretation: _____

22.

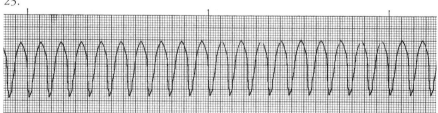

Rate: _____
Rhythm: _____
P wave: _____
PR interval: _____
QRS: _____
Interpretation: _____

23.

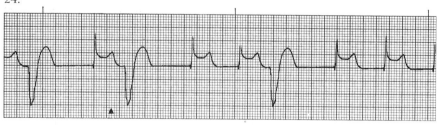

Rate: _____
Rhythm: _____
P wave: _____
PR interval: _____
QRS: _____
Interpretation: _____

24.

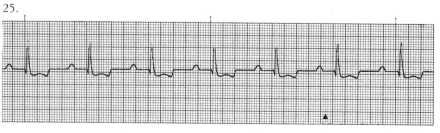

Rate: _____
Rhythm: _____
P wave: _____
PR interval: _____
QRS: _____
Interpretation: _____

25.

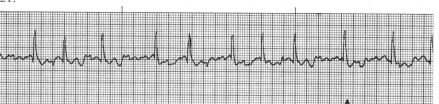

Rate: _____
Rhythm: _____
P wave: _____
PR interval: _____
QRS: _____
Interpretation: _____

BIBLIOGRAPHY

American Heart Association: *Advanced cardiac life support,* Cummins RO, editor, Dallas, 1997, AHA.

Connover M: *Understanding electrocardiography: arrhythmias and the 12-lead ECG,* ed 6, St Louis, 1996, Mosby.

Goldberger AL, Goldberger E: *Clinical electrocardiography: a simplified approach,* ed 6, St Louis, 1998, Mosby.

Huff J: *ECG Workout: exercises in arrhythmia interpretation,* ed 4, Philadelphia, 2002, Lippincott-Williams & Wilkins.

Huszar R: *Basic arrhythmias,* ed 2, St Louis, 1996, Mosby.

Kinney R, Packa D: *Comprehensive cardiac care,* ed 8, St Louis, 1996, Mosby.

Lochaas T, Newell L: *Learning ECGs workbook,* St Louis, 1994, Mosby.

Mulholand G, Brewer B: *Improving your skills in 12-lead ECG interpretation,* Baltimore, 1995, Lippincott, Williams & Wilkins.

Phalen T: *The 12-lead ECG in acute myocardial infarction,* St Louis, 1996, Mosby.

Tait C: *Learning ECGs instructor's manual,* St Louis, 1994, Mosby.

Thaler MS: *The only ECG book you'll ever need,* ed 2, Philadelphia, 1995, Lippincott-Raven.

CHAPTER
11

Douglas D. Deming

Assessment of Neonatal and Pediatric Patients

LEARNING OBJECTIVES

Upon completion of this chapter, the reader should be able to accomplish the following:

1. Identify the type of information found in the pregnancy history, labor history, and delivery history and the clinical significance of common findings.
2. Identify the value of the Apgar scoring system and the five physical criteria used in this scoring system.
3. Identify the Apgar scores that indicate normal status, moderate depression, and severe depression of the newborn.
4. Identify normal values for the vital signs in newborns and the clinical implications of abnormalities.
5. Identify the clinical implications of retractions, nasal flaring, and grunting.
6. Identify the normal time for capillary refill and the clinical significance of poor capillary refill in the infant.
7. Identify the clinical significance of abdominal distention in the infant.
8. Recognize true statements regarding the technique for auscultation of the infant.
9. Identify the clinical implications of abnormal breath sounds in the infant.
10. Identify potential causes of murmurs heard during auscultation of the infant precordium.
11. Identify normal values for the white and red blood cell count and partial differential for the infant at birth, 7 days of age, and 14 days of age.
12. Identify the possible causes of abnormalities in the white blood cell and red blood cell counts in the infant.
13. Identify the clinical implications for abnormalities in blood glucose, total protein and albumin, serum enzymes, and electrolytes.
14. Identify normal values for arterial pH, Po_2, Pco_2, HCO_3^-, and base excess at birth, 24 hours after birth, and 1 month to 2 years after birth.
15. Identify which blood gas parameter is significantly different between capillary blood and arterial blood.
16. Identify the factors that can lead to misleading results from the transcutaneous oxygen monitor.
17. Identify the lung volumes that can be measured in the newborn and the clinical value of such measurements.
18. Identify the clinical findings that suggest the need for a chest radiograph in the infant.

CHAPTER OUTLINE
Assessment of the Newborn
History
Physical Examination
Techniques of Examination
Clinical Laboratory Data
Newborn Blood Gases
Pulmonary Function Testing
Radiographs
Assessment of Critically Ill Infants
Airway
Hemodynamic Assessments
Assessment of the Older Infant and Child
History
Physical Examination
Clinical Laboratory Data
Blood Gases
Pulmonary Function Testing
Radiographs

KEY TERMS
abortion
acrocyanosis
Apgar score
apnea
ascites
bradycardia
bradypnea
bronchopulmonary
  dysplasia (BPD)
bruit
chronologic age
coarctation of the aorta
cranial sutures
croup
crying vital capacity (CVC)
epiglottitis
estimated date of
  confinement (EDC)
fetal hemoglobin (Hb F)
gestational age
gravida
grunting
hepatomegaly
hyperdynamic precordium

hyperglycemia
hyperthermia
hypoglycemia
hypothermia
hypotonia
interrupted aortic arch
    syndrome
intraventricular
    hemorrhage (IVH)
last menstrual period
    (LMP)
lecithin/sphingomyelin
    (L/S) ratio
leukocytosis
leukopenia
long apnea
meconium
meconium aspiration
    syndrome (MAS)
nasal flaring
neutral thermal
    environment (NTE)
neutropenia
osteopenia of the
    premature
para

patent ductus arteriosus
    (PDA)
periodic breathing
phosphatidylglycerol
    (PG)
phosphatidylinositol
    (PI)
pneumoperitoneum
polycythemia
postterm infants
preterm infants
respiratory distress
    syndrome (RDS)
retractions
short apnea
sinus bradycardia
splenomegaly
spontaneous abortion
tachycardia
tachypnea
term infant
therapeutic abortion
thrombocytopenia
thrombocytosis
transient tachypnea of the
    newborn (TTNB)

CHAPTER OVERVIEW

The fundamentals for assessing the newborn and pediatric patient are a good history, thorough physical examination, and careful attention to selected laboratory and radiographic information. Although the basic principles that apply to adult patients also apply here, certain characteristics make assessment of the newborn and pediatric patient unique. These characteristics include lack of verbal communication skills, the tendency to be afraid of strangers (particularly people in white coats), and inability or reluctance to follow directions. This chapter reviews the assessment of the newborn and pediatric patient with respiratory disease.

For the purposes of this chapter, a *young infant* is younger than 3 months old, an *older infant* is between 3 and 12 months old, and a *child* is between 12 months old and adolescence. A young infant's age can be defined as either chronologic or gestational. Chronologic age is the age of the infant computed from the date of birth. Gestational age is the age of the infant computed from the date of conception. Gestational age usually is assigned based on the history and physical examination. Term infants are born between 37 and 42 weeks of gestational age, preterm infants are born at fewer than 37 weeks of gestational age, and postterm infants are born at 43 or more weeks of gestational age.

ASSESSMENT OF THE NEWBORN

History

The newborn's history is obtained from several sources and covers more than just the medical history of the infant. Sources include the parents, the mother's labor and delivery chart, and the infant's own chart.

Maternal History

The newborn's history begins with the mother's history. Was the mother healthy before she was pregnant? Does she have chronic diseases? Is she taking medications or illicit drugs? For example, infants born to mothers with diabetes mellitus often are maturationally delayed and may be susceptible to diseases of prematurity such as respiratory distress syndrome (RDS). Conversely, infants born to mothers who have chronic hypertension may be maturationally advanced for their gestational age.

The mother's previous pregnancy history can give the historian valuable information. Obstetricians note this information in the mother's medical record using the terms gravida, para, and abortion. *Gravida* is a pregnant woman, *para* is a woman who delivers a live infant, and *abortion* is the delivering of a dead infant. These terms will most likely be abbreviated and followed by numbers (e.g., G2, P1, Ab0, meaning this woman is in her second pregnancy, has delivered a living infant, and has not had any abortions). Abortions can be further subdivided into therapeutic and spontaneous; these are abbreviated as TAb and SAb, respectively. If the mother has had multiple pregnancies that have ended with spontaneous abortions rather than living infants, there is the possibility of chromosomal or metabolic disease that can have serious consequences for the current pregnancy, or the mother may have an incompetent cervix that is associated with chronic preterm deliveries. If the mother has had multiple pregnancies that have ended with therapeutic abortions, the historian should think about the possibility of maternal drug abuse. Finally, for a mother who has had multiple pregnancies that have ended with the delivery of living children, the historian should inquire about the perinatal health of those children, because severity of diseases tends to be similar in families.

Family History

It is important to inquire about family history, as well as maternal history. Is there a history of prematurity? Have there been other infants with respiratory problems? The incidence and severity of diseases such as RDS are similar among siblings. There may also be an increased tendency for the recurrence of pneumonias caused by group B β-hemolytic streptococcus in siblings.

Pregnancy History

In evaluating the infant with respiratory disease, valuable information can be found in the pregnancy, labor, and delivery histories. In the pregnancy history, the interviewer records information about the mother and the fetus. Did the mother have any illnesses during gestation? Congenital viral infections that profoundly affect the infant may have produced only mild or even no symptoms in the mother. Did the mother have any vaginal bleeding? The mother usually is the source of vaginal bleeding, but occasionally the baby is bleeding, and these infants must be evaluated for hypovolemia (low blood volume). Did the mother note any evidence of amniotic infection or urinary tract infection? An infant delivered in the presence of infection has an increased risk of infection-caused respiratory difficulty. Did the mother have traumatic injury? A traumatic injury may compromise the uteroplacental interface and thus decrease transfer of oxygen and other nutrients to the baby. Did the mother's uterus grow appropriately during pregnancy? If not, the infant may not have grown and could have pulmonary hypoplasia, severe malformations, or congenital infection. Any of these diseases may cause significant respiratory distress in the newborn.

Because the incidence of respiratory disease varies with different gestational ages, determining when the infant was actually due it is important. The interviewer should attempt to identify the date of the mother's last menstrual period (LMP), her estimated date of delivery (this appears as the estimated date of confinement (EDC) on the mother's chart), her obstetric record of uterine growth, and any reports from ultrasound examinations that she may have had.

Infants born in early gestation are more susceptible to RDS, pulmonary interstitial emphysema, intracranial hemorrhage, and bronchopulmonary dysplasia. Infants born in late gestation are more susceptible to severe perinatal asphyxia, meconium aspiration, and the development of persistent pulmonary hypertension.

Fetal History

Useful information about the infant can be determined from the prenatal assessment of the fetus. This information could include the following: fetal movement monitoring, biophysical profile, lecithin/sphingomyelin (L/S) ratio, presence of phosphatidylinositol (PI) and phosphatidylglycerol (PG), fetal monitoring tracings, and non-stress tests (NSTs).

Fetal movement monitoring is easily accomplished using three widely available tools: maternal observation, fetal ultrasound, and fetal Doppler ultrasound. The simplest of these tools is having the mother keep a log of the timing, strength, and duration of the fetal movements for a period of time. Fetal ultrasound and Doppler ultrasound provide more quantifiable data but for shorter periods. Having a history of decreased fetal movement should alert the clinician of the possibility of the fetus being in trouble. This could be prenatal asphyxia and impending death or the possibility of severe neuromuscular disease, in which the newborn will be unable to support spontaneous independent respiration.

The biophysical profile is an ultrasound evaluation of fetal breathing, body movement, tone, reactive heart rate, and amniotic fluid volume. Like the Apgar score, each of these parameters has a maximal score of 2 and a minimal score of 0. The score for a normal fetus is 8 or 10. With lower biophysical profile scores, the chance of significant fetal and newborn problems increases (Table 11-1). These potential problems include intrauterine growth retardation, significant fetal acidosis, stillbirth, and neonatal death.

The L/S ratio is the ratio of two phospholipids: lecithin and sphingomyelin. Increasing levels of lecithin indicate improving maturation of the lung's surfactant system. Like lecithin, PI and PG become present with advancing maturation of the lung. Their presence is usually indicative of lung maturation.

Fetal monitoring is a continuous graphic method of recording the fetal heart rate and uterine contractions. Various patterns (fetal tachycardia, variable decelerations, and late decelerations) are signs that fetus may be in trouble in the uterine environment. Knowing that a fetus has any of these heart rate patterns should alert the care team that this infant may need a more extensive resuscitation and more careful evaluation after birth.

The NST is a method of evaluating the stability of the fetus's physiology within the uterine environment. The test monitors

Table 11-1 Biophysical Profile

Biophysical variable	Normal (score = 2)	Abnormal (score = 0)
Fetal breathing	One or more episodes of ≥30 seconds in 30 minutes	No breathing or <30 seconds in 30 minutes
Fetal body movement	Three or more discrete movements in 30 minutes	No movement or less than three movements in 30 minutes
Fetal tone	At least one episode of flex-extend-flex movements of limb	Absent or incomplete flex-extend-flex movements
Reactive fetal heart rate	Two or more accelerations of ≥15 beats/min in 30 minutes	Less than two such accelerations in 30 minutes or <15 beats/min
Amniotic fluid volume	One or more amniotic fluid pockets measuring ≥10 mm in two perpendicular planes	No amniotic fluid pocket or pockets <10 mm in two planes

From James D: *Br J Hosp Med* 49:561, 1993.

the acceleration of the fetal heart rate in response to fetal movement. A healthy fetus has a minimum of an increase in heart rate of at least 15 beats/min. To be considered reactive, the fetus needs to have a minimum of two accelerations in 20 minutes. A fetus is considered nonreactive when it fails to have heart rate response in two consecutive 20-minute periods. A fetus that is nonreactive is at greater risk of fetal death. This will prompt the obstetrician to consider the possibility of an accelerated or operative delivery (cesarean section). A fetus with a nonreactive NST is potentially quite distressed, and there is urgency to evaluating its problems and intervening. Knowing that a fetus has a nonreactive NST should alert the care team that this infant may need a more extensive resuscitation and more careful evaluation after birth.

Labor History

The labor history is obtained to evaluate the well-being of the infant during the transition from intrauterine to extrauterine life. The infant must successfully deal with cyclic decreases in uterine blood flow, as well as compression of his/her body. The interviewer should evaluate the available obstetric information. This might include fetal heart rate tracings, fetal activity, biophysical profile, and fetal ultrasound. Information that suggests perinatal asphyxia might include variable or late heart rate decelerations, low biophysical profile, decrease in fetal movement, presence of meconium (first feces of an infant) in the amniotic fluid, long labor, and abnormal vaginal bleeding. The interviewer should also look for information that might suggest an infection in the infant. This might include maternal fever, high maternal white blood cell (WBC) count, tender uterus, rupture of the amniotic membranes for more than 24 hours, foul-smelling amniotic fluid, and fetal tachycardia.

Delivery History

The delivery history should include the method of delivery for the infant: vaginal or cesarean section; spontaneous, forceps, or vacuum extraction; or low, middle, or high forceps. Infants who are successfully dealing with the labor process are born by spontaneous or low forceps vaginal deliveries and usually are normal. Infants who are in trouble during delivery are more likely to be delivered by vacuum extraction, middle or high forceps, or cesarean delivery. (Some cesarean deliveries are performed because the infant is positioned in such a manner that vaginal delivery would be high risk, not because the infant is in trouble.) These infants are at greater risk for respiratory disease. It is also helpful to know what type of anesthetic the mother had for delivery (e.g., narcotics, local, epidural, spinal, or general). Narcotics and general anesthetics may enter the infant's bloodstream and produce respiratory depression in the infant. Spinal anesthetics may lower the mother's blood pressure, thus compromising the oxygen supply to the infant.

At the time of delivery, there is usually a great deal of excitement and tension that may hinder critical powers of observation that are important in determining the well-being of the newborn. The most standard objective measurement of the newborn's well-being is the Apgar score. This is a simple, quick, and reliable means of assessment. It assigns the infant points for the presence of five specific physical criteria (Table 11-2). Most infants are evaluated and assigned Apgar scores at 1 and 5 minutes. However, if the infant is having difficulty during the transition to extrauterine life, Apgar scores can be assigned more often and over a longer time span. For example, a sick infant may have 1-, 2-, 5-, 10-, 15-, and 20-minute Apgar scores. Of course, the process of assigning an Apgar score must not delay the initiation of resuscitative measures. If an infant is becoming asphyxiated, the signs measured by the Apgar score generally decline in a particular order (color, reflex irritability, muscle tone, respiratory effort, and heart rate). Conversely, the signs improve in a similar order (heart rate, respiratory effort, reflex irritability, color, and muscle tone) when the infant is recovering.

The Apgar score is useful in identifying infants who need resuscitation. Infants who are adjusting well to extrauterine life usually have 1-minute scores of 7 to 10. They may show acrocyanosis, irregular respirations, or hypotonia (lack of muscle tone). They usually require only routine newborn care such as drying, temperature maintenance, and clearing of the airway. They may occasionally require supplemental oxygen for a brief period. Moderately depressed infants have 1-minute scores of 4 to 6. They need more than routine care and often need an increased FIO_2 (fraction of inspired oxygen) with bag and mask ventilation. Most infants respond well to this therapy and improve in a few minutes. Infants who have 1-minute scores of 0 to 3 are severely depressed and need extensive medical care such as intubation and mechanical ventilation.

Although the 1-minute Apgar score is a useful tool in screening infants who might require resuscitation, the 5-minute

Table 11-2	Apgar Scores		
Sign	Score 0	Score 1	Score 2
Heart rate	Absent	<100/min	>100/min
Respiratory effort	Absent	Gasping, irregular	Good
Muscle tone	Limp	Some flexion	Active motion
Reflex irritability	No response	Grimace	Cry
Color	Body pale or blue, extremities blue	Body pink, extremities blue	Completely pink

Apgar score is a better predictor of the infant's neurologic outcome. Infants who have 5-minute Apgar scores of less than 5 have a greater risk of neurologic impairment at 1 year of age.

SIMPLY STATED

Newborns are evaluated at 1- and 5-minute intervals after birth with the Apgar scoring system. This system calls for evaluation of the infant's color, heart rate, respiratory rate, muscle tone, and reflex irritability (normal score = 7 to 10, moderate depression = 4 to 6, and severe depression = 0 to 3).

Postnatal History

After the delivery, the historian should document the magnitude of the infant's resuscitation, present diseases, treatment of the diseases, length of the hospital stay, condition at discharge, and problems that have developed since the infant was last seen. For most infants, all of this information is normal, and the postnatal history is brief. All infants require some form of resuscitation. The simplest resuscitation required is clearing the airway and drying the skin. It is important to document whether the infant required only this simple intervention; a more significant intervention with oxygen, manual ventilation with bag and mask, or intubation; or chemical resuscitation with the administration of drugs to support cardiac output. How did the infant respond to resuscitation? Was the response immediate or slow?

If the infant is still hospitalized, the only further information needed for an adequate assessment is what diseases the infant has, what treatment has been initiated, and what the response to treatment has been. If the infant has been discharged and is now being readmitted, seen again in a practice office, or seen at home, the historian must inquire about the infant's condition since discharge. Was the infant still sick at the time of discharge? Did the infant require continuing treatment at home? How is the infant doing with the current treatment? What kind of problem does the infant have now?

Physical Examination

The skills for physical examination of a newborn are not difficult to learn. As previously emphasized (see Chapter 5), abnormalities can be detected only by examiners who recognize normal respiratory function. Beginning examiners should develop the techniques of physical examination on well babies to understand the complex subtleties of abnormalities in sick infants.

Examination of a newborn is based on three of the four classic principles of physical examination: inspection, palpation, and auscultation. Percussion is rarely used in examining newborns because of small cavity and organ sizes. Therefore percussion is not described in this chapter. However, transillumination is a useful tool in the assessment of newborns and is discussed later in this chapter.

Careful inspection reveals clues about the type and severity of respiratory disease. It is important to inspect the overall appearance of the infant carefully because respiratory diseases in the newborn often are manifested by many extrapulmonary signs. Palpation is useful in determining the cause of respiratory distress and the severity of side effects from the lung disease and its treatment. As in the adult, auscultation is used to define characteristics of the disease process occurring in the lung. However, statements about the internal location of the pathologic process must be made with greater caution in newborns because localization by auscultation is difficult in the small chest cavity.

Gestational Age Assessment

Gestational age is assigned by the maternal dates, fetal ultrasound, and gestational assessment examination. Most women know approximately when they conceive. This is frequently confirmed by an early fetal ultrasound examination. Unless there is a significant discrepancy between these two dating assessments, the mother's dates are usually accepted. Sometimes the mother does not know the date of conception or there is significant disagreement between the maternal dates and the fetal ultrasound. In those situations, the gestational age assessment can be done with a gestational assessment tool.

The original assessment tools were developed by Dubowitz and Dubowitz. These tools have been modified and validated over many years. Most nurseries currently use a Ballard examination (Figure 11-1), which is a modification of the Dubowitz examination. A gestational age assessment should be performed for any infant who is small, who was born prematurely, or for whom there is uncertainty about the gestational age.

The Ballard examination is divided into two sections: Neuromuscular Maturity and Physical Maturity. The infant is scored for various neuromuscular and physical attributes. The infant's neuromuscular and physical characteristics are scored by matching the infant's characteristics to the table's descriptions and then marking the table. Each column of the table has a numerical value ranging from -1 to 5. The numerical values for all of the marked cells are added together. It is important that a cell is marked in each row. The sum is then compared with the maturity scale and a gestational age is assigned. The Ballard examination is accurate to within 2 weeks of the gestational age.

Vital Signs

Body temperature

The range of normal body temperature in the newborn does not differ from that in the adult. Humans maintain body temperature by balancing heat production with heat loss. The newborn loses much more heat to the environment than the older child or adult, largely because heat loss is determined by the ratio of the surface area of the body to the total body mass (Table 11-3). The average adult male has a surface area of 1.7 m^2 and a body mass of 80 kg. This results in a body surface area/body mass

NEWBORN MATURITY RATING & CLASSIFICATION

ESTIMATION OF GESTATIONAL AGE BY MATURITY RATING
Symbols: X - 1st Exam   O - 2nd Exam   Side 1

Gestation by Dates _____ wks

Birth Date _____ Hour _____ am/pm

APGAR _____ 1 min _____ 5 min

NEUROMUSCULAR MATURITY

	-1	0	1	2	3	4	5
Posture							
Square Window (wrist)	>90°	90°	60°	45°	30°	0°	
Arm Recoil		180°	140°-180°	110°-140°	90°-110°	<90°	
Popliteal Angle	180°	160°	140°	120°	100°	90°	<90°
Scarf Sign							
Heel to Ear							

PHYSICAL MATURITY

Skin	sticky; friable; transparent	gelatinous; red; translucent	smooth; pink; visible veins	superficial peeling &/or rash; few veins	cracking; pale areas; rare veins	parchment; deep cracking; no vessels	leathery; cracked; wrinkled
Lanugo		none	sparse	abundant	thinning	bald areas	mostly bald
Plantar Surface	heel-toe 40-50 mm: -1 <40 mm: -2	>50 mm; no crease	faint red marks	anterior transverse crease only	creases ant. 2/3	creases over entire sole	
Breast		imperceptible	barely perceptible	flat areola; no bud	stippled areola; 1-2 mm bud	raised areola; 3-4 mm bud	full areola; 5-10 mm bud
Eye/Ear	lids fused loosely: -1 tightly: -2	lids open; pinna flat; stays folded	sl. curved pinna; soft; slow recoil	well-curved pinna; soft but ready recoil	formed & firm; instant recoil	thick cartilage; ear stiff	
Genitals male	scrotum flat; smooth	scrotum empty; faint rugae	testes in upper canal; rare rugae	testes descending; few rugae	testes down; good rugae	testes pendulous; deep rugae	
Genitals female	clitoris prominent; labia flat	prominent clitoris; small labia minora	prominent clitoris; enlarging minora	majora & minora equally prominent	majora large; minora small	majora cover clitoris & minora	

Scoring system: Ballard JL, Khoury JC, Wedig K, Wang L, Eilers-Walsman BL, Lipp R. New Ballard Score, expanded to include extremely premature infants. J Pediatr. 1991;119:417-423.

MATURITY RATING

score	weeks
-10	20
-5	22
0	24
5	26
10	28
15	30
20	32
25	34
30	36
35	38
40	40
45	42
50	44

SCORING SECTION

	1st Exam=X	2nd Exam=O
Estimating Gest Age by Maturity Rating	_____ Weeks	_____ Weeks
Time of Exam	Date _____ Hour _____ am/pm	Date _____ Hour_____ am/pm
Age at Exam	_____ Hours	_____ Hours
Signature of Examiner	_____ M.D./R.N.	_____ M.D./R.N.

Figure 11-1 Ballard gestational age scoring system. (From Ballard et al: New Ballard Score, expanded to include extremely premature infants, *J Pediatr* 119:417-423, 1991.)

ratio of 0.02 m²/kg. The average term infant has a body surface area of 0.25 m² and a body mass of 3.5 kg, which results in a surface area/mass ratio of 0.07 m²/kg. This is more than three times the surface area/mass ratio of an adult male. For infants younger in gestational age, the problem becomes even more significant. A 28-week-gestational-age infant has a body surface area of approximately 0.15 m² and a body mass of 1 kg. This results in a surface area/mass ratio of 0.15 m²/kg, which is more than six times greater than that of an adult male. Because of this, newborn term and preterm infants lose heat easily and are extremely dependent on the environment to help them maintain body temperature. Infants, like all physical objects, lose heat to the environment by one of four mechanisms: conduction (touching a cold or wet object), convection (gas blowing over the skin surface), evaporation (liquid evaporating from the skin surface), and radiation (attempting to warm a cold surface not in contact with the skin). All of these mecha-

nisms must be considered when helping infants deal with their environment.

SIMPLY STATED
Newborns are very prone to heat loss because of their high ratio of surface area to mass. A neutral thermal environment is essential to avoid stressing the infant.

Hyperthermia is a core body temperature of more than 37.5° C. Hyperthermia in the newborn usually is caused by environmental factors. The infant may be wrapped in too many clothes, placed close to a heater, or placed in too warm an isolette or radiant warmer. It is uncommon, although not rare, for an infant with hyperthermia to have an infection.

Table 11-3	Ratio of Surface Area to Mass		
	Surface Area (m²)	Mass (kg)	Surface Area/Mass (m²/kg)
Adult male	1.7	80	0.02
Term infant	0.25	3.5	0.07
28-week-old infant	0.15	1.0	0.15

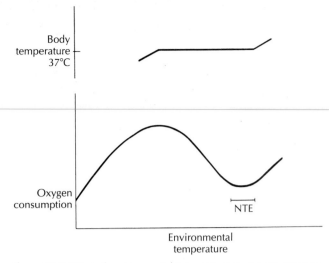

Figure 11-2 Effect of environmental temperature on oxygen consumption and body temperature. *NTE,* Neutral thermal environment.

Hypothermia is a core body temperature of less than 36.5° C. Hypothermia is a more common sign of infection in the newborn than in the older child or adult. Hypothermia probably occurs because the infant is unable to maintain normal heat production during an acute infection. The infant, in contrast to the adult, does not shiver when hypothermic.

Measurement of body temperature

Several methods are used to obtain body temperature in infants. The most common of these are axillary and rectal temperatures. Axillary temperature is approximately 0.5° C lower than oral temperature, and rectal temperature (closest approximation of core body temperature) is approximately 0.5° C higher. Other methods of measuring skin temperature are becoming more widely available, including infrared reflectance and liquid crystal thermography. Infrared reflectance is used to measure tympanic membrane temperature, which may be an indicator of core temperature. Liquid crystal thermography measures skin heat and is useful for screening but is not particularly accurate.

In addition to noting body temperature, the examiner should also note the temperature of the infant's environment. Most sick infants are placed in a neutral thermal environment (NTE), which is the environmental temperature at which the infant's metabolic demand and therefore oxygen consumption is the least (Figure 11-2). If the environmental temperature leaves the neutral thermal range, the infant usually can maintain a stable body temperature, but at the cost of a significant increase in oxygen consumption. Neutral thermal environments are defined for an infant based on weight and gestational and chronologic age.[1]

Pulse

The normal pulse rate for infants is between 100 and 160 beats/min and is a function of the developmental age of the infant. The normal resting heart rate is higher in young-gestational-age infants. The resting heart rate also decreases with increasing chronologic age. Infants cannot significantly change their cardiac output by increasing stroke volume (volume of blood ejected from the heart with ventricular contraction), because their stroke volume at rest is normally more than 90% of maximal stroke volume. Infants increase their cardiac output by increasing their heart rate.

Tachycardia in the newborn is a heart rate greater than 160 beats/min, and bradycardia is a heart rate of less than 100 beats/min. Tachycardias in the newborn can be caused by crying, pain, decrease in the circulating blood volume, drugs, hyperthermia, and heart disease. Bradycardias can be caused by hypoxia, Valsalva maneuver (often occurs during crying), heart disease, hypothermia, vagal stimulation (e.g., passing a nasogastric tube), and certain drugs. In addition, there are a few infants with sinus bradycardia (a normal variant) who have resting heart rates of 70 to 100 beats/min.

Assessment of pulse rate

Because of the small size of the radial arteries, the pulse usually is evaluated at the brachial or femoral artery. The examiner's index finger pad is used to assess either of these pulses. To evaluate the brachial pulse, the examiner places his/her index finger pad over the brachial artery on the medial superior surface of the arm just proximal to the medial epicondyle of the elbow, with the baby in a supine position. The femoral artery pulse can be assessed at the groin, about halfway across the thigh, just below the inguinal ligament (Figure 11-3).

Respiratory rate

The normal respiratory rate for infants is between 30 and 60 breaths/min and is a function of the developmental age of the infant. The normal respiratory rate decreases as gestational age increases. Infants' respiratory rates are higher than those of older children and adults because of mechanical properties of their chest walls and airways. *Functional residual capacity (FRC)* is maintained by the opposition of two forces: outward spring of the chest wall and recoil of the alveoli. Infants have a lower FRC than older children or adults, because infants' chest walls are more compliant. This in turn places their *closing volume* (the lung volume at airway collapse) within their tidal volume. Should the

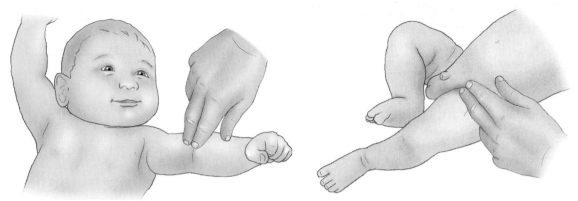

Figure 11-3 Position of brachial and femoral pulses in the newborn.

infant with collapsed airways attempt to inhale a large tidal volume, the chest wall would collapse inward (retract). Conversely, a forced exhalation against collapsed airways would trap gas in the lung. Infants breathe rapidly and shallowly to avoid chest wall collapse and gas trapping in the lung.

Tachypnea is a respiratory rate of greater than 60 breaths/min, and bradypnea is a respiratory rate of less than 30 breaths/min. In newborns, tachypnea can be caused by hypoxemia, metabolic and respiratory acidosis, congenital heart disease, anxiety, pain, hyperthermia, and crying. Bradypnea is not a normal physiologic response in newborns. Bradypnea can be caused by certain medications (e.g., narcotics), hypothermia, and central nervous system diseases, and it may be an important clinical sign of the imminent decompensation of the newborn with lung disease. Nonintubated infants with lung disease usually are tachypneic. As the disease progresses and the infant tires from the increasing work of breathing, bradypnea occurs just before total respiratory collapse.

Another common respiratory pattern of infants is apnea, or the cessation of respiratory effort. The cessation of breathing for more than 15 to 20 seconds is long apnea, for 6 to 14 seconds is short apnea, and for less than 6 seconds is a **respiratory pause.** A phenomenon known as periodic breathing also exists in newborns. During periodic breathing, the infant has multiple episodes of respiratory pauses or short apnea interspersed with normal-appearing ventilation. This pattern of breathing may continue for several minutes to several hours. Long apnea is always a pathologic state. Small numbers of short apneas and respiratory pauses and short spells of periodic breathing (Figure 11-4) are normal in preterm and term infants up to 3 months of age.

Assessment of respiratory rate

The respiratory rate can be obtained by visually observing chest motion or counting respiration while listening with a stethoscope. Visual observation provides a respiratory rate closer to the infant's resting rate. However, because the normal infant breathes rapidly with a small tidal volume, visualization of all of the true breaths may be difficult. If the examiner thinks this is a possibility, the respiratory rate should be assessed by listening with a stethoscope. The examiner must recognize that the infant is likely to respond to the touch of the stethoscope with a temporary increase in respiratory rate.

The infant's respirations are assessed for rate, as well as for regularity and depth. Many immature infants have normal rates but very irregular breathing patterns, which may consist of periodic respiration or even apnea interspersed with periods of normal respiration. In addition, infants with significant lung disease may have normal respiratory rates but tidal volumes so small that they have minimal effective ventilation.

Blood pressure

The normal values for blood pressure depend on the size of the infant, with pressures decreasing with lower weights (Table 11-4). Usually, a term infant's systolic blood pressure should be no higher than 70 mm Hg, with diastolic pressure no higher than 50 mm Hg. Normal pulse pressure (the difference between systolic and diastolic blood pressure) in a term infant is between 15 and 25 mm Hg.

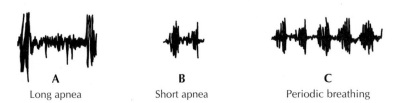

A	B	C
Long apnea	Short apnea	Periodic breathing

Figure 11-4 Respiratory patterns showing chest wall motion during long apnea **(A)**, short apnea **(B)**, and periodic breathing **(C)**.

Table 11-4	Normal Newborn Blood Pressures in the First Hours of Life	
Birth Weight (g)	Systolic (mm Hg)	Diastolic (mm Hg)
501-750	50-62	26-36
751-1000	48-59	23-36
1001-1250	49-61	26-35
1251-1500	46-56	23-33
1501-1750	46-58	23-33
1751-2000	48-61	24-35
2001-3000	59	35
>3000	66	41

Adapted from Hegyi T et al: *J Pediatr* 124:630, 1994; and Kitterman JA, Phibbs RH, Tooley WH: *Pediatrics* 44:959, 1969.

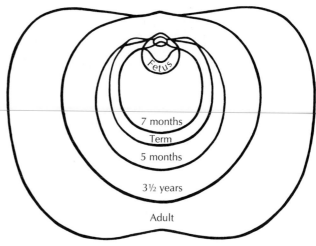

Figure 11-5 Changes in anteroposterior chest configuration with age.

Measurement of blood pressure

There are two common methods of determining blood pressure in newborns: blood pressure cuff (sphygmomanometer) and direct arterial pressure. The more common method is to use a blood pressure cuff. Four techniques can be used for determining blood pressure with a cuff. The auscultatory methods used in adults are technically difficult to perform in newborns and are rarely used. Two other methods that reflect systolic pressure are the flush technique and the palpation technique. In the flush technique, the examiner compresses the extremity beyond the blood pressure cuff, inflates the cuff to above the expected systolic pressure, and deflates the cuff, watching for the return of normal skin color to the blanched extremity. In the palpation technique, the examiner palpates an artery distal to the blood pressure cuff, inflates the cuff to above the expected systolic pressure, and allows the cuff to deflate, noting when pulsations return. The fourth method, using an oscillometric noninvasive blood pressure monitoring machine, provides the most reliable blood pressure information of the four techniques mentioned.

The other common method for obtaining blood pressure in newborns is direct measurement of pressure through an arterial cannula. This is discussed in greater depth later in this chapter.

Morphometric Measurements

In newborns, there are three important measurements that usually are not thought of in the physical examination of adults: weight, length, and head circumference. There are standard tables of normal growth for all gestational and developmental ages for these measurements.[2,3] These measurements provide important clues to assessing the infant's past nutritional environment and current state and predicting the infant's long-term growth.

Lung Topography

The infant's lungs are situated in the chest much as in the adult, but the infant's chest has a greater anteroposterior (AP) dia-

meter than the adult's. The AP diameter of the infant's chest decreases proportionally and becomes more like the adult configuration with growth (Figure 11-5). The imaginary lines and thoracic cage landmarks are the same in infants as in adults (see Chapter 5).

Techniques of Examination

Inspection

Inspection is probably the most important and often the most neglected portion of the physical examination of a newborn. The infant should be nude and in a supine position initially. The examiner should look first at the infant's overall appearance to identify level of illness, presence of malformations, and whether the infant's body position is appropriate for the gestational age (Figure 11-6). The term infant at rest flexes his/her arms and legs into a fetal position. Infants at earlier gestational ages have less muscle tone, and their extremities are less flexed at rest.

The examiner should look at the infant's skin to see whether the infant is cyanotic. Some caution must be used in interpreting these findings. Infants with hypothermia or infants with polycythemia (hematocrit levels greater than 65%) may have bluish extremities (acrocyanosis), yet they are not really hypoxemic. Infants who are preterm and immature with thin skin can look quite pink when they are really hypoxemic. The careful examiner looks at the color of the mucous membranes in the mouth and tongue and of the nail beds in the extremities. These locations give a more reliable indication of the infant's true level of oxygenation.

The effort involved in breathing and the breathing pattern should be noted, especially the regularity of respirations. An infant with respiratory distress characteristically exhibits tachypnea (discussed earlier), retractions, nasal flaring, and sometimes, grunting.

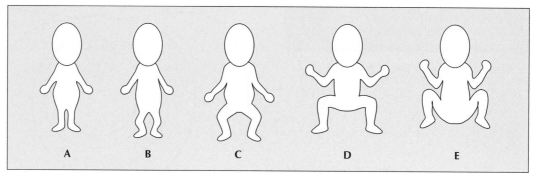

Figure 11-6 Progression in body position with gestational age. **A**, 26-week infant. **B**, 28-week infant. **C**, 32-week infant. **D**, 36-week infant. **E**, 40-week term infant.

Retractions

Retractions (sinking inward of the skin around the chest wall during inspiration) occur when the lung's compliance is less than the compliance of the chest wall or when there is a significant airway obstruction. Thus retractions are a sign of an increase in the work of breathing. The diaphragm contracts during inspiration, increasing the negative pressure in the intrapleural space. In the normal respiratory system, the lung is the most compliant structure and will inflate to relieve this negative pressure. However, in a healthy infant, the chest wall is only slightly less compliant than the lung. Any lung disease that causes a decrease in compliance can cause the lung to become less compliant than the chest wall. The chest wall then represents the most compliant structure in the respiratory system and collapses inward in response to the increasing negative intrathoracic pressure generated by diaphragmatic contraction.

Three common points of collapse are the *intercostal* area (between the ribs), the *subcostal* area (below the lower rib margin), and the *substernal* area (below the bottom of the sternum) (Figure 11-7). A fourth point of collapse is the *supraclavicular* area (above the clavicles).

Retractions tend to be in different locations depending on the cause of the respiratory distress. Infants with lung disease tend to have retractions toward the center of the body (substernal and subcostal). Infants with heart disease tend to have intercostal retractions on the sides of their bodies, because their large hearts prevent backward motion of the sternum. Finally, infants with obstructed airways tend to have large suprasternal retractions with accessory respiratory muscle contractions. Although scoring systems have historically been used to evaluate the severity of retractions, they are not in widespread use currently.

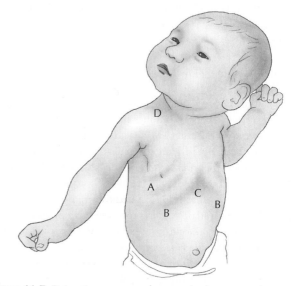

Figure 11-7 Retractions commonly occur in these areas: intercostal *(A)*, subcostal *(B)*, substernal *(C)*, and supraclavicular *(D)*.

Nasal flaring

Nasal flaring is the dilation of the alae nasi during inspiration. Nasal flaring is an attempt by the infant to achieve airway dilation to decrease airway resistance, increase gas flow, and achieve a larger tidal volume. Infants are obligate nose breathers, and the minute ventilation they require must be achieved through their noses.

Grunting

Grunting is a sound heard at the end of expiration just before rapid inspiration. Grunting is the infant's attempt to increase the gas volume in the lung. It is typically heard in infants with diseases that decrease lung volume (e.g., RDS). Adults and older children with normal FRC typically increase their lung volume from their resting FRC with inspiration. However, infants who have a disease that decreases FRC attempt to increase their lung volume by holding their tidal volume at end-inspiration. The infant accomplishes this by

---

SIMPLY STATED

Retractions in the infant indicate a serious increase in the work of breathing, and further assessment and monitoring are mandatory.

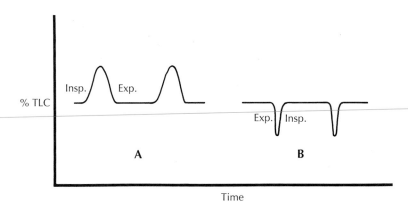

Figure 11-8 Comparison of lung volumes during tidal breathing: **A**, Adult. **B**, Grunting infant. *exp.*, Expiratory; *insp.*, inspiratory; *TLC*, total lung capacity.

occluding the airway with glottic closure and actively exhaling against the closed glottis after the end of inspiration. The grunting sound is produced when the infant suddenly opens the glottis and quickly exhales, inhales, and again closes the glottis (Figure 11-8).

Precordium

While observing the respiratory pattern and effort, the examiner should look at the precordium (area over the heart) for any increase in motion. Increased motion is present if the examiner can see the chest wall lifting or moving as the heart contracts. This increase in motion, or hyperdynamic precordium, is an indication of increased volume load on the heart, usually secondary to a left-to-right shunt of blood through the ductus arteriosus. When an infant has a patent ductus arteriosus (PDA), the anatomic connection between the aorta and pulmonary artery remains open and blood from the aorta flows into the pulmonary artery, which can cause congestive heart failure and pulmonary edema. The presence of a hyperdynamic precordium is a clue that the infant's respiratory distress may not be completely of pulmonary origin and requires further evaluation.

Palpation

In infants, palpation is an important tool for physical assessment. However, the use of palpation in the physical examination of infants is directed less at the lungs than at other organ systems that may influence pulmonary function.

The easiest organ to palpate is the skin. Palpation of the skin can give the examiner valuable information about the infant's cardiac output and fluid volume status, both of which are clinically important in the evaluation of the infant's pulmonary status.

The three aspects of the skin that are useful in evaluating cardiac output are the skin perfusion, skin temperature, and peripheral pulses. To check the skin perfusion, or capillary refill, the examiner should blanch the infant's skin with a finger and note how long it takes for the blanched skin to recover its color. Capillary refill is checked on the trunk and extremities. Capillary refill will be longer than 3 seconds if the infant has a low cardiac output. The examiner should keep in mind that other pathologic states, such as acidosis, hypoxemia, hypo-

glycemia, and hypothermia, can decrease blood flow to the skin and prolong capillary refill.

An approximation of the infant's skin temperature can be determined by feeling the skin. The dorsum, or back side, of the hand and fingers is more sensitive to temperature than the front side or palmar surface. Infants with low cardiac output or any abnormality that decreases skin blood flow have skin that feels cool.

Comparing the central and peripheral arterial pulses gives the examiner valuable clues about the infant's cardiac output. A careful examiner should be able to palpate the pulses of the radial, brachial, posterior tibial, and dorsalis pedis arteries. The infant should be examined closely for a decrease in cardiac output if these pulses are not easily palpable or if there is a big discrepancy between them and the central arterial pulses of the femoral or axillary arteries. The examiner should also look for any discrepancies between the pulses in the upper and lower extremities. If pulses in the lower extremity are weaker than those in the upper, the infant may have an aortic obstruction such as coarctation of the aorta or interrupted aortic arch syndrome.

> ### SIMPLY STATED
> Palpation of the infant for skin temperature, capillary refill, and quality of peripheral pulses is helpful in determining the general quality of cardiac output.

Finally, the examiner can achieve a rough idea about the fluid volume of the infant by feeling the turgor or fullness of the infant's skin. Infants with low fluid volumes have a loss of skin turgor. This is manifest by "tenting" or gathering of the skin when it is lightly pinched together.

Palpation of the abdomen may be of help in assessing an infant's pulmonary status. An infant's abdomen and abdominal organs move significantly with respiration because the diaphragm is the major source of power for respiration and the abdominal wall musculature is relatively weak. Anything that impedes the motion of the abdomen or its organs hinders the infant's respiration. Liver or spleen enlargement (hepatomegaly or splenomegaly, respectively); enlargement of other organs such as kidneys, bladder, or bowel; or intraabdominal tumors can impede abdominal motion. Distention of the abdomen by fluid (ascites) or air *(gaseous bowel distention)* or pneumoperitoneum (free air in the abdomen) also impedes abdominal motion.

Gentleness is important when palpating an infant's abdomen. Many examiners fail to feel enlarged organs or masses because their vigor pushes the organ or mass away from their fingers. Examiners should gently place their second and third fingers on the skin of the lower abdomen perpendicular to the spine and then slowly slide their fingers up toward the costal margin. The liver should be soft and mobile, palpable on the right side of the abdomen parallel to and 1 to 2 cm below the costal margin. The spleen may be palpable as a soft tip below the left costal margin at the anterior axillary line. The kidney may be palpated in the immediate newborn period by compressing it between one hand placed under the posterior flank and the other hand firmly pressing in from the anterior abdominal wall.

Major central nervous system diseases, such as intraventricular hemorrhage (IVH) and *hydrocephalus,* are causes of respiratory problems in preterm infants. The examiner should evaluate the tautness of the **anterior fontanel** (the soft spot on top of the infant's head). Infants who have had a major IVH or hydrocephalus may have a full, tense fontanel. In addition, the cranial sutures (junctions between two skull bones) may be widely separated in these conditions.

Auscultation

The last of the classic techniques routinely used in infant examination is auscultation. Auscultation is the least definitive of the three examination techniques discussed, but this does not mean it is unimportant. Auscultation yields the best information if the infant is quiet. Because of this, auscultation is the first thing done after inspection. Auscultation should be performed with a warm chest piece that has a small (1.0- to 1.5-cm diameter) diaphragm and bell. This allows for maximal localization of the findings. For auscultatory examination of the lungs, the infant is ideally in the prone position. However, because most infants are in a supine position or on their side, the examiner should try to complete most of the examination before moving the infant. If the infant's position does not allow an adequate examination, the examiner should gently move the infant to a more desirable position. Normal infant breath sounds are bronchovesicular in character and harsher than in the adult. The techniques for use of the stethoscope and the types of adventitious lung sounds heard are the same as in the adult (see Chapter 5).

The clinical significance of breath sounds in the infant is similar to that in the adult. Because the infant's thoracic cage is small and sound is transmitted easily, breath sounds usually are not entirely absent. A decrease in breath sounds implies a decrease in gas flow through the airways, as in RDS, atelectasis, pneumothorax, or pleural effusion. Wheezing implies gas flow through constricted airways; infants with bronchopulmonary dysplasia (BPD) may have wheezing. Crackles usually imply excess fluid or secretions in the lung (pulmonary edema) or the presence of pneumonia. A loud ripping sound like the separa-

tion of Velcro often is associated with the presence of pulmonary interstitial emphysema.

In addition to listening for the breath sounds, the examiner should also listen for the presence of cardiac murmurs. The presence of a murmur does not mean that the infant has heart disease, but it may mean that the infant requires further diagnostic evaluation. Almost all infants have physiologic murmurs such as physiologic pulmonary stenosis or venous hum. The pathologic murmurs that are characteristic of the newborn period are caused by PDA, ventricular septal defect, tricuspid insufficiency, and major congenital heart disease.

The abdomen is another area of the body where auscultation may help in pulmonary assessment. The abdomen should be auscultated when there is a question about whether an infant is properly intubated. Loud sounds of air movement are heard over the stomach during inspiration if the endotracheal tube is in the esophagus. The presence of a bruit (a murmur-like sound) in the liver or neck should raise the question of whether the infant has an arteriovenous malformation in the liver or head. This type of malformation can cause respiratory distress because of high-output heart failure.

Transillumination

Transillumination is a technique often used in examining infants but not older patients. It can be used in infants because their chest wall is thin enough to shine a light through. The source is usually a bright fiberoptic light, which is placed against the chest wall in a dark room. Normally, this produces a lighted halo around the point of contact with the skin. In the presence of a pneumothorax or pneumomediastinum, the entire hemithorax lights up. This technique is rapid and allows quick treatment of a serious condition. The procedure should be performed by an examiner who is familiar with the technique, because some fiberoptic lights can cause cutaneous burns and it is possible to be misled by the area of transilluminance.

Clinical Laboratory Data

Two crucial issues face anyone who wants to use the clinical laboratory in pulmonary assessment of newborns. The first and most obvious issue is that the normal values for clinical laboratory tests may be different between newborns and adults. The magnitude of these differences depends on the laboratory test in question. However, to complicate this issue further, the normal values may depend on the gestational or chronologic age of the newborn. The second, less obvious issue is the relationship between the test sample volume and the infant's blood volume.

An infant's blood volume is approximately 80 to 110 mL/kg of body weight, with young-gestational-age infants tending to have higher volume per weight. Depending on the severity of the illness, most infants can tolerate an acute blood loss of no more than 10% of their blood volume. This means that for a 0.5-kg infant, all of the laboratory tests should require no more than 5.5 mL of blood. The infant will need replacement volume if the laboratory tests require more than this amount.

A corollary of this issue is that even if the infant can tolerate the volume loss, it may not be practical or technically feasible to withdraw the sample volume. Infants have small vessels that tend to be fragile, and it often is not possible to draw large volumes by venipuncture or arterial puncture.

Hematology

The WBC count in infants tends to be higher than in older patients. Normal values vary with the chronologic age of the infant (Table 11-5). In general, infants closer to delivery have higher WBC counts. Over the first week of life, total WBCs tend to fall to a plateau that is just slightly higher than the normal values for adults.

Leukocytosis, or a WBC count greater than 15,000/mm³, usually is a reflection of the infant's environment rather than of infection, as in the older patient. When evaluating an infant with a high WBC count, the examiner should consider infection, as well as crying, hyperthermia from excess wrapping or high environmental temperature, and other environmental stresses. Leukopenia, particularly neutropenia (an absolute neutrophil count of less than 2000 neutrophils/mm³), is a more ominous sign. Usually, neutropenia indicates an infection and implies that the infant is being overwhelmed. The neutropenia from infection can be caused by one of two mechanisms: peripheral consumption of neutrophils or failure to produce and release neutrophils from the bone marrow.

There is still a great deal of debate about whether the newborn's leukocytes function as well as those of an older person. It is fair to say that even a term newborn's response to infection is not optimal, but why this is and what cellular or immunologic functions are involved are still being investigated.

> ### SIMPLY STATED
> In the infant, significant leukocytosis (WBC >15,000/mm³) is more often the result of environmental stress (e.g., hyperthermia) rather than infection, as it is in the older child or adult. Neutropenia (absolute neutrophil count <2000 neutrophils/mm³) is a serious condition and needs to be evaluated immediately.

The normal values for the red blood cell (RBC) count, hematocrit, and hemoglobin depend on chronologic age. In utero, the fetus is stimulated to produce a large number of RBCs by the low partial pressure of arterial oxygen (Pao_2). This stimulus is withdrawn at the time of birth. The normal newborn severely limits or ceases the production of RBCs until a new stimulus is received. Anemia is the normal physiologic stimulus for this. In healthy term infants, this "physiologic anemia" occurs at approximately 6 weeks of age. In preterm infants, it usually occurs between 8 and 12 weeks of age. Infants who have received transfusions have a 4- to 6-week delay in the onset of RBC production. After an infant begins RBC production, hematocrit and hemoglobin levels rise to slightly above the level of an adult and remain there throughout childhood (Table 11-6).

Platelet counts often are obtained in newborns and infants when they are being evaluated for thrombocytopenia, disseminated intravascular coagulation, or other bleeding disorders (see Table 11-6). Normal values are between 100,000 and 350,000/mm³; however, most clinicians will not transfuse infants with platelets unless the count is less than 25,000/mm³ and the infant is bleeding. Thrombocytopenia (platelet count

Table 11-5 White Blood Cell, Neutrophil, and Platelet Counts of Very-Low-Birthweight Infants During the First 6 Weeks of Life

| Day of Life | n | Percentiles | | | | |
		10	25	50	75	90
WBCs (10⁹/L)						
3	376	4.8	7.1	9.5	14.4	24.5
12-14	180	8.1	9.7	12.3	15.2	19.8
24-26	233	7.2	8.5	10.4	12.4	14.6
40-42	212	6.8	7.7	9.1	11.0	13.0
Neutrophils (10⁹/L)						
3	334	1.5	2.7	4.7	8.2	14.8
12-14	161	2.2	3.1	4.6	6.8	10.6
24-26	205	1.3	1.9	2.9	4.0	5.3
40-42	175	1.0	1.4	2.2	3.1	4.6
Platelets (10⁹/L)						
3	558	95	140	204	285	355
12-14	372	142	216	318	414	499
24-26	394	171	242	338	443	555
40-42	370	189	275	357	456	550

Modified from Fanaroff AA, Martin RJ, editors: *Behrman's neonatal-perinatal medicine: Diseases of the fetus and infant,* ed 7, St Louis, 2002, Mosby.

| Table 11-6 | Red Blood Cell Parameters of Very-Low-Birthweight Infants During the First 6 Weeks of Life |

Day of Life		Percentiles				
	n	10	25	50	75	90
Hemoglobin (g/dL)						
3	559	12.5	14.0	15.6	17.1	18.5
12-14	203	11.1	12.5	14.4	15.7	17.4
24-26	192	9.7	10.9	12.4	14.2	15.6
40-42	150	8.4	9.3	10.6	12.4	13.8
Hematocrit (%)						
3	561	39	43	47	52	56
12-14	205	34	39	44	48	53
24-26	196	29	32	39	44	48
40-42	152	26	28	33	38	44
Corrected reticulocytes (%)						
3	283	1.9	4.2	7.1	12.0	20
12-14	139	0.5	0.8	1.7	2.7	5.7
24-26	140	0.5	0.8	1.5	2.6	4.7
40-42	114	0.6	1.0	1.8	3.4	5.6

Modified from Fanaroff AA, Martin RJ, editors: *Behrman's neonatal-perinatal medicine: Diseases of the fetus and infant*, ed 7, St Louis, 2002, Mosby.

less than 100,000/mm^3) may be a sign of disseminated intravascular coagulation from severe infection or one of many other causes. Thrombocytosis (platelet count greater than 350,000/mm^3) usually is not a clinical problem in the newborn. Thrombocytosis can be seen in infants with iron-deficiency anemia or hemolytic anemia, during recovery from thrombocytopenia, and in infants whose mothers have inflammatory collagen-vascular disease. A high normal value in infants is not well established, but clinical symptoms are not seen until the platelet count exceeds 1 million.

The values for partial thromboplastin time, prothrombin time, fibrinogen, mean corpuscular volume, mean corpuscular hemoglobin, mean corpuscular hemoglobin concentration, and reticulocyte count are close to the normal values for adults (see Tables 11-6 and 11-7). Mean corpuscular volume and reticulocyte counts are higher in the immediate newborn period but decrease over the first few months of life to normal adult levels.

Blood Chemistry

Blood glucose probably is the most frequent blood chemistry determination made in newborns. This simple test is of tremendous importance because hypoglycemia, or low serum glucose, is as detrimental to the developing newborn's brain as hypoxia is. Because the exact levels and length of time necessary to cause damage to the central nervous system have not been determined, most physicians treat an infant with a glucose level of less than 40 mg/dL. There are easy methods for approximating serum glucose at the bedside. These methods are used as screening tests, and any abnormalities found are confirmed with serum glucose levels obtained in the clinical laboratory.

Hypoglycemia can be caused by a variety of metabolic disturbances including infection, hyperinsulinism secondary to maternal diabetes mellitus, and inadequate glycogen stores secondary to being small for gestational age. Although only symptomatic treatment is usually needed, an extensive evaluation of the infant's glucose control mechanisms is often necessary. Hyperglycemia, or blood glucose greater than 160 mg/dL, is most often iatrogenic. However, hyperglycemia is also one of the early signs of septicemia in infants. The problems with hyperglycemia from diabetes mellitus are rare in this age group.

Total protein and albumin are useful tools in evaluating the nutritional status of the ill newborn. They may also give helpful clues for evaluating the cause of pulmonary edema (Table 11-8). Colloid osmotic pressure usually is not measured in infants, because the sample volume required is large.

The serum enzymes that are so useful in adults are much less useful in newborns and the pediatric age group. For many of the enzymes, normal values have not yet been established, and the clinical significance of abnormal values often is unknown. *Lactate dehydrogenase (LDH), aspartate transaminase (AST),* and *alanine transaminase (ALT)* are used when evaluating liver function. *Creatinine phosphokinase (CPK)* and its isoenzymes are useful in determining myocardial injury. *Alkaline phosphatase* is useful in evaluating bone growth and the adequacy of an infant's nutrition.

Serum drug level determinations are becoming increasingly useful during the newborn period. Because infants are small, there is a narrow difference between therapeutic and toxic doses of most medications. The need to obtain drug levels has always been present, but it has been practical only as improving technology has permitted smaller sample volumes. Drug levels for

Table 11-7	Normal Coagulation Test Values		
Category	Fibrinogen (mg/dL)	Partial Thromboplastin Time (sec)	Prothrombin Time (sec)
Preterm infant (1500-2500 g)	233	90	17 (12-21)
Term infant, cord blood	216	71	16 (13-20)
Term infant, 48 hours	210	65	17.5 (12-21)
Normal child	190-420	37-50	12-14

Modified from Fanaroff AA, Martin RJ, editors: *Behrman's neonatal-perinatal medicine: diseases of the fetus and infant,* ed 3, St Louis, 1982, Mosby.

Table 11-8	Normal Values for Blood Chemistries
Determination	Value
Sodium (mEq/L)	133-149
Potassium (mEq/L)	5.3-6.4
Chloride (mEq/L)	87-114
Total carbon dioxide (mEq/L)	19-22
Total protein (g/dL)	4.8-8.5
Albumin (g/dL)	2.9-5.5
Bilirubin (mg/dL)	
24 hours	1.0-6.0
48 hours	6.0-8.0
3-5 days	4.0-15.0

Modified from Fanaroff AA, Martin RJ, editors: *Behrman's neonatal-perinatal medicine: Diseases of the fetus and infant,* ed 5, St Louis, 1992, Mosby; and Meites S, editor: *Pediatric clinical chemistry: A survey of normals and instrumentation, with commentary,* Washington, DC, 1992, American Association for Clinical Chemistry.

antibiotics (vancomycin, gentamicin, and other aminoglycosides), anticonvulsants (phenobarbital, phenytoin), antiarrhythmics, caffeine, and theophylline are often used. Digitalis and cyclosporine levels are used less often.

Serum bilirubin determination is often used in evaluating newborns. Probably more than 70% of infants have a bilirubin determination during the first week of life. There are many causes for **hyperbilirubinemia** during the newborn period. Some abnormalities in bilirubin metabolism are likely to affect pulmonary function. First is hyperbilirubinemia from any cause that requires treatment by phototherapy. Phototherapy is associated with tachypnea in the newborn, although the exact mechanism of the tachypnea is not known. Second is hyperbilirubinemia treated with an exchange transfusion. An exchange transfusion is a procedure in which the infant's blood is replaced with donor blood by cyclically withdrawing the infant's blood and transfusing aliquots of donor blood. Usually, exchange transfusions are used to treat hyperbilirubinemia caused by hemolytic diseases. Finally, the most severe and rarest is hyperbilirubinemia associated with severe hemolytic disease and hydrops fetalis. In this disorder, the hyperbilirubinemia is not the fundamental problem. The infant has *anasarca* (massive total body edema) with pleural effusions and abdominal ascites that cause profound respiratory failure.

Electrolytes, blood urea nitrogen (BUN), and serum creatinine determinations are all useful laboratory tests for newborns. The normal values (see Table 11-8) depend on the infant's chronologic age, nutritional status, and fluid status. They are generally similar to adult values, with serum potassium being slightly higher and BUN and creatinine levels lower. These values are useful in a variety of clinical situations, from assessing the infant's fluid status to evaluating renal function.

Calcium and *phosphorus* levels are of indirect importance in the evaluation of a newborn with chronic lung disease. Infants with BPD or other chronic lung diseases have increased work of breathing and increased metabolic and nutritional needs. The metabolism of calcium and phosphorus is a valuable clue to the nutritional status of the chronically ill infant. A chronically ill infant with poor nutrition has low levels of calcium and phosphorus and an increased risk of developing rickets. Osteopenia of the premature (a rickets-like disease caused by chronically low phosphorous intake) may worsen the infant's pulmonary status by increasing the chest wall compliance secondary to a decrease in the mineralization of the ribs and decreasing the infant's depth of respiration secondary to pain from rib fractures.

Microbiology

The sputum analysis that is useful in adults is not possible in newborns. Until a child is approximately 6 years old, sputum is swallowed and not expectorated. However, if the infant is intubated, samples can be obtained with sterile suction catheters through the endotracheal tube. In an older infant or young child, samples may be obtained from the stomach through nasogastric tubes. Samples obtained from the stomach should be interpreted with caution. Even samples obtained through the endotracheal tube may reflect bacterial colonization rather than infection. In addition to the Gram stain, culture, and sensitivity, a polymorphonuclear neutrophil (PMN) count is useful. High PMN counts in the tracheal or stomach samples are strongly suggestive of infection rather than colonization.

Newborn Blood Gases

Monitoring the blood gas status of newborns is done either by analysis of the gas in a blood sample or by transcutaneous monitoring. Analysis of blood samples is performed on blood obtained from arterial, capillary, or venous sources. Transcutaneous measurements of oxygen (PO_2) and carbon dioxide (PCO_2) tension, oxygen saturation (SaO_2), or near-infrared niroscopy can be made.

Fetal Hemoglobin

The newborn's oxygen-carrying mechanism is significantly different from that of the older infant, child, or adult. The presence of fetal hemoglobin (Hb F) has significant effects on the transport of oxygen. Fetal hemoglobin meets the needs of the fetus in the oxygen-poor environment of intrauterine life. The fetal hemoglobin curve is shifted to the left of the adult hemoglobin (Hb A) curve (Figure 11-9). Thus fetal hemoglobin has a higher affinity for oxygen than adult hemoglobin. This means that fetal hemoglobin absorbs oxygen more readily but also releases it more slowly. The half-life for RBCs with fetal hemoglobin is approximately 45 days. Thus a newborn infant who is not transfused will have a significant portion of the RBC population with fetal hemoglobin until approximately 60 to 90 days of life.

Arterial Blood Gases

Arterial blood samples are the most reliable source for blood gas analysis in newborns. Normal values in newborns depend on the age of the infant when the blood is drawn (Table 11-9). Once infants are beyond the transitional period after delivery (usually 4 to 12 hours), their arterial oxygen (PaO_2), carbon dioxide ($PaCO_2$), and pH values should be similar to those of the older child or adult. During the transitional period, PaO_2 is lower, $PaCO_2$ is higher, and pH is lower as compared with later. Sick infants who require supplemental oxygenation or mechanical ventilation often have values for PaO_2, $PaCO_2$, and pH that are not quite normal for this age but are accepted because of the complications that result from such treatment.

The fact that an arterial blood sample provides the most reliable source for blood gas analysis in newborns must be weighed

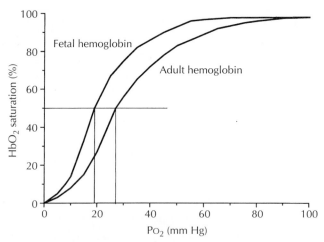

Figure 11-9 Oxygen hemoglobin dissociation curves for fetal and adult hemoglobins. Fetal hemoglobin P_{50} is approximately 18.6. Adult hemoglobin P_{50} is approximately 27.

against the problems associated with arterial puncture in newborns and young infants. Arterial puncture is technically possible, but it requires good technique and, often, extra assistance. Newborns and young infants have small arteries and are notoriously uncooperative, moving their extremities and making the arterial puncture difficult. This also increases the risk of arterial damage. In addition, arterial blood does not always reflect the resting state for the newborn or young infant, because the discomfort associated with the puncture usually causes the baby to cry. Infants who are crying change their ventilation in one of two patterns: They either hyperventilate or hold their breath and stop ventilating. Either of these changes in ventilation rapidly alters the values for oxygen, carbon dioxide, and pH in the blood.

The placement of an umbilical arterial catheter allows the clinician to obtain arterial blood samples without altering the infant's physiology in the immediate newborn period. This is useful in evaluating sick infants without causing them the pain and discomfort of percutaneous arterial puncture. Umbilical arterial catheters are widely used in neonatal intensive care units. The use of these catheters presents some significant risks such as embolization, thrombosis, vasospasm, and infection. Their use by experienced personnel minimizes these risks.

Table 11-9	Normal Values for Arterial Blood Gases in Infants				
Age	pH	Pao$_2$	Paco$_2$	HCO$_3^-$	Base Excess
Newborn	7.25-7.35	50-70	26-40	17-23	(−10 – −2)
24 hours	7.30-7.40	60-80	26-40	18-25	(−4 – +2)
2 days to 1 month	7.32-7.43	85-95	30-40	16-25	(−6 – +1)
1 month to 2 years	7.34-7.46	85-105	30-45	20-28	(−4 – +2)

Unpublished data from author's laboratory; and data from Meites S, editor: *Pediatric clinical chemistry: A survey of normals, methods and instrumentation, with commentary,* Washington, DC, 1982, American Association for Clinical Chemistry.

Capillary Blood Gases

Because of the risk and the technical expertise involved in obtaining arterial blood gas samples, many nurseries and pediatric wards obtain blood gas samples by capillary puncture. Although the results require special consideration, less technical expertise and fewer people are required to do a capillary puncture than an arterial puncture. In general, capillary samples are obtained by puncturing the skin of the infant's warmed heel. Fingers and earlobes are less commonly used sites for obtaining capillary samples.

When the values of capillary carbon dioxide tension (P_cCO_2) and pH are compared with those obtained by arterial sample, carbon dioxide is 2 to 5 mm Hg higher, and pH is 0.01 to 0.03 units lower. These small differences are inconsequential in most clinical situations. However, when the values of the capillary oxygen tension (P_cO_2) are compared with those obtained by arterial samples, the difference is not so slight. Unfortunately, there is not a fixed ratio for P_aO_2/P_cO_2. An infant with a P_cO_2 of 50 mm Hg may have a PaO_2 of 50 to 90 mm Hg or higher. The only statement that can be made about PaO_2 by knowing only P_cO_2 is that PaO_2 is no lower than P_cO_2.

When capillary blood gas sampling is appropriate, the person drawing the sample and the person evaluating the results need to remember the underlying problems that must be overcome in obtaining the sample. A capillary sample that closely reflects arterial blood must be obtained from a warmed extremity (skin temperature should be approximately 103° F). Caution must be used in warming the extremity so that the infant is not burned and the warming device does not cool and secondarily cool the extremity. All of the values will be unreliable if the extremity is edematous, acrocyanotic, or not warmed or if the infant has poor peripheral circulation. In addition, because this procedure is painful, like arterial puncture, it reflects the infant's condition during crying, which may be vastly different from rest. Finally, if there is difficulty obtaining the sample, the results may reflect air or tissue contamination rather than the infant's true status.

> **SIMPLY STATED**
> Capillary blood samples from the infant usually reflect P_{CO_2} and pH values reasonably close to those of arterial blood; however, the P_{O_2} of capillary blood is often significantly below that of arterial blood.

Venous Blood Gases

Venous blood samples can also be obtained for gas analysis. These are useful in computing the oxygen extraction or carbon dioxide production of tissues (see Chapter 13).

Noninvasive Monitors

One of the most significant recent advances in monitoring sick patients has been the development of transcutaneous oxygen and carbon dioxide monitors. These monitors give staff members up-to-date information that they otherwise would not have. In newborn intensive care units, these devices are being used around the clock to monitor sick infants.

Transcutaneous oxygen monitors

Transcutaneous oxygen pressure ($tcPO_2$) monitors measure electrical current that is directly proportional to the number of oxygen molecules present in the electrode. The $tcPO_2$ electrode measures oxygen present in the capillaries and tissue of the skin and not PaO_2, but $tcPO_2$ usually approximates PaO_2, with $tcPO_2$ slightly lower than PaO_2. Any condition that decreases blood flow under the electrode, such as acidosis, shock, hypovolemia, or hypoglycemia, can cause a $tcPO_2$ that is falsely lower than PaO_2.

The $tcPO_2$ monitor is a good method of evaluating the physiologic changes that occur with blood gas sampling. The pain of blood gas sampling can cause changes in the infant's resting condition. The infant can produce an increase in $PaCO_2$ and a decrease in PaO_2 by becoming apneic. If the infant cries and hyperventilates, the $PaCO_2$ might decrease and the PaO_2 might increase. The person obtaining the sample should note the $tcPO_2$ value three times: before disturbing the infant, at the beginning of blood flow, and 40 to 60 seconds after completion of sampling. These three values can then be used to assess the infant's resting condition, the physiologic changes the procedure caused, and the correlation between PaO_2 and $tcPO_2$.

Transcutaneous carbon dioxide monitors

Transcutaneous carbon dioxide pressure ($tcPCO_2$) electrodes are sometimes used clinically. Similar to the $tcPO_2$ electrodes, they measure the gas present in the skin and not that in the blood. The $tcPCO_2$ electrode has merit as a trend monitor for carbon dioxide.

There are still problems with both $tcPO_2$ and $tcPCO_2$. Both techniques use heated electrodes, which must be repositioned every 2 to 4 hours. The heater in the electrode can cause burns. The tape used to secure the electrode may tear the fragile skin of a preterm infant during repositioning. The monitors have slow response times and are subject to multiple skin perfusion artifacts.

Pulse oximeters

Pulse oximetry has become a useful monitoring tool in the past few years. Pulse oximeters measure the changing transmission of red and infrared light through a pulsating capillary bed to identify the saturation of hemoglobin with oxygen. They overcome many of the problems of the transcutaneous monitors. The oximeter is not heated; therefore it does not require repositioning and does not cause burns. It has a much faster response time, and it does not require tight taping to the skin. (See Chapter 13 for a further discussion of pulse oximeters.)

Niroscopy

Near-infrared **niroscopy** is a monitoring technique that is being evaluated for assessing tissue oxygenation. This technique measures the oxidation reduction state of cytochrome aa_3, which is thought to be a marker of tissue oxygenation status. Although niroscopy is beginning to be used clinically, it is still mainly a research tool.

Pulmonary Function Testing

Volumes

Pulmonary function can be tested in newborns. In the past few years, standard computerized equipment for neonatal and young infant pulmonary function testing has become available. This has taken pulmonary function testing in this age group out of the realm of the research laboratory and made it available to the clinician. Although nurseries that measure pulmonary function usually are still found in major teaching and research institutions, now small institutions without major research support can be involved in pulmonary function testing. A variety of technologies that compute pulmonary functions exist. These devices are capable of traditional lung mechanics, active and passive exhalation mechanics, and FRC measurements using either helium dilution or nitrogen washout techniques.

The fundamental difference between newborn and adult pulmonary function testing is the patient's ability to cooperate. The pulmonary function tests for adults and older children depend on the patient's ability to follow simple commands. The tests performed on infants must be reproducible without patient cooperation.

Three volumes can be measured easily in newborns independent of their cooperation: FRC, thoracic gas volume (TGV), and crying vital capacity (CVC). A certain degree of caution must be exercised when interpreting the results of these tests, however. The range of normal values is great, and all three tests are subject to error. To compare the results of these tests for two babies or even for the same baby at different times, the results must be described against a standard unit. Usually, this is done with the body weight in kilograms (e.g., milliliters of gas per kilogram) or body length in centimeters (e.g., milliliters of gas per centimeter).

FRC is measured by two methods: closed-system helium dilution and open-system nitrogen washout. Both methods are becoming available with the computerized pulmonary function machines. TGV (method of DuBois[4,5]) requires the use of a plethysmograph and measures all of the gas in the thoracic cavity whether or not it is communicating with the airway. By comparing the TGV with the FRC, the clinician can determine the presence of trapped gas in the thorax.

CVC is the measurement of tidal volume while the infant is crying. It is useful in following infants who have lung diseases that cause changes in FRC (e.g., RDS), in whom it is difficult to measure FRC. CVC does require that the infant be able to cry vigorously, which may be difficult for sick infants.

A method of measuring distribution of ventilation is available using a nitrogen washout curve. The pulmonary clearance delay (PCD)[6,7] divides the lung into fast, intermediate, and slow ventilating areas based on calculations from expired nitrogen concentrations obtained during a nitrogen washout. The PCD can be used to evaluate what percentage of the lung is ventilating effectively.

The most important clinical lung volume measurement is the FRC. Because the lung mechanics are affected if the FRC is either too high or too low, it is imperative that clinicians be able to regulate FRC. When the FRC is high, the compliance is lower, resistance is higher, and $PaCO_2$ is significantly elevated. When the FRC is low, compliance is very low, resistance is very high, PaO_2 is decreased, and $PaCO_2$ is increased.

RDS causes the FRC to be decreased. Meconium aspiration syndrome (MAS) is a disease in which FRC is increased. Diseases such as pneumonia and BPD may have either decreased or increased FRCs depending on the current stage of the disease and the respiratory support that is being used.

Mechanics

Compliance

Compliance is a measure of the distensibility of the lung. It is calculated by dividing change in volume by change in pressure and requires measurement of tidal volume and transpulmonary pressure. Tidal volume can be measured in newborns by either pneumotachography or plethysmography. Plethysmographs are tricky to use with infants, because making an airtight seal around the face is difficult. In addition, plethysmographs for infants are all custom-made. Therefore most nurseries measure tidal volume by pneumotachography.

Transpulmonary pressure is the difference between airway pressure and pleural pressure. It is approximated by measuring airway and esophageal pressure in intubated infants and esophageal pressure in nonintubated infants. Either an air-filled balloon or saline-filled catheter in midesophagus can be used. Tidal volume is integrated from the pneumotachometer signal, a pressure-volume loop is constructed, and the compliance of the lung is calculated. The compliance of the chest wall can also be measured by changing the two pressure sources from airway minus esophageal to esophageal minus atmospheric pressure.

Compliance is significantly lower in infants with RDS. This begins to improve dramatically with the return of surfactant function in the lung. Compliance is also lower in infants with BPD and pneumonia.

Resistance

Resistance is a measure of the inhibition of gas flow through airways. It is calculated by dividing change in transpulmonary pressure by change in flow. These measurements are obtained with the same equipment used for compliance.

Resistance is elevated in infants with MAS and BPD. The airway resistance in infants with MAS remains elevated for several weeks until the chemical phase of the disease is resolved.

Infants with BPD will probably have increased airway resistance for all of their lives.

Work of breathing

The work of breathing is the cumulative product of the pressure generated and the volume at each instant of the respiratory cycle. It is usually calculated by planimetry of the pressure-volume curve or by electrically integrating the pressure and volume signals.

Because airway resistance is the major contributor to the planimetric area of a pressure-volume loop, work of breathing is increased in the diseases that have major resistive components: MAS and BPD.

Lung mechanics with mechanical ventilators

Recently, more sophisticated infant ventilators have been developed that can measure the mechanical properties of the respiratory system in the newborn during mechanical ventilation. These machines allow the clinician to match the settings of the ventilator with the individual needs of the infant. It is possible to diagnose overdistention (Figure 11-10), air leak (Figure 11-11), short inspiratory time (Figure 11-12), and other dysfunctional ventilator–patient interactions. These machines are capable of synchronizing the mechanical cycle with the infant's spontaneous breaths.

Chemoreceptor Response

Sudden infant death syndrome has stimulated a tremendous amount of research into the way infants control respiration. Some

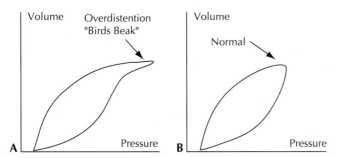

Figure 11-10 Pressure-volume loops of a mechanically ventilated infant showing overdistention **(A)** and normal inflation pressures **(B)**.

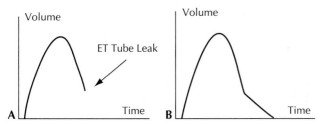

Figure 11-11 Volume-time curves of a mechanically ventilated infant show air leak around the endotracheal (ET) tube **(A)** and no air leak **(B)**.

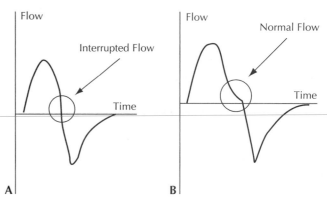

Figure 11-12 Flow-time curves of a mechanically ventilated infant show interrupted inspiratory flow secondary to inadequate inspiratory time **(A)** and normal inspiratory flow with adequate inspiratory time **(B)**.

investigators have shown that newborns have a blunted response to hypercapnia and a severely diminished or paradoxical response to hypoxia. Many nurseries have the ability to look at carbon dioxide and oxygen responses. These studies are usually performed by measuring tidal volume, minute ventilation, end-tidal oxygen and carbon dioxide, and transcutaneous oxygen. The infant's minute ventilation is then plotted against $PaCO_2$ or FIO_2.

Radiographs

Radiographic views and the methods for obtaining radiographs are significantly different between infants and older patients. In the older patient, the x-ray beam passes from the back of the patient to the front (posteroanterior [PA]). This minimizes distortion from the divergence of the x-ray beam as it passes through the body. In addition, the preferred patient position for taking x-ray films in adults is upright. Infants cannot be placed upright easily, and they dislike being forced to lie on their stomachs; thus most chest x-ray films are taken with the infant in the supine position, lying on the x-ray film. The x-ray beam passes from the front of the infant to the back (AP view).

The typical views used to evaluate an infant's lung are AP and lateral chest films. As in the older patient, these two views allow the examiner to see all areas of the lung in a standard presentation. It is important that the viewer approach the reading of these films systematically. The viewer should evaluate the airways—including the larynx, trachea, and major bronchi—for deviation from external masses or pressure, for filling defects from internal masses or hypoplasia, and for normal location in the chest.

Occasionally, decubitus films of the chest and abdomen are helpful in evaluating the status of the newborn or young infant. They can be useful in detecting the presence of fluid or air in the pleural space and in evaluating the presence of fluid from a foreign body. In older patients, this is done with a combination of inspiration and expiration chest films. Because newborns cannot cooperate for these views, right and left lateral decubitus views show an obstruction by not collapsing. For example, if the infant has a mechanical obstruction in the right mainstem bronchus, the left lung will collapse if the infant is lying left side down, but the right lung will not collapse when the infant is lying right side down.

Chest radiographs should be done in infants who have unexplained tachypnea, cyanosis, abnormal breath sounds, malformations of the chest or airway, or a sick appearance. In addition, any infant who has a significant worsening of his/her clinical status should have a chest radiograph. This might include infants who suddenly have an increase in respiratory rate, the appearance or worsening of retractions, or a sudden increase in $Paco_2$. Less obvious, but equally important, is the need to obtain a chest radiograph in mechanically ventilated infants who suddenly improve clinically. This is especially true for infants who are being mechanically ventilated with high-frequency ventilators, which can make physical assessment much more difficult (e.g., cannot evaluate breath sounds).

The two diseases that are classic newborn lung diseases are respiratory distress syndrome (RDS) and meconium aspiration syndrome (MAS). RDS is a disease of inadequate surfactant production. The immature alveoli have increased surface tension and collapse. The chest radiograph of these infants is fairly typical. It includes diffuse hazy, ground-glass appearance; air bronchograms extending out to the periphery of the lungs; and low lung volumes (Figure 11-13). MAS is primarily an airway disease. The stressed mature fetus passes meconium into the amniotic fluid and then with gasping

respirations inhales the meconium-laden amniotic fluid into its lungs. The disease has two phases: an early mechanical phase and a late chemical phase. The chest radiograph shows a typical pattern of mixed atelectasis and local emphysema (Figure 11-14).

Transient tachypnea of the newborn (TTNB) is another disease that has diagnostic radiographs. In TTNB, the amniotic fluid in the lung is incompletely resorbed at the time of delivery. The characteristic chest radiograph shortly after birth shows diffuse streakiness and fluid in the major and minor fissures. This is impossible to distinguish from the chest radiograph of pneumonia. The characteristic of TTNB is the rapid resolution of the disease. By 24 hours of age, the newborn's chest radiograph is typically normal (Figure 11-15).

ASSESSMENT OF CRITICALLY ILL INFANTS

Airway

Evaluation of airway patency in newborns is not as easy as it is in adults and older children. Infants with obstructed airways still have chest wall motion, and with chest auscultation they may even have noises that could be misinterpreted as breath sounds. The examiner needs a thorough knowledge of normal newborn breath sounds and chest wall motion to be able to evaluate airway patency in infants.

Even experienced examiners can be deceived about the adequacy of the airway in intubated infants, because the signs usually used in the older patient may not be reliable in the newborn. For example, an infant whose right mainstem

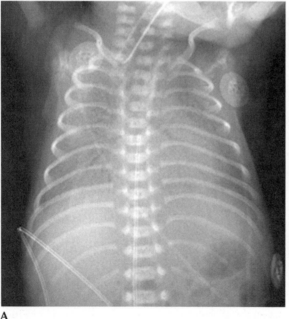
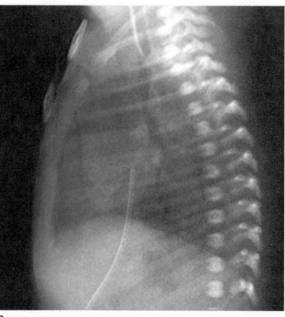

A

B

Figure 11-13 Anteroposterior (**A**) and lateral (**B**) chest radiographs of a preterm infant with respiratory distress syndrome. Both views show diffuse hazy, ground-glass appearance, air bronchograms, and low lung volumes.

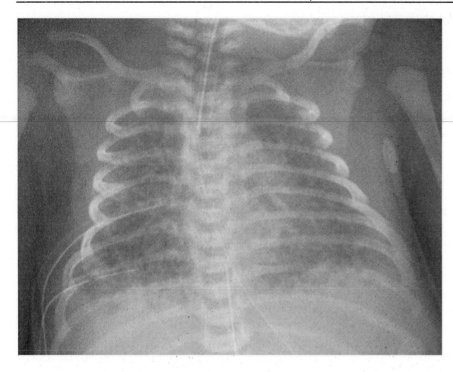

Figure 11-14 Anteroposterior chest radiograph of a term infant with meconium aspiration syndrome. This view shows the typical pattern of mixed atelectasis and local emphysema.

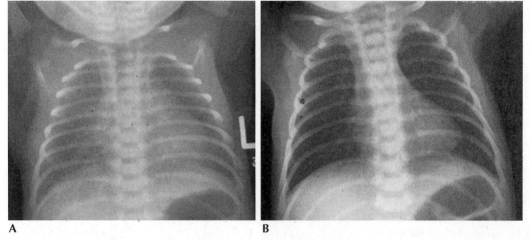

A   B

Figure 11-15 Two anteroposterior chest radiographs of an infant with transient tachypnea of the newborn: **A,** First day of life. **B,** Second day of life.

bronchus is intubated may still have breath sounds in the left hemithorax, as well as left chest wall motion. This can occur because of the short tracheal lengths (less than 10 cm) and the increased compliance of the chest wall. The examiner must be careful to compare all of the lung fields when auscultating. A misplaced endotracheal tube creates a subtle difference in breath sounds, particularly in the apices, which can be picked up by the careful examiner.

The synchrony of spontaneous ventilation rate compared with mechanical ventilation rate is more important than its frequency in the newborn. An infant who exhales during the inspiratory cycle of the ventilator can generate tremendous intrathoracic pressures, potentially damaging the lung. Asynchronous breathing between the infant and the ventilator usually is seen during the hours and days immediately following intubation and the start of mechanical ventilation. The examiner must watch the infant's chest wall motion while listening to the ventilator cycle to document this asynchronous breathing. An inward motion of the chest or absence of an outward motion of the chest wall during mechanical inspiration may indicate that the infant is breathing asynchronously with the ventilator.

A significant improvement in infant mechanical ventilators has been the development of synchronization. Two forms are currently available: synchronized intermittent mandatory ventilation (SIMV) and assist control. SIMV delivers the prescribed number of breaths but in synchrony with the infant's spontaneous breathing. Assist control delivers assistance in synchrony with each breath the infant takes.

Synchronous mechanical ventilators use a variety of triggers for the infant to control the initiation of the breath. These triggers are volume (through either pneumotachography or hot-wire anemometry), abdominal wall motion (Graseby capsule), or thoracic impedance. The important characteristics that must be present for any of the systems to be useful are sensitivity to small change and rapid response time.

The airway pressures monitored in infants are the peak airway pressure, mean airway pressure, positive end-expiratory pressure, and occasionally, esophageal pressure. These pressures are interpreted like their counterparts in the adult intensive care unit (see Chapter 13).

Static airway pressure, intrapleural pressure, lung volume, and expired gas analysis generally are not used in the clinical management of newborns. Airway resistance and lung compliance are being used clinically more often with the advent of reproducible, easy-to-use neonatal pulmonary function equipment. Equipment that uses measurement of expired carbon dioxide and nitrogen pressures is being developed for use in newborns and may become clinically useful in the future.

Hemodynamic Assessments

Hemodynamic monitoring in the critically ill infant is in some ways easier and in other ways more difficult than in the adult. The presence of patent umbilical vessels makes cannulation of the aorta and inferior vena cava simple.

However, cannulation of the pulmonary artery is difficult and usually must be performed in a cardiac catheterization laboratory. In addition, the newborn may have varying degrees of right-to-left shunt, depending on the pulmonary vascular resistance, with the presence of a PDA and a patent foramen ovale. This makes calculation of cardiac output difficult if not impossible.

Cannulation of the umbilical artery and vein is routine practice in almost every nursery in the country. The technique for such a cannulation is easy, and although there are risks to indwelling central catheters, they can be minimized by using a good technique and appropriate indications. In addition, many nurseries are now using percutaneous puncture to cannulate radial arteries and subclavian veins. The indications for umbilical artery catheterization include a source for frequent arterial blood gas (ABG) sampling, continuous blood pressure monitoring, and large-scale blood replacement (e.g., exchange transfusion). The indications for umbilical venous catheterization include central venous pressure monitoring and large-scale blood replacement. The course of the umbilical artery and vein is shown in Figure 11-16.

These two methods of hemodynamic monitoring are susceptible to many of the same problems that exist in adults and older children. Signal damping is a major concern for several reasons: the small internal lumina of the catheters involved, softer materials used in catheter production, and development of fibrin sleeves. Infections, thrombus formation, embolization,

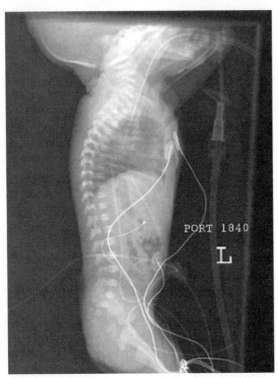
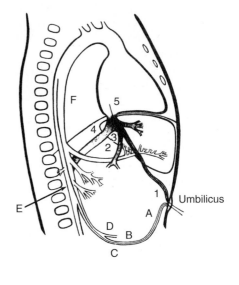

Figure 11-16 Lateral radiograph and diagram of the course of umbilical venous and arterial catheters. Umbilical venous catheter enters through umbilicus, passes through *1,* umbilical vein; *2,* portal vein; *3,* ductus venosus; and *4,* inferior vena cava and stops in *5,* right atrium. Umbilical arterial catheter enters through umbilicus, passes through *A,* umbilical artery; *B,* hypogastric artery; *C,* internal iliac artery; *D,* common iliac artery; and *E,* abdominal aorta and stops in *F,* thoracic aorta.

and arteriospasm are also major concerns when using these monitoring methods.

ASSESSMENT OF THE OLDER INFANT AND CHILD

History

The history of the older infant and the child combines that of the newborn and the adult. The parents remain the major source of information about the infant or child until adolescence. Until the age of 2 years, it is important to include the birth history as part of the evaluation of these patients. The historian assessing the patient must begin to include a review of systems in the historical assessment at 3 months of age. The review of systems is not of great benefit before this.

It is important to differentiate acute from chronic problems. When did the symptoms begin? How rapidly have the symptoms progressed? Is the child truly sick or just not feeling well?

The historian inquiring about the pulmonary symptoms in an older infant or child is limited to signs that are visible or audible to the parent. Historical information about coughing, wheezing, cyanosis, purulent nasal discharge, frequent colds or infections, and change in behavior is easy to obtain. Dyspnea, chest pain, night sweats, and other symptoms that are not observable by the parent may be impossible to document. It should be remembered that hemoptysis and sputum expectoration do not occur in children. Most children swallow any mucus, blood, or purulent material that might be generated by the upper or lower airway.

In addition to experiencing the usual respiratory symptoms, the older infant and child often have extrapulmonary symptoms caused by pulmonary disease. The careful historian queries parents about these symptoms. The most obvious of these signs is general activity. Infants and children who are sick act differently from well babies and children. The parents or guardians are the best judges of an infant's or child's normal behavior. The clinician must be alert to a parent's statement that the child is acting differently. Similarly, infants and children who are sick do not eat well. The interviewer should inquire about the infant's feeding habits if the parents do not bring this up.

Gastrointestinal upset is a common complaint in infants and children. Vomiting and diarrhea are major causes for hospitalization in this age group. Many people who take care of infants and children forget that vomiting and diarrhea may be manifestations of pneumonia or other pulmonary diseases. In addition, diseases such as cystic fibrosis and gastroesophageal reflux may have gastrointestinal and pulmonary symptoms.

Finally, an infant or child who does not maintain growth appropriate for developmental age (failure to thrive) should be investigated for an underlying chronic pulmonary disease. In this age group, such diseases include asthma, cystic fibrosis, gastroesophageal reflux, foreign body aspiration, chronic infection (e.g., sinusitis, cytomegalovirus, tuberculosis, sarcoidosis, histoplasmosis, coccidioidomycosis, bronchiectasis, lung abscess, empyema), nonasthmatic allergic pulmonary diseases, neuromuscular disease affecting the chest wall, and immotile cilia syndrome.

Physical Examination

The components of the physical examination discussed in Chapter 5 are the basis for the physical examination of an older infant or child. Observation, palpation, percussion, and auscultation should be used to localize the disease process within the patient's body. The uniqueness of the physical examination in the older infant or child is in the order in which the examination progresses. It is most important to gain the infant or child's trust and cooperation. The examiner should first examine the parts that upset or frighten the infant or child the least, saving for last the parts of the examination that are upsetting or frightening. If possible, the clinician should make a game out of the examination.

Two of the major respiratory diseases in the young child are croup and epiglottitis. Croup is usually a viral disease affecting the trachea and small airways. The child may have cold symptoms such as a stuffy or runny nose for a few days. He/she may also have a fever. These symptoms progress to a loud, seal-like barking cough; rapid and/or difficult respiration; and grunting or wheezing while breathing. In severe cases, the child may develop stridor (high-pitched squeaking noise during inspiration) and/or cyanosis. The symptoms of croup often worsen when the infant is upset or crying and at night. Scoring systems have been developed to help quantify the degree of illness with croup. These scoring systems often can be used with minimal disturbance of the sick and often anxious child. A scoring system developed by Leipzig et al.[8] has been widely used for children with croup (Table 11-10). It has been validated independently and has been shown to be a reliable score.[9] A score greater than 5 is an indication of impending airway obstruction.

Epiglottitis is usually a bacterial disease that causes significant edema and inflammation of the epiglottis. The child presents with drooling dysphasia and respiratory distress. All of these symptoms come from the swelling and inflammation of the epiglottis. These children are usually febrile and appear sick and anxious. They often have stridor. They usually do not cough. Epiglottitis can be a life-threatening disease that should be treated as an emergency.

Asthma is an increasingly prevalent disease in children of all ages beyond infancy. Asthma is a chronic airway disease that is caused by airway inflammation and hyperresponsiveness to irritants. The typical symptoms include intermittent dry cough and/or expiratory wheezing. Young children may report nonfocal chest pain. Older children may report shortness of breath and chest tightness. Severe exacerbations may include airflow obstruction that can be life-threatening. A scoring system developed by Wood et al.[10] has been used to evaluate children with asthma (Table 11-11). A score of 5 or higher indicates *impending* respiratory failure. A score of 7 or higher with a $PaCO_2$ of 65 mm Hg or more indicates *existing* respiratory failure.

Table 11-10	**Croup Assessment Scoring System**			
	Croup Score			
	0	1	2	3
Stridor	None	Faintly audible	Easily audible	—
Sternal retraction	None	Minimal	Obvious	—
Respiratory rate (breaths/min)				
0-5 kg	<35	36-40	41-45	>45
5.1-10 kg	<30	21-24	25-30	>30
>10 kg	<20	21-24	25-30	>30
Pulse rate (beats/min)				
<3 months	<150	151-165	166-190	>90
3-6 months	<130	131-145	146-170	>170
7-12 months	<120	120-135	136-150	>150
1-3 years	<110	111-125	126-140	>140
3-5 years	<90	91-100	101-120	>120

The respiratory rate is adjusted for body weight and the pulse rate for age.
From Jacobs S et al: *Anaesthesia* 49:903, 1994.

Table 11-11	**Status Asthmaticus Clinical Scoring System**		
	Asthma Score		
	0	1	2
PO_2 or cyanosis	70-100 (RA)	70 (RA)	≤70 (40% FIO_2)
Inspiratory breath sounds	Normal	Unequal	Decreased to absent
Accessory muscles used	None	Moderate	Maximal
Expiratory wheezing	None	Moderate	Marked
Cerebral function	Normal	Depressed or agitated	Coma

From Wood DW et al: *Am J Dis Child* 123:227, 1972.
RA, Radial artery.

Clinical Laboratory Data

Older infants, children, and adolescents tend to have a narrower range of normal values on both clinical laboratory and blood gas laboratory tests. Their normal values tend to reflect the normal values seen in adults. Although some laboratory tests show a wide divergence from adult values (e.g., growth hormone and others), in most clinical situations, the normal values for adults can also be used for the pediatric population.

Other special tests are occasionally used in this age group for the diagnosis of diseases that have a major pulmonary component. Sweat chloride is the most prominent of these. This test is used to diagnose cystic fibrosis. It is simple to perform, but lab-oratories often obtain erroneous results because of poor methods or techniques.

Blood Gases

The older infant and child present a unique problem in obtaining and interpreting blood gases. Their arteries are still small, and arterial puncture is not easy. Most of these patients vigorously object to having an arterial puncture performed even if they are sick. Because of this, more than one person is usually required to obtain the sample. As in the newborn, the older infant and child can quickly change ABG values by crying and hyperventilating. The clinician interpreting the ABG sample should be aware of the patient's disease, as well as what conditions existed when the sample was obtained.

Pulse oximetry is more reliable in this age group than is transcutaneous monitoring. Because of the increased thickness of the skin and subcutaneous tissue, there is a greater difference between arterial and transcutaneous gas values. However, transcutaneous monitoring is still useful as a trending device to identify changes in the patient's status. It is also useful in estimating the true arterial gas value, because the value may have changed during the sampling process. The greatest problem with pulse oximeters in this age group is motion artifact. Manufacturers are working on solutions to this problem.

Pulmonary Function Testing

Beyond the newborn and young infant stage, standard pulmonary function testing is not possible until the child is between 5 and 6 years of age. There are two important points to remember when doing pulmonary function tests on a child. First, the validity of the results is directly related to the child's cooperativeness.

Children in the 5- to 8-year range can have remarkably short attention spans and be frustratingly uncooperative. Second, the lungs of the child are still growing, and the results of pulmonary function tests must be adjusted to body size.

Pulmonary function testing is particularly useful in children with asthma. Machines are now available for clinical use in the outpatient setting. These allow rapid diagnosis of expiratory collapse. Most of these systems use a forced exhalation, measuring peak expiratory flow. With increasing bronchospasm, the child has decreasingly lower peak flows and a scooped rather than linear expiratory flow pattern (Figure 11-17).

Radiographs

As the infant becomes older and progresses through childhood, radiographs become easier to obtain and interpret. After the child can sit erectly, it becomes possible to take a PA chest film. One of the major problems in the young ambulating child is foreign body aspiration. When a child can follow simple instructions, after the age of 2 to 3 years, inspiratory-expiratory films can be taken to evaluate this problem. Before the age of 2 to 3 years, right and left lateral decubitus films can be obtained that yield essentially the same information as inspiratory-expiratory films.

A lateral view of the neck can help distinguish between croup or laryngotracheobronchitis and epiglottitis. Subglottic narrowing is present in laryngotracheobronchitis, and supraglottic narrowing with a large thumb-shaped epiglottis is present with epiglottitis (Figure 11-18).

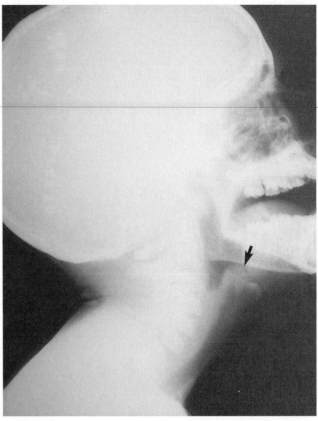

Figure 11-18 Lateral neck radiograph demonstrating an enlarged epiglottis *(arrow)*. (Courtesy Lionel Young, MD, Loma Linda University Medical Center, Loma Linda, California. From Wilkins RL, Dexter JR: *Respiratory disease: Principles of patient care,* Philadelphia, 1993, FA Davis.)

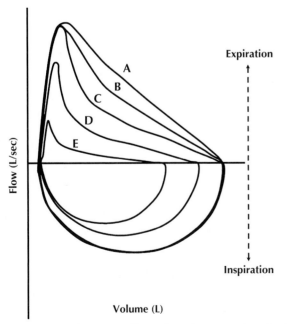

Figure 11-17 Forced expiratory flow-volume loops in asthmatic children showing *(A)* normal flow and *(B to E)* progressive worsening of flow with airway constriction.

REVIEW QUESTIONS

1. Infants born in late gestation are more susceptible to:
   a. Respiratory distress syndrome.
   b. Pulmonary interstitial emphysema.
   c. Intracranial hemorrhage.
   d. Meconium aspiration.

2. What Apgar parameter usually deteriorates first in the hypoxic infant?
   a. Respiratory effort
   b. Heart rate
   c. Muscle tone
   d. Skin color

3. Infants needing extensive medical resuscitation at birth will have Apgar scores in the range of:
   a. 7-10
   b. 4-6
   c. 0-3
   d. None of the above

4. T   F   Hypothermia is a common sign of infection in the newborn.

5. T   F   Hyperthermia in a newborn usually is caused by environmental factors.

6. What is the upper limit of normal range for heart rate in the newborn?
   a. 120 beats/min
   b. 140 beats/min
   c. 160 beats/min
   d. 180 beats/min

7. Which of the following is not a typical cause of tachypnea in the newborn?
   a. Hypothermia
   b. Hypoxemia
   c. Respiratory acidosis
   d. Pain

8. What is the upper limit for normal systolic blood pressure in the term newborn?
   a. 60 mm Hg
   b. 70 mm Hg
   c. 80 mm Hg
   d. 90 mm Hg

9. What is indicated by the presence of retractions in the newborn?
   a. A stiff chest wall
   b. Stiff lungs
   c. Reduced airway resistance
   d. Heart failure

10. What is indicated by a capillary refill greater than 3 seconds in the infant?
    a. Normal cardiopulmonary function
    b. Respiratory failure
    c. Circulatory failure
    d. Renal failure

11. What effect does abdominal distention have on respiration?
    a. It impedes diaphragm movement.
    b. It increases the chance of ventilatory failure.
    c. It may cause respiratory failure.
    d. All of the above.

12. What abnormal finding during chest auscultation is associated with BPD in the infant?
    a. Bronchial breath sounds
    b. Inspiratory fine crackles
    c. Wheezing
    d. Stridor

13. What is the normal leukocyte count for newborns?
    a. 5000-15,000/mm^3
    b. 9000-30,000/mm^3
    c. 15,000-40,000/mm^3
    d. 21,000-35,000/mm^3

14. What is indicated by leukopenia in the infant?
    a. Overwhelming infection
    b. Chronic infection
    c. Acute infection
    d. Local infection

15. What clinical problem is associated with low serum levels of calcium and phosphorus?
    a. Acute hypoxia
    b. Liver failure
    c. Poor nutrition
    d. Renal failure

16. What is the normal range for Pao_2 at birth?
    a. 40-60 mm Hg
    b. 50-70 mm Hg
    c. 60-80 mm Hg
    d. 70-90 mm Hg

17. What parameter demonstrates the largest difference when comparing capillary blood with arterial blood?
    a. Po_2
    b. Pco_2
    c. pH
    d. None of the above

18. Which of the following conditions is least likely to cause a falsely low $tcPo_2$ reading?
    a. Acidosis
    b. Shock
    c. Hypovolemia
    d. Hyperthermia

19. What lung volume is not easily measured in the newborn?
    a. Thoracic gas volume
    b. Residual volume
    c. Functional residual capacity
    d. Crying vital capacity

20. Which of the following clinical findings suggest the need for a chest radiograph in the infant?
    a. Cyanosis
    b. Unexplained tachypnea
    c. Abnormal breath sounds
    d. All of the above

REFERENCES

1. Klaus MH, Fanaroff AA, editors: *Care of the high-risk neonate,* ed 4, Philadelphia, 1993, WB Saunders.
2. Smith DW: *Growth and its disorders,* Philadelphia, 1977, WB Saunders.
3. Fanaroff AA, Martin RJ, editors: *Behrman's neonatal-perinatal medicine: Diseases of the fetus and infant,* ed 7, St Louis, 2002, Mosby.
4. DuBois AB, Botelho SY, Comroe JH: A rapid plethysmographic method for measuring thoracic gas volume: A comparison with a nitrogen washout method for measuring functional residual capacity in normal subject, *J Clin Invest* 35:322, 1956.
5. Klaus MH and others: Lung volume in the newborn infant, *Pediatrics* 30:111, 1962.
6. Strang LB, McGrath MW: Alveolar ventilation in normal newborn infants studied by air wash-in after oxygen breathing, *Clin Sci* 23:129, 1962.
7. Fowler WS, Cornish ER Jr, Kety SS: Lung ventilation studies VIII: Analysis of alveolar ventilation by pulmonary N_2 clearance curves, *J Clin Invest* 31:40, 1952.
8. Leipzig B and others: A prospective randomized study to determine the efficacy of steroids in treatment of croup, *J Pediatr* 94:194, 1979.
9. Jacobs S and others: Validation of a croup score and its use in triaging children with croup, *Anaesthesia* 49:903, 1994.
10. Wood DW, Downes JJ, Lecks HI: A clinical scoring system for the diagnosis of respiratory failure, *Am J Dis Child* 123:227, 1972.

BIBLIOGRAPHY

Burgess WR, Chernick V: *Respiratory therapy in newborn infants and children,* New York, 1982, Thieme-Stratton.

Fanaroff AA, Martin RJ, editors: *Behrman's neonatal-perinatal medicine: diseases of the fetus and infant,* ed 7, St Louis, 2002, Mosby.

Wilkins RL, Hodgkin JE, Lopez B: *Fundamentals of lung and heart sounds,* ed 3, St Louis, 2004, Mosby. (Includes audio CD with neonatal lung sounds.)

Assessment of Older Adult Patients

LEARNING OBJECTIVES

Upon completion of this chapter, the reader should be able to accomplish the following:

1. Identify several techniques for reducing communication barriers with older adult patients.
2. Discuss how patient loss of vision and hearing affect geriatric assessment efforts.
3. Describe techniques healthcare providers can use to compensate for hearing or vision loss in patients.
4. Identify age-related structural and physiologic changes in the cardiovascular and pulmonary systems.
5. Discuss reasons why older adults have a depressed immune system.
6. Describe pulmonary and cardiac assessment techniques.
7. Identify specific diagnostic tests that have altered, age-related normal values.
8. Explain how functional ability relates to level of health, both actual and perceived.

KEY TERMS

ageism	presbycusis
immunosenescence	presbyopia
isolated systolic hypertension (ISH)	pseudohypertension
ototoxicity	tinnitus

CHAPTER OVERVIEW

The purpose of this chapter is to introduce the respiratory therapist to many age-related changes in older adult patients. Gradual decline and chronic illness characterize aging. Many healthcare professionals are focused on treatment of acute illnesses and conditions. Clinicians may need to gain a different perspective when assessing and managing elderly patients and the chronic conditions associated with old age.

Communicating with older adults in the healthcare environment can be challenging, but it is a necessary component of patient care. Treatment in today's healthcare arena takes teamwork. Getting patients involved and having them take a share of the responsibility by communicating with us can lead to better outcomes.

Assessing vital signs, interpreting diagnostic tests, and understanding age-related physiologic and structural changes in organ systems are all important. Realizing that older adults have depressed immune systems and may present with unusual signs and symptoms is key to appropriate disease management.

Assessment of the functional performance of an older adult patient may uncover a potential source of disability or impairment or a special need. A systematic inventory of functional abilities can lead to improved diagnostic evaluation and choice of interventions. Functional ability can be directly correlated with the index of health.

The "graying of America" will increase the number of older adults seeking medical attention. A Center for Disease Control and Prevention survey on visits to physician offices revealed that although Americans visited the doctor at about the same rate from 1985 to 1999, adults over age 65 increased their rate of office visits by over 20%.[1] The U.S. Census Bureau reveals similar statistics. Between 1995 and 1999, there was a 14.5% increase in visits to office-based physicians and hospital out-patient departments in the over-65 age bracket.[2] Those choosing healthcare as a profession today will spend about 75% of their professional lives taking care of older people.[3] The need for clinicians that are knowledgeable about aging and aged people will be critical in future years.

SIMPLY STATED

More than 50% of patients requiring the services of cardiopulmonary professionals are aged 65 years and older.

THE IMPORTANCE OF PATIENT-CLINICIAN INTERACTION

The importance of patient-clinician interaction cannot be overstated. Chapter 1 discusses the stages of patient-clinician interaction. The same general techniques for establishing rapport with patients holds true for older adults, but one important difference that must not be overlooked with older patients is time. Gathering data from older patients takes more time. Wise and efficient use of time can make a difference between just recording vital signs and really assessing the patient. Having a plan before making contact with the patient allows the clinician to gather better history and physical data. Keep in mind: older adults who are institutionalized may be weakened by chronic or acute conditions. Asking an older patient to do unnecessary repeated maneuvers, performing unnecessary manipulations, and exposing his/her skin for long periods of time may exacerbate these conditions. Performing a structured assessment in a calm, unhurried, and respectful manner is fundamental to good geriatric patient assessment.

SIMPLY STATED

To conserve the patient's energy, organize your assessment.

Principles of Communication

As discussed in Chapter 2, principles of communication are key factors in information gathering. Patient data that have not been gathered cannot be assessed.

Many young clinicians in their daily lives are segregated from older adults. There may be a tendency to associate aging with illness and death. The connection of aging with chronic illness and death may lead to ageism, or discrimination against old people. Ageism in the healthcare setting can lead practitioners to listen to older patients less carefully, spend less time addressing their concerns, and treat them mechanically, without compassion. If clinicians approach their patients with an ageist attitude, communication is hindered.

Reducing Communication Barriers in Older Adults

Communication implies two things: the message has been delivered, and the message has been understood. When older patients know what practitioners are asking and why, they are usually more compliant.

There are many potential barriers that hinder patient/caregiver communication. Sensory deficit, such as hearing or visual impairment, are obvious barriers. Physical barriers related to poorly fitted dentures, nonfunctional hearing aids, or surgical removal of vocal chords may make it impossible for patients to talk. Aphasia, related to stroke, head trauma, or Alzheimer's disease, might affect both speech and processing of language, as can the adverse effects of many medications. Emotional barriers often manifested as depression can block communication efforts. Other emotional events such as the loss of a loved one, the death of a spouse, or even being relocated to a healthcare institution against the patient's wishes may be obstacles to effective communication.

Although determining the exact cause of the communication barrier is beyond the scope of therapists, there are a few interventions that may help bridge the gap. It is always important to approach older adults in a caring manner. A smile, a pat on the hand, and a kind word while making eye contact are usually successful forms of nonverbal communication. When addressing the patient, use his/her last name preceded by the appropriate title (e.g., Mrs., Miss, Mr., Dr., Father). Using the patient's last name shows respect and promotes an atmosphere of equality. Call the patient by his/her first name only if you are given permission. Calling patients "sweetie" or "dear" is too familiar and may be interpreted as condescending.

Be aware of the environment. If the room is too hot, too cold, or too dark, or if sunlight from a window is blinding your patient, his/her discomfort may affect your assessment efforts and thus assessment results. Introduce yourself clearly, both by name and by department. Give the patient your full attention. Let him/her know that you are performing an important job. Tell the patient you look forward to working with him/her and encourage him/her to ask questions as they arise. If the patient seems confused, a gentle reminder of your role and goal may reassure him/her. Eliminate or reduce background noise and interruptions when possible. Taking a few seconds to do this up front will save time later.

Approach the patient and position yourself at eye level (Figure 12-1). Maintain an unhurried pace but keep the assess-

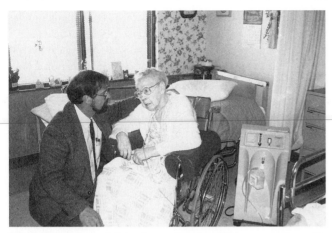

Figure 12-1 Patient-clinician interaction: the elderly may need very little, but they need that little so much. (From Sorenson HM, Thorson JA: *Geriatric respiratory care.* Albany, NY, 1997, Delmar.)

ment structured in a logical manner so that all subjective and objective data can be recorded. An unorganized, unstructured, and hurried approach to assessment can be counterproductive. When soliciting patient responses, wait for an answer. Try not to put words in the patient's mouth. Older adults function better when they do not feel rushed.

AGE-RELATED SENSORY DEFICIT

Research confirms the presence of age-related decremental changes in vision and hearing. Young people tend to have sharper eyesight and the ability to hear greater ranges of sound than older people do. Older adults, however, are not all hard of hearing or visually impaired.

Hearing Impairment

Presbycusis, an age-related, progressive, bilateral hearing loss, is the most common cause of auditory impairment in the United States. This condition affects about 23% of adults between the ages of 65 and 75 years.[4] In the 70- to 80-year-old age group, as many as 50% of older adults have hearing impairment which actually affects their communication skills.[5] Statistics on the exact number of older adults with impaired hearing varies depending on the source of information. A prospective patient evaluation and retrospective analysis from 576 consecutive frail elders found hearing impairment in 64% of those tested.[6] The burden of hearing loss in older adults is considerable and is often associated with diminished functional independence.

Tinnitus, defined as a symptom rather than a disease, is also more prevalent in the elderly.[7] Tinnitus is an auditory perception not caused by external sounds. It may be described as ringing, buzzing, roaring or chirping. Depending on the severity of symptoms, tinnitus can result in mental status changes ranging from mild irritation to depression and suicidal thoughts.

Because tinnitus can be a result of ototoxicity, drug-induced hearing impairment should always be considered in older adults. Ototoxicity is defined as a damaging effect on the eighth cranial nerve or in the organs of hearing or balance. The diminished hearing capacity that healthcare practitioners observe in institutionalized patients may be inflated by ototoxicity. Commonly prescribed pharmacologic agents including aminoglycoside antibiotics (streptomycin, kanamycin, neomycin, gentamicin and viomycin), salicylates, diuretics (ethacrinic acid and furosemide), and quinine or chloroquinine are particularly notorious for causing ototoxicity.[8]

Assessing for Hearing Impairment

There are simple and accurate methods to assess the presence or absence of hearing loss. Some that are commonly used are the whispered voice, a tuning fork, finger rub, a portable audioscope and the Hearing Handicapped Inventory for the Elderly-Screening (HHIE-S) questionnaire.[9] For a therapist at the bedside, however, a quick way to assess whether your patient has adequate hearing is to whisper a simple question while standing nearby and out of the patient's direct view. This simple test will help you determine whether you need to consider compensatory modifications.

Compensating for Hearing Impairment

If a hearing loss is suspected, ask clearly, "Can you hear me?" while facing the patient. If no documented hearing loss exists on the chart, discuss with the nurse the possibility of accumulated earwax or ototoxicity. If the patient has a hearing aid, make sure that it works and that it is in place. If there is no hearing aid, consider using an amplification device if available. Speak clearly, keeping the entire mouth visible. (If you need to wear an isolation mask or if a mustache is present, patients may be at a disadvantage.)

If comfortable with the patient and the situation, you may use your stethoscope as an amplification device by placing the earpieces in the patient's ears and speaking through the bell.

Vision Impairment

Presbyopia, a normal age-related change in the lens of the eye, usually results in correctable farsightedness. Although presbyopia can occur in adults as early as age 40, it is much more common in older adults. More serious disorders of the eye that frequently affect older patients include cataract, glaucoma, diabetic retinopathy, and macular degeneration. Age is the major risk factor for developing cataract, an opacity of the lens that reduces visual acuity. Patients that live to an advanced age are likely to develop cataract.

Because visual impairment has been identified as the second most prevalent disability in adults over age 65 years,[10] and studies also reveal that sensory impairment diminishes functional status,[6] respiratory therapists need to be aware of assessment techniques and compensatory strategies when caring for patients with vision loss.

Assessing for Vision Impairment

To determine the level of vision loss in older adults, evaluation by an optometrist or ophthalmologist who specializes in low vision is necessary. An evaluation of visual acuity, however, is probably not necessary for providing many forms of respiratory care.

In institutionalized patients, vision problems that put patients at high risk for falls necessitate intervention.

Compensating for Vision Loss or Impairment

Of primary importance for hospitalized patients with low vision is consistency and safety. The old adage "a place for everything and everything in its place" is critical for those with visual impairment.[11] Waste baskets, chairs, and bedside tables that are moved around the room for the convenience of the caregivers may pose a hazard. Paper handkerchiefs, a hairbrush, or a telephone moved away from where the patient has placed them will be missed. If the patient wears eyeglasses, make sure they are clean and properly positioned. Older adults with low vision may be able to read words that are enlarged and in a bold print. Medicine bottle lids can be marked with a single large letter indicating the name of the medication for when they are discharged from the hospital. Words written with puff paint, available at craft stores, can help patients distinguish between different metered-dose inhalers. Older patients with low vision will require increased illumination. Halogen lighting, if available, provides more illumination than incandescent bulbs. Enhancing contrast also enables elders with low vision to locate and identify objects. The use of coping strategies by older adults with age-related vision loss is associated with better adaptive outcomes.[10]

When patients are blind, verbal communication is extremely important. Speak clearly, and thoroughly explain the procedures you are going to perform until comprehension is evident. If it becomes necessary to move a patient with vision loss, tell him/her what you are going to do, offer an arm as a support and guide, and let the patient initiate the movement.

SIMPLY STATED

Communication barriers that result from sensory deficit may hinder geriatric assessment and compromise patient safety.

AGING OF THE ORGAN SYSTEMS

The effect of aging on specific organ systems varies widely from one person to another. We spend about one fourth of our lives growing up and another three fourths growing old. Simple observation will attest to the fact that we do not all age at the same rate. Organ systems age independent of one another also. Lifestyle choices and environmental factors influence organ system functioning. The combination of these external factors, along with aging and disease processes, alter the body's organ systems both in structure and function.

Age-Related Changes

A brief review of age-related changes in the cardiovascular and pulmonary systems might be helpful before the assessment of an older adult patient. Keep in mind that the following information reflects average changes with age. In older adults, deviation from average is not uncommon. Aging and disease processes also tend to overlap in producing similar signs and symptoms. When evaluating older patients, it is important to understand and recognize the differences.

Cardiovascular System

Diseases of the heart and blood vessels are common in elderly patients. The widespread prevalence of coronary artery disease has presented a challenge for researchers engaged in studying the effect of normal aging on the heart. Evidence regarding aging and human cardiovascular function is generally limited by the need to measure serial cardiac anatomy and physiology noninvasively.[12] Cardiovascular changes have been studied invasively in aging animals; however, translation of animal data to humans cannot be presumed. Many older adults do have some measure of cardiac hypertrophy but it is generally accepted that in the absence of disease, there is minimal alteration in the size of the heart. Because of decreased contractile properties in the heart and blood vessels, there is an age-related increase in systolic blood pressure and an elevated left ventricular afterload, which results in left ventricular wall thickening. Arterial walls stiffen with age. Blood vessels lose elastin and smooth muscle fibers and gain collagen and calcium deposits. Left ventricular systolic function remains relatively stable with no significant changes in resting left ventricular ejection fraction, cardiac output, or stroke volume.[12] Left ventricular diastolic function, however, is reduced; this is most likely due to structural changes in the left ventricular myocardium. The early left ventricular diastolic filling rate progressively slows after the age of 20 years. By the age of 80 years, the rate may be reduced by up to 50%.[8]

There is an age-related increase in elastic and collagen tissue in the cardiac conducting system. Researchers have noted a pronounced reduction in the number of pacemaker cells in the sinoatrial (SA) node,[12] estimated by one author to be as high as a 90% decline in SA node cell numbers.[13] The consequence of these age-related losses is an increase in cardiac arrhythmias. Atrial fibrillation is the most common cardiac arrhythmia, occurring in up to 5% of adults older than 80 years of age.[14] Pressure receptor sensitivity declines with age. As a result, older adults have a blunted compensatory response to both hypertensive and hypotensive stimuli.

Calcification of heart valves is more prevalent in the elderly. In elderly patients, the predominant causes of valvular heart disease are degenerative calcification, myxomatous degeneration, papillary muscle dysfunction, and infective endocarditis. One third of patients older than 70 years of age have calcium deposits in the aortic or mitral valves.[8]

BOX 12-1	Symptoms of Left-Sided Versus Right-Sided CHF

Left-Sided Failure	Right-Sided Failure
Exertional dyspnea, orthopnea	Edema
Possible nocturnal dyspnea	Distended neck veins
Cheyne-Stokes breathing	Cyanosis
Pale, cool skin	Dyspnea
Dysrhythmias	Dysrhythmias
Fatigue	Hepatomegaly
Restlessness, irritability	Occasional ascites
Shortened attention span	

Congestive heart failure (CHF) may result from valvular disease, hypertension, cardiomyopathy, or ischemic heart disease. The incidence of CHF doubles for each decade of life between 45 and 75 years.[3] The pressure the ventricles must overcome to pump blood out of the heart can lead to left ventricular failure, right ventricular failure, or biventricular failure. Left- and right-sided failures will both result in reduced cardiac output and an increased heart rate. Some other CHF symptoms are more typically associated with the damaged ventricle, either left or right (Box 12-1).

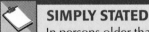

SIMPLY STATED

In persons older than 65 years of age, CHF is the most common medical diagnosis.

Pulmonary System

There are a number of age-related physiologic changes in the pulmonary system. Structurally, the trachea and bronchi become more rigid with age. Smooth muscle fibers in the lungs are progressively replaced with fibrous connective tissue. Alveolar septa gradually deteriorate. Although the number of alveoli does not change, loss of alveolar walls increases the size of the alveoli and reduces surface area for gas exchange. The alveolar-capillary membrane thickens, causing a reduction in diffusion of pulmonary gases. Aging lungs have less elastic recoil. The chest wall becomes stiffer, probably as a result of ossification of the cartilage-rib juncture and progressive dorsal kyphosis. Although loss of elasticity of lung tissue actually increases lung compliance, the rigidity of the thoracic cage reduces compliance enough to result in an overall decrease in lung compliance. The stiffer chest wall and reduction in elastic recoil are factors in an age-related increase in functional residual capacity and residual volume.

Physiologically, aging alters both ventilation and gas exchange. Changes in ventilation and gas distribution are primarily related to the altered lung and chest wall compliance. The balance of inward forces (elastic recoil) and outward forces (chest wall and muscles of ventilation) determine

lung volumes at rest. At about age 55 years, respiratory muscle strength begins to weaken.[8] The diaphragm may be reduced to about 75% of the strength normal for healthy young adults. The important functional changes that take place with aging of the pulmonary system are reductions in elastic recoil and ventilatory muscle strength. The central control of these activities also changes with increasing years. Cardiac and pulmonary responses to decreased oxygen and elevated carbon dioxide levels diminish with age. Thus, the changes in ventilation and respiration with aging emerge as a complex picture.[15] In the absence of disease, age-related changes in the lungs are inconsequential. However, the combination of age-related and disease-related pulmonary changes puts the patient at risk for increased morbidity and mortality.

Pulmonary Defense Mechanisms

Aging not only alters physiologic functioning of the lung (ventilation and respiration) but also affects the protective function of the lungs. With increasing age, the epithelial cells of the mucous membrane that line the tracheobronchial tree show degenerative changes. Ciliary activity slows down. There is a decrease in the phagocytic activity of the macrophages in the mucous membrane. Combined, these changes lead to a reduction in mucociliary clearance. In addition, the loss of an effective cough reflex contributes to the increased susceptibility of older patients to lung infections.

Institutionalized older adults are subject to some conditions that may result in a reduced level of consciousness. Neurologic disorders and pharmacologic agents such as narcotics or sedatives can effectively blunt the cough reflex. Aspiration is always a concern. Patients with dysphasia, impaired esophageal motility, or reflux disease are at added risk when the cough mechanism is not working properly.

Immunity

Humoral immunity, which takes place in bodily fluids, is associated with antibody production and B lymphocytes. T cells are primarily related to cell-mediated immunity and constitute about 70% of the lymphoid pool in the blood. Cell-mediated immunity involves a variety of activities designed to restrain or destroy cells that the body recognizes as harmful. With age comes a decrease in cell-mediated immunity. This age-related decline in cellular immunity correlates with an increased frequency of secondary (reactivation) tuberculosis in elderly patients. The acute antibody response to extrinsic antigens, such as pneumococcal and influenza vaccines, is also reduced in old age. Immunizations, although not as effective in older adults, are still strongly recommended.

Research regarding the clinical implications of immunosenescence, aging of the immune system, is confounded by a number of factors. Within subpopulations of older adults, there is considerable heterogeneity of the immune response. Genetic factors may play a role, as may environmental pollutants, socioeconomic status, and nutrition. Even efforts to increase immune function (nutritional supplements, booster vaccines) may not be equally effective in older adults. Although increased rates of infection and malignancy are associated with the dysregulated immune response common in older adults, these changes have not been causally related to the increased incidence of disease.[16] What does seem reasonable to presume, however, is that the age-related changes in the immune system may impair the older patient's ability to effectively repel bacterial infections and may make them more susceptible to increased morbidity and mortality from pneumonia, sepsis, or other bacterial growths.

Unusual Presentations of Illness

What you see in a 40-year-old presenting with an acute process or exacerbation of a chronic disease may differ from the presenting symptoms of an 80-year-old with the same disease. The variations in signs and symptoms can make it difficult to diagnose such common occurrences as pneumonia or a heart attack.

Some older adults will downplay their symptoms, assuming the aches and pains are simply "old age." However, research indicates that in some cases aging neurons may decrease peripheral sensitivity, causing a reduced sense of pain.[17]

Immune system changes, as previously discussed, put older adults at a higher risk for harboring infectious agents. Changes in the cardiac system may result in blunting of the tachycardic response to hypoxia or sepsis. Some aging organ systems lose the ability to compensate for injury to other organ systems.

Inflammation is one of the body's first responses to infection or injury. It was once believed that in older adults the diminished febrile response, mild leukocytosis, and weakened local inflammatory response were related to the aging process. New evidence has shown that, in younger adults with multiple illnesses, the same lack of immune response occurs. Recent data supports the theory that it is the accumulation of diseases, not the age of the patient, that impairs immunity.[8]

Pneumonia

In a patient with pneumonia, typical presentations are cough, fever, and purulent sputum production. These signs can be deceptively subtle in older adults, particularly a lack of an elevated temperature. With a lower base temperature and a reduced ability to mount a febrile response, older adults with pneumonia may be quite ill before the cause is detected. Some older patients with an infection may simply complain of a poor appetite, lack of ability to perform daily activities, and a generalized weakness. Extrapulmonary symptoms such as nausea, vomiting, diarrhea, myalgia, and arthralgia are common. The most sensitive sign of pneumonia in an elderly adult is an increased respiratory rate (greater than 28 breaths/min).[16]

Chest x-rays may be helpful in diagnosing pneumonia, but this is not the case if the patient is dehydrated. The pneumonic infiltrate may be obscured by pulmonary edema or may not be detectable on the chest film until 24 to 48 hours after the patient has been rehydrated.[18]

Sputum specimens collected for culture and sensitivity are recommended to avoid empiric therapy with a broad-spectrum antibiotic. Unfortunately, obtaining a good sputum specimen from an older debilitated patient is the exception, not the rule. For patients who do not respond to therapy or who relapse after an initial response to therapy, collecting sputum via transtracheal aspiration or a bronchoscopy may be considered. Depending on the pathogenic organism, blood cultures have a diagnostic yield of only about 10% to 20%.[16]

Heart Failure

In the United States, heart failure is a major source of chronic disability and the leading indication for hospitalization in adults over the age of 65 years.[19] Although the incidence of death from myocardial infarction (MI) has been reduced over the past 30 years, it remains an important cause of morbidity in the older population. About 50% of patients who die from MI are older than 75 years of age.[19] Unfortunately, clinical presentation of heart attack may be altered by advanced age. The most common symptom is chest pain, but the pain may be referred. Complaints of shoulder, throat, and abdominal pain are common. Some patients may complain of bilateral elbow pain. Other atypical symptoms that can accompany a heart attack are syncope, acute confusion, weakness, fatigue, and restlessness. In the case of silent MIs, pain is not a symptom. A prospective study, part of the Bronx Aging Study, showing the magnitude of unrecognized or silent MIs, revealed that the annual incidence of recognized MI was 3.2/100 person years whereas the incidence of unrecognized MI was 2.4/100 person years.[20] Although atypical presentation may cause diagnostic difficulty, there are many subtle clues that should alert practitioners. Because of the degeneration of the cardiac conduction fibers, if an older patient complains of dizziness, the healthcare professional should suspect heart problems. Cough and wheezing may indicate early left-sided heart failure. Hemoptysis in an older adult may be indicative of heart failure or a pulmonary embolus. Shortness of breath should put the clinician on alert. Dyspnea associated with new-onset congestive cardiac failure may be the only presenting complaint.[19]

An awareness of how and why disease can present with unusual symptoms will reduce the chances of missing a diagnosis. Informed clinicians performing good assessments can make a difference in the patient outcome.

 SIMPLY STATED
Dyspnea and lethargy may be presenting symptoms of MI; be alert.

Asthma

In older adults, the diagnosis of asthma is not uncommon. It has been estimated that 5% of adults older than 60 years[21] and 7% to 9% of adults older than age 70 have asthma.[22]

Asthma, unfortunately, is often misdiagnosed and/or under-diagnosed in our older patient population. Reasons for this are unclear. Perhaps it is because asthma has historically been considered a disease common to children and young adults. Other potential confounding factors may be associated with normal age-related pulmonary changes and a blunted perception of symptoms. It is possible that when asthma and chronic obstructive pulmonary disease (COPD) occur simultaneously, only the COPD is diagnosed. The classic symptoms of asthma—shortness of breath, wheezing, and cough—are also common in such diseases as CHF, emphysema, chronic bronchitis, gastroesophageal reflux, and transbronchial tumors.[21]

Because asthma is more common than presumed in older adults, therapists need to be aware that some presenting symptoms may be atypical. Elderly asthmatics are less likely to have a history of allergic disease, less likely to have nocturnal or early morning symptoms, more likely to have a poor immediate response to bronchodilator therapy, and more likely to have a later onset of symptoms. Wheezing, however, remains common. A diagnosis of asthma should be considered in elderly patients with wheezing or dyspnea.

Underdiagnosis of asthma may be more related to the underuse of objective measurement instruments, spirometry and peak flow meters. Functional ability to do reproducible maneuvers may have been a concern in the past, but according to Enright et al,[23] about 90% of the elderly participants in the Cardiovascular Health Study Research Group were capable of performing good-quality spirometry tests within 10 minutes. Older adults who experience symptoms and have not been previously assessed for asthma should be considered candidates for pulmonary function screening.

SIMPLY STATED
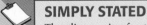

The diagnosis of asthma should be considered in older adults who are wheezing.

PATIENT ASSESSMENT

Patient assessment represents a skill that is crucial to caring for the elderly. Vital signs such as temperature, pulse, blood pressure, and respiratory rate, along with lung sounds and breathing pattern, are noninvasive windows to the health status of the patient. Assessment is truly an art. Given today's climate of managed care, protocols, and clinical practice guidelines, strong assessment skills are vital to good patient care and cost-effective disease management. Because patient assessment is the foundation, the information gathered must be accurate.

One component of assessment that is occasionally overlooked is taking a patient's history. A thorough health history should tell you 80% of what a physical assessment will reveal.[3] Another means of facilitating physical assessment is to try and conceptualize the anatomy. Having a basic knowledge of anatomy and understanding how disease alters both anatomy and physiology are key to accurate assessment.

Vital Signs

Temperature

Because of decreased metabolism, the loss of muscle mass, and a reduction in vasoconstriction, older adults have an altered ability to regulate body heat. Older adults usually have lower body temperatures. In patients older than 90 years, body temperatures of 96° and 97° F are not uncommon. Simply taking temperatures in older adults may be a challenge. Oral thermometers are not useful if the elderly patient cannot easily keep his/her mouth closed for 2 or 3 minutes. If an oral thermometer is used, shake the mercury down to at least 94° F before starting.

The axillary method may not be accurate, particularly in a thin, older adult with a loss of underarm body tissue. Rectal temperatures are accurate but necessitate turning the patient completely to one side, a maneuver that could result in a fractured hip. Tympanic membrane thermometers, although more expensive, are accurate, easy to use, and able to record temperatures within seconds.

Regardless of the method used, it is important to establish a norm for each patient and assess for trends. Once the norm is established, an increase in temperature alerts the healthcare professional to the possibility of infection. A 95-year-old patient with a temperature of 101° F (whose normal body temperature is 96° F) is in trouble. That is equivalent to 103.6° F in a person whose normal temperature is 98.6° F.

Because the thermoregulatory mechanism in older adults is blunted, environmental temperatures may be more influential. During room temperature extremes (hot or cold), monitor the patient's body temperature on a regular basis.

Pulse

The heart rate at rest is regulated by sympathetic and, to a greater degree, parasympathetic tone. In healthy men, the supine resting heart rate does not change with age. In a sitting position, the heart rate in the same individual will drop slightly from the rate exhibited when supine. In an inactive older adult, the pulse rate may decrease to 50 to 55 beats/min. In active older adults, although heart rates vary, a normal pulse may range between 60 and 100 beats/min. Arrhythmias that produce a rapid heart rate are not tolerated well by elderly patients, who may already have a decreased functional capacity. If there are any new (not previously noted) irregularities in pulse volume or rhythm, consult a nurse or physician about a follow-up assessment. To most accurately assess pulse in an older patient, use a stethoscope and count beats at the apex.

Blood Pressure

The measurement of blood pressure is essential. Hypertension is an important cardiovascular risk factor in the elderly. Blood pressure and pulse pressure increase progressively with age. In most populations, average diastolic blood pressure increases with age until the sixth decade then stabilizes, whereas systolic blood pressure continues to rise. As a result, the pulse pressure (the difference between systolic and diastolic pressures) may widen. A normal pulse pressure is anywhere between 50 and 100 mm Hg in older adults. If when documenting blood pressure you note a narrowing of the pulse pressure, it might be wise to monitor the patient. A narrowing pulse pressure might be an early sign of a slow leak tamponade and can be present up to 2 days before a tamponade crisis.[3]

Systolic blood pressure rises with aging as a consequence of the loss of elasticity in the peripheral vessels. It is estimated that 60% of older adults have either elevated systolic or diastolic blood pressures or both. Elevation of only the systolic pressure is termed isolated systolic hypertension (ISH). The Systolic Hypertension in the Elderly Program (SHEP) demonstrated that treating ISH in older patients decreased the incidence of stroke.[24] Historically, a sustained systolic pressure of more than 160 mm Hg or a diastolic pressure over 90 mm Hg was thought to constitute hypertension.

Recently, the U.S. National Heart Lung and Blood Institute (NHLBI) published the latest guidelines for classifying and managing high blood pressure (Table 12-1). The document is known as the Seventh Report of the Joint National Committee on Prevention, Detection, Evaluation and Treatment of High Blood Pressure, or the JNC-7 Report.[25,26]

According to a national survey, 70% of Americans with hypertension are aware of their problem. Fifty-nine percent are being treated for the condition, and 34% of those being treated have their blood pressure under control.[25] The new guidelines focus on improving these statistics by recommending interventions/treatments designed to help people regain control of their disease. The recommended treatment guidelines include medication management and lifestyle change.

Blood pressure may be falsely high in older adults because of arterial stiffness. An overestimated blood pressure (pseudohypertension) should be suspected in patients with elevated systolic and diastolic pressures but no end-organ damage.

Blood pressure must be measured accurately. Ask the patient to sit quietly for 3 to 5 minutes before taking a measurement, and use a cuff large enough to cover at least one third of the patient's upper arm. Measure pressure in both arms, and note any significant difference. Both supine and standing (or sitting)

blood pressures, taken 1 to 3 minutes after the positional change, may reveal the presence of orthostatic hypotension. (Exercise caution, however, when testing volume-depleted patients.) A drop of 20 mm Hg systolic or 10 mm Hg diastolic, or an increased heart rate of 20 beats/min, is abnormal. Orthostatic hypotension in older adults is often associated with syncope and falls. Failure to check both supine and standing blood pressure is an oversight in potentially diagnosing an important and often correctable problem. Clearly, obtaining accurate blood pressures is important in the treatment and management of hypertension in the elderly. Remember that emergency room blood pressures are not baseline data. They are measured under less than optimal conditions. Check blood pressure again before acting on a single measurement. Also, document blood pressure trends. Safe drug therapy may depend on accurate daily blood pressure measurement.

SIMPLY STATED
ER blood pressure measurements are not baseline.

Respiratory Rate

Residual volume increases almost 50% by the age of 70 years. Because the total lung capacity remains relatively stable, the increase in residual volume comes at the expense of the vital capacity. In older adults, the respiratory rate may increase as a result of a decreased depth of ventilation. Normal respiratory rate in elderly patients ranges from 16 to 25 breaths/min.

Tachypnea or hyperpnea may be the result of exercise, for example, in a patient who just ambulated in the hallway or returned from therapy. Other factors that could result in an increased rate or depth of breathing are anxiety, fever, pneumonia, hypoxemia, acidemia, or lesions in the pons and medulla. Bradypnea might be secondary to pharmacologic respiratory depressants, or the patient may just be sleeping. When an abnormally slow rate of breathing is noted, other causes could be alkalosis, hypothermia, or hypoglycemia. Older adults are more susceptible to hypothermia. Additionally, older patients with diabetes have a sixfold greater risk of hypothermia, most likely due to vascular disease that alters the body's thermoregulatory mechanism.[8] In patients being treated with oral antidiabetic agents (sulfonylureas), the incidence of hypoglycemia increases with age and/or concomitant use of aspirin or sulfonamide antibiotics.[27] Accurate respiratory rates, documented in a timely manner, can assist caregivers in looking for trends and can lead to additional diagnoses. If shallow breathing is noted, respiration may be easier to count by watching the rise and fall of the abdomen instead of the chest.

Dyspnea in older adults is abnormal. If the patient exhibits shortness of breath at rest, only 20% of his/her lung structure may be functioning.[3] Next to pain, dyspnea is the symptom most feared by patients and caregivers alike. A respiratory rate greater than 25 breaths/min may signal a lower respiratory tract

Table 12-1	NHLBI Categories of High Blood Pressure		
Category	Systolic BP (mm Hg)		Diastolic BP (mm Hg)
Normal	Below 120	and	Below 80
Prehypertension	120-139	or	80-89
Hypertension stage 1	140-159	or	90-99
Hypertension stage 2	160 and above	or	100 and above

From Griffith RW: High blood pressure: new guidelines are out! *Health and Age* June 5, 2003. Available at http://www.healthandage.com.

infection, CHF, or another disorder prior to the appearance of other clinical signs.[8]

Inspection and Palpation

Generally defined as a visual examination of the patient, inspection can be done while taking a patient history, checking vital signs, or auscultating lung sounds.

Breathing Patterns

Note the pattern of breathing. Is Cheyne-Stokes or periodic breathing perceptible? If so, document the length of the apnea episodes. Older adults with heart disease may demonstrate this pattern of irregular breathing while sleeping. The more common etiologic factors of Cheyne-Stokes include CHF, uremia, decreased blood flow to the respiratory center of the brain, drug-induced respiratory depression, or brain damage. Biot's breathing, an irregular breathing pattern, also has characteristic periods of apnea. Again, document the apnea in seconds. Biot's breathing occurs most often in patients with brain damage and increased intercranial pressure (see Chapter 5).

Cyanosis

Look for cyanosis. If the extremities (i.e., fingers, toes, tip of nose, earlobes) are bluish in color, the patient has peripheral cyanosis. Peripheral cyanosis is often related to inadequate circulation but may be noted in patients who are cold, anxious, or have some measure of venous obstruction.

Central cyanosis results from a decreased concentration of oxygen in arterial blood and may be a result of advanced lung disease or CHF.

In older adults, two other manifestations of cyanosis may be noted. *Small vessel syndrome* can present as local areas of cyanosis or necrosis in a hand or foot that generally has adequate circulation. A number of predisposing conditions can result in small vessel syndrome, such as disseminated intravascular coagulation, essential thrombocytosis, polycythemia, scleroderma, or emboli from arterial aneurysms.[8] *Raynaud's phenomenon* is another syndrome that can present with intermittent cutaneous pallor or cyanosis. It is typically caused by exposure to cold or emotional stimuli and related to peripheral vasospasm. However, older adults may experience the pallor and cyanosis at room temperature.

Skin Turgor

Diminished skin turgor or fullness of the skin is a normal age-related integumentary change. The loss of subcutaneous fat and water, deterioration of elastin, and decreased vascularity can result in wrinkling and loose skin. Pinching the skin to check for tenting used to be a quick check for the presence of dehydration. Now that the age-associated structural changes are understood, tenting is no longer used as a valid indicator of dehydration. The condition of the tongue may be a better marker of dehydration than the skin.[28] If dehydration in an elderly patient is suspected, consult a physician.

SIMPLY STATED
Dehydration can be life threatening and should not be disregarded.

Clubbing

The abnormal enlargement of the distal phalanges, most easily noted in the fingers, is not age related. However, the conditions that lead to clubbing are chronic, and older adults have a higher incidence of chronic disease. COPD alone, even in the presence of hypoxemia, does not lead to clubbing. If older adult patients with COPD have clubbing, something other than obstructive lung disease is occurring, such as pulmonary manifestations of connective tissue disease.[15]

Edema

The visible signs of fluid accumulation can signal the presence of a variety of diseases. Check the patient's lower extremities for the presence of edema or swelling. Ask about or check the chart for any recent sudden weight gain. A gain of more than 2 lb in a day or more than 5 lb in a week may be fluid retention and could signal CHF.[29] A rapid onset of unilateral leg swelling and dependent edema suggests a diagnosis of deep venous thrombosis.

Unfortunately, because they more commonly exhibit atypical presentations, peripheral edema is not always a reliable indicator of heart failure in the elderly.

Jugular Venous Distention

Peripheral edema may not be a reliable indicator of heart failure, but jugular venous distention (JVD) in older adults is very suggestive of right heart failure. Chapter 5 contains a detailed description of estimating jugular venous pressure. Hepatojugular reflux, or distention of the jugular vein induced by manual pressure over the liver, is also a reliable indicator of right heart insufficiency in the elderly.[8] When performing the inspection portion of the physical examination, be sure to make a neck vein assessment.

Palpation

Touching the patient to evaluate for the presence of pathology can assist in the process of assessment. Normally, palpation includes an evaluation for fremitus, an estimation of thoracic expansion and feeling for crepitus. In older patients, palpation may initially be a scouting maneuver for skin condition, scars, signs of infection, and the presence of bumps or bruises.

When assessing patients whose respiration is being aided with mechanical ventilators, those who have had thoracic surgery, or those who have sustained trauma, palpate first for sub-cutaneous emphysema. Start assessing at the neck and, using fingertips, gently "walk" down the sides of the neck from the jaw to the clavicle. Crepitus feels like crackling under the skin. Crepitus associated with subcutaneous emphysema is more common in patients who have sustained intrathoracic trauma or barotrauma.

Fremitus consists of palpable vibrations felt on the chest wall when the patient is repeating a sound. The vibrations caused by sound increase over areas of consolidation. Evaluating for fremitus requires a cooperative patient. Likewise, estimating thoracic expansion by palpation requires deep inspiratory and expiratory maneuvers. These maneuvers may be physically difficult for elderly patients to perform. Palpate for chest excursion on a case-by-case basis.

Pulmonary Auscultation

Assessing lung sounds can generate very useful diagnostic information. Abnormal or added lung sounds are referred to as *adventitious* and can be classified as *crackles* or *wheezes*. A few simple questions can be used to classify lung sounds and guide the diagnosis.

Questions to Ask Yourself About LUNG SOUNDS

Is the sound continuous or discontinuous?
Is the sound on one side or both?
Is the sound on inspiration or expiration?
Does the sound clear with coughing?

Older adult patients may not be able to sustain good-quality deep breathing. They may only be able to give you three to four good, deep breaths before they tire. In a quiet environment, with the patient leaning forward, assess posterior lobes first. Position your stethoscope (on skin) midway between the patient's waist and scapula, and get four good bilateral breaths. Listen for a full inspiratory/expiratory (I/E) cycle. Moving the stethoscope from side to side, compare sounds; then, proceed with anterior and lateral chest assessment. Because the patient will be taking deeper breaths during the examination, caution must be exercised to prevent hyperventilation. Ask the patient to report any feelings of dizziness.

Auscultation may reveal diminished breath sounds even in older patients with healthy lungs. An increased anteroposterior diameter and shallow breathing are common in the elderly and add to the difficulty of hearing normal vesicular breath sounds. However, pathologic conditions still produce characteristic wheezes and crackles. Fine, inspiratory crackles are more likely to represent atelectasis, pulmonary fibrosis, or an acute inflammatory process in elderly patients.[16] When present, coarse crackles heard on both inspiration and expiration that do not clear with a cough may indicate severe pulmonary edema or severe pneumonia. CHF or asthma may cause wheezing.

SIMPLY STATED

During auscultation, start on the back, place the stethoscope on the patient's skin, and listen for a full I/E cycle.

Cardiac Auscultation

The growing population of older patients is presenting a unique challenge for healthcare providers. Care of adult patients requires at least a working knowledge of cardiac assessment. Cardiac conduction defects, disease, and valvular incompetence can all result in altered heart sounds and murmurs.

Heart Sounds

In about 30% to 40% of elderly patients, you may note an audible splitting of the second heart sound (S_2). Significant splitting of the S_2 that increases with inspiration suggests the presence of right bundle branch block. An S_3 is indicative of ventricular disease in the elderly and can be auscultated in the same vertical line as S_2, but about 2 inches lower at the fourth intercostal space. It may be one of the earliest markers of CHF. S_4 sounds, when present, can be heard best at the fifth intercostal space, midclavicular line, left side. An S_4 is a sign of ventricular disease, as in the patient with CHF or recent MI.

Heart Murmurs

Heart murmurs are a swooshing sound also described as sustained noises (e.g., blowing, harsh, rough, or rumbling sounds). Heart murmurs are most often the result of valvular heart disease and can be caused by stenosis, regurgitation, or valvular incompetence. Murmurs can be further classified as systolic or diastolic. Systolic ejection murmurs, usually in the aortic valve, are detected in about 50% of elderly patients.[16] Some murmurs indicate life-threatening illness. Trauma, infective endocarditis, aortic dissection, papillary muscle, or septal rupture are all acute, severe heart problems and may cause harsh regurgitant murmurs. Urgent attention is indicated.

Infective endocarditis has become more prevalent in older adults despite advances in antibiotic therapy. The increased numbers of older adults accounts for some of the statistical increases. Also factoring into the picture are an increase in the number of older adults with prosthetic valves, a higher prevalence of hospital-acquired bacteremia, and longer survival of persons with a history of rheumatic heart disease. Cardiac murmurs are found in more than 90% of patients with infective endocarditis.[8]

Heart sounds are usually softer in older adults. This may be the result of weakened myocardial function or an increased AP diameter. An increased AP diameter increases the distance between the heart and chest wall and will make detection of the heart sounds more difficult. Take time to listen to heart sounds. The more you listen, the more skilled you will become at distinguishing subtle abnormalities.

DIAGNOSTIC TESTS

Physiologic and structural changes in the pulmonary system will be manifested as alterations in common diagnostic tests. Arterial blood gases, pulse oximetry, and pulmonary function studies reveal age-associated changes. Age-appropriate norms should be taken into consideration when interpreting diagnostic tests.

Gas Exchange

The effects of pulmonary aging result in a reduced vital capacity and expiratory flow rates, an increase in closing volume, and reduced partial pressure of arterial oxygenation (PaO_2). To a certain degree, gas exchange is altered even in healthy older adults.

Changes in closing volume and closing capacity affect gas exchange. Closing volume is the volume of gas in the lungs in excess of residual volume at end exhalation. This additional volume is the result of small airway closure in the dependent, lower portions of the lungs that occurs during maximal exhalation. Closing capacity is simply closing volume added to residual volume. The closing capacity increases from about 30% of total lung capacity at age 20 years to about 50% of total lung capacity at age 70. This closure reduces ventilation to lower lung regions and shifts the distribution of ventilation to upper lung regions. Although perfusion increases slightly in the upper regions of aged lungs, the majority of blood flow still perfuses the lower lung regions. These physiologic alterations, ventilation shifting to upper lung segments, and perfusion remaining in the gravity-dependent lower lung segments result in an increased ventilation/perfusion $\dot{V}/\dot{Q}$ mismatch.

As was stated earlier, there is an age-associated loss of alveolar surface area. The alveolar-arterial oxygen partial pressure gradient ($P[A - a]O_2$) is also increased in older adults; this could be a consequence of either intrapulmonary shunting, diffusion limitation of oxygen/carbon dioxide gas exchange, or $\dot{V}/\dot{Q}$ abnormalities. A study was conducted on normal subjects (lifetime nonsmokers with normal spirometry) aged 18 to 71 years. The age-related increase in $\dot{V}/\dot{Q}$ mismatching was confirmed, but it was not as great as expected. The amount of intrapulmonary shunting was almost negligible (less than 1% of cardiac output in 90% of cases), and the PaO_2 was reduced but only slightly.[30]

Arterial Blood Gases

Arterial partial pressure of oxygen (PaO_2) declines with age. The linear deterioration of arterial oxygen tension associated with aging is now projected to be about -0.245 mm Hg/year.[32]

The age-associated decline in PaO_2, although predictable, has been the subject of recent investigation. Some of the traditional arterial oxygenation reference studies did not include adequate samples of subjects older than 60 years, yet these studies were used to extrapolate beyond age 60.[31] A newer study conducted in 1995 included a large sample of subjects' aged 40 to 90 years. This investigation demonstrated that PaO_2 values clearly declined up to age 75 and then tended to rise (Figure 12-2). The mean PaO_2 value for adults older than 75 years was demonstrated to be approximately 83 mm Hg.[32] A more recent study (1999) measured PaO_2 on more than 330 healthy subjects aged 18 to 81 years at two different barometric pressures—sea level and 1400 meters. The decline in PaO_2 in this study[33] (-0.245 mm Hg/year) was consistent with the decline in other studies.[34,35]

Based on a decline of -0.245 mm Hg/year, Table 12-2 provides a new estimate of age-related PaO_2 changes.

Even though the PaO_2 is reduced as a result of aging, in the absence of disease the PaO_2 is adequate to provide for tissue oxygenation. Oxygen consumption declines with age in both males and females as a result of reduced metabolism and the replacement of lean tissue with fat.

Some hypercapnia is occasionally noted in elderly patients, but there does not seem to be a consistent age-related alteration in $PaCO_2$. This could be the result of a greater diffusibility of carbon dioxide through the alveolar-capillary membrane and the differences in the oxygen and carbon dioxide dissociation curves.[36]

Pulse Oximetry

The mild reduction in PaO_2 common to older adults will be consistent with lower oxygen saturation as measured by pulse oximetry (SpO_2). A PaO_2 of 60 mm Hg corresponds to a SpO_2 of 90%. As long as the patient's PaO_2 values remain on the flat

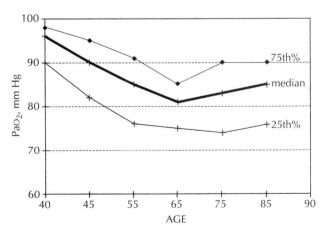

Figure 12-2 In healthy people, arterial oxygen (PaO_2) decreases throughout middle age, but stabilizes beyond age 65 years. (From Hazzard WR, Blass JP, Halter JB, et al, editors: *Principles of geriatric medicine and gerontology*, ed 5, New York, Pa, 2003, McGraw-Hill.)

Table 12-2	Estimated Age-Associated Change in Pao$_2$ by Decade

Age (years)	Estimated Pao$_2$ (mm Hg)
10	100
20	97.55
30	95.1
40	92.65
50	90.2
60	87.75
70	85.30
80	82.85
90	80.4
100	77.95

BOX 12-2	Age-Associated Pulmonary Function Test Changes

Reduced vital capacity, both slow and forced
Reduced peak expiratory flows
Reduced inspiratory capacity
Reduced forced expiratory flows ($FEF_{25\%-75\%}$)
Reduced forced expiratory volume in 1 second
Decreased diffusing capacity
Increased residual volume
Increased functional residual capacity

portion of the oxyhemoglobin dissociation curve, the aging process does not significantly decrease the SpO$_2$.

Some of the factors that cause pulse oximeters to inaccurately record SpO$_2$ are severe or rapid desaturation, hypotension, hypothermia, abnormal hemoglobin, and low perfusion.[37] The presence of a good, measurable pulse is essential to the measurement of SpO$_2$. Unfortunately, in some older patients with poor perfusion/circulation, obtaining a reading can be a problem.

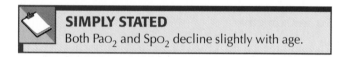

SIMPLY STATED
Both Pao$_2$ and SpO$_2$ decline slightly with age.

Pulmonary Function Studies

After the age of 25 years, pulmonary function in adults starts to decline gradually. The loss of elastic recoil and stiffening of the chest wall shift the balance of lung volumes and capacities. The total lung capacity and tidal volume remain relatively stable throughout the adult life span. The big change is in the residual volume, which almost doubles with advanced age.

The effect of senescence on pulmonary function measurements has been well documented. When trying to diagnose functional impairment of airflow by performing pulmonary function studies in older adults, it is important that age-appropriate norms be used as a standard (see Box 12-2).

The effect of changes in lung and chest wall mechanics cause forced vital capacity (FVC) and forced expiratory volume in 1 second (FEV$_1$) to diminish as early as age 20. The mean rate of decline is approximately 30 mL/year for men and 23 mL/year for women.[8]

Diffusing capacity of the lung for carbon monoxide (DLCO) peaks in persons in their early 20s and then gradually decreases. The reduction is estimated to be 2.03 mL/min/mm Hg/year in men.[8] Women normally have a 10% lower diffusing capacity than men of equal height and weight. Because of age-related changes in V̇/Q̇ and loss of alveolar surface area, the

age-related decline in DLCO is not linear. Decremental changes in total pulmonary diffusing capacity become more prominent after the age of 40 years.[8]

Standard pulmonary function testing in the elderly requires significant coordination and cooperation on the part of the therapist and patient. Explaining the procedure to the patient may take additional time and require more demonstration. Frequent maneuvers such as repeated breath holding and timed effort-dependent exhalations are required. The extra exertion may be difficult for some patients. After obtaining the best data possible, a consultation with the pulmonologist concerning the patient's level of comprehension and performance may assist in the interpretation of results.

Prediction regression formulas for pulmonary function tests and prediction nomograms for spirometric values are available. The formulas are both age variable and gender specific. The nomograms can accommodate persons aged 20 to 90 years and are also gender specific.

It is important to remember that the predicted values are derived from a statistical analysis of "normal" subjects. These test subjects are classified as normal based on the absence of history or symptoms of lung disease in themselves or their families. Minimal exposure to environmental risk factors (e.g., smoking, pollution) would also be a criterion in selecting these subjects.[38]

Older adults being seen by pulmonary specialists rarely are without a component of lung disease or environmental risk factors. When interpreting pulmonary function studies as part of a geriatric assessment, the age-related deviation from normal must be taken into consideration.

Laboratory Values

Many factors are responsible for the alteration in laboratory values of older adults. Diet, exercise, multisystem disease, and physiologic and structural age-related changes are all variables, which make determination of "normal" a challenge. The normal value for a laboratory test is its mean value +/−2 standard deviations in a population of healthy persons.[8] An abnormal result does not necessarily confirm the presence of disease or disorder. The likelihood of disease is estimated by knowing the test's specificity and sensitivity. Clinicians do not always have precise information on the specificity and sensitivity of tests in the elderly, and the prevalence of disease often differs in older populations.[8] Box 12-3 shows some laboratory values and the increases/decreases that can result from the aging process.

Hematology

Total hemoglobin in both males and females may remain in the normal range or decrease slightly with age. The decrease is related to the reduced formation and development of blood cells in the bone marrow. In men, reduced hemoglobin may also be a factor of a drop in androgen. Hematocrit may also decrease slightly, related to reduced hematopoiesis (see Chapter 6). Aging is not associated with significant changes in the white cell count; however, leukopenia, most frequently neutropenia, occurs in conjunction with a broad spectrum of medical problems. In older adults, leukopenia is likely the result of acquired or secondary disorders, either reactive (e.g., medications, nutritional deficits, infections, diminished T and B lymphocytes) or malignant.[16]

Blood Chemistry

Age-related albumin reduction is related to a reduced liver size, blood flow, and enzyme production. Low serum albumin can also be a factor of malnutrition. Blood urea nitrogen may remain unchanged or may increase when related to compromised renal function. Creatinine clearance declines, but serum creatinine levels remain stable because elderly persons have less muscle mass. Creatinine clearance as a measure of kidney function is useful information in prescribing drugs for the elderly. Formulas and nomograms are available for determining age-adjusted normal values for clearance of creatinine. In patients with a reduced creatinine clearance, some drugs need to be modified as to dosage to prevent the development of a drug toxicity. Serum calcium levels will be slightly decreased, whereas potassium will be slightly increased. Fasting glucose increases with age, but values usually remain within the normal range. Glucose tolerance decreases gradually with age. The lack of exercise, obesity, and some medications, however, can exert more influence on glucose tolerance than age alone. When testing for glucose tolerance, there will be a higher peak in 2 hours with a slower decline to base in older adults.[28]

Because variability is a hallmark of aging, it is difficult to extrapolate norms with confidence in the elderly. Of more use would be the establishment of norms for each individual when healthy, to compare with laboratory values when diagnosing a new condition or disease. This, of course, is not feasible with anything except routine tests performed at the time of annual physical examinations. The value of doing an occasional blood-screening test in healthy elderly adults would be appreciated, however, when facing a challenging disease or diagnosis.

> **SIMPLY STATED**
> In older adults, do not assume that variations from the norm are always abnormal or that normal values are always an indicator of health.

COMPREHENSIVE GERIATRIC ASSESSMENT

Performing a comprehensive geriatric assessment has become an established component of medical practice, given the growing population of older adults. The needs of many frail elderly patients are too broad to be met by an assessment based only on diagnosis. Because the symptoms that cause the patient to seek medical attention are not always directly related to the disease, a more thorough investigation is warranted. For example, a patient may seek help because of an unstable gait and an inability to walk. The underlying diagnosis may be CHF that has produced peripheral edema, causing problems with locomotion before the obvious shortness of breath is noticeable.

Comprehensive geriatric assessment is considered by most geriatricians to be an important and effective form of secondary and tertiary care for the elderly.[16] Recently, some managed care organizations have realized the potential benefits of preventive intervention. The principle forces driving the managed care of older patients in the United States are Congress and the Health Care Financing Administration (HCFA). The Congressional Balanced Budget Act of 1997 mandated that Medicare managed care organizations no longer be called "risk contractors," but rather "coordinated care plans."[39] Coordinated care planning opens the door to an opportunity to apply principles of geriatric assessment to a large population of older adults.

BOX 12-3	Effect of Aging on Laboratory Values

Increased Values	Decreased Values
Sedimentation rate (mild elevation)	Creatinine clearance
Serum glucose	Albumin
Serum cholesterol	Serum calcium
Serum triglycerides	Serum iron
Serum uric acid	Serum phosphorus
Serum fibrinogen	Serum zinc
Serum copper	Serum vitamins B_6, B_{12}, and C
Serum norepinephrine	
Prostate-specific antigen	
Serum potassium (slight increase)	

Unchanged Values

Hemoglobin
Red blood cell count
White blood cell count
Blood urea nitrogen
Serum creatinine
Serum electrolytes (sodium, chloride, and bicarbonate)

References: Abrams WB, Beers MH, Berkow R, editors: *The Merck manual of geriatrics*, ed 2, Whitehouse Station, NJ, 1995, Merck; and Lamy PP: *Prescribing for the elderly*, New York, 1980, PSG.

An improvement in functional ability, rather than a cure, is often the most important goal of geriatric assessment. Geriatric assessment is time consuming. It involves not only looking at physical health but also upper and lower extremity function, nutrition, and mental status. Screening for depression, urinary incontinence, a social support network, the adequacy of the home environment, and functional ability are all components of the comprehensive geriatric assessment.

Functional Ability

Although not usually assessed by respiratory therapists, the functional ability of older adults is closely related to a perceived index of health. As a general rule, health in late life is usually not defined as staying out of the hospital so much as it is retaining the ability to perform daily activities.[40] An often-heard statement from older adults is "I don't feel old as long as I can get around and do things."

Because "health" is so closely correlated with "ability" in older patients, perhaps a brief review of patient's abilities would be beneficial. How often, as clinicians, do we deal with older patients suffering from hospital psychosis? Because patients are out of their familiar environment, away from their usual caregivers, and sick, depression often becomes a problem. Asking simple questions about their abilities may put a more positive focus on what the patients can do versus the temporary losses they are suffering. A positive attitude can have a large impact on a patient's outlook for recovery.

Activities of Daily Living

A number of instruments have been developed for measuring the older adult's ability to complete activities of daily living (ADLs). The basic ADLs usually assessed are mobility and the ability to participate in personal hygiene/grooming, to feed oneself, to carry out toileting, and to dress oneself. To carry out these ADLs, patients must have sufficient range of motion, strength, and endurance.

Instrumental Activities of Daily Living

Some measurement tools have been designed to evaluate more complex skills, known as *instrumental activities of daily living* (IADL). Household management skills, money management, the ability to use the telephone, writing skills, and the ability to shop are categorized as IADLs.

Since only about 5% of adults older than 65 years in the United States are residents of nursing homes, the hospitalized patient population includes a large percent of noninstitutionalized older adults with a relatively high degree of functional ability.

Deterioration of functional ability in previously unimpaired elderly persons is an early, subtle sign of illness and is often not accompanied by typical disease signs and symptoms. As soon as functional impairment develops, a thorough clinical evaluation will best serve the patient in maintaining quality of life.

SUMMARY

Older adults live with multiple chronic conditions. Many of these conditions require intermittent hospitalization. Because of age-related changes in the body's organ systems, older adults do not respond as quickly as younger adults, and recovery time is lengthened. An accurate and timely patient assessment can facilitate early entry into appropriate disease management. Geriatric assessment can be time consuming and challenging to perform. Age-associated sensory, physical, and psychological decremental changes in older adults must be taken into consideration. Unusual presenting signs and symptoms occasionally mask disease processes in elderly patients. Comprehensive geriatric assessment, which encompasses a wide variety of systems assessment, is becoming more common as managed care organizations realize the benefits of preventive intervention.

Respiratory therapists, as members of the healthcare team, must be skilled at and involved in geriatric patient assessment. The patient's own assessment of his/her health status is often the best predictor of survival. It is a wise clinician who understands, accepts, and works with this information.

REVIEW QUESTIONS

1. Communicating with older adults is which of the following?
   a. A waste of time if they can't respond
   b. Unnecessary; just check their ID band
   c. A time-consuming task if done appropriately
   d. Impossible when they can't see or hear well

2. Which of the following statements might reflect an ageist attitude?
   a. Many older adults have poor vision.
   b. Most older adults are sick and frail.
   c. Many older adults have some measure of hearing loss.
   d. Most older adults have some degree of cardiac hypertrophy.

3. Which of the following medications might precipitate ototoxicity?
   a. Theophylline
   b. Atropine sulfate
   c. Antihistamines
   d. Aspirin

4. Which of the following is the major risk factor associated with development of cataract?
   a. Age
   b. Smoking
   c. Alcohol consumption
   d. Overexposure to bright light

5. Normal age-related restructuring of the heart results in an enlarged _____ wall.
   a. left ventricular
   b. right ventricular
   c. left atrial
   d. right atrial

6. Typical symptoms of right-sided heart failure include all of the following *except*:
   a. jugular venous distention.
   b. Cheyne-Stokes breathing.
   c. cyanosis.
   d. hepatomegaly.

7. Which of the following is *not* an age-related pulmonary change?
   a. Loss of elastic recoil
   b. Increase in functional residual capacity
   c. Increase in total lung compliance
   d. Decrease in vital capacity

8. Blunted cell-mediated immunity in older adults is one factor in the increased incidence of which of the following?
   a. Pneumonia
   b. Leukemia
   c. Emphysema
   d. Tuberculosis

9. List four atypical symptoms of acute myocardial infarct in older adults.

10. A 90-year-old patient is admitted to the hospital with a diagnosis of pneumonia. Based on your knowledge of pneumonia in older adults, you would most likely expect the patient to present with which of the following?
    a. An increased respiratory rate
    b. A productive cough
    c. An elevated body temperature
    d. Radiating chest pain

11. Which of the following is the definition of pulse pressure?
    a. A palpable apical pulse
    b. A pulse felt over the point of maximal impulse
    c. The sum of systolic and diastolic pressures
    d. The difference between systolic and diastolic pressures

12. Syncope associated with standing up quickly may be the result of which of the following?
    a. Hyperthermia
    b. Orthostatic hypertension
    c. Orthostatic hypotension
    d. Pulmonary hypertension

13. Which of the following is an abnormal heart sound in older adults that may be an early sign of CHF?
    a. S_1.
    b. S_2.
    c. S_3.
    d. S_4.

14. Which serum value may decrease as a result of the normal aging process?
    a. Glucose
    b. Calcium
    c. Creatinine
    d. Cholesterol

15. Which of the following activities would be classified as an independent activity of daily living (IADL)?
    a. Combing one's own hair
    b. Walking from the bedroom to the kitchen
    c. Calling the neighbor on the telephone
    d. Getting dressed by oneself

16. Based on current data, what is the estimated PaO_2 of a healthy 74-year-old?
    a. 74.4 mm Hg
    b. 80.8 mm Hg
    c. 84.2 mm Hg
    d. 87.2 mm Hg

17. Approximately what percent of adults older than 65 years of age in the United States live in a nursing home?
    a. 5%
    b. 10%
    c. 15%
    d. 20%

18. T F Functional ability can be directly correlated with the index of health.

19. T F Immunizations for older adults are a waste of time.

20. T F Ageism is a process of stereotyping and discriminating against people because they are old.

REFERENCES

1. National Center for Health Statistics. Physician visits increase for older patients. News Release, July 17, 2003, Hyattsville, Md.
2. U.S. Census Bureau: Statistical Abstract of the United States; Health and Nutrition, Table 159, 2001.
3. Townsend D: Geriatric Patient Assessment (conference) Omaha, Neb, 1998, Debra's Concepts of Care, Inc.
4. Siedman MD, et al: Molecular mechanisms of age-related hearing loss. *Ageing Research and Reviews* 1(3):331-343, 2002.
5. Davis A: Prevalence of hearing impairment. In Davis A, editors: *Hearing in adults*. London, 1994, Whurr Publishers Ltd.

6. Keller BK, et al: The effect of visual and hearing impairment on functional status. *J Am Geriatr Soc* 47(11):1319-1325, 1999.

7. Noell CA, Meyerhoff WL: Tinnitus: diagnosis and treatment of this elusive symptom. *Geriatrics* 58(2):28-34, 2003.

8. Beers MH, Berkow R, editors: *The Merck manual of geriatrics*, ed 3. Whitehouse Station, NJ, 2000, Merck & Company.

9. Mulrow CD, Lichtenstein. MJ: Screening for hearing impairment in the elderly: rationale and strategy. *J Gen Intern Med* 6:249-258, 1991.

10. Brennan M, Cardinali G: The use of preexisting and novel coping strategies in adapting to age-related vision loss. *Gerontologist* 40:327-334, 2000.

11. Warnecke P: A caregiver's eye on elders with low vision. *CARING Magazine* January:12-15, 2003.

12. Oxenham H, Sharpe N: Cardiovascular aging and heart failure. *Eur J Heart Failure* 5:427-434, 2003.

13. Kaloustian K: Effects of exercise on the cardiovascular system. Presented at the AGHE Annual Meeting, San Jose, Calif. February 22-25, 2001.

14. Waktare JEP: Atrial fibrillation. *Circulation* 106:14-16, 2002.

15. Connolly MJ, editor: *Respiratory disease in the elderly*. London, 1996, Chapman & Hall.

16. Hazzard WR and others, editors: In *Principles of geriatric medicine and gerontology*, ed 5. York, Pa, 2003, McGraw-Hill.

17. Emmett KR: Nonspecific and atypical presentation of disease in the older patient. *Geriatrics* 53(2):50-60, 1998.

18. Feldman C: Pneumonia in the elderly. *Clin Chest Med* 20:563,1999.

19. Ham RJ, Sloane PD, Warshaw GA, editors: *Primary care geriatrics*, ed 4. St. Louis, 2002, Mosby.

20. Nadelmann J, et al: Prevalence, incidence, and prognosis of recognized and unrecognized myocardial infarction in people aged 75 and older: the Bronx Aging Study. *Am J Cardiol* 66:533, 1990.

21. Huss K, Travis P: Prevalence, severity of asthma continues to rise in the elderly. *Academy News* February/March 1997, American Academy of Allergies, Asthma & Immunology.

22. Braman SS: Asthma in the elderly. *Clin Geriatr Med* 19: 57-75, 2003.

23. Enright PL and others: Underdiagnosis and undertreatment of asthma in the elderly. *Chest* 116:603-613, 1999.

24. Perry HM and others: Effect of treating isolated systolic hypertension on the risk of developing various types and subtypes of stroke: the Systolic Hypertension in the Elderly Program (SHEP). *JAMA* 284:465-471, 2000.

25. Griffith RW: High blood pressure: new guidelines are out! *Health and Age* June 5, 2003. Available at http://www.healthandage.com.

26. Chobanian AV and others: The Seventh Report of the Joint National Committee on Prevention, Detection, Evaluation, and Treatment of High Blood Pressure. *JAMA* 289:2560-2571, 2003.

27. Spratto GR, Woods AL: *Nurses drug reference*. Albany, NY 1994, Delmar.

28. Hogstel MO: *Nursing care of the older adult*. Albany, NY, 1994, Delmar.

29. Emlet CA and others: *In home assessment of older adults*. Gaithersburg, Md, 1996, Aspen Publishers.

30. Cardús J and others: Increase in pulmonary ventilation-perfusion inequality with age in healthy subjects. *Am J Respir Crit Care Med* 156:648-653, 1997.

31. Hazzard WR, editor: *Principles of geriatric medicine*. New York, 1998, McGraw-Hill.

32. Cerveri I and others: Reference values of arterial oxygen tension in the middle-aged and elderly. *Am J Respir Crit Care Med* 152:934-941, 1995.

33. Crapo RO, et al: Arterial blood gas reference values for sea level and an altitude of 1,400 meters. *Am J Respir Crit Care Med* 160:1525-1531, 1999.

34. Raine JM, Bishop JM: A-a difference in O_2 tension and physiologic dead space in normal man. *J Appl Physiol* 18:284-288, 1963.

35. Marshall BE, Millar RA: Some factors influencing postoperative hypoxemia. *Anesthesia* 20:408-428, 1965.

36. Levitsky MG: *Pulmonary physiology*, ed 3. New York, 1991, McGraw-Hill.

37. Jensen LA, et al: Meta-analysis of arterial oxygen saturation monitoring by pulse oximetry in adults. *Heart Lung* 27:387-408, 1998.

38. Ruppel GL: *Manual of pulmonary function testing*, ed 8. St. Louis, Mo, 2003, Mosby.

39. Fillit HM, et al: How the principles of geriatric assessment are shaping managed care. *Geriatrics* 53:76, 1998.

40. Thorson JA: *Aging in a changing society*. Belmont, Calif, 1995, Wadsworth.

13

Michael H. Terry

Respiratory Monitoring in the Intensive Care Unit

LEARNING OBJECTIVES

Upon completion of this chapter, the reader should be able to accomplish the following:

1. Identify the methods, normal values, and significance of measuring the following lung volumes in the intensive care unit:
   a. Tidal volume
   b. Vital capacity
   c. Functional residual capacity
2. Recognize the methods, normal values, and significance of measuring the following airway pressures or related indices in the intensive care unit:
   a. Peak pressure
   b. Plateau pressure
   c. Compliance
   d. Airway resistance
   e. Mean airway pressure
   f. Maximum inspiratory pressure
3. Recognize the definition, methods of detection, and methods of minimizing auto-PEEP.
4. Recognize the value of monitoring pressure, volume, and flow tracings in mechanically ventilated patients.
5. Recognize the methods and significance of measuring the fraction of inspired oxygen and exhaled carbon dioxide in the intensive care unit.
6. Identify the components of oxygen transport and their significance.
7. Identify the components involved in the clinical evaluation of oxygenation and their significance.
8. Recognize how the following parameters can be used to evaluate tissue oxygen delivery and utilization:
   a. Oxygen delivery and availability
   b. Oxygen consumption
   c. Mixed venous oxygen tension
   d. Venous saturation
   e. Arterial to mixed venous oxygen content difference
   f. Oxygen extraction ratio
   g. Blood lactate
9. Recognize the value and limitations of pulse oximetry in monitoring oxygenation and oxygen delivery.

CHAPTER OUTLINE
Ventilatory Assessment
    Lung Volumes and Flows
    Airway Pressures
    Integrating Pressure, Flow, and Volume
    Fractional Gas Concentrations
Evaluation of Oxygenation
    Evaluation of Oxygen Transport
    Monitoring the Adequacy of Arterial Oxygenation
    Monitoring Tissue Oxygen Delivery and Utilization

KEY TERMS
airway resistance
alveolar dead space
anatomic dead space
arterial-mixed venous oxygen content difference $[C(a - \bar{v})O_2]$
auto-PEEP
capnography
capnometry
carbon dioxide production $(\dot{V}CO_2)$
compliance
dead space–tidal volume ratio (V_D/V_T)
dynamic compliance
dynamic hyperinflation
end-tidal P_{CO_2} ($P_{ET}CO_2$)
Fick principle

fractional saturation
functional residual capacity (FRC)
functional saturation
intrapulmonary shunt $(\dot{Q}S/\dot{Q}T)$
lower inflection point
maximum inspiratory pressure ($P_{I\,max}$)
mean airway pressure
mixed venous oxygen tension ($P\bar{v}O_2$)
mixed venous oxygen saturation ($S\bar{v}O_2$)
monitoring
oxygen consumption
oxygen content
oxygen delivery (DO_2)

Tom Malinowski, BS, RRT, RCP, contributed this chapter in the previous edition.

oxygen extraction ratio
  $[C(a - \bar{v})O_2/CaO_2]$
oxygen transport
oxyhemoglobin
  dissociation curve
  (ODC)
PaO_2/PAO_2 ratio
peak pressure
physiologic dead space

plateau pressure
pressure-volume loop
pulse oximetry
rapid-shallow breathing
  index (RSBI)
static compliance
upper inflection point
volutrauma

CHAPTER OVERVIEW

Monitoring has been defined as "repeated or continuous observations or measurements of the patient, his or her physiologic function, and the function of life support equipment, for the purpose of guiding management decisions, including when to make therapeutic interventions, and assessment of those interventions."[1]

Respiratory monitoring refers to the process of continuously evaluating the cardiopulmonary status of patients for the purpose of improving clinical management. The goals of monitoring include alerting clinicians to changes in the patient's condition and improving our understanding of pathophysiology, diagnosis, and cost-effective clinical management. This is accomplished through the use of physical examination, measurements and calculations, and alarms.

The goals of this chapter are to introduce the tools available for the most common forms of respiratory monitoring, describe the information they can provide, and state when they should and should not be used. This chapter describes primarily ventilatory and oxygenation assessment. Some of the information that normally would be included under respiratory monitoring, such as physical assessment and blood gas interpretation, is reviewed in other chapters of this book.

VENTILATORY ASSESSMENT

Arterial PCO_2 is traditionally thought of as the standard for assessing ventilation[2] (see Chapter 7). However, changes in the patient's metabolism, lung mechanics, ventilatory efficiency, and equipment function will occur before changes are seen in the blood gases. It is therefore important to monitor the ventilatory parameters in addition to the blood gases.

The ventilatory measurements that can be monitored at the bedside in the intensive care unit (ICU) routinely include the following:
- Lung volumes and flows
- Airway pressures
- Fractional gas concentrations

Lung Volumes and Flows

Ventilation is the process of moving gases between the atmosphere and the lung. These gases occupy spaces commonly called *lung volumes*. Lung volumes have been described and their meas-

urement discussed in Chapter 8, but their importance to the critical care clinician is emphasized here.

Why Monitor Lung Volumes?

There are four reasons why lung volumes are important to the clinician:
- They affect gas exchange in the lung.
- They reflect changes in patient's clinical status (improvement or deterioration).
- They indicate response to therapy.
- They signal problems with patient/ventilator interface (i.e., circuitry, ventilator settings)

Who Should Be Monitored for Lung Volumes?

Following is a list of the most common circumstances in which patients will benefit from the monitoring of lung volumes:
A. Intubated patients
  1. Patients being considered for mechanical ventilation
  2. Patients receiving and being weaned from mechanical ventilation
  3. Patients with an abnormal breathing pattern
B. Nonintubated patients
  1. Preoperative evaluation (especially upper abdominal and thoracic surgery)
  2. Adult patients with respiratory rates greater than 30 breaths per minute
  3. Patients with neuromuscular disease
  4. Patients with central nervous system (CNS) depression
  5. Patients with deteriorating blood gases
  6. Patients receiving noninvasive positive-pressure ventilation

What Do We Measure?

Tidal volume (V_T) is defined as the volume of air inspired or passively exhaled in a normal respiratory cycle. V_T for a healthy person varies with each breath but is usually 5 to 7 mL/kg of ideal body weight.

V_T has two components: alveolar volume (V_A), or the portion of V_T that effectively exchanges with alveolar-capillary blood, and dead space volume (V_D), or the portion of V_T that does not exchange with capillary blood. The V_D is normally about 2 mL/kg of ideal body weight, or about 25% to 30% of the V_T, and consists of the conductive airways and alveolar units that are ventilated but not perfused. This is the true or physiologic dead space.

In healthy, spontaneously breathing persons, the V_T occasionally increases to three or four times normal levels. These larger tidal breaths are known as *sighs* and normally occur about six to ten times each hour. In acutely ill patients there is often a loss of the sigh, and the size of the patient's V_T tends to diminish.[3] In addition, the V_T does not vary from breath to breath.[4] Impending respiratory failure causes V_T to become more irregular. If shallow breathing without occasional sighing is maintained for prolonged periods, atelectasis and pneumonia may result, especially in patients breathing high oxygen concentrations or in patients with a compromised mucociliary clearance mechanism.

Conditions that may cause the V_T to be reduced include pneumonia, atelectasis, the postoperative period following chest and abdominal surgery, chest trauma, acute exacerbation of chronic obstructive pulmonary disease (COPD), congestive heart failure (CHF), pulmonary edema, acute restrictive diseases such as acute respiratory distress syndrome (ARDS), neuromuscular diseases, and CNS depression (especially of the respiratory centers).

Larger-than-normal V_T may be seen with metabolic acidosis or severe neurologic injury.

Critically ill patients without an artificial airway may not tolerate the measurement of V_T. To get accurate measurements, the use of a face mask or mouthpiece is required. Patients often change their breathing patterns when a mask or mouthpiece is applied, thereby altering their V_T.

Patients receiving continuous mechanical ventilation (CMV) are routinely ventilated with tidal volumes of 10 to 12 mL/kg, two to three times the normal spontaneous V_T (5 to 7 mL/kg). When normal spontaneous V_T is used during CMV without positive end-expiratory pressure (PEEP), there is a reduction in functional residual capacity (FRC), an increase in intrapulmonary shunt, and a fall in partial pressure of arterial oxygen (PaO_2). These potentially harmful conditions can be reversed in part or totally by increasing the V_T to 10 to 12 mL/kg or by applying PEEP.[5]

The use of higher V_T ventilation can induce iatrogenic complications, particularly in patients with severe respiratory failure.[6,7] Considerable experimental evidence exists that lung injury may occur with high V_T that increases peak alveolar pressures (plateau pressure) beyond 30 cm H_2O.[8-10] The use of high-V_T ventilation may predispose patients to volutrauma, a lung injury that occurs from overdistention of the terminal respiratory units. Volutrauma often develops in nondependent lung regions and is a main reason why lung damage persists after recovery from severe protracted ARDS.[11] Consequently, patients at risk for developing ARDS should be ventilated with mechanical V_T of 6 to 8 mL/kg instead of 10 to 12 mL/kg.[12]

The application of PEEP in combination with smaller V_T maintains FRC and prevents the fall in PaO_2. This may suggest that an increase in mean lung volume is more important than larger V_T.[5,13]

Monitoring the V_T of the mechanically ventilated patient is crucial. Discrepancies between set and measured V_T are often seen in mechanically ventilated patients. Most of the time the differences are not clinically significant, and the clinician can make small adjustments in the V_T settings to adjust for the patient demands. The differences are often caused by the compressible volume of the ventilator circuit or environmental factors at the different locations of the inspiratory and expiratory flow sensors (i.e., heated, humidified gases, differing flow profiles). Compressible volume is an important consideration, particularly in patients with higher peak airway pressures and lower V_T. Other sources include pneumothorax, leaks in the

ventilator circuit, or a leaky endotracheal (ET) tube cuff. A low measured V_T can also be caused by "stacking" or dynamic hyperinflation, a problem seen with severe airway obstruction. If not enough time is allowed for exhalation before the next breath is initiated by the ventilator, the subsequent V_T will "stack" on top of the previous breath. Reduction of ventilator rate, increased inspiratory flows, bronchodilators and decreased V_T may help resolve the problem, which, if not corrected, can lead to severe barotrauma.

Where V_T is monitored often plays an important role in data interpretation. Proximal volume monitoring eliminates the compressible volume factor of tubing circuits and may more accurately reflect delivered V_T than does expiratory limb monitoring. This is particularly true during conditions of low V_T, low lung compliance, and high airway resistance. Proximal monitoring is not without drawbacks. Proximal sensing makes the measuring device more susceptible to condensate and secretions, potentially reducing reliability and accuracy. It may also increase circuit resistance and dead space, increasing the respiratory work for the patient.

Air trapping and dynamic hyperinflation often occur in mechanically ventilated patients with severe airway obstruction. One technique that can measure the degree of dynamic hyperinflation is to measure the volume of gas exhaled during a prolonged apnea (20 to 40 seconds) following a tidal breath from the ventilator. This maneuver measures the additional trapped gas above the patient's normal FRC. Ventilatory adjustments that reduce minute ventilation ($\dot{V}_E$) and lengthen expiratory time will reduce the degree of air trapping.

SIMPLY STATED

V_T for mechanically ventilated patients should be adjusted for clinical conditions. Some patients should be ventilated with a lower V_T of 6 to 8 mL/kg. These include those at risk of air trapping and dynamic hyperinflation or ARDS.

Patients receiving intermittent mandatory ventilation (IMV) and synchronized IMV (SIMV) are allowed to breathe spontaneously through the ventilator circuit between mechanical breaths. As a result, their spontaneous V_T may differ in size from the mechanical V_T being delivered by the ventilator. It is important for the clinician to distinguish between spontaneous and mechanical V_T during weaning so that a true assessment of the patient's ventilatory status can be made.

Before and during weaning from mechanical ventilation, spontaneous V_T should be monitored frequently. The adult patient's spontaneous V_T should be at least 300 mL if weaning is to be successful.[14] If V_T falls more than 25% during weaning, the clinician should be alerted to the possibility of impending respiratory muscle fatigue. This finding is often accompanied by a concurrent rise in the respiratory rate.

The rapid-shallow breathing index (RSBI) incorporates this spontaneous breath rate change and measures the ratio of respiratory frequency (f) to V_T.

$$RSBI = f\,(breaths/min)\,/\,V_T\,(liters)$$

RSBI values greater than 100 have been reported to be strong prognostic indicators of weaning failure. More predictive than a single measurement is the progressive change in RSBI. Patients who demonstrate a significant increase in their RSBI upon ventilator discontinuation are very likely to fail weaning.[15,16] Serial measurements of the RSBI index during a period of spontaneous breathing can more accurately predict the ability to be successfully weaned from mechanical ventilator support.[17]

$\dot{V}_E$ is the product of V_T and respiratory rate or frequency and represents the total volume of gas inspired or exhaled by the patient in 1 minute. The average $\dot{V}_E$ for a normal healthy adult is 4 to 8 L/min. As with V_T, approximately 25% to 30% of $\dot{V}_E$ is in the form of dead space ventilation. $\dot{V}_E$ is often increased in the early stages of respiratory failure; it is not until later stages of failure that $\dot{V}_E$ begins to fall.

Arterial carbon dioxide pressure ($PaCO_2$) is considered an indicator of the adequacy of ventilation. The relationship of $\dot{V}_E$ to $PaCO_2$ indicates the efficiency of ventilation. A $\dot{V}_E$ of 6 L/min is usually associated with a $PaCO_2$ of approximately 40 mm Hg in a healthy person with a normal metabolic rate. If a higher-than-normal $\dot{V}_E$ is associated with a normal $PaCO_2$ in a patient with a normal metabolic rate, there must be an increase in wasted or dead space ventilation. This is usually associated with hypovolemia, a decrease in lung perfusion as seen with pulmonary embolism, or reduced V_T.

An increase in carbon dioxide production caused by an increased metabolism (as occurs with trauma or fever) or high carbohydrate loading accompanying glucose administration via parenteral feedings may cause an increase in $\dot{V}_E$ with a normal $PaCO_2$ (see Chapter 17). The elevated production of carbon dioxide requires an increase in ventilation to maintain the $PaCO_2$ in normal range. The $PaCO_2$ of patients mechanically ventilated in the control mode varies with changes in metabolism. Patients with varying metabolic rates should be ventilated with modes that allow them to set their own respiratory rates and thereby increase $\dot{V}_E$ to clear higher levels of carbon dioxide produced.

When a $\dot{V}_E$ greater than 10 L/min is needed for a mechanically ventilated patient to maintain a normal $PaCO_2$, weaning is not likely to be successful. The elevated $\dot{V}_E$ indicates that the patient's respiratory muscles will probably fatigue when the mechanical ventilation is discontinued. A resting spontaneous $\dot{V}_E$ of 10 L/min or less during a T-piece trial is often considered an acceptable weaning criterion. Although spontaneous $\dot{V}_E$ is often used as a weaning criterion, it is often unreliable.[18,19]

$\dot{V}_E$ may fluctuate widely both during traditional T-piece weaning and during IMV and therefore should be monitored frequently before and during weaning. A rapid rise or a sudden drop in $\dot{V}_E$ should be investigated quickly because both may signal ventilatory failure.[14]

Many therapeutic activities can alter $\dot{V}_E$. A good example is the postoperative administration of opiates to control pain. Opiates can blunt the respiratory drive sufficiently to cause a sudden onset of hypoventilation.

Vital capacity (VC) is the maximum volume of gas that can be expired from the lungs following a maximal inspiration.

Normal values for healthy persons range from 60 to 80 mL/kg of ideal body weight. The VC maneuver is position dependent, the largest values usually being recorded with the patient in the upright position.

The VC is an excellent measurement of ventilatory reserve in the cooperative patient. It reflects the respiratory muscle strength and volume capacity of the lung while the patient is performing a sustained maximal inspiratory or expiratory maneuver. These are of paramount importance in maintaining an adequate cough to clear secretions and in guaranteeing periodic inflation of alveoli that may be prone to collapse.

VC can be measured as either a forced maneuver (forced vital capacity [FVC]) or a slow expiratory maneuver (slow vital capacity [SVC]). An FVC maneuver also provides expiratory flow values and an indication of airway resistance (Rāw). The SVC maneuver may be much easier for the patient to perform, especially if the patient is lethargic, is medicated, is experiencing pain, or has obstructive airway disease.

The accuracy and repeatability of the values depend on the patient's effort and the coaching skills of the clinician. It is important that the patient understand how to perform the maneuver correctly. A tight seal around the mouthpiece or mask is crucial. The patient may perform better if able to observe the tracing generated by the effort or to receive some similar visual feedback.

During preoperative evaluation of a patient's lung function, findings of a reduction in forced expiratory volume in 1 second (FEV_1/FVC%) to less than 50% of normal, or an FVC of less than 20 mL/kg, because of nonreversible obstructive or restrictive disease indicate that the patient is at high risk for developing pulmonary complications in the postoperative period. Factors that influence the degree of decrease in VC during the postoperative period and the incidence of postoperative pulmonary complications include the surgical site, smoking history, age, nutritional status, obesity, pain, type of anesthesia, and type of narcotics used for pain control.

> **SIMPLY STATED**
> Serial, not individual, measurements of weaning indices (RSBI, VC, V_T) are most likely to predict success or failure.

Although many factors can contribute to a reduction in VC postoperatively, one of the most important is the incision site. Thoracoabdominal incisions are associated with the highest incidence of postoperative morbidity, followed by upper abdominal incisions, then transsternal surgery. Thoracic and upper abdominal surgery produce a significant fall in VC within the first day postoperatively. This reduction may persist for up to 2 weeks.[20] Operative procedures below the umbilicus are associated with fewer pulmonary complications, even in patients with preexisting pulmonary disease.

A VC of 10 to 15 mL/kg is usually needed for effective deep breathing and coughing. Values of less than 10 mL/kg are usually associated with impending respiratory failure.

Values greater than 10 mL/kg usually indicate adequate ventilatory reserve and the possibility of discontinuing CMV and extubation.

VC is also measured in order to follow the responsiveness of the patient to various respiratory therapies, such as incentive spirometry or intermittent positive-pressure breathing (IPPB). A common goal of both these maneuvers is to promote lung expansion.

Functional residual capacity (FRC) is the volume of gas remaining in the lungs at the end of a normal passive exhalation. It is rarely measured in the ICU. The FRC is continuously in contact with pulmonary capillary blood and thereby undergoing gas exchange. It is composed of a combination of residual volume (RV) and expiratory reserve volume (ERV). Normally, FRC is about 40 mL/kg of ideal body weight, or approximately 35% to 40% of total lung capacity (TLC).

FRC can vary from breath to breath by as much as 300 mL in healthy persons.[21] Changes in body position affect FRC, with the greatest values being recorded in the upright position.[22-24] Using lung models, it has been estimated that 25% of a 500-mL V_T comes in contact and mixes with the FRC during each breath, thereby continuously supplying fresh oxygen-enriched air to the gas exchange units.[25] Prolonged changes in FRC can have a dramatic effect on gas exchange.

When alveolar volume falls, as with atelectasis, FRC is reduced and there are regional changes in alveolar pressure-volume curves. Initially, as FRC decreases, dependent alveoli collapse and require higher distending pressures to reinflate. Because the apical alveoli remain at least partially open, they are more compliant and require less pressure to reinflate. Subsequently, during mechanical ventilation, the inspired volumes are preferentially distributed to the apices. Unfortunately these apical alveoli are poorly perfused with blood. This distribution of inspired volumes to nondependent, poorly perfused alveoli contributes to the abnormal gas exchange seen in patients with decreased FRC. Experimental evidence now demonstrates that repeated collapse and reinflation of alveoli leads to alveolar damage, capillary rupture, and considerable lung injury. The application of PEEP prevents alveolar collapse and may reduce the extent of acute lung injury.[26-28]

Therapeutic modalities such as PEEP or continuous positive airway pressure (CPAP) increase FRC.[29,30] This is a primary benefit to patients with atelectasis and refractory hypoxemia. The increase in FRC occurs within seconds of the application of PEEP, but the PaO_2 may take longer to increase.[31]

In healthy adults, 5 cm H_2O of PEEP results in a total increase in FRC of approximately 400 to 500 mL. In patients with restrictive lung diseases (low compliance), the increase in FRC with 5 cm H_2O of PEEP is much lower. Some patients may require an FRC that exceeds the predicted normal volumes to achieve adequate oxygenation.[30]

Airway Pressures

It is important to monitor airway pressures for the following reasons:

- To help determine the need for mechanical ventilation and the patient's readiness for weaning
- To help determine the site and thereby the cause of impedance to mechanical ventilation
- To evaluate elastic recoil and compliance of the intact thorax
- To help estimate the amount of positive airway pressure being transmitted to the heart and major vessels
- To help assess the patient's respiratory muscle strength

Airway pressures should be measured as closely as possible to the ET tube. This prevents resistance caused by the ventilator circuit from influencing the peak pressure measurement. On certain occasions, as when using high-frequency ventilation or tracheal gas insufflation (TGI), the pressure should be measured at the distal tip of the ET tube.

Distal ET tip measurements may prove useful in triggering inspiratory and expiratory cycling during pressure support ventilation.[32] Distal measurement will eliminate sensing problems associated with the added Rāw of the ET tube. Distal measurement of airway pressure is not without problems. Repeatable accuracy and reliability can be confounded by humidification, secretions, and limitations in the cannula diameter size.

Peak Pressure

Peak pressure is the maximum pressure attained during the inspiratory phase of mechanical ventilation. It reflects the amount of force needed to overcome opposition to airflow into the lungs. Causes of this opposition to flow include resistance generated by the ventilator circuit, the artificial airway (ET tube), and the patient's airways and elastic recoil of the thoracic cage and the lungs. Sudden increases in peak airway pressure should alert the clinician to the possible presence of a patient-ventilator interface problem. Potential causes of an increase in peak pressure are listed in Box 13-1.

If the peak pressure increases while the plateau pressure (explained later) is unchanged, an increase in Rāw is probably occurring. Common causes include bronchospasm, airway secretions, and mucus plugging. As a result of the relationship between peak pressure and Rāw, monitoring the peak pressure provides valuable information about the bronchodilator-induced changes in lung function of the mechanically ventilated patient.[33,34] It is important to note that whenever changes in the peak pressure are used for evaluating Rāw, no changes in the inspiratory flow, flow pattern, or V_T should be made.

High peak airway pressure is often considered the cause of barotrauma.[35] However, evidence suggests that high peak alveolar pressures from overdistention lead to alveolar rupture, or volutrauma.[6,7,36] Conditions that raise the peak airway pressure may not affect alveolar pressure because of increased inspiratory resistance during mechanical ventilation. Static pressure more accurately reflects alveolar pressure than does peak pressure and should be used as the primary indicator for the risk of alveolar rupture.[36]

BOX 13-1 Potential Causes of Increased Peak Pressure

Resistance Factors

Patient Airways

Bronchospasm
Peribronchiolar edema
Retained secretions
Airway obstruction caused by foreign body

Artificial Airway

Internal diameter of tube too small
Kinking of ET tube
Mucus plugging
Cuff herniation
Tube impinging on tracheal wall

Ventilator Circuit

Water in tubing
Kinking of circuit tubing
High inspiratory flow rates (mechanical)

Elastic Recoil

Thoracic Cage

Chest wall deformity
Obesity
Abdominal distention, compression, or herniation
Diaphragmatic and intercostal muscle discoordination
Active expiration, restlessness, pain
Patient placement in lateral or prone position
Chest wraps or casts

Lung Involvement

Acute respiratory failure
Pneumonia
Adult respiratory distress syndrome
Atelectasis
Pneumothorax
Fibrosis

Plateau Pressure

One way to determine the cause of an elevated peak pressure is to separate the resistance component from the elastic recoil of the combined lung and chest wall. This can be accomplished by measuring the plateau pressure. The plateau pressure (also referred to as *static pressure*) is the pressure required to maintain a delivered V_T in a patient's lungs during a period of no gas flow. Plateau pressure is measured by occluding an exhalation valve immediately after the onset of the inspiratory breath and holding the exhalation valve closed throughout a portion of the expiratory phase until a plateau pressure is observed. In patients with airway obstruction, plateau pressure may take several seconds to be achieved. Another technique incorporates a shutter valve that intermittently stops flow during the expiratory phase.[37]

During the period of no gas flow, the $\bar{R}aw$ component of ventilation is eliminated, leaving the elastic recoil component as the force required to maintain inflation. If the volume maintained inside the lungs during this plateau period is known, the effective static compliance can be determined.

Mechanically ventilated patients with status asthmaticus may have low levels of measured auto-PEEP (discussed later) despite obvious signs of dynamic hyperinflation. Plateau pressure has been suggested to be superior to auto-PEEP for determining the degree of dynamic hyperinflation in these patients.[38] Consequently, patients with severe dynamic hyperinflation at risk of barotrauma who demonstrate low auto-PEEP may be better evaluated by using plateau pressures.

Mean Airway Pressure (MAP)

Mean airway pressure is the average pressure recorded during the positive-pressure and spontaneous phases of a respiratory cycle. MAP is calculated to determine the average airway pressure being applied to the lungs. Ventilator measurements affecting MAP include CPAP and PEEP levels, inspiratory time (flow rate, flow patterns), peak pressure, and rate. Increases in MAP are usually associated with an improvement in PaO_2, but can cause barotrauma and a reduction in cardiac output. Some studies indicate that PEEP and CPAP levels affect oxygenation more than variation in inspiratory flow rates and inspiratory times, even though they both increase MAP.[39] MAP is often considered to be equivalent to mean alveolar pressure, but these values are not always equal. Discrepancies between the two values may be caused by imbalances in inspiratory and expiratory resistance, variable flow resistance, leakage of gas volume, and measurement error.[40] Despite the absence of reported studies that show a correlation between specific levels of MAP and barotrauma, MAP levels greater than 30 cm H_2O appear to greatly enhance the risk of lung injury. Currently, no studies have shown a correlation between specific levels of MAP and barotrauma in the adult population.

Clinicians may need to adjust MAP levels when switching from one ventilator brand or modality to another. This is particularly important when switching to high-frequency oscillation (HFO) ventilation. Typically, we use a MAP of 4 to 8 cm H_2O higher when switching to HFO.

Maximum Inspiratory Pressure (P$_{Imax}$)

P_{Imax}, sometimes called the negative inspiratory force (NIF), is the maximum inspiratory pressure the patient's ventilatory pump is capable of generating against a closed airway. Several factors influence the patient's ability to produce a normal P_{Imax}:
• Respiratory muscle strength
• Patient effort
• Ventilatory drive
• Lung volume
• Phrenic nerve function
• Nutritional status
• Oxygenation status
• Acid-base status

Because P_{Imax} is intended to be a measure of respiratory muscle strength, these variables must be considered when interpreting P_{Imax}.

P_{Imax} can be measured even if an artificial airway is not in place by using a mask or mouthpiece and an external pressure manometer. The alert patient should be asked to exhale to a volume between FRC and RV because this will improve the mechanical advantage of the inspiratory muscles. At the end of exhalation, the airway is occluded while the patient makes a maximal inspiratory effort.

Marini and associates[41] have reported a standardized approach to measuring P_{Imax} in uncooperative critically ill patients. The patient is prepared for the maneuver by careful explanation of the procedure, proper positioning, and thorough suctioning with hyperoxygenation. Next, a one-way valve is placed in the expiratory path of a rigid T-tube to allow exhalation but not inhalation. This technique reduces lung volume to a level between RV and FRC. P_{Imax} is usually generated within 20 seconds of occlusion. Careful explanation of the procedure is important because occlusion of the airway can be frightening.

A normal P_{Imax} is approximately 80 to 110 cm H_2O. A P_{Imax} of 30 cm H_2O has been shown to predict successful weaning[2]; however, there is some debate as to its usefulness.[42] Although P_{Imax} is useful in measuring the patient's respiratory muscle strength, it provides little information about muscle endurance. P_{Imax} should not be the sole respiratory factor used to predict the patient's ability to wean.

Auto-PEEP

Mechanically ventilated patients may develop a condition called auto-PEEP. This can be seen if airway obstruction is present.[34,43] If there is insufficient time for exhalation, the lung is unable to return to its relaxed state before the next mechanical breath. Therefore exhalation of each successive V_T is incomplete, and a positive alveolar pressure occurs. The alveolar pressure slowly rises and results in a PEEP-like effect, hence the term *auto-PEEP*. Auto-PEEP is not detected by the ventilator pressure manometer unless the expiratory limb is occluded. When the flow is stopped at end-exhalation, pressure equilibrates throughout the closed system and registers on the ventilator manometer.

Auto-PEEP is defined as the difference between total-PEEP (obtained by expiratory hold maneuver) and the set-PEEP on the ventilator.[44]

All patients receiving mechanical ventilation should be assessed for the presence of auto-PEEP. It can be detected through physical examination by observation, palpation, and auscultation of the patient's chest during exhalation to determine if flow ends prior to the onset of the next inhalation. More accurately, the flow-time scalar can be examined to determine if expiratory flow returns to baseline prior to the subsequent inhalation.

If auto-PEEP is detected, measurement of total-PEEP should be attempted. It is not always possible to make accurate measurements of total-PEEP because the patient must be totally passive and the circuit cannot have any leaks. Many modern ventilators incorporate the ability to impose an expiratory pause that allows the measurement of total-PEEP.

When auto-PEEP is caused by dynamic airway compression, the patient may be unable to trigger ventilator breaths despite spontaneous efforts. Forceful inspiratory efforts or inability to trigger the ventilator will be seen. Titrating PEEP in this case may reduce the inspiratory efforts needed to trigger inspiratory breaths. There are negligible increases in peak inspiratory pressure during application of PEEP in such cases.

Auto-PEEP varies with the time allowed for exhalation, the elastic recoil of the lung, and the resistance to flow of the airways, ET tube, and expiratory limb (exhalation valve) of the ventilator circuit. Bronchodilator therapy, higher ventilator inspiratory flow rates, and a reduction in the mechanical rate have been shown to reduce the auto-PEEP effect. The most effective method to reduce auto-PEEP during conventional ventilation is through the reduction of $\dot{V}_E$. Strategies that alter V_T, ventilator rate, or inspiratory time without reducing $\dot{V}_E$ do little to reduce auto-PEEP.

Compliance

Compliance is defined as volume change per unit of pressure change, or the amount of lung volume achieved per unit of pressure. Two forms of compliance are commonly reported: effective dynamic compliance and static compliance. Dynamic compliance represents the total impedance to gas flow into the lungs, and it is determined by dividing mechanical V_T by the peak airway pressure minus the end expiratory pressure (EEP):

$$Dynamic\ compliance = \{VT - [(Ppk - EEP) \times CV]\}/Ppk - EEP$$

where:

    V_T = Tidal volume
    Ppk = Peak airway pressure
    EEP = Total-PEEP (defined later)
    CV = Tubing compliance correction factor

Dynamic compliance incorporates both the flow-resistive characteristics of the airways and ventilator circuit and the elastic components of the lung and chest wall. Dynamic compliance curves are seen most commonly on ventilator graphic screens via the pressure/volume tracings.

Static compliance is the lung volume change per unit of pressure during a period of no gas flow. It is calculated clinically by dividing V_T by the plateau pressure minus EEP:

$$Static\ compliance = V_T - [(P_{plat} - EEP) \times CV] / P_{plat} - EEP$$

where:

    V_T = Tidal volume
    P_{plat} = Plateau pressure
    EEP = Total-PEEP
    CV = Tubing compliance correction factor

In practice, static calculations should be based on at least three breaths. The measured values include not only the lung-thorax unit, but also the compliance of the ventilator circuit.

Compliance of the adult ventilator circuit varies with the structure and diameter of the tubing but is generally 1 to 3 mL/cm H_2O/L of the circuitry volume. If the patient is being ventilated with high airway pressures, a significant portion of the V_T is lost to tubing expansion, and erroneous compliance measurements can be computed if this loss is not considered.

Effective static compliance measurements can be valuable in monitoring patients receiving mechanical ventilation.[45] Lung diseases such as pulmonary edema, pneumothorax, pneumonia, and ARDS increase lung recoil and the observed static pressure. As a result, the static compliance is reduced in such situations.

The textbook normal values for thoracic compliance of 100 mL/cm H_2O are rarely seen in mechanically ventilated patients because even patients with normal lungs usually develop a decrease in lung volume and compliance after receiving positive-pressure ventilation for a few hours. Thus normal compliance values in patients receiving mechanical ventilation range from 60 to 80 mL/cm H_2O. Compliance values of less than 25 mL/cm H_2O are not usually associated with successful weaning attempts[2,13] or PEEP withdrawal.

Airway Resistance (Rāw)

Rāw is the opposition to airflow by the nonelastic forces of the lung. True Rāw is not measured routinely in the ICU. A reliable estimate of the flow-restrictive components of Rāw can be made by subtracting the static or plateau pressure from the peak pressure and dividing by flow in liters per second. Normal values are 2 to 3 cm H_2O/L/sec.

$$R\bar{a}w = \frac{\text{Peak pressure (cm } H_2O) - \text{Plateau pressure (cm } H_2O)}{\text{Flow (L/sec)}}$$

Rāw can be elevated by numerous factors (discussed earlier). Increased Rāw can cause problems not only during positive-pressure breathing, but also during spontaneous breathing. A small-diameter ET tube will significantly increase the work of breathing for a spontaneously breathing patient. High flow rates from a continuous-flow IMV system can increase expiratory work by forcing the patient to exhale the mechanically delivered V_T against the expiratory valve of both the machine and the continuous flow of the IMV system.

Integrating Pressure, Flow, and Volume

Evaluating the Patient/Ventilator Interface

The critical care practitioner is often called upon to evaluate the integration of the ventilator to the patient. Most often this consists of a sequential evaluation starting at the airway (type, size, integrity, stability), progressing down both limbs of the ventilator circuit (leaks, temperature, condensate), and terminating with the ventilator settings and patient-monitoring panel. The practitioner can also observe the synchrony of the patient's breathing pattern and respiratory effort. This approach is beneficial at the beginning of the shift, after any ventilator-related event, and before the adjustment of ventilator settings. The practitioner should then focus on the ventilator settings

and, when available, the graphic display of pressure, flow, and volume data.

Monitoring Pressure, Flow, and Volume in the ICU

Most ventilators manufactured during the past 5 years are equipped with a graphic display screen. This screen allows the clinician to review large amounts of patient ventilation data. Three of the most important parameters to follow are the pressure, flow, and volume tracings of mechanically ventilated patients. The data can be displayed as a single parameter in a continuous tracing over time, called a *scalar*, or in combination with other parameters, called a *loop*. The individual parameters may be indexed to each other, as in a pressure-volume loop or a flow-volume loop. The integration of these three parameters provides a wealth of information important for proper ventilator management.

Pressure-Time Waveforms

The continuous display of the airway pressure waveform provides the opportunity to visually evaluate the following (Figure 13-1):
- Airway pressure levels
- Characteristics of the airway pressure curve during all breath cycles
- Mode of ventilation
- Estimations on the respiratory work
- Adequacy of inspiratory flow pattern and peak flow
- Inspiratory resistive load (peak — plateau pressures)
- Gross estimates of patient inspiratory effort
- Estimations of the level of synchrony between the patient and ventilator

The pressure display on a ventilator graphic screen traces the rise and fall in airway pressure as measured within the ventilator circuit. The clinician must remember that this tracing is a reflection of airway circuit pressure (including ventilator circuit and ET tube resistance), not necessarily the airway pressure within the lung (intrapulmonary). In fact, only during a period of zero airflow (inspiratory or expiratory hold) does the ventilator airway pressure waveform reflect the actual intrapulmonary pressure (Figure 13-2).

Volume-Time Waveforms

The volume-time waveform is most often used to compare the inspiratory and expiratory delivered volumes. This can be particularly useful in checking for leaks within the ventilator circuit system or in determining the amount of leak around the ET tube or through a chest tube (Figure 13-3).

Flow-Time Waveforms

The flow-time waveform allows the clinician to evaluate the following:
- Both inspiratory and expiratory flow rates
- Characteristics of the flow profile during all breath cycles
- Presence of air trapping (i.e., auto-PEEP) (Figure 13-4)

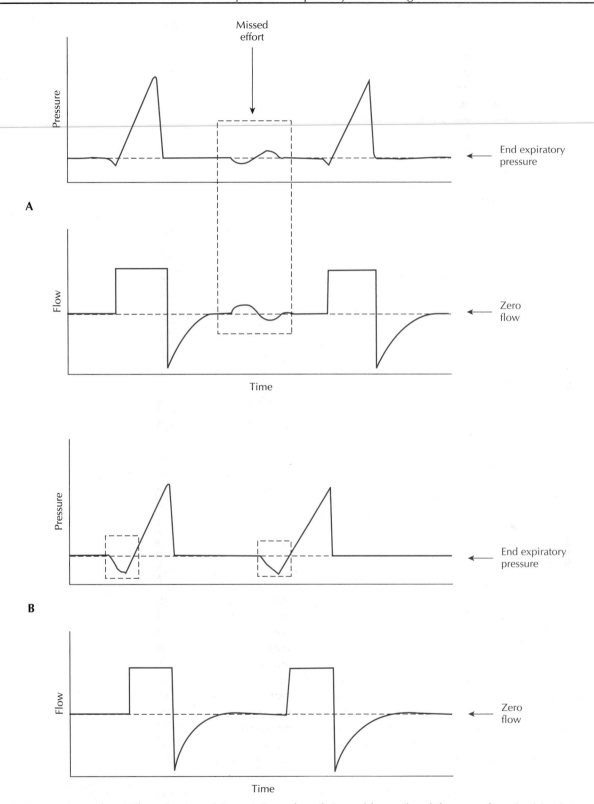

Figure 13-1 Pressure-time scalars. **A,** The patient is receiving assist/control ventilation and the ventilator fails to sense the patient's inspiratory effort on the second attempt – missed effort. The trigger method and sensitivity should be adjusted to avoid missed efforts. **B,** Delayed onset of flow resulting from lack of sensitivity results in excessive trigger work.

Continued

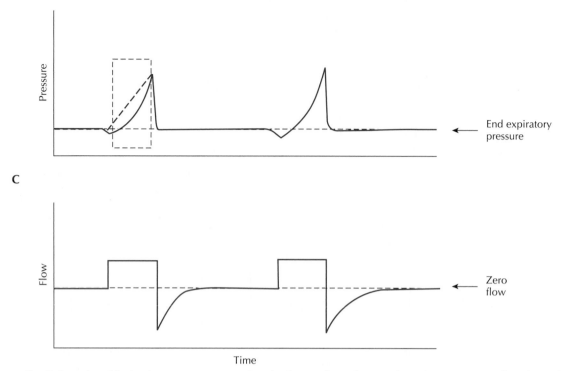

Figure 13-1 cont'd.   C, Scooping of the inspiratory pressure curve from inadequate flow relative to the patient's inspiratory flow demand. The dotted line represents the expected path of rise in inspiratory pressure.

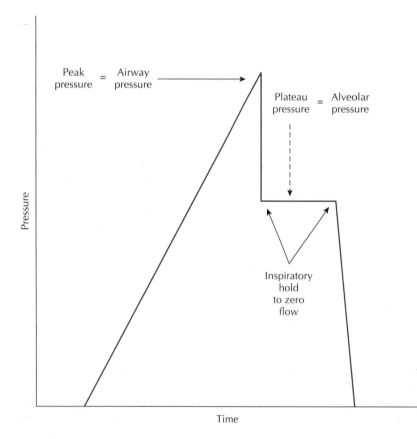

Figure 13-2 Pressure-time scalar. A theoretical inspiratory ventilator pressure tracing. The solid-lined arrow indicates peak airway pressure; the dotted lined arrow indicates theoretical alveolar pressure. The difference between the dotted and solid line is the resistive component of the ventilator circuit, endotracheal tube, and airways. Notice that alveolar pressure equates to airway pressure only during the static, no-flow period.

- Estimations of inspiratory effort
- Estimations of the level of synchrony between the patient and ventilator

The inspiratory flow profile provides information about how the ventilator breath is entering the patient. This profile is influenced not only by the flow pattern selected and mode of ventilation being used, but also by the resistive and elastic forces of the chest and the level of patient effort. The inspiratory flow rate and pattern should match the patient's efforts and breathing demands, demonstrating patient/ventilator syn-

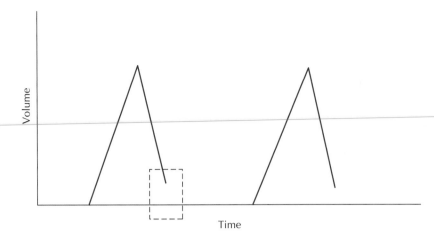

Figure 13-3 Volume-time scalar. The inspiratory volume is greater than the expiratory volume due to a leak in the patient/ventilator system, possibly from a bronchopleural fistula, endotracheal tube leak or ventilator circuit leak.

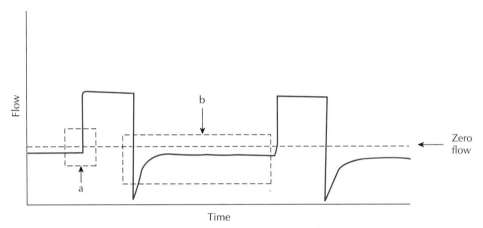

Figure 13-4 Flow-time scalar. The expiratory flow fails to return to baseline prior to the onset of the next inhalation. This demonstrates the presence of flow trapping and auto-PEEP. The shape of the expiratory tracing demonstrates a prolonged expiratory time with low expiratory flow consistent with significant expiratory resistance in either the patient or the ventilator circuit.

chrony. The inspiratory profile of the flow waveform should demonstrate a smooth, consistent rise up to the maximal flow rate. If the flow rate is too slow, the profile will show a dip or become concave. Too high a flow rate creates a sharp, sudden rise. Some patients, particularly those with significant dyspnea, may require a higher inspiratory flow rate. Flow rate and flow profiles are particularly important to monitor during volume-limited modes of ventilation because they require the practitioner to set a pattern and determine a finite flow rate. The practitioner should evaluate the inspiratory flow profile periodically and make necessary adjustments to the flow rate when using volume-limited modes of ventilation.

During pressure-limited ventilation (PS, PC, PRVC, VAPS),* the inspiratory flow rate is determined by the resistive and elastic forces of the lungs and patient inspiratory effort. The flow rate and flow pattern are not altered by the practitioner. This flow pattern shows a rapid rise to a maximal flow rate, followed by a gradual tapering to a point of flow termination. This pattern is usually well matched to any changes in patient effort and allows the patient to determine the rate of the inspiratory phase of the breath.

The expiratory flow profile displays how gas is leaving the lung and indicates the level of expiratory resistance and expiratory time required to return to a point of zero flow.

The expiratory flow profile is used routinely to determine the presence of air trapping. When air trapping occurs, flow continues throughout expiration and is terminated abruptly by the onset of the next inflation. However, a quantitative calculation of total-PEEP cannot be made from an examination of the expiratory flow profile unless accompanied by a pressure/time tracing with an expiratory hold to zero flow.

Pressure/Volume Curves

The integration of pressure and volume data produces a useful tool known as the *pressure/volume loop*. Pressure is most often displayed on the x-axis, with volume on the y-axis. The angle of the inspiratory and expiratory curves is known as the *slope of the tracings*. The pressure/volume curve is a display of the dynamic compliance, the resistive and elastic components of the circuit/patient interface. A typical tracing during constant inspiratory flow reveals a slightly concave inspiratory tracing, with the expiratory curve being slightly convex. The flatter the slope, the less compliant the system. Lower compliance tracings are most often seen with restrictive conditions such as ARDS and lung consolidation. The more "square" the tracing, the greater the degree of resistance (Figure 13-5). During nonconstant inspiratory flow, the inspiratory arm may have an exaggerated bulge because of the high degree of resistance during the initial burst of flow (Figure 13-6).

---

*PS, Pressure support; PC, pressure control; PRVC, pressure-regulated volume control; VAPS, volume-assured pressure support.

Titrating PEEP and Tidal Volume with the Pressure/Volume Curve

Some investigators have advocated using a static pressure-volume curve to titrate PEEP and tidal volume. It is not routinely used in the ICU, mainly because it is time-consuming and cumbersome, but it can be very valuable for some patients, particularly those with acute lung injury. This technique,

incorporating a supersyringe and pressure manometer, requires the sequential delivery of specific volumes to the ET tube. The volumes are delivered to the lung and held for a few seconds to allow equilibration and a static condition to occur. Sometimes the lung is inflated to a maximal level and then allowed to empty to the desired volume levels. The corresponding pressures are recorded and compared with the volumes to form a curve. The initial points of the curve are fairly flat, indicating increasing pressure with minimal alveolar recruitment. As one moves up the curve, the compliance points change their slope. This is seen as a greater change in lung volume per unit of pressure. The point on the curve at which this upslope occurs is known as the lower inflection point. This is considered to be the minimal PEEP that should be applied to the lung. As the volume delivered into the lung increases, the corresponding slope increases. Eventually, the slope flattens again, indicating

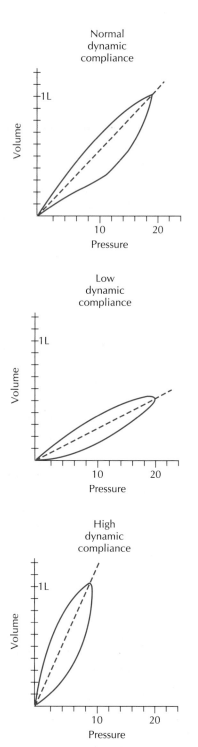

Figure 13-5 Dynamic pressure-volume loops. The slope of the curve represents the dynamic compliance of the system *(dashed lines)*.

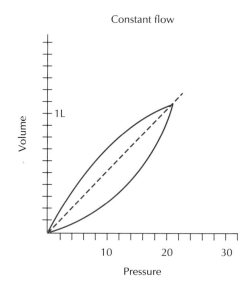

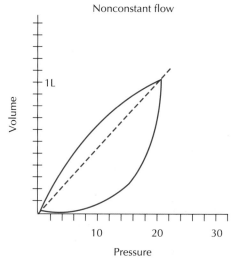

Figure 13-6 Dynamic pressure-volume loops. Nonconstant flow (decelerating ramp) changes the appearance of the pressure-volume loop. The decelerating inspiratory flow seen with pressure-limited ventilation will cause the inspiratory curve to bow outward.

that more pressure is being required to deliver the given volume. This upper flattening characteristic is known as a *beak* and it commences at the upper inflection point. Its presence indicates overdistention of the lung. The static pressure/volume curve therefore can be used to adjust the minimal PEEP required to recruit and maintain open alveoli (lower inflection point) and to determine the maximal pressure level to limit the possibility of overdistention (upper inflection point) (Figure 13-7).

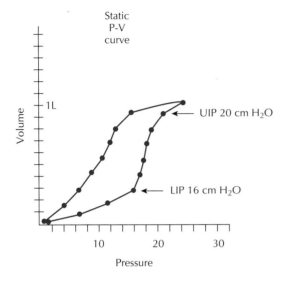

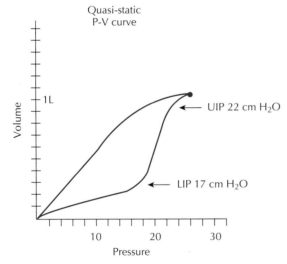

Figure 13-7 Static and quasi-static pressure-volume loops. The static pressure-volume loop is constructed by serial injection of aliquots of volume with a pause to zero flow and recording the resultant pressure. The volume and pressure data points are plotted through both inhalation and exhalation. The lower and upper inflection points can often be determined by this method. It can be difficult to accomplish on the unstable, critically ill patient. The quasi-static method uses a constant, low flow (<10 L/min), inhalation with continuous recording of the volume and pressure data points. Although there is a small error related to the pressure being recorded during flow, the error is fairly constant and the inflection points can be approximated with this method. For both methods the patient must remain completely passive and attention to detail is critical in obtaining reliable results.

The dynamic pressure-volume curves commonly displayed on ventilators in the ICU are different from the static curves just described. Because the pressure volume points are being taken while the ventilator is delivering the breath, the ventilator tracings are incorporating the resistive and elastic characteristics of the entire ventilator circuit. Consequently, the inflection point is typically higher than the minimal level of PEEP.

Quasi-static pressure-volume curves using specific settings have been advocated as a simple and reliable technique to determine the lower and upper inflection points.[46] Inflation of the lungs is accomplished with a constant, low flow (< 10 L/min) from FRC through the tidal volume range. The pressure-volume curve for this inflation is frozen on the screen for assessment. Some ventilator manufacturers are pursuing incorporating this as an executable maneuver in their software.

> **SIMPLY STATED**
> Graphic displays of ventilator pressure, volume, and flow waveforms are invaluable in the titration of ventilator settings and the assessment of patient/ventilator synchrony.

Fractional Gas Concentrations

The ability to monitor delivered oxygen concentrations is crucial for many respiratory procedures, and exhaled gases, sampled either intermittently or continuously, provide information about changes in equipment function, blood gases, tissue perfusion, ventilation-perfusion ($\dot{V}/\dot{Q}$) relationships, and metabolic rate. This section deals with oxygen concentration and carbon dioxide analysis and their use in the ICU.

Fraction of Inspired Oxygen Concentration

Measurement of the fraction of inspired oxygen (FIO_2) is essential to the modern ICU. Various oxygen delivery devices require at least intermittent analysis of FIO_2 to ensure that the appropriate oxygen concentration is being delivered and to interpret blood gases. If the FIO_2 is inappropriately low, hypoxia may result; an inappropriate elevation of FIO_2 may lead to oxygen toxicity. Variations in delivered oxygen concentrations may make metabolic evaluations impossible.[47]

Exhaled Carbon Dioxide

Carbon dioxide is one of the by-products of tissue metabolism, and its elimination is a prime function of ventilation. Monitoring of exhaled carbon dioxide with either capnometry, simple measurement, or capnography, graphing the measurement against time, can detect changes in the following:

- Metabolic rate as a result of cardiac output and body temperature changes, shivering, seizures, trauma, and high carbohydrate infusion
- Ventilator function such as a patient disconnection or apnea

- Efficiency of ventilation (by looking at the increase and decrease in alveolar and dead space ventilation)
- Transport of carbon dioxide as a result of changes in perfusion

Carbon dioxide elimination depends on cardiac output and on the regional $\dot{V}/\dot{Q}$ ratios and the emptying times of different regions of the lung. Nondependent lung regions open first and empty last and usually have high $\dot{V}/\dot{Q}$ ratios and subsequently low alveolar carbon dioxide concentrations. Dependent lung regions have low $\dot{V}/\dot{Q}$ ratios, with alveolar carbon dioxide values approaching mixed venous values. Exhaled alveolar carbon dioxide concentrations are often at their highest at the end of exhalation, so the term end-tidal Pco_2 ($PETco_2$) may be used to indicate the highest exhaled carbon dioxide concentrations attained. In normal subjects, the $PETco_2$ is an accurate estimate of $Paco_2$, but conditions that alter $\dot{V}/\dot{Q}$ relationships, such as mechanical ventilation, pulmonary disease, and a decrease in perfusion, increase the arterial-$PETco_2$ gradient.[48]

Capnometry has also been applied in the operating room, emergency department, and prehospital care setting for determination of ET tube placement, airway disconnect, and systemic perfusion monitoring during cardiopulmonary resuscitation (CPR). The last application may prove to be useful as a noninvasive prognostic indicator of CPR effectiveness (Figure 13-8).[49]

Analysis may be done on a breath-by-breath basis or by sampling mean concentration. The systems currently used include infrared analysis, which detects absorption of a specific wavelength of infrared radiation, partial-pressure analyzers, and mass spectrometry. Sampling may be done either by aspiration through a sample line or by placement of the sensor around the dead space of a ventilator circuit. Carbon dioxide tracings can be plotted against time or, by incorporating a flow transducer, volume. The latter technique allows the practitioner to measure breath-by-breath dead space.

SIMPLY STATED

End-tidal CO_2 as a predictor of $Paco_2$ has application in patient populations with minimal $\dot{V}/\dot{Q}$ imbalance or circuit leaks.

A single breath tracing for carbon dioxide concentration over time is illustrated in Figure 13-9. The tracing has three phases. Phase I contains no carbon dioxide (pure dead space). Phase II shows a rapid increase in carbon dioxide concentration. Phase III rises as a result of sequential lung emptying and the continual release of carbon dioxide into the alveoli during expiration.

Carbon dioxide production ($\dot{V}co_2$) is the carbon dioxide produced and excreted over 1 minute. The $\dot{V}co_2$ values provide information about changes in metabolic rate and transport of carbon dioxide. The formula for calculating $\dot{V}co_2$ is as follows:

$$\dot{V}co_2 = F\bar{E}co_2 \times \dot{V}_E$$

where

$F\bar{E}co_2$ = Mean fraction of expired carbon dioxide

$\dot{V}_E$ = Minute volume exhaled at STPD (a volume of gas at standard temperature and pressure that contains no water vapor)

The formula assumes that there is no carbon dioxide in inspired air. $\dot{V}co_2$ is often increased in fever (10% increase per 1° C increase), trauma, peritonitis (25% to 50% increase), head trauma, rewarming after hypothermia, and high carbohydrate loading with total parenteral nutrition. $\dot{V}co_2$ increases with carbohydrate loading as a result of oxidation of carbohydrates and carbohydrate conversion to fats (lipogenesis). $\dot{V}co_2$ may increase by 75% because of carbohydrate overloading (see section on respiratory quotient in Chapter 17.)

A rapid decrease in $\dot{V}co_2$ or elimination accompanies a low cardiac output and a fall in tissue perfusion, decreased right ventricular output, decreased venous return, or pulmonary embolism.

Dead Space-Tidal Volume Ratio (V_D/V_T). V_D is the inspired volume that does not come in contact with pulmonary capillary blood. The V_D/V_T ratio expresses the relationship between V_D and total V_T, or the portion of the V_T that is "wasted." V_D has two components: anatomic dead space and alveolar dead space. Anatomic dead space is made up of the conducting airways and is normally about 2 mL/kg of ideal body weight. Alveolar dead space is classically defined as alveoli that are ventilated but not perfused. The combination of anatomic and alveolar dead space is called physiologic dead space. V_D/V_T is traditionally calculated by the Englehoff modification of the Bohr equation, as follows:

$$V_D/V_T = \frac{Paco_2 - P\bar{E}co_2}{Paco_2}$$

where

$Paco_2$ = Arterial Pco_2

$P\bar{E}co_2$ = Pco_2 of mixed exhaled gas

The patient is stabilized for 20 minutes, and arterial blood and exhaled gases are sampled simultaneously. The exhaled gases may be collected in a Douglas bag or sampled at the outlet of a mixing box. Factors that may contaminate or dilute the $P\bar{E}co_2$, such as compressible gas volume from the patient ventilator circuit or gases from a continuous flow IMV system, should be eliminated by double exhalation valves.[50] A correction factor for patients on the assist/control mode of CMV can also eliminate compressible volume. The correction factor does not work during IMV because spontaneous and mechanical tidal volumes can vary in IMV modes.[51]

$$P\bar{E}co_2 \text{ corrected} = \frac{V_T}{V_T - CV} \times P\bar{E}co_2$$

where

CV = Compressible volume in tubing

V_T = Mechanical tidal volume

The use of the V_D/V_T in patients on IMV may be misleading as a result of variations in $P\bar{E}co_2$ between mechanical and spontaneous breaths.

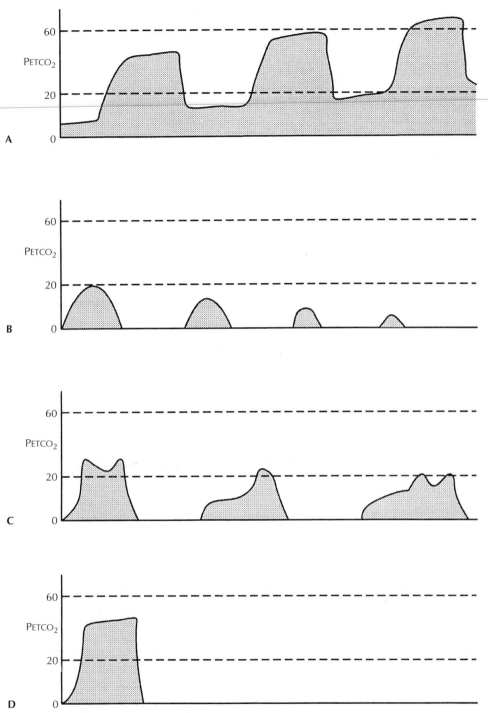

Figure 13-8 Examples of abnormal capnograms. **A,** Progressive rebreathing causing a rise in baseline $PETCO_2$. **B,** Placement of endotracheal (ET) tube in esophagus, causing a drop in $PETCO_2$ to 0. **C,** Leak in sample line or around ET tube cuff, resulting in low and variable $PETCO_2$ levels. **D,** Ventilator disconnect, causing an abrupt drop in $PETCO_2$ to 0.

The normal V_D/V_T for healthy persons is between 25% and 35% and is position dependent. Patients receiving positive-pressure ventilation usually have a higher V_D/V_T while they are upright or in the lateral position than when they are in the supine position.[51] During anesthesia, V_D/V_T is usually increased because of an overall reduction in lung volume. In patients receiving mechanical ventilation, faster inspiratory flow rates or small tidal volumes usually are associated with an increase in V_D/V_T.[48,52] Variations in the inspiratory waveforms, tapered wave, sine waves, and end-inspiratory pause maneuvers may decrease V_D/V_T.[53] Changes in the pulmonary perfusion caused by emboli, hypoperfusion, and precapillary constriction may result in an increased V_D/V_T.

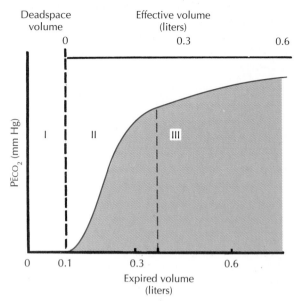

Figure 13-9 Single-breath tracing for exhaled carbon dioxide.

EVALUATION OF OXYGENATION

Inappropriate oxygenation is a common occurrence in patients in the ICU. The recognition and correction of this problem are crucial to the patient's well-being. Respiratory care maneuvers, pharmacologic and fluid support, and diagnostic procedures often affect tissue oxygenation. The bedside clinician must be able to monitor and determine the effect of these activities.

This section describes the concepts and techniques used in the assessment of oxygenation: first the components of oxygen transport and the measurements used to monitor oxygenation, then the indices of pulmonary gas exchange and indicators of systemic oxygenation and when they should be used.

The potential causes of hypoxemia and hypoxia are diverse. Hypoxic episodes can be iatrogenic in origin, as with suctioning or equipment failure. Progressive disease or a new problem can make oxygenation more difficult. Therefore, the bedside clinician must be able to identify the causes of these problems, select the appropriate therapy or therapies, and monitor the outcome. Causes of impaired oxygenation in critically ill patients are listed in Box 13-2. Haldane, the physiologist, said it best almost a century ago: "Anoxia not only stops the machine but wrecks the machinery."[53a]

Evaluation of Oxygen Transport

Oxygen transport is the essential mechanism by which oxygen is carried from the lungs to the capillary bed. Equally important is how oxygen is used by the tissues, a process known as oxygen consumption. The majority of cellular oxygen is used for the production of adenosine triphosphate (ATP). Recent evidence shows that other activities such as cell wall sta-

---

BOX 13-2   Causes of Impaired Oxygenation in Critically Ill Patients

Equipment-related problems, low/high flow oxygen delivery devices
Loose tubing connection, cannula
Loose humidifier, nipple connector
Inadequate flow to meet patient peak inspiratory flow, air entrainment
Blender malfunction

Ventilator-Related Problems

Endotracheal: tracheostomy tube malfunctions
Ventilator and circuit malfunctions
Improper settings, modes of ventilation

Progression of Underlying Disease Process

Acute respiratory distress syndrome
Cardiogenic pulmonary edema
Pneumonia
Airway obstruction, asthma/chronic obstructive pulmonary disease

Onset of a New Clinical Problem

Pneumothoraces: simple, tension, loculated
Lobar atelectasis
Gastric aspiration
Artificial airway problems: stenosis, fistula, malacia
Nosocomial pneumonia
Fluid overload
Microatelectasis
Bronchospasm
Retained secretions
Shock
Sepsis
Additional organ failure

Interventions and Procedures

Endotracheal suctioning
Position changes
Chest physiotherapy
Bronchoscopy
Thoracentesis
Peritoneal dialysis
Hemodialysis
Transport
Diagnostic procedures
Line/tube placement

Medications

Bronchodilators
Vasodilators
Inotropic agents

Miscellaneous

Leukocytopenia
Intralipids

Data from Glauser R and others: Worsening oxygenation in the mechanically ventilated patient, *Am Rev Respir Dis* 138:458, 1988.

bilization and chemical synthesis are extremely oxygen dependent and sensitive to minor fluctuations in oxygen tension. Box 13-3 lists some of the crucial factors that determine oxygen delivery (DO_2) and oxygen utilization.

Oxygen Reserves

In the critically ill patient, an increase in oxygen consumption or an impairment in DO_2 to the tissues must be compensated for by an increase in one or more of the reserve systems:

- Cardiac output and distribution
- PaO_2 and SaO_2 values
- Sufficient levels of functional hemoglobin

Patients with two compromised reserve systems are at high risk for inadequate DO_2 and subsequent tissue hypoxia. Patients in the ICU often have compromised reserve systems. Low cardiac output (shock), blood flow maldistribution, anemia, and ventilatory failure do not allow adequate compensation to occur. As the abnormal situation persists, it becomes more difficult to correct. The longer oxygenation is compromised, the more profoundly the "machinery" is damaged.

Oxygen content is defined as the total amount of oxygen carried in the blood and is the sum of oxygen bound chemically to hemoglobin (Hb) plus oxygen dissolved in plasma. Under normal conditions Hb is responsible for carrying 99% or more of the oxygen in the blood. The remaining oxygen (<1%) is dissolved in plasma and is measured as PaO_2. PaO_2 is important because it reflects the degree of saturation of hemoglobin and the driving pressure of oxygen between systemic capillary blood and the tissues:

$$O_2 \text{ content} = (Hb \times 1.34 \times \% \text{ Saturation}) + (PaO_2 \times 0.003)$$

Traditional respiratory care has focused on the physiologic mechanisms that result in inadequate oxygenation of the pulmonary capillary blood. These mechanisms include:

- $\dot{V}/\dot{Q}$ mismatch (most common cause)
- Diffusion block (rare cause)
- Hypoventilation
- Shunt (extreme $\dot{V}/\dot{Q}$ mismatch)

SIMPLY STATED

Oxygen transport depends primarily on three reserve components:
  Cardiac output and distribution
  PaO_2 and SaO_2 values
  Sufficient levels of functional hemoglobin
A compromise in any of the three parameters must be compensated for by the other components. Patients with two compromised reserve systems are at high risk for inadequate DO_2 and subsequent tissue hypoxia.

Cardiac Output

The techniques used to assess cardiac output are described in Chapter 14. DO_2 is extremely dependent on cardiac output and systemic distribution of blood flow. The major determinant of cardiac output is metabolic activity, whereas peripheral distribution of blood flow depends on regional oxygen consumption, temperature, humoral agents, and other factors. Cardiac output is not sensitive to moderate changes in oxygen tension (PO_2) and usually does not increase until the PaO_2 drops below 50 mm Hg.[54] In the patient with shock, blood flow to the low-oxygen-consuming regions of the body (i.e., the skin) is reduced as a protective mechanism in response to an increase in sympathetic tone.

Oxyhemoglobin Dissociation Curve

Another factor influencing DO_2 is the oxyhemoglobin dissociation curve (ODC). The ODC graphically depicts the relationship between PaO_2 and the oxygen content or hemoglobin saturation. The clinical significance of the curve is that large changes in PaO_2 may have little effect on the oxygen content or hemoglobin saturation of arterial blood on the upper, flat portion of the curve ($PaO_2 > 70$ mm Hg), but dramatic changes occur in oxygen content or hemoglobin saturation at the steep portion of the curve ($PaO_2 = 40$ to 70 mm Hg). At this part of the curve, large volumes of oxygen can be unloaded at the cellular level with small changes in PaO_2. Shifting the curve to the right or left may profoundly affect oxygen availability to the tissues.[55]

Clinically the position of the curve is measured by tonometry or calculated at a point where the oxygen's partial pressure has saturated 50% of the hemoglobin (P-50). The normal P-50 value is a PO_2 of approximately 27 mm Hg. Many factors can affect the position of the curve. A shift to the left decreases the P-50. This indicates an increase in oxygen affinity or a tendency for the hemoglobin not to release oxygen to the tissues. A shift to the right (increased P-50) indicates a reduction in oxygen-hemoglobin affinity, resulting in oxygen being released more readily to the tissues.

A left-shifted ODC can be caused by massive transfusion of acid-citrate-dextrose–stored blood, rapid correction of acidosis that has been present for hours or days, or severe

---

BOX 13-3	Factors that Determine Oxygen Delivery and Utilization

Oxygen Transport

Oxygen content of the blood
Cardiac output
Distribution of cardiac output
Oxyhemoglobin dissociation curve

Oxygen Utilization

Metabolic rate (disease, trauma, sepsis, nutrition)
Cell integrity (organ injury, sepsis)
Oxygen availability
Level of cellular toxins, by-products (organ injury, sepsis)

hyperventilation resulting in respiratory alkalosis. Other less commonly seen causes of a left-shifted ODC are hypothermia and hypophosphatemia.

The normal compensatory mechanism for a left-shifted curve is an increase in the cardiac output. Patients with compromised reserve systems who are not capable of increasing cardiac output or who cannot tolerate a further reduction in tissue oxygenation are at great risk for hypoxia if they have a significantly left-shifted ODC.

To show how efficient the position of the ODC is in improving Do_2, consider the following theoretical clinical situation. A patient with a normal fixed oxygen consumption of 250 mL/min, a cardiac output of 5.4 L/min, a mixed venous oxygen tension ($P\bar{v}o_2$) of 36 mm Hg, and a P-50 of 27 mm Hg develops a clinical condition in which the ODC shifts to the left and reduces P-50 so severely that P-50 falls to 20 mm Hg. This patient would need to increase cardiac output by 50% to deliver the equivalent volume of oxygen to the tissues. However, if P-50 were increased from 27 mm Hg to 30 mm Hg, the patient would require 20% less cardiac output.[25] If this theoretical patient had a damaged heart and was unable to increase cardiac output, the significant shift to the left of ODC could be very serious.

In most patients, a rightward shift of the ODC is advantageous for oxygen transport except under the most extreme hypoxemic conditions (Pao_2 = 30 to 35 mm Hg).

Monitoring the Adequacy of Arterial Oxygenation

Partial Pressure of Arterial Oxygen

Pao_2 is used universally in the ICU as a measure of pulmonary gas exchange, but it is not specific or sensitive enough to be used exclusively in the estimation of oxygen transport. Practitioners must keep this in mind when treating the critically ill patient who is hemodynamically unstable. For managing a pulmonary gas exchange problem (e.g., asthma) that is not associated with other complications, Pao_2 is an excellent value to follow to identify which therapies are effective. It should not be relied on in assessing systemic oxygen transport for the following reasons. First, it is a gas tension and does not directly reflect delivered oxygen. Second, Pao_2 reflects partial pressure available at the systemic bed, not what is used. Third, factors that may improve oxygen transport by improving cardiac output may cause Pao_2 to fall because of an increase in intrapulmonary shunt.[56,57] It is not uncommon for multiple deficiencies to exist that adversely affect the oxygen transport system but are not directly related to pulmonary gas exchange.

Under most clinical conditions, Pao_2 should be kept within a range of 60 to 80 mm Hg. This usually ensures an arterial saturation of at least 90%. Pao_2 values greater than 80 mm Hg are usually unnecessary except in situations such as carbon monoxide poisoning and during periods of severe anemia or cardiogenic shock. Hyperoxic Pao_2 does not necessarily improve oxygen transport. A Pao_2 greater than 125 mm Hg has been shown to cause a reduction of blood flow to both the kidneys and the brain, probably as a result of vasoconstriction.[55]

Alveolar-Arterial Oxygen Tension Difference

$P(A - a)o_2$ has commonly been used as an indication of gas exchange efficiency. Its major limitation is that it changes with adjustments in Fio_2.[58] See Chapter 7 for a description of how $P(A - a)o_2$ is calculated.

Arterial-Alveolar Tension Ratio

The Pao_2/Pao_2 ratio is a more useful index of pulmonary gas exchange than the $P(A - a)o_2$ because it remains more stable with changes in Fio_2. It is most stable when Fio_2 is greater than 0.30 and Pao_2 is less than 100 mm Hg. For example, a Pao_2 of 60 mm Hg and a $Paco_2$ of 40 mm Hg while breathing an Fio_2 of 0.4 can be calculated as follows:

$$\frac{Pao_2 (60)}{Pao_2 (245)\{[(760 - 47) \times Fio_2 (0.4)] - Paco_2 (40)\}} = 0.24$$

It can also be used to predict the Fio_2 required for a desired Pao_2.[59]

Pao_2/Fio_2 Ratio

The Pao_2/Fio_2 ratio is similar to the Pao_2/Pao_2 ratio but easier to use because it does not require calculation of Pao_2. This may lead to an increase in error because it does not compensate for changes in $Paco_2$. A Pao_2/Fio_2 ratio of 200 or greater has been identified as an indication that the patient may be ready for a reduction in the PEEP level.[60]

Oxygenation Index

The oxygen index (OI) was initially developed as an index of ventilatory-oxygenation support for a human surfactant trial[61] and was more recently adapted as a prognostic index for morbidity and mortality for infants requiring extracorporeal membrane oxygenation (ECMO).[62] The OI is calculated by the following formula:

$$\frac{MAP \times Fio_2 \times 100}{Pao_2}$$

where
MAP = Mean airway pressure
Fio_2 = Fraction of inspired oxygen
Pao_2 = Postductal Pao_2

The advantage of the OI over other indices is that it incorporates MAP, a ventilation value that is strongly related to the degree of ventilatory support (and lung injury) and oxygenation. Infant ECMO candidates with severe respiratory failure often have OI values greater than 40, indicative of a high predicted mortality (greater than 80%). OI values greater than 20 to 25 indicate a predicted mortality greater than 50%.[62,63]

Intrapulmonary Shunt

Intrapulmonary shunt ($\dot{Q}S/\dot{Q}T$) is a major contributor to hypoxemia in most patients in the ICU. It is defined as perfusion without ventilation and theoretically should be differentiated from another cause of hypoxemia: low $\dot{V}/\dot{Q}$ ratios, or perfusion greater than ventilation. Clinical states that often produce an increase in $\dot{Q}S/\dot{Q}T$ are atelectasis, pneumonia, ARDS, pulmonary edema, and, rarely, congenital heart anomalies or arteriovenous anastomosis. The $\dot{Q}S/\dot{Q}T$ and $\dot{V}/\dot{Q}$ relation may be measured by tracer gas techniques[29] or radioactive gas and microsphere techniques,[24] but the calculation most often used in the ICU is the following classic shunt equation:

$$\dot{Q}S/\dot{Q}T = \frac{C\acute{c}o_2 - Cao_2}{C\acute{c}o_2 - C\bar{v}o_2}$$

where

$C\acute{c}o_2$ = End-capillary oxygen content
Cao_2 = Arterial oxygen content
$C\bar{v}o_2$ = Mixed venous oxygen content

Shunt fraction determination with 100% oxygen.

$\dot{Q}S/\dot{Q}T$ is often measured while the patient is breathing 100% oxygen. However, breathing 100% oxygen for 30 minutes can lead to nitrogen washout and collapse of low $\dot{V}/\dot{Q}$ units.[64-66] This phenomenon of alveolar collapse appears to be caused by poor ventilation of low $\dot{V}/\dot{Q}$ units so that oxygen uptake by the blood exceeds Do_2 to the alveoli via ventilation. The resulting microatelectasis increases shunt. Regional blood flow is usually reduced to areas of the lung with low $\dot{V}/\dot{Q}$ as a protective mechanism.[65] Breathing 100% oxygen alters this natural autoregulation,[66,67] causing increased shunt.

Pulmonary vasodilation[67] and inotropic agents (e.g., dopamine) increase cardiac output but can also increase intrapulmonary shunt.[56,57] If oxygen transport is improved with this pharmacologic support, its use may be indicated regardless of the increased shunt.

In patients without pulmonary artery catheters, an estimation of intrapulmonary shunt can be made by substituting the measured arteriovenous difference in the denominator with the value 3.5 vol%. This is a typical value in a critically ill patient with acceptable cardiac reserves.

The estimated shunt has been compared with the other oxygen tension indices described and to the gold standard, the measured shunt. The estimated shunt fraction has a stronger correlation to measured shunt than the other indices.[68]

Pulse Oximetry

Pulse oximetry is a noninvasive technique for measuring oxygen saturation of hemoglobin in the blood. The oximeter uses the spectrophotometric principle of light absorption. Pulse oximeters transmit two wavelengths of light—red and infrared—through arterialized capillary beds, such as the ear lobe or digit. Some of the light is absorbed by skin, fat, muscle, and venous blood, which are constant sources of absorption.

Some of the light is absorbed by the blood that flows through the arterioles in a pulsatile manner typical of arterial blood flow. As a result, there is a variable source of absorption. The pulse oximeter ignores the constant sources and focuses on the pulsatile absorption. The light absorption of oxygenated hemoglobin is different from that of reduced hemoglobin, and the pulse oximeter reads the differences to determine the degree of oxygen saturation. This process is rapid and provides measurement of heart rate as well as oxygen saturation.

The co-oximeters commonly used in blood gas laboratories transmit many wavelengths of light and can detect the amount of methemoglobin (MetHb), carboxyhemoglobin (CoHb), deoxyhemoglobin, and oxyhemoglobin. Pulse oximeters and co-oximeters therefore measure saturation differently. The pulse oximeter value is called functional saturation because it looks only at hemoglobins capable of binding with oxygen. It compares the amount of hemoglobin that is saturated with the amount of hemoglobin that is capable of being saturated:

$$\text{Pulse oximeter saturation} = \frac{\text{Hb saturated}}{\text{Hb saturated} + \text{Hb unsaturated}}$$

The co-oximeter value is called fractional saturation. It compares the amount of hemoglobin that is saturated with the total amount of hemoglobin that is present, including the forms of hemoglobin that do not bind with oxygen, the dyshemoglobins (e.g., CoHb, MetHb):

$$\frac{\text{Co-oximeter}}{\text{saturation}} = \frac{\text{Hb saturated}}{\text{Hb saturated} + \text{Hb unsaturated} + \text{Dyshemoglobins}}$$

As a result, in clinical conditions where dysfunctional hemoglobin levels are elevated (e.g., carbon monoxide poisoning, increased MetHb), the pulse oximeter will overestimate the true saturation.

Because pulse oximetry is quick and noninvasive and can be used for continuous monitoring, it has become extremely popular in recent years. As many as 28 companies manufacture pulse oximeters. Many studies have been performed to compare the accuracy and responsiveness of these different oximeters to direct measures of saturation.[69,70] Studies of healthy and critically ill patients with adequate cardiac outputs generally show a high degree of accuracy and correlation when compared with direct arterial saturation, as long as saturation is greater than 65%. The ability of oximeters to accurately measure severe desaturation (<65%) varies widely between instruments. Conditions that can cause erroneous values include abnormal perfusion levels from low cardiac output or peripheral shunting, hypothermia, elevated bilirubin concentrations (>10 mg/dL), elevated COHb or MetHb levels, and indocyanine green (Cardio-Green) or methylene blue dye.

Oximetry has been shown to be helpful in multiple settings, including the operating room or emergency room, during transport, and during special procedures such as bronchoscopy, computed tomography (CT) scanning, sleep studies, exercise testing, weaning from supplemental oxygen and mechanical ventilation, and pulmonary rehabilitation.[71,72] Oximetry can also be helpful in prescribing home oxygen therapy.

Selecting the monitoring site can be crucial to obtaining accurate results. Motion and states of low tissue perfusion interfere with signal acquisition. Pulse oximetry sensors are primarily applied to the thumb or a finger of the hand if available. Secondarily the great toe of either foot, an ear lobe, or the forehead can be used with the appropriate equipment. The ear lobe and forehead sensors are specifically manufactured for those sites and should not be applied elsewhere. Recent evidence of greater accuracy and precision of the forehead sensor during various states of oxygenation during exercise is encouraging.[73] One of the main limitations of pulse oximetry has been its lack of accuracy during hypothermia and shock. Since the forehead tissue is primarily perfused by arteries that originate centrally, it is theorized there will be adequate perfusion in this tissue even when peripheral circulation is compromised.

Pulse oximetry can be a useful tool in the ICU, but it is also prone to overuse and misinterpretation. Normal pulse oximetry values do not guarantee adequate DO_2 to the tissues. The anemic patient may be adequately saturated, but hypoxia may be present because of the low CaO_2.

Improvements in pulse oximetry technology have resulted in better artifact filtration and pulse signal recognition. These changes enable pulse oximeters to more accurately trace SpO_2 readings during periods of movement and during low flow, low perfusion states.

MONITORING TISSUE OXYGEN DELIVERY AND UTILIZATION

Oxygen Delivery/Availability

Oxygen delivery (DO_2) is calculated by the following equation:

$$\text{Cardiac output} \times CaO_2 \times 10^* = O_2 \text{ delivery}$$

The delivered oxygen value reflects the total amount of oxygen carried in the blood per unit of time. Normal values range from 550 to 650 mL/min/m². The delivered oxygen often is elevated with hyperdynamic states such as septic shock. Reduced values indicate low cardiac output, or decreased CaO_2. Increases in mean airway pressure may increase oxygen content but decrease cardiac output. Measuring DO_2 is one way to see whether the overall effect of a specific therapy is positive or negative. It could be argued that DO_2 as defined earlier does not accurately reflect the oxygen made available to the tissues. For example, oxygen bound to hemoglobin at a partial pressure of less than 20 mm Hg is typically considered to be unavailable to support aerobic metabolism. This occurs because, at a PaO_2 less than 20 mm Hg, there is an insufficient partial pressure gradient for oxygen to diffuse to the tissues. Hence the total amount of oxygen carried in the blood at a PO_2 of 20 mm Hg is unavailable for tissue consumption. The amount of oxygen available would be the oxygen that could be extracted by the tissues:

$$O_2 \text{ available} = CO \times (CaO_2 - C_{20}O_2)$$

where

CO = Cardiac output

CaO_2 = Arterial oxygen content

$C_{20}O_2$ = Oxygen content at a PO_2 of 20 mm Hg

The amount of $C_{20}O_2$ is significantly influenced by the position of the ODC as measured by the P-50. Left shifts in the ODC (low P-50) result in higher levels of $C_{20}O_2$ and less oxygen available to the tissues (Figure 13-10).

> **SIMPLY STATED**
> Roughly 30% to 50% of oxygen carried in the blood is not available to the tissues, but serves to keep the oxygen reservoir filled.

Oxygen Consumption

Oxygen consumption ($\dot{V}O_2$) is defined as the oxygen consumed by the entire body in milliliters per minute. The normal range is 2.86 to 4.29 mL/min/kg at STPD or 100 to 140 mL/min/m² of body surface area. If one thinks of DO_2 as supply, then $\dot{V}O_2$ is utilization. Adequate supply does not always ensure proper utilization.

Many factors determine tissue $\dot{V}O_2$. $\dot{V}O_2$ can be limited by decreased oxygen availability because of a decrease in regional perfusion or a decrease in oxygen content.[74,75] Demand may exceed supply, as in a hypermetabolic state, or cellular metabolism may be impaired, as in cyanide poisoning.

$\dot{V}O_2$ can be measured directly, through the analysis of inspired and exhaled gas volumes and concentrations, or indirectly, by multiplying the cardiac output by the arteriovenous oxygen content difference (Fick calculation). The formula for calculating $\dot{V}O_2$ using the direct method is as follows:

$$\dot{V}O_2 = \left(\left[\left(\frac{1 - F\bar{E}O_2}{1 - FIO_2} \right) \times FIO_2 \right] - F\bar{E}O_2 \right) \times \dot{V}_E$$

All volumes are converted to STPD conditions. Fraction of exhaled gas that is oxygen ($F\bar{E}O_2$) is measured directly. The formula assumes that nitrogen is an inert (nonreactive) gas and that no other gases are present. The presence of nitrous oxide (a gas used in surgery by anesthesiologists) may introduce a considerable error if the patient's $\dot{V}O_2$ is measured immediately after anesthesia.

Another direct technique requires that the patient breathe a specific concentration of gas through a closed circuit system that incorporates a carbon dioxide absorber. $\dot{V}O_2$ can be measured by the following formula:

$$\dot{V}O_2 = \text{Change in volume at STPD} \times FIO_2$$

Direct $\dot{V}O_2$ measurement techniques are extremely demanding. The circuit must be completely free of leaks. Gas volumes and concentrations must be accurately collected and measured. The FIO_2 must remain stable with minimal fluctuation. Recent technologic advances allow $\dot{V}O_2$ to be monitored continuously

---

*Change vol% to ml/L.

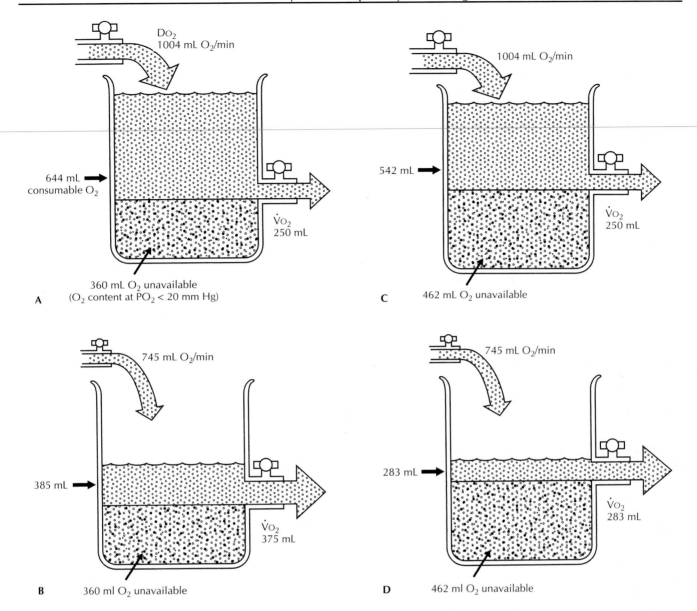

Figure 13-10 Interactions of oxygen delivery, oxygen consumption, and consumable oxygen. **A,** Do_2 (cardiac output × Cao_2) and $\dot{V}o_2$ (metabolic rate) are normal. The amount of O_2 carried in blood but not available to tissues for aerobic metabolism (O_2 carried at a Po_2 of 20 mm Hg) is represented by the hatched area below the spigot. Consumable oxygen (Do_2unavailable O_2) exceeds $\dot{V}o_2$. **B,** A typical occurrence in trauma. There is a reduction in Do_2 (fall in Hb, Pao_2/Sao_2, cardiac output) and an increase in $\dot{V}o_2$ (tissue injury, sepsis, etc.). Despite the fall in Do_2, Cons O_2 exceeds $\dot{V}o_2$, ensuring adequate oxygen availability. **C,** An increase in oxygen unavailable for consumption (i.e., left shift in oxygen demand curve [ODC]). Consequently, there is a reduction in Cons O_2, but sufficient O_2 remains available to exceed $\dot{V}o_2$. **D,** Collapse of oxygen reserves (reduced Do_2, low Cons O_2). $\dot{V}o_2$ is limited by Cons O_2. $\dot{V}o_2$ may rise if Cons O_2 is increased, either by increasing Do_2 or by right shifting the ODC. If metabolic demands continue to exceed O_2 availability, lactic acidosis results. *Cons O_2,* Oxygen available at a Po_2 20 mm Hg (see text); *Do_2,* delivered oxygen; *$\dot{V}o_2$,* oxygen consumption.

in critically ill patients during continuous mechanical ventilation.[76] The indirect calculation of $\dot{V}o_2$ is based on the Fick principle:

$$\dot{V}o_2 = \text{Cardiac output} \times C(a-\bar{v})O_2$$

The Fick principle is used often in the ICU, because of its convenience more than its accuracy. Variations between Fick calculations and direct measurement of $\dot{V}o_2$ may be as high as 20%, primarily because of errors in venous gas sampling and cardiac

output analysis.[77] This error is greatest in patients with high cardiac output.

Interpretation of $\dot{V}o_2$

When Do_2 is adequate, $\dot{V}o_2$ is determined by the metabolic demands of the patient. $\dot{V}o_2$ will stay constant as long as the delivered oxygen is greater than a critical threshold of approximately 8 to 10 mL/min/kg in anesthetized humans.[78] This critical threshold is significantly elevated in ARDS and sepsis[79] (Figure 13-11). In patients with ARDS, $\dot{V}o_2$ is linearly related to Do_2 up to 21 mL/min/kg.[80]

ICU patients often exhibit alterations in $\dot{V}o_2$ caused by trauma, sepsis, shock, changes in body temperature, anesthesia, therapeutic modalities such as chest physiotherapy, and ventilator settings. $\dot{V}o_2$ has been shown to be an excellent predictor of survival in patients with trauma and shock and is helpful in determining the adequacy of resuscitation.[75,79] It has also been advocated as an index of the cost of breathing in terms of oxygen use and therefore is useful in predicting the patient's ability to be weaned from mechanical ventilation.[81]

$\dot{V}o_2$ values of 100% to 150% of normal following trauma or shock are associated with a better prognosis and have been identified as appropriate therapeutic goals for the high-risk surgical patient.[82] Values less than 100% may be the result of decreased oxygen availability, as with low cardiac output or oxygen content, or with decreased use, as in hypothermia. In patients with severe injury, values greater than 150% may indicate a poor prognosis. If Do_2 is increased for any reason, increased availability may lead to increased consumption. This phenomenon has been observed in patients with ARDS, cardiogenic pulmonary edema, COPD, and pneumonia.[73,83]

📋 **SIMPLY STATED**

Oxygen consumption is partially influenced by oxygen availability. In many critically ill patients, as Do_2 goes, so goes oxygen consumption.

Mixed Venous Oxygen Tension

$P\bar{v}o_2$ is a measure of the partial pressure of oxygen in mixed venous blood and is an indication of oxygen usage by the entire body. Factors that influence oxygen transport and consumption invariably affect $P\bar{v}o_2$. The normal range is 38 to 42 mm Hg. Low $P\bar{v}o_2$ may result from the following:

- Inadequate cardiac output
- Anemia
- Significant hypoxia
- "Affinity" hypoxia (low $P\bar{v}o_2$ with increased $S\bar{v}o_2$)

A $P\bar{v}o_2$ of less than 27 mm Hg is usually associated with lactic acidosis. Increased $P\bar{v}o_2$ (> 45 mm Hg) may result from the following:

- Poor sampling technique
- Left-to-right shunt
- Septic shock
- Increased cardiac output
- Cyanide poisoning

Because $P\bar{v}o_2$ reflects the components of the supply-demand balance in perfused tissues, it is possible to have normal values of $P\bar{v}o_2$ and still have inadequate Do_2 to certain organs (e.g., kidneys). Organs with poor perfusion make a minimal contribution to venous return; therefore $P\bar{v}o_2$ may remain in the normal range even though an oxygen deficit exists, as in the vasodilated, septic patient with normal cardiac output.

$P\bar{v}o_2$ may not reflect changes in Do_2 and cardiac output. Because variations in $\dot{V}o_2$ also affect the balance between supply and demand, elevated $P\bar{v}o_2$ may indicate inadequate tissue oxygen utilization and marked maldistribution in systemic blood flow. This is common in septic shock. Low $P\bar{v}o_2$ may be expected when the tissues are using the available oxygen effectively, but the supply is inadequate.[84]

Table 13-1 shows that $\dot{V}o_2$ is high for the heart and the brain, so the $P\bar{v}o_2$ of these organs is extremely critical. A fall in perfusion would require a compensatory mechanism to maintain blood flow and oxygen to these organs.

The mixed venous sample is obtained by slowly aspirating, over approximately 1 minute, 3 to 5 mL of blood from the distal port of a pulmonary artery catheter. Central venous blood samples may trend well if the catheter is properly positioned, but generally there is a difference of 2 to 3 mm Hg between the Po_2 of central venous and pulmonary artery samples. The technique

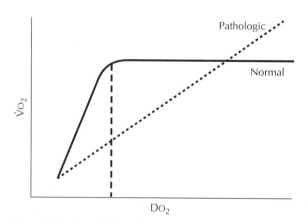

Figure 13-11 Supply dependence of oxygen consumption. Under normal conditions *(solid line)*, oxygen consumption ($\dot{V}o_2$) will increase until a critical threshold *(dashed line)* of delivered oxygen (Do_2) is reached. Beyond this critical threshold, $\dot{V}o_2$ remains stable, despite the increase in Do_2. In pathologic conditions *(dotted line)*, such as ARDS, $\dot{V}o_2$ may not plateau but will continue to rise, as Do_2 increases, until well past the normal critical threshold.

Table 13-1	**Basal Tissue Oxygen Exchange**	
	$P\bar{v}o_2$ (mm Hg)	Arteriovenous Oxygen Difference (vol%)*
Heart	23	11.4 (11)
Muscle	34	8.4 (30)
Brain	33	6.3 (20)
Viscera	43	4.1 (25)
Kidney	56	1.3 (7)
Skin	60	1.0 (2)

Modified with permission from Finch CA, Lenfant C: *N Engl J Med* 286:407, 1972.

*The number in parentheses represents the percentage of total oxygen delivery.

used for mixed venous gas analysis is important because errors in sampling may result in erroneous readings. The pressure waveform should be inspected before the sample is aspirated to ensure that the catheter is not wedged. Wedging may result in aspirating postcapillary blood and thus produce an erroneously high measurement of $P\bar{v}O_2$. Air bubbles in the sample are also a possible cause of falsely elevated values.

Mixed Venous Oxygen Saturation

Mixed venous oxygen saturation ($S\bar{v}O_2$) is measured from a mixed venous blood sample. Small changes in $P\bar{v}O_2$ lead to large changes in $S\bar{v}O_2$ and therefore large changes in $C\bar{v}O_2$. As a result, the $S\bar{v}O_2$ measurement is a sensitive index of cardiac output and tissue perfusion if $\dot{V}O_2$ is stable (Table 13-2). Like $P\bar{v}O_2$, $S\bar{v}O_2$ is a means of monitoring the general supply-and-demand differences in DO_2, not the use of oxygen at a specific site.

$S\bar{v}O_2$ may be monitored continuously through a fiberoptic reflectance oximetry system incorporated in a five-lumen pulmonary artery catheter. The system incorporates the principle of reflection spectrophotometry. Traditional oximetry uses transmission spectrophotometry. An optical module transmits light through the blood via a fiberoptic monofilament. Reflected light is transmitted by a separate monofilament to a photodetector in the module. Because reduced hemoglobin and oxygenated hemoglobin absorb different wavelengths of light, a microprocessor can quantify the reflected wavelengths and calculate $S\bar{v}O_2$ (Figure 13-12). When the catheter is properly positioned and calibrated, values correlate well with benchmark saturation measurements.[85] Continuous monitoring has the advantage of providing immediate feedback for purposes of evaluating therapy.

Various factors such as suctioning, shivering, pharmacologic intervention, extubation, weaning, and positive-pressure therapy can decrease the $S\bar{v}O_2$ measurement, signifying a deterioration in pulmonary gas exchange, an increase in $\dot{V}O_2$, or a reduction in cardiac output.

Arterial–Mixed Venous Oxygen Content Difference

The arterial–mixed venous oxygen content difference, $C(a - \bar{v})O_2$, reflects the difference in oxygen content between arterial and venous blood. It is derived after simultaneous arterial and mixed venous blood gases are drawn. Normal range is 4 to 6 vol%.

Values greater than 6 vol% may be the result of the following:
- Low cardiac output
- Increasing $\dot{V}O_2$

Values less than 4 vol% may be the result of the following:
- Septic shock
- Increased cardiac output
- Anemia
- Increased oxygen affinity caused by a left-shifted ODC

The $C(a - \bar{v})O_2$ is useful in determining the effects of mechanical ventilation and PEEP on cardiac output[86] and evaluating the need for additional circulatory support. It has a slight advantage over the $P\bar{v}O_2$ measurement in that it reflects content differences instead of partial pressure.

> ## SIMPLY STATED
> Traditional parameters such as pulse oximetry and PaO_2 reflect the adequacy of pulmonary oxygenation, not tissue oxygenation.

Oxygen Extraction Ratio

The oxygen extraction ratio $[C(a - \bar{v})O_2 / CaO_2]$ expresses the relationship between available oxygen (oxygen content of arterial blood) and oxygen extracted ($C(a - \bar{v})O_2$. The normal value is 25% to 30%. Values greater than 30% indicate one of the following:
- Increased extraction caused by low cardiac output
- Increased $\dot{V}O_2$
- Decreased oxygen availability caused by decreased CaO_2

Values less than 25% indicate that supply is out of proportion to demand, which may be a result of the following:
- High cardiac output
- Sepsis with systemic shunts

The oxygen extraction ratio identifies the portion of the delivered oxygen actually consumed and is therefore an index of the efficiency of circulation.

Blood Lactate

If oxygen transport or its use by the tissues is insufficient for metabolic demands, anaerobic metabolism occurs and lactic acid is produced. Clinically this is seen as a metabolic acidosis with an elevation in blood lactate concentrations. The degree of lactic acidosis corresponds to the severity of oxygen deficit and is therefore a good indicator of prognostic outcome in patients with shock.[87,88] Normal values for blood lactate are less than 1.7 to 2.0 mM/L. In patients with shock, lactate levels greater than 3.83 mM/L are associated with 67% mortality, and values greater than 8 mM/L are associated with greater than 90% mortality.[88,89] Beta-adrenergic stimulator drugs increase lactate levels because of glycolysis, and beta blockers decrease

Table 13-2	Interpretation of Venous Saturation ($S\bar{v}O_2$)
$S\bar{v}O_2$	Interpretation
68%-77%	Normal
>77%	Sepsis, left-to-right shunt, excessive cardiac output, hypothermia, cell poisoning, wedged catheter
<60%	Cardiac decompensation
<50%	Lactic acidosis
<30%	Unconsciousness
<20%	Permanent damage

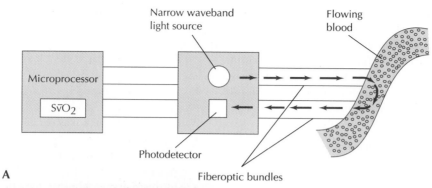

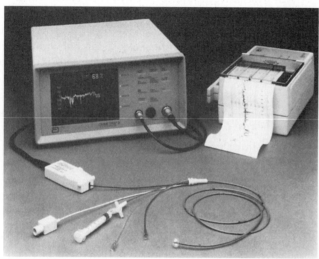

Figure 13-12 A, Principles of reflection spectrophotometry. **B,** Fiberoptic catheter system used for continuous monitoring of venous oxygen saturation. (**A,** From Ruppel GL: *Manual of pulmonary function testing,* ed 8, St Louis, 2003, Mosby. **B,** Courtesy Hospira, Inc., Lake Forest, IL.)

blood lactate levels.[90] Patients with lactic acidosis are often treated with alkaline solutions such as sodium bicarbonate. This alkalinization may increase blood lactate levels because of a redistribution of extracellular and intracellular lactate levels but does not indicate a worsening metabolic acidosis.[91]

Patients with cirrhosis have a reduced ability to clear peak lactate concentrations after periods of increased production. As a result, lactate is useful in confirming the presence of tissue hypoxia in these patients, but it is not a useful prognostic index.[92]

SIMPLY STATED

Parameters that incorporate ventilator settings (oxygenation index) are helpful in determining severity of illness and can guide the initiation of other forms of care (i.e., if OI ≥ 25 for 4 hours, consider lung-protective ventilation strategies).

REVIEW QUESTIONS

1. Which of the following is true regarding the measurement of tidal volume as a means of ventilatory assessment in the intensive care unit?
   a. It is normally 3 to 4 mL/kg of ideal body weight.
   b. It should be at least 450 mL before weaning from mechanical ventilation.
   c. It may decrease after abdominal or thoracic surgery.
   d. All of the above.

2. Which of the following would minimize the chance of stacking of mechanical tidal volumes (air trapping) during mechanical ventilation?
   a. Increasing inspiratory flow
   b. Increasing mechanical respiratory rate
   c. Increasing the set tidal volume
   d. None of the above

3. An increased $\dot{V}_E$ with a normal $PaCO_2$ indicates which of the following?
   a. Shunt
   b. Decreased metabolic rate
   c. Increased dead space
   d. Atelectasis

4. T   F   An increased metabolic rate results in an increased production of carbon dioxide.

5. Which of the following is true regarding the measurement of vital capacity in the intensive care unit?
   a. The value obtained depends on patient position and effort.
   b. It reflects the ventilatory reserve of the patient.

c. A value of less than 10 mL/kg suggests pending respiratory failure.

d. All of the above.

6. Which of the following modalities increases functional residual capacity?
   a. Prolonging expiratory time (expiratory retard)
   b. PEEP/CPAP
   c. Pressure-controlled ventilation
   d. Volume-controlled ventilation

7. Which of the following would cause peak airway pressures to increase on a mechanical ventilator?
   a. Partial obstruction of an artificial airway
   b. Tension pneumothorax
   c. High inspiratory flow setting
   d. All of the above

8. T F The measurement of plateau pressure during mechanical ventilation is a better index of the elastic recoil of the lung than peak pressure.

9. Given a peak pressure of 50 cm H_2O, a static pressure of 35 cm H_2O, a PEEP of 5 cm H_2O, and a measured tidal volume of 850 mL, what is the effective static compliance?
   a. 12 mL/cm H_2O
   b. 18 mL/cm H_2O
   c. 24 mL/cm H_2O
   d. 28 mL/cm H_2O

10. Which of the following is true regarding auto-PEEP?
    a. It normally is not detected on the ventilator manometer.
    b. It can be reduced by decreasing inspiratory flow.
    c. Bronchodilators exacerbate the condition.
    d. All of the above.

11. Given a peak airway pressure of 40 cm H_2O, a static pressure of 32 cm H_2O, a PEEP of 7 cm H_2O, a tidal volume of 675 mL, and an inspiratory flow of 60 L/min what is the airway resistance?
    a. 2 cm H_2O/L/sec
    b. 5 cm H_2O/L/sec
    c. 8 cm H_2O/L/sec
    d. 12 cm H_2O/L/sec

12. T F Increases in mean airway pressure usually cause a reduction in PaO_2.

13. T F A MIP of 30 cm H_2O has been shown to be a predictor of successful weaning.

14. Which of the following might be useful in adjusting the level of PEEP applied to a patient with acute lung injury?
    a. Flow-pressure loop
    b. Volume-time scalar
    c. Pressure-volume loop
    d. Pressure-time scalar

15. The pressure-time scalar can be used to assess which of the following?
    a. Peak airway pressure
    b. Mode of ventilation
    c. Estimate of patient effort
    d. Adequacy of inspiratory flow
    e. All of the above

16. Which of the following is true regarding the measurement of V_D/V_T in the intensive care unit?
    a. It is calculated using the PaO_2 and $PaCO_2$.
    b. It is often increased during mechanical ventilation.
    c. It is normally 50% to 60%.
    d. None of the above.

17. Which of the following would most likely result in a decrease in oxygen transport?
    a. Cardiac output of 6 L/min
    b. Arterial saturation of 75%
    c. Hemoglobin level of 15 g/dL
    d. All of the above

18. T F A left-shifted oxyhemoglobin dissociation curve may result in a decreased oxygen delivery to the tissues.

19. Which of the following clinical indices denotes poor oxygenation?
    a. PaO_2 of 80 mm Hg
    b. PaO_2/F_IO_2 ratio of 400
    c. $P(A-a)DO_2$ of 55 on 21% oxygen
    d. All of the above

20. T F Oxygen consumption is an excellent predictor of survival in patients with shock and trauma.

21. Which of the following would cause a low $P\bar{v}O_2$?
    a. Left to right shunt
    b. Increased cardiac output
    c. Septic shock
    d. Hypoxia

22. T F A $C(a-\bar{v})O_2$ of 8 vol% could be caused by a reduced cardiac output.

23. Which of the following is true regarding the measurement of blood lactate?
    a. It corresponds to the level of oxygen deficit.
    b. It is usually a result of anaerobic metabolism.
    c. It can be increased by the administration of beta-adrenergic agonist drugs.
    d. All of the above.

24. What does pulse oximetry measure?
    a. PaO$_2$
    b. Functional saturation
    c. Oxygen content
    d. Blood pH

REFERENCES

1. Hudson LD: Monitoring of critically ill patients: conference summary, *Respir Care* 30:628, 1985.

2. Tobin MJ: Respiratory monitoring in the intensive care unit, *Am Rev Respir Dis* 138:1625, 1988.

3. Askanazi J and others: Patterns of ventilation in postoperative and acutely ill patients, *Crit Care Med* 7:41, 1979.

4. Engoren M: Approximate entropy of respiratory rate and tidal volume during weaning from mechanical ventilation, *Crit Care Med* 26(11):1817, 1998.

5. Hedley-Whyte J and others: The response of patients with respiratory failure and cardiopulmonary disease to different levels of constant volume ventilation, *J Clin Invest* 45:1543, 1966.

6. Meade MO and others: How to use articles about harm: the relationship between high tidal volumes, ventilating pressures, and ventilator-induced lung injury, *Crit Care Med* 25(11):1915, 1997.

7. Hickling KG and others: Low mortality rate in adult respiratory distress syndrome using low-volume, pressure-limited ventilation with permissive hypercapnia: a prospective study, *Crit Care Med* 22(10):1568, 1994.

8. Carlton DP and others: Lung overexpansion increases pulmonary microvascular protein permeability in young lambs, *J Appl Physiol* 69:577, 1990.

9. Dreyfuss D and others: High inflation pressure pulmonary edema, respective effects of high airway pressure, high tidal volume, and positive end-expiratory pressure, *Am Rev Respir Dis* 137:1159, 1988.

10. Hernandez LA and others: Chest wall restriction limits high airway pressure–induced lung injury in young rabbits, *J Appl Physiol* 66:2364, 1989.

11. Finfer S, Rocker G: Alveolar overdistension is an important mechanism of persistent lung damage following severe protracted ARDS, *Anaesth Int Care* 24(5):569, 1996.

12. ARDS Network: Ventilation with lower tidal volumes as compared with traditional tidal volumes for acute lung injury and the acute respiratory distress syndrome, *N Engl J Med* 342(18):1301-1308, 2000.

13. Neumann P and others: Effect of different pressure levels on the dynamics of lung collapse and recruitment in oleic-acid–induced lung injury, *Am J Respir Crit Care Med* 158(5):1636, 1998.

14. DeHaven CB and others: Evaluation of two extubation criteria: attributes contributing to success, *Crit Care Med* 14:92, 1986.

15. Vassilakopoulos T, Zakynthinos S, Roussos C: The tension-time index and the frequency/tidal volume ratio are the major pathophysiologic determinants of weaning failure and success, *Am J Respir Crit Care Med* 158(2):378, 1998.

16. Jubran A, Tobin MJ: Pathophysiologic basis of acute respiratory distress in patients who fail a trial of weaning from mechanical ventilation, *Am J Respir Crit Care Med* 155(3):906, 1997.

17. Krieger BP and others: Serial measurements of the rapid-shallow-breathing index as a predictor of weaning outcome in elderly medical patients, *Chest* 112(4):1029, 1997.

18. Yang KL, Tobin MJ: A prospective study of indexes predicting the outcome of trials of weaning from mechanical ventilation, *N Engl J Med* 324:1445, 1991.

19. Capdevila X and others: Changes in breathing pattern and respiratory muscle performance parameters during difficult weaning, *Crit Care Med* 26(1):79, 1998.

20. Craig DG: Postoperative recovery of pulmonary function, anaesthesia and analgesia, *Anaesthesia* 60:46, 1981.

21. Wessell HV and others: Breath-by-breath variation of FRC: effect on VO$_2$ and VCO$_2$ measured at the mouth, *J Appl Physiol* 46:1122, 1979.

22. Kaneko JK and others: Regional distribution of ventilation and perfusion as a function of body position, *J Appl Physiol* 21:767, 1966.

23. West JB: *Regional differences in the lung,* New York, 1977, Academic Press.

24. West JB: Regional differences in the lung, *Chest* 74:426, 1978.

25. Scadding JG, Cumming G: *Scientific foundations of respiratory medicine,* Philadelphia, 1981, WB Saunders.

26. Webb H, Tierney D: Experimental pulmonary edema due to intermittent positive pressure ventilation with high inflation pressures: protection with PEEP, *Am Rev Respir Dis* 110:556, 1974.

27. Corbridge T and others: Adverse effects of large tidal volume, and low PEEP in canine acid aspiration, *Am Rev Respir Dis* 142:311, 1990.

28. Muscedere J and others: Tidal ventilation at low airway pressures can cause pulmonary edema (abstract), *Am Rev Respir Dis* 145:A454, 1992.

29. Dantzker DR and others: Ventilation-perfusion distributions in the adult respiratory distress syndrome, *Am Rev Respir Dis* 120:1039, 1979.

30. Shapiro BA and others: Positive end expiratory pressure therapy in adults with special reference to acute lung injury: a review of the literature to suggested clinical correlations, *Crit Care Med* 12:127, 1984.

31. Rose DM and others: Temporal responses of FRC and oxygen tension to changes in PEEP, *Crit Care Med* 9:79, 1981.

32. Warters RD, Allen SJ, Tonnesen AS: Intratracheal pressure monitoring during synchronized intermittent mandatory ventilation and pressure-controlled inverse ratio ventilation, *Crit Care Med* 25(2):227, 1997.

33. Gay PC and others: Evaluation of bronchodilator responsiveness in mechanically ventilated patients, *Am Rev Respir Dis* 138:880, 1987.

34. Morina P and others: Effects of nebulized salbutamol on respiratory mechanics in adult respiratory distress syndrome, *Intens Care Med* 23(1):58, 1997.

35. Haake R and others: Barotrauma: pathophysiology, risk factors, and prevention, *Chest* 91:608, 1987.

36. Pierson DJ: Alveolar rupture during mechanical ventilation: role of PEEP, peak airway pressure, and distending volume, *Respir Care* 33:472, 1988.

37. Gottfried SB and others: Interrupter technique for measurement of respiratory mechanics in anaesthetized humans, *J Appl Physiol* 59:647, 1985.

38. Leatherman J and others: Does measured auto-PEEP accurately reflect the degree of dynamic hyperinflation during mechanical ventilation of status asthma? (abstract), *Am Rev Respir Dis* 147:A877, 1993.

39. Berman LS and others: Inspiration expiration ratio: is mean airway pressure the difference? *Crit Care Med* 9:775, 1981.

40. Marini JJ, Ravenscraft SA: Mean airway pressure: physiologic determinants and clinical importance—part 2: clinical implications, *Crit Care Med* 20:1604, 1992.

41. Marini JJ and others: Estimation of inspiratory muscle strength in mechanically ventilated patients: the measurement of maximal inspiratory pressure, *Crit Care Med* 1:32, 1986.

42. Tahvanai J and others: Extubating criteria after weaning from IMV and CPAP, *Crit Care Med* 11:702, 1983.

43. Marini JJ: The role of the inspiratory circuit in the work of breathing during mechanical ventilation, *Respir Care* 32:419, 1987.

44. Brouchard L: Intrinsic (or auto-) PEEP during controlled mechanical ventilation, *Int Care Med* 28:1376-1378, 2002.

45. Bone RC: Compliance and dynamic characteristics curves in acute respiratory failure, *Crit Care Med* 4:173, 1976.

46. Lu Q, Rouby JJ: Measurement of pressure-volume curves in patients on mechanical ventilation: methods and significance, *Crit Care* 4:91-100, 2000.

47. Browning JA and others: Effect of a fluctuating FIO_2 on metabolic measurement in mechanically ventilated patients, *Crit Care Med* 10:82, 1982.

48. Fletcher R: *The single breath test for carbon dioxide,* Lund, Sweden, 1980, University of Lund.

49. AARC Clinical Practice Guideline, Capnography/Capnometry during mechanical ventilation – 2003 revision and update, *Resp Care* 48(5):534-539, 2003.

50. Craig K, Pierson DJ: Expired gas collections for deadspace calculations: a comparison of two methods, *Respir Care* 24:435, 1979.

51. Reidek K and others: Regional intrapulmonary gas distribution in awake and anaesthetized paralyzed man, *J Appl Physiol* 42:391, 1977.

52. Fairley HB, Blenkarm GD: Effect on pulmonary gas exchange of variations in inspiratory flow rate during IPPV, *Br J Anaesth* 38:320, 1966.

53. Dammann JF and others: Optimal flow pattern for mechanical ventilation of the lungs, *Crit Care Med* 6:293, 1978.

53a. Haldane JS: Symptoms, causes, and prevention of anoxemia. *Br Med J* 65-72, 1919.

54. Finch CA, Lenfant C: Oxygen transport in man, *N Engl J Med* 286:407, 1972.

55. Bryant-Brown CW: Blood flow to the organs: parameters for function and survival in critical illness, *Crit Care Med* 16:170, 1988.

56. Berk JL and others: The use of dopamine to correct the reduced cardiac output resulting from positive end expiratory pressure, *Crit Care Med* 5:269, 1977.

57. Jardin F and others: Dobutamine: a hemodynamic evaluation in human septic shock, *Crit Care Med* 9:329, 1981.

58. Kanber GJ and others: The alveolar-arterial oxygen gradient in young and elderly men during air and oxygen breathing, *Am Rev Respir Dis* 97:376, 1968.

59. Maxwell C and others: Use of the arterial/alveolar oxygen tension ratio to predict the inspired oxygen concentration needed for a desired arterial oxygen tension, *Respir Care* 29:1135, 1984.

60. Luterman A and others: Withdrawal from positive end-expiratory pressure, *Surgery* 83:328, 1981.

61. Hallman M and others: Exogenous human surfactant for treatment of severe respiratory distress syndrome: a randomized prospective clinical trial, *J Pediatr* 106:963, 1985.

62. Bartlett H and others: Extracorporeal membrane oxygenation (ECMO) in neonatal respiratory failure, *Ann Surg* 204:236, 1986.

63. Cane RD: Minimizing errors in intrapulmonary shunt calculations, *Crit Care Med* 8:294, 1980.

64. West JB: Pulmonary gas exchange in the critically ill patient, *Crit Care Med* 2:171, 1974.

65. Suter PM and others: Shunt, lung volume and perfusion during short periods of ventilation with oxygen, *Anesthesiology* 43:617, 1975.

66. Quan SF and others: Changes in venous admixture with alterations of inspired oxygen concentration, *Anesthesiology* 52:477, 1980.

67. Domino KB and others: Influence of mixed venous oxygen tension on blood flow to atelectatic lung, *Anesthesiology* 59:428, 1983.

68. Cane RD and others: Unreliability of oxygen tension-based indices in reflecting intrapulmonary shunting in critically ill patients, *Crit Care Med* 16:1243, 1988.

69. Severinghaus JW, Naifeh KH: Accuracy of response of six pulse oximeters to profound hypoxia, *Anesthesiology* 67:551, 1987.

70. Nickerson BG and others: Bias and precision of pulse oximeters and arterial oximeters, *Chest* 93:515, 1988.

71. Chapman KR and others: The accuracy and response characteristics of a simplified ear oximeter, *Chest* 83:860, 1983.

72. Scoggin C and others: Clinical evaluation of a new ear oximeter, *Heart Lung* 6:121, 1977.

73. Yamaya Y and others: Validity of pulse oximetry during maximal exercise in normoxia, hypoxia, and hyperoxia, *J Appl Physiol* 92: 162-168, 2002.

74. Mohsenifar Z and others: Dependence of oxygen consumption on oxygen delivery in patients with chronic congestive heart failure, *Chest* 92:447, 1987.

75. Shoemaker WC and others: Tissue oxygen debt as a determinant of lethal and nonlethal postoperative organ failure, *Crit Care Med* 16:1117, 1988.

76. Nelson LD and others: Clinical validation of a new metabolic monitor suitable for use in critically ill patients, *Crit Care Med* 15:951, 1987.

77. Nelson LD and others: Vo_2 and PEEP in acute respiratory failure, *Crit Care Med* 10:857, 1982.

78. Cain SM: Peripheral oxygen uptake and delivery in health and disease, *Clin Chest Med* 4:139, 1983.

79. Astiz ME and others: Relationship of oxygen delivery and mixed venous oxygenation to lactic acidosis in patients with sepsis and acute myocardial infarction, *Crit Care Med* 16:655, 1988.

80. Moshsenifar Z and others: Relationship between O_2 delivery and O_2 consumption in ARDS, *Chest* 84:267, 1983.

81. Harpin RP and others: Correlation of the oxygen cost of breathing and length of weaning from mechanical ventilation, *Crit Care Med* 15:807, 1987.

82. Shoemaker WC and others: Prospective trial of supranormal values of survivors as therapeutic goals in high-risk surgical patients, *Chest* 94:1176, 1988.

83. Danek SJ and others: The dependence of oxygen uptake on oxygen delivery in ARDS, *Am Rev Respir Dis* 122:387, 1980.

84. Dantzker DR: Oxygen transport and utilization, *Respir Care* 33:874, 1988.

85. Divertie MB, McMichan JC: Continuous monitoring of mixed venous oxygen saturation, *Chest* 85:423, 1984.

86. Downs JB and others: The effect of incremental PEEP on Pao_2 in patients with respiratory failure, *Anesth Analg* 52:210, 1973.

87. Broder G, Weil MH: Excess lactate: an index of reversibility of shock in human patients, *Science* 143:1457, 1964.

88. Rashkin MC and others: Oxygen delivery in critically ill patients: relationship to blood lactate and survival, *Chest* 87:580, 1985.

89. Cady LD and others: Quantitation of severity of critical illness with special reference to blood lactate, *Crit Care Med* 1:75, 1973.

90. Berk J, Sampliner JE: *Handbook of critical care medicine,* ed 2, Boston, 1982, Little, Brown.

91. Pichette C and others: Elevation of the blood lactate concentration by alkali therapy without requiring additional lactic acid accumulation: theoretical considerations, *Crit Care Med* 10:323, 1982.

92. Rinke C: Controversies in lactic acidosis: implications in critically ill patients, *JAMA* 258:49, 1988.

CHAPTER

14

Michael L. Lum

Assessment of Cardiac Output

LEARNING OBJECTIVES

Upon completion of this chapter, the reader should be able to accomplish the following:

1. Define cardiac output, *cardiac index, stroke volume, and venous return.*
2. Recognize the following regarding cardiac output:
   a. Method of calculation
   b. Range of normal values
   c. Effect of sympathetic nervous stimulation
3. Recognize the following regarding the distribution of blood flow:
   a. Effect of metabolism and reduced oxygen availability on the regulation of blood flow through organs
   b. Percentage of total blood volume in venous system
   c. Effect of blood loss (hypovolemia) on circulatory function
   d. Basal distribution of blood flow to organs versus distribution during cardiac failure
   e. Effect of mechanical ventilation
4. Define and identify significance of the following indicators of cardiac output:
   a. Cardiac index
   b. Ejection fraction
   c. Stroke volume
   d. End-diastolic volume
   e. Cardiac work
   f. Ventricular stroke work
5. Recognize the following regarding preload:
   a. Definition
   b. Values used to measure preload of the left and right ventricles
   c. Factors affecting
   d. Clinical value of ventricular function curves
   e. Effect of mechanical ventilation
6. Recognize the following for afterload:
   a. Definition
   b. Factors affecting
   c. Measurement

d. Effect of vasodilators
e. Calculation of systemic and pulmonary vascular resistance
f. Effect of mechanical ventilation
7. Identify the following regarding contractility:
   a. Definition
   b. Factors affecting
   c. Assessment
8. Recognize the technique for obtaining cardiac output via the following invasive methods:
   a. Thermodilution
   b. Fick
   c. Pulse contour
   d. Doppler ultrasonic transducers
9. Recognize the noninvasive methods for evaluating cardiac performance:
   a. Transthoracic electrical bioimpedance
   b. Echocardiography
   c. Radionuclide cardiac imaging
   d. Partial CO_2 rebreathing

CHAPTER OUTLINE
Cardiac Output
Venous Return
Measures of Cardiac Output and Pump Function
    Cardiac Index
    Cardiac Work
    Ventricular Stroke Work
    Ventricular Volume
    Ejection Fraction
Determinants of Pump Function
    Heart Rate
    Preload
    Afterload
    Contractility
Methods of Measuring Cardiac Output
    Invasive Methods
    Noninvasive Methods

Susan Jones Krider, RN, MS, contributed this chapter in the previous edition.

KEY TERMS

afterload

cardiac index (CI)

cardiac output

cardiac work

cardiac work index

central venous pressure (CVP)

contractility

ejection fraction (EF)

end-diastolic pressure (EDP)

end-diastolic volume (EDV)

negative inotropic effect

positive inotropic effect

preload

pulmonary capillary wedge pressure (PCWP)

pulmonary vascular resistance (PVR)

rate-pressure product

stroke volume (SV)

systemic vascular resistance (SVR)

venous return

ventricular compliance

ventricular function curves

ventricular stroke work

CHAPTER OVERVIEW

Hemodynamic monitoring of the critically ill is an essential function in the intensive care unit. Adequacy of perfusion is the most important factor in the assessment of the cardiovascular system's ability to meet the body's metabolic demands. Early detection of key circulatory function derangements allows the clinician to begin proactive therapeutic interventions. This is important because most patients do not succumb to their disease but to vital organ failure.[1]

In this chapter, we introduce the fundamental concepts related to assessment of perfusion. The chapter centers around the definition of cardiac output and related physiologic measurements. In addition, the factors that affect cardiac output and the techniques for measuring it are described. Chapter 15 describes the specific hemodynamic parameters used in the ICU to monitor patients with circulatory issues.

CARDIAC OUTPUT

The amount of blood pumped out of the left ventricle in a minute is known as cardiac output (Box 14-1). It is the product of heart rate (HR) and stroke volume (SV), the volume of blood ejected by the ventricle by a single heart beat. Normal SV for adults is 60 to 130 mL/beat and is roughly equal for both the left and right ventricles. The average cardiac output for men and women of all ages is approximately 5 L/min at rest (normal range is 4 to 8 L/min); however, the normal cardiac output for an individual varies with age, sex (10% higher in men), body size, blood viscosity (hematocrit), and the tissue demand for oxygen.

The normal heart, when not stimulated by the autonomic nervous system, is capable of pumping approximately 10 to 13 L/min and twice that amount when stimulated by the sympathetic nervous system. A well-trained athlete's heart enlarges sometimes as much as 50% and is capable of pumping up to 35 L/min.[2,3] Under normal conditions, the heart plays a passive role in cardiac output and pumps whatever amount of blood is returned to it. When the diseased or damaged heart can no

---

BOX 14-1   Cardiac Output: An Overview

Cardiac output (CO):

Amount of blood pumped by the heart per minute
$$CO = Heart\ Rate \times Stroke\ Volume$$
Varies with age, sex, body size, blood viscosity, and tissue demand for oxygen
Normal adult cardiac output: 4-8 L/min
cardiac index: 2.5-4 L/min/m^2

Stroke volume (SV):

Volume of blood ejected with each beat, determined by:
Preload: stretch on ventricle at filling before contraction volume, venous return, compliance
Afterload: resistance to ventricular emptying vasoconstriction versus vasodilation, blood viscosity, ventricular wall tension, negative intrathoracic pressure
Contractility: strength of ventricular contraction sympathetic stimulation, inotropes, depressants, coronary flow, heart muscle damage

Frank-Starling mechanism (ventricular function curve):

Defines a characteristic relationship between:
Volume filling the ventricle (end diastolic volume) and volume ejected per contraction (ventricular stroke volume) ↑ filling volume → ↑ muscle stretch → ↑ energy → ↑ output
If the ventricle becomes too large, overdistention → ↓ SV

Ventricular filling volume and filling pressure are closely related:

Filling pressure is used to evaluate ventricular filling volume
Atrial pressures approximate ventricular end-diastolic pressure
Right atrial pressure (RAP or CVP) for right heart filling
Left atrial pressure (LAP) for left heart filling
Pulmonary wedge pressure approximates LAP and left heart filling pressure in most patients. (See Chapter 15.)

Cardiac output can be used to determine vascular resistance:

$$Resistance = \frac{Pressure}{Flow} \quad (See\ Table\ 14\text{-}3.)$$
↑ Vascular resistance → ↑ heart work
↓ Vascular resistance (vasodilation) → ↓ heart work and potentially to hypovolemia
Right heart: Pulmonary vascular resistance (PVR)
Left heart: Systemic vascular resistance (SVR)
Ventricular filling pressure, volume, vascular resistance, and blood pressure can be manipulated by fluids and drugs to optimize cardiac output and perfusion of oxygen and nutrients to the tissues.

---

longer pump the amount of blood returned to it, it is said to be *failing*.

VENOUS RETURN

The volume of blood returning to the right atrium is known as the venous return. The resting blood flow through an organ is determined by the metabolic needs of the organ. As the organ's demand for oxygen increases, perfusion to the organ increases. The muscles, liver, and kidneys receive the greatest amount of blood flow in the resting state because of their high metabolic needs (Table 14-1). When the metabolic activity of the tissue increases (as seen with exercise) or when the availability of oxygen to the tissues decreases (as occurs at high altitudes or with carbon monoxide or cyanide poisoning), vasodilation allows more blood to flow to the tissues.

The muscle fibers of the precapillary sphincters and the metarterioles in the capillary beds are controlled by the concentration of oxygen, carbon dioxide, hydrogen ions, electrolytes, and other humoral substances. When oxygen is low and hydrogen ions and carbon dioxide levels are increased at the tissue level, vasodilation occurs. The greater the vasodilation, the more blood flows to the area. (Hypoxia has the opposite effect on the pulmonary vasculature, causing vasoconstriction, which shunts the greatest amount of blood flow to the oxygenated alveoli, thus maintaining the best oxygenation.)

In addition to providing tissue regulatory control of cardiac output, the venous system acts as a reservoir of blood to maintain flow to the vital organs when blood volume is lost. Approximately 64% of the total blood volume is normally in the venous system.[3] When blood volume decreases, the veins as well as the venous reservoirs (spleen, liver, abdominal veins, and even heart and lungs) constrict and redistribute volume to maintain venous return and cardiac pressures. In fact, 20% to 25% of the total blood volume can be lost without altering circulatory function and pressures.[3] If blood flow is decreased to the point that central nervous system (CNS) compensatory mechanisms come into play, sympathetic stimulation causes vasoconstriction and the blood flow to certain organs is further decreased. Table 14-1 shows that as the heart fails, the CNS will reduce blood flow to the liver, kidneys, and other body areas to maintain perfusion to the most vital organs (heart and brain).

> ### SIMPLY STATED
> - The adequacy of perfusion is the most important factor in the assessment of the cardiovascular system's ability to meet the body's metabolic demands.
> - Blood flow to tissues can be inadequate when blood pressure is too low, but a normal blood pressure does not always indicate optimal blood flow to the tissues.
> - The ability to measure cardiac output as well as blood pressure enables the clinician to assess and manipulate the abnormal cardiovascular system in a rational fashion to improve blood flow to tissues.

MEASURES OF CARDIAC OUTPUT AND PUMP FUNCTION

Cardiac Index

Because cardiac output, like most other hemodynamic measurements, varies with body size, cardiac index may be used to describe flow output. Cardiac index (CI) is *cardiac output divided by body surface area (BSA)* and is reported as liters per minute per square meter (L/min/m²). *Body surface area (BSA)* is calculated using the patient's weight and height and a nomogram (Figure 14-1). When a straight line is drawn connecting the patient's weight and height, it intersects the center line and shows the patient's BSA in square meters. The advantage of using an index is that the normals are standardized and comparisons can be made among patients of different heights and weights.

A normal resting cardiac index for patients of all ages is 2.5 to 4.0 L/min/m², with the average for adults approximately 3.0 L/min/m² (Table 14-2). The cardiac index is highest at 10 years of age and decreases with age to approximately 2.4 L/min/m² at age 80 years.[3]

> ### SIMPLY STATED
> The advantage of using an indexed measurement such as cardiac index is that the normals are standardized and comparisons can be made among patients of different sizes.

Cardiac Work

Cardiac work is a measurement of the energy the heart uses to eject blood against the aortic or pulmonary pressures (resistance) and increases as the end-diastolic ventricular size increases. Cardiac work correlates well with the oxygen requirements of the heart. Although the left and right ventricles eject the same volume of blood, the left ventricle must eject against the mean aortic pressure (MAP), which is about six times the mean pulmonary artery pressure (MPAP); therefore the measures of cardiac work are much higher for the left ventricle. The

Table 14-1	Distribution of Blood Flow					
	Basal		**Cardiac Failure**		**Exercise**	
	L/min	%	L/min	%	L/min	%
Brain	0.75	13	0.5	15	0.75	3.0
Heart	0.25	4	0.3	9	1.0	4.0
Muscle	1.2	21	1.2	35	22.0	88.0
Liver	1.4	24	0.8	24	0.3	1.2
Kidney	1.1	19	0.35	10	0.25	1.0
Skin	0.5	9	0.05	1	0.6	2.4
Other	0.6	10	0.2	6	0.1	0.4
	5.8		3.4		25.0	
O₂ uptake	240 mL/min		300 mL/min		2000 mL/min	

Adapted from Finch CA, Lenfant C: Oxygen transport in man, *N Engl J Med* 286:407, 1972.

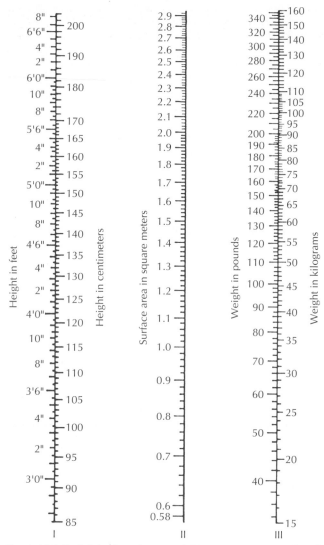

Figure 14-1 DuBois body surface area (BSA) nomogram. BSA is found by locating the patient's height on scale I and weight on scale III and placing a straightedge between the two points. The line intersects scale II at patient's BSA. (From DuBois EF: *Basal metabolism in health and disease*, Philadelphia, 1936, Lea & Febiger.)

cardiac work index (*LCWI and RCWI*) measures the work per minute per square meter for each ventricle and is calculated using the following formulas:

$$LCWI = CI \times MAP \times 0.0136 = 3.4 - 4.2 \ kg / min/m^2$$

$$RCWI = CI \times MPAP \times 0.0136 = 0.4 - 0.66 \ kg / min /m^2$$

where 0.0136 is a conversion factor for changing pressure to work.

Ventricular Stroke Work

Ventricular stroke work is a measure of myocardial work per contraction. It is the product of the SV times the pressure across the vascular bed. Normal indexed values are as follows:

Left ventricular stroke work index (LVSWI) =
43 – 61 g/min/m²/beat

Right ventricular stroke work index (RVSWI) =
7 – 12 g/min/m²/beat

Ventricular Volume

End-diastolic ventricular size can be assessed by the end-diastolic volume (EDV), defined as the amount of blood in the ventricle at the end of filling (diastole). The most common indirect method of measuring the end-diastolic ventricular size is the measurement of the end-diastolic pressures (EDP). Further discussion of the EDV and EDP relationship is found in this chapter under the "Ventricular Function Curves" section.

Ejection Fraction

Ejection fraction (EF) represents the percentage of the end-diastolic volume that is ejected with each beat. Normal ejection fraction is 65% to 70%. Ejection fraction is either measured directly or calculated from the following formula:

$$EF = SV/EDV$$

The ejection fraction declines as cardiac function deteriorates. When the ejection fraction falls to the 30% range, a patient's exercise tolerance is severely limited because of the heart's inability to maintain an adequate cardiac output.

DETERMINANTS OF PUMP FUNCTION

The performance ability of the heart (cardiac output) is determined by both HR and SV. SV is determined by three factors: preload, afterload, and contractility (Figure 14-2).

Heart Rate

HR normally does not play a large role in control of cardiac output in the adult except when it is outside the normal range or when arrhythmia is present.

Bradycardia is a HR less than 60 beats/min in an adult. Low HR does not drop cardiac output if the heart can compensate with increased SV; the best example is the well-trained athlete with a resting pulse rate below 50 but a normal blood pressure. However, if a patient has a damaged heart that cannot alter SV to compensate for bradycardia, cardiac output will fall.

Tachycardia (adult HR > 100 beats/min) is the body's compensation to maintain cardiac output when compensatory mechanisms to increase SV are inadequate. In the resting patient, cardiac output may begin to decline at rates of 120 to 130 beats/min. Because diastole is shortened by increased rates, the time for ventricular filling is decreased with tachycardia. In addition, maintaining the higher rate requires an increased oxygen consumption that the patient with coronary artery disease may not be able to provide. With exercise and sympathoadrenal stimulation, cardiac output does not decline until approximately 180 beats/min. *Premature heart beats* (pre-

Table 14-2 Hemodynamic Variables, Normal Values, and Formulas

Variable	Normal Range*	Formula
Cardiac output (CO)	4-8 L/min	CO = direct measurement
Cardiac index (CI)	2.5-5.0 L/min/m^2	CI = CO/BSA
Stroke volume (SV)	60-130 mL/beat	SV = CO/HR or EDV − ESV
Stroke index (SI)	30-50 mL/m^2	SI = CI HR or SV/BSA
Ejection fraction (EF)	65%-75%	EF = SV/EDV or direct measurement
End-diastolic volume (EDV)	120-180 mL/beat	EDV = direct measurement
End-systolic volume (ESV)	50-60 mL	ESV = direct measurement
Rate-pressure product (RPP)	<12,000 mm Hg	RPP = systolic BP × HR
Coronary perfusion pressure (CPP)	60-80 mm Hg	CPP = diastolic BP − PCWP
Left cardiac work index (LCWI)	3.4-4.2 kg/min/m^2	LCWI = CI × MAP × 0.0136†
Right cardiac work index (RCWI)	0.4-0.66 kg/min/m^2	RCWI = CI × MPAP × 0.0136†
Left ventricular stroke work index (LVSWI)	50-62 g/min/m^2/beat	LVSWI = SI × MAP × 0.0136‡
Right ventricular stroke work index (RVSWI)	7.9-9.7 g/min/m^2/beat	RVSWI = SI × MPAP × 0.0136‡
Pulmonary vascular resistance (PVR)	<2 units 110-250 dynes/sec/cm^5	PVR = (MPAP − PCWP)/CO PVR = (MPAP − PCWP)/CO × 80§
Pulmonary vascular resistance index (PVRI)	225-315 dynes/sec/cm^5/m^2	PVRI = (MPAP − PCWP)/CI × 80§
Systemic vascular resistance (SVR)	15-20 units 900-1400 dynes/sec/cm^5	SVR = (MAP − CVP)/CO SVR = (MAP − CVP)/CO × 80§
Systemic vascular resistance index (SVRI)	1970-2400 dynes/sec/cm^5/m^2	SVRI = (MAP − CVP)/CI × 80§

BP, Blood pressure; *CVP*, central venous pressure (mm Hg); *MAP*, mean arterial pressure (mm Hg); *MPAP*, mean pulmonary artery pressure (mm Hg); *PCWP*, pulmonary capillary wedge pressure (mm Hg).

*Normal values for adults. Sources vary in normal values reported, but values are within the same general range.

†Conversion factor to convert L/mm Hg to kg min/m^2; 0.0144 is used by some sources.[28]

‡Conversion factor to convert mL/mm Hg to g/min/m^2; 0.144 is used by some sources.[28] An alternative version of the formula includes subtraction of the filling pressures: LVSWI = SV × (MAP − PCWP) × 0.0136; RSWI = SV × (MPAP − CVP) × 0.0136.[29,30]

§Conversion factors of 79.92 and 79.96 may also be used.[28,29]

Data from Shoemaker WC: Monitoring of the critically ill patient. In Shoemaker WC and others: *Textbook of critical care medicine*, ed 2, Philadelphia, 1989, WB Saunders; Pollard E, Seliger E: *An implementation of bedside physiological calculations*, Waltham, Mass, 1985, Hewlett-Packard; and Daily EK, Schroeder JS: *Techniques in bedside hemodynamic monitoring*, ed 4, St. Louis, 1989, Mosby.

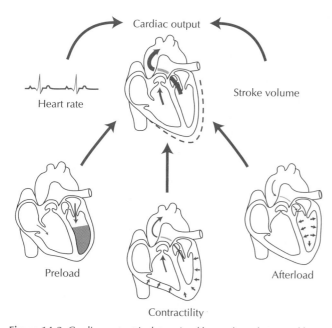

Figure 14-2 Cardiac output is determined by stroke volume and heart rate. Stroke volume is determined by preload, afterload, and contractility.

mature ventricular [PVCs] and atrial [PACs] contractions) also alter the time for ventricular filling and may decrease cardiac output.

Preload

Preload is the stretch on the ventricular muscle fibers before contraction. *Preload* is created by the *end-diastolic volume*. In 1914, Starling found that up to a critical limit, the force of a muscle contraction was directly related to the initial length of the muscle prior to contraction. His theory has come to be known as *Starling's law* of the heart. Simply stated, the greater the stretch on the resting ventricle, the greater the strength of contraction within physiologic limits. When the physiologic limits are exceeded, greater stretching of the muscles does not result in an increased force of contraction.

Ventricular Function Curves

Figure 14-3 shows ventricular function curves (often called *Starling curves*) for the right and left ventricles. The horizontal axis represents the volume (preload), and the vertical axis is a measure of the heart's output: cardiac output, cardiac index, SV, stroke index, or ventricular stroke work index. Increasing the volume increases output. When the pump becomes over-stretched, it is no longer able to eject all of its blood efficiently and cardiac output begins to fall.

Continuously measured end-diastolic volume is the ideal but time-consuming way to assess preload. Most critical care units only measure ventricular volumes on a periodic basis using echocardiography or radionuclide imaging. Therefore atrial pressures, which can be measured continuously, are used to reflect end-diastolic volume. During diastole, the atrioventricular valves (tricuspid and mitral) are open. If there is no narrowing or dysfunction of the valves, the pressures in the atrium and ventricle should be the same at end-diastole. The filling pressure for the right heart is right atrial pressure, commonly measured as central venous pressure (CVP). The filling pressure for the left heart is left atrial pressure, commonly measured as pulmonary capillary wedge pressure (PCWP). How these pressures are measured and used to represent preload is discussed in Chapter 15. Because a nonlinear relationship exists between the *end-diastolic volume* and *end-diastolic pressure*, filling pressure does not always reflect ventricular volume in the critically ill patient when ventricular compliance is altered. An example in which end-diastolic pressure does not accurately reflect end-diastolic volume is in patients with increased ventricle chamber stiffness (e.g., myocardial infarction). End-diastolic pressure may remain constant as end-diastolic volume decreases.

Ventricular Compliance

It is important to understand that pressure is the result of the volume, space, and compliance of the chamber the volume is entering. Forcing 100 mL of water into a small, rigid chamber takes more pressure than filling a compliant balloon with 100 mL of water. Figure 14-4 shows how ventricular pressure is affected by changes in volume and ventricular compliance (elasticity, stretchability, distensibility). When compliance is reduced, a much higher pressure is generated for a given volume. Pressure also increases more rapidly as the ventricle fills; thus the ends of the curves rise more abruptly as the ventricle becomes full and tension is developed in the ventricular walls.

Factors that *decrease ventricular compliance* and therefore cause the pressure to increase out of proportion to the volume include the following:

- Myocardial ischemia and infarction
- Hemorrhagic and septic shock
- Pericardial effusions
- Right ventricular dilation and overload (causing the septum to shift to the left and impinge on the left ventricle)

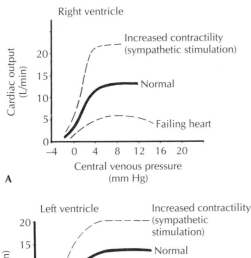

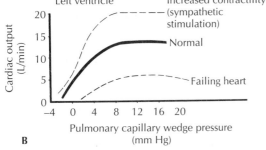

Figure 14-3 Ventricular function curves for right and left ventricles. Note that filling pressures are used to represent end-diastolic volume. **A,** Ventricular function curves for right ventricle. Upstroke of curve shows rapid change in cardiac output for small change in end-diastolic volume initially, but the curve then plateaus, with little change in output for large changes in right atrial pressure. Dashed curves show change in output for given pressure occurring with altered contractility from sympathetic stimulation (as occurs with exercise or fear) and heart failure. **B,** Ventricular function curves for left ventricle. End-diastolic volume can be used for plotting horizontal axis. Cardiac index, stroke volume, or left ventricular stroke work index can be graphed on the vertical axis rather than cardiac output. Output begins to decline after pulmonary capillary wedge pressure reaches 20 mm Hg unless ventricular compliance is altered.

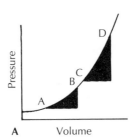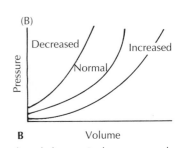

Figure 14-4 Compliance can be altered along a single pressure volume relationship or by a change in the rate of increase in diastolic pressure. **A,** Small rise in pressure (point A to point B) for given change in end-diastolic volume is in contrast to large increase in pressure seen from point C to point D with the same (or smaller) change in end-diastolic volume. Therefore the ventricle described by A to B is more compliant than the ventricle described by C to D. **B,** Ventricular compliance curves. Not only may compliance fall along the ascending curve, but disease and drugs may also effect a change in the compliance curve up and to the left (reduced compliance) or down and to the right (increased compliance). (From Sibbald WJ, Driedger AA: Right and left ventricular preload and diastolic ventricular compliance: implications for therapy in critically ill patients. In Shoemaker WC, Thompson WL, editors: *Critical care: state of the art*, vol 3, Fullerton, Calif, 1982, Society for Critical Care Medicine.)

- Positive end-expiratory pressure (PEEP)
- Continuous positive airway pressure (CPAP)
- Inotropic drugs (increase the strength of myocardial contraction)

Factors that *increase ventricular compliance* include:
- Relief of ischemia
- Vasodilator drugs (nitroprusside, nitroglycerin)
- Cardiomyopathies

Factors That Affect Venous Return, Preload, and Cardiac Output

The three main factors affecting the amount of blood returned to the heart are the following:
- Changes in circulating blood volume
- Changes in the distribution of the blood volume
- Atrial contraction

Circulating blood volume

Circulating blood volume is obviously altered by bleeding but is also decreased by loss of other body fluids. Large amounts of urine output (as occurs with diuretics), wound drainage, diarrhea, perspiration, and gastric secretions can result in a large decrease in blood volume (hypovolemia). Fluid can also shift into the interstitial space. Sepsis, burns, and shock may result in tremendous amounts of fluid being moved into this so-called *third space*. On the other hand, fluids ingested or given intravenously increase the circulating blood volume. Administration of colloids (large-molecular-weight solutions) pulls water from the interstitial space to "dilute out" the large molecules, resulting in an increase in blood volume. Small children can also have large increases in blood volume from respiratory care humidification, especially ultrasonic nebulizers.

Distribution of the blood volume

Distribution of the blood volume is altered not only by third-spacing, but also by changes in *body position, venous tone, intrathoracic pressure*, and, rarely, by obstruction of the large veins returning to the heart. As the body changes position, blood tends to move to dependent areas. Standing decreases venous return; conversely, raising the legs of a patient who is lying down increases venous return.

Venous tone also alters the distribution of blood in the body. Venous tone may increase (vasoconstriction) as a compensatory mechanism and shift more blood to the core (heart, lungs, and brain). Vasodilation therapy resulting from therapy with nitrates, nitroprusside (Nipride), or furosemide (Lasix) relaxes vascular tone and may decrease venous return.

Raised intrathoracic pressure decreases venous return. Tension pneumothorax, the Valsalva maneuver, breath-holding in children, prolonged bouts of coughing, and positive-pressure ventilation increase intrathoracic pressure and thereby decrease venous return.

Atrial contraction

Atrial contraction contributes approximately 30% of the total cardiac output by loading the ventricle at the end of diastole. When a patient develops atrial fibrillation, atrioventricular dissociation, or third-degree heart block, or is being paced by a ventricular pacemaker, this so-called *atrial kick* is lost, and cardiac output may fall.

Clinical Applications of Ventricular Function Curves

Preload is the major determinant of contractility, but ideal filling pressures vary greatly with cardiac compliance and the patient's condition. *Ventricular function curves* may be constructed to find a patient's ideal filling pressure at a given time and provide information about ventricular compliance. Most commonly, they are used when large amounts of fluid are administered; however, they may also be used to monitor cardiac output response to changes in filling pressure resulting from volume unloading (diuresis) and administration of intravenous cardiopulmonary drugs such as inotropes and vasodilators.

To construct a ventricular function curve, cardiac index, cardiac output, SV, or another measure of heart output is plotted on the vertical axis. Filling pressure (usually pulmonary artery diastolic or pulmonary capillary wedge pressure) is plotted on the horizontal axis. A baseline cardiac output measurement is obtained, and the point corresponding to the cardiac output reading and simultaneous pressure reading is plotted (Figure 14-5, *A*). A *fluid challenge* is administered, and another set of output and pressure measurements is obtained. Pressure is again plotted against output. As the plotting continues, a Starling (or ventricular function) curve is created. When satisfactory cardiac output is achieved or when cardiac output begins to decline as the filling pressure increases, the fluid challenge is stopped. The pressure that corresponds to the highest cardiac output reading obtained is used to indicate optimal preload. Volume can then be administered as needed to maintain this optimal pressure. It is important to remember that the venous system will begin to "relax" and expand as the volume status is corrected, so it is necessary to follow the patient carefully and reassess the need for additional volume.

Effects of Mechanical Ventilation on Preload and Venous Return

Normal spontaneous breathing

During normal spontaneous *inspiration*, contraction of the diaphragm and enlargement of the thoracic cage reduces the intrapleural pressure to approximately −6 cm H_2O. The decrease in intrapleural pressure enlarges the normally negative gradient between the intrathoracic and extrathoracic vessels and favors the movement of blood into the chest and heart, thus increasing venous return. These negative inspiratory pressures are also transferred to the heart. The resulting fall in intracardiac pressures pulls more blood into the heart, which augments preload.

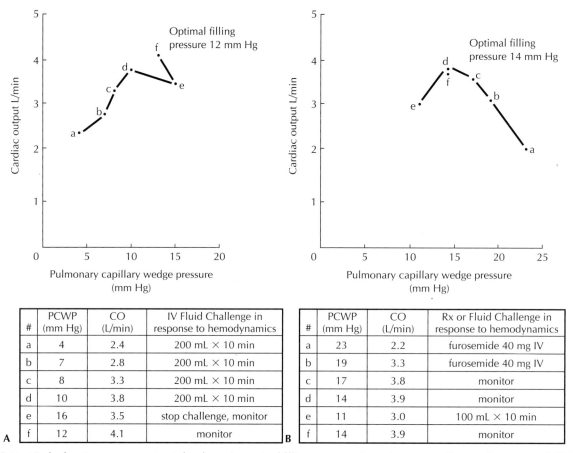

#	PCWP (mm Hg)	CO (L/min)	IV Fluid Challenge in response to hemodynamics
a	4	2.4	200 mL × 10 min
b	7	2.8	200 mL × 10 min
c	8	3.3	200 mL × 10 min
d	10	3.8	200 mL × 10 min
e	16	3.5	stop challenge, monitor
f	12	4.1	monitor

A

#	PCWP (mm Hg)	CO (L/min)	Rx or Fluid Challenge in response to hemodynamics
a	23	2.2	furosemide 40 mg IV
b	19	3.3	furosemide 40 mg IV
c	17	3.8	monitor
d	14	3.9	monitor
e	11	3.0	100 mL × 10 min
f	14	3.9	monitor

B

Figure 14-5 Ventricular function curves constructed to determine optimal filling pressure using pulmonary capillary wedge pressure (PCWP, mm Hg) as the filling pressure measurement, and *cardiac output* (CO, L/min) as the heart output measurement. **A,** *Fluid challenge curve for a patient with low output (CO 2.4 L/min) and low filling pressure (PCWP 4 mm Hg)* treated with 4 IV fluid challenges. Administrations of the first three fluid challenges *(a-c)* were followed by increases in filling pressure and output (↑ PCWP to 10, ↑ CO to 3.8). After the fourth challenge *(d)*, filling pressure continued to increase but output began to fall *(e)* (↑ PCWP to 16, ↓ CO to 3.5), suggesting volume overload. The fluid challenge was stopped. Subsequent measurements confirmed that output increased as the filling pressure dropped back toward normal *(f)* (↓ PCWP to 12, ↑ CO to 4.1). An optimal filling pressure near 12 mm Hg using PCWP was suggested. **B,** *Diuresis curve for a heart failure patient with low cardiac output (2.2 L/min) and high filling pressure (PCWP 23 mm Hg)* treated with two doses of intravenous (IV) furosemide. Diuresis following the first dose of furosemide decreased the filling pressure with a corresponding improvement in heart output *(b)* (↓ PCWP to 19, ↑ CO to 3.3). A second dose of furosemide was given to further unload the ventricle and improve pulmonary congestion. Filling pressure decreased toward the normal range and output improved *(c-d)* (↓ PCWP to 14, ↑ CO to 3.9). However, continuing diuresis caused the filling pressure and the output to drop *(e)* (↓ PCWP to 11, ↓ CO to 3.0). A fluid challenge was given to increase filling pressure and output improved *(f)* (↑ PCWP to 14, ↑ CO to 3.9). An optimal filling pressure near 14 mm Hg using PCWP was suggested.

During spontaneous *expiration*, the reverse occurs. Recoil of the thoracic cage causes the intrathoracic pressure to rise, augmenting cardiac output and creating the slight rise in arterial blood pressure that is normally seen with expiration. Thus spontaneous inspiration functions as a circulatory assist pump for the heart. During *labored breathing*, these pressure changes are increased and may result in a *paradoxical pulse:* a drop in blood pressure during inspiration of more than 10 mm Hg.

Increased intrapleural pressure

Increased intrapleural pressure, as occurs during the Valsalva maneuver, decreases venous return, and thereby may decrease cardiac output. Increased intrapleural pressure also occurs with

loss of spontaneous breathing, disruption of the chest wall, collection of fluid or air in the pleural space, or positive-pressure ventilation.

Positive-pressure ventilation and compliance

The effect positive pressure breathing has on venous return depends on how much of the airway pressure is transferred to the pleural space. When lung and thorax *compliances are equal,* only about half of the change in airway pressure is transmitted to the pleural space. If the lung compliance decreases, as occurs with certain types of respiratory failure, less positive pressure is transmitted to the pleural space; thus these patients can better tolerate positive-pressure ventilation with little effect on cardiovascular function.

When *chest wall compliance decreases*, more airway pressure is transmitted to the pleural space. This is commonly seen with abdominal distention or following surgery, when patients splint their chests and abdomens because of pain. If *chest wall compliance is decreased while lung compliance is increased* (e.g., chronic obstructive pulmonary disease [COPD]), even more of the raised airway pressure is transmitted to the pleural space. These patients are more likely to develop problems of both decreased venous return and increased pulmonary vascular resistance, resulting in decreased cardiac output during positive pressure ventilation.

PEEP and CPAP

Positive expiratory pressures including auto-PEEP (inadvertent PEEP) not only exaggerate the inspiratory effects of positive-pressure ventilation, but also maintain increased intrapleural pressure throughout expiration, thus having an even greater potential of decreasing venous return. It has been shown that *venous return* is affected most by continuous mechanical ventilation (CMV) with PEEP, less by CPAP, and least by spontaneous breathing ambient inspiratory pressure and PEEP.

Cardiac output is affected less by positive airway pressure (e.g., CMV, PEEP, CPAP) if intravascular volume is maintained or increased to offset the ventilator-induced reduction in venous return. The effect of mechanical ventilation on pulmonary artery pressure measurement is discussed in Chapter 15.

SIMPLY STATED

Because the heart is inside the chest, it is subject to the pressure changes occurring in the chest:
- Positive pressures around the heart push on the heart, making it harder for blood to enter the heart (decrease venous return) but easier for blood to be ejected.
- Negative pressures around the heart pull blood toward the heart (increase venous return and preload) but make it more difficult for blood to leave the heart.

Afterload

Afterload, the resistance or sum of the external factors that oppose ventricular ejection, has two components:
- Tension in the ventricular wall
- Peripheral resistance (sometimes called *impedance*)

Ventricular Wall Tension

Cardiac factors that deter ventricular emptying include the following:
- Distention of the ventricle
- Increased intraventricular pressure
- Thin ventricular wall
- Negative intrathoracic pressure

Resistance to ventricular emptying is even greater when both ventricle distention and intraventricular pressure are increased at the same time.

Increased afterload

When the ventricle is distended from too much volume and pressure, tension in the muscle increases and more oxygen and energy are required for contraction. Thus afterload increases. Similarly, as intrathoracic pressure becomes more negative, the vacuum-like effect favors the opening and filling of the ventricle but increases resistance to ventricular emptying.

Decreased afterload

Positive intrathoracic pressure favors compression of the ventricle, decreases the pressure gradient across the ventricular wall, and decreases resistance to ventricular emptying, but opposes right ventricular filling. Intermittent positive pressure breathing (IPPB) with PEEP may compress the heart during inspiration, reducing diastolic filling but at the same time enhancing systolic emptying, a perfect combination for many patients in congestive heart failure. Afterload also decreases as the size of the ventricular muscles increases.

Peripheral Resistance

The peripheral component of afterload is determined by the following:
- Elasticity (compliance) of the vessels
- Size (radius) of the vessels
- Viscosity of the blood
- Changes in pressure from one end of the vessel to the other

Increased vascular resistance

The *radius* of the vessels is the greatest determinant of peripheral resistance to blood flow. When the vessels are constricted, the heart must exert more energy to eject the blood. Vasoconstriction further increases afterload because the constricted vessels are less compliant. As afterload increases, the *myocardial oxygen demands* on the heart also increase. When the heart is receiving an inadequate supply of oxygen (as occurs with coronary artery disease), it is not able to produce the amount of energy needed to eject efficiently against the afterload, and failure worsens. A downward cycle of cardiac failure ensues if afterload is not decreased; inadequate cardiac output causes vasoconstriction, which causes increased work for the heart, which results in less cardiac output and more vasoconstriction, and so on. The cycle is broken by maximizing cardiac oxygenation and performance and decreasing the afterload, either by vasodilator therapy or with a cardiac assist device such as an intraaortic balloon pump.

Afterload also increases as the *viscosity* of the blood increases. This is an important consideration in patients with chronic pulmonary disease because the concentration of red blood cells in their blood often is abnormally high to increase their oxygen-carrying capacity. When hematocrit levels significantly exceed about 60%, cardiac output often decreases. Conversely, one of the causes of high cardiac output (hyperdynamic state) is anemia (low hematocrit).

Blood flow is also dependent on a pressure gradient. When the backpressure in the venous system increases, as occurs when the right heart is not able to pump blood efficiently, the pressure gradient across the capillary beds decreases. Flow from the arteries through the capillaries to the venous system slows. This damming effect causes the afterload to increase.

Decreased vascular resistance

It is important to remember that although vasodilator therapy decreases afterload and therefore decreases the energy demands on the heart, it also increases the size of the "vascular container." If the container is made larger but the volume in the container stays the same, the amount of blood returning to the heart (venous return) decreases, and preload decreases. Conversely, when the volume in the ventricle is more than the ventricle can pump effectively, decreasing the preload can unload the ventricle and improve cardiac output. However, if the venous return decreases too much, the stretch on the ventricle (preload) will be inadequate and cardiac output will fall. In addition, if vasodilation causes the arterial diastolic pressure to fall below 50 mm Hg or mean arterial pressure (MAP) to fall below 60 mm Hg, perfusion to the coronary arteries may decrease, and cardiac output will be compromised even further.

Calculating Systemic and Pulmonary Vascular Resistance

Calculation of systemic vascular resistance (SVR) and pulmonary vascular resistance (PVR) provides numbers that can be used to evaluate the vascular component of afterload for each of the ventricles. As the numbers increase, afterload is increasing; decreasing numbers mean that afterload is decreasing. There are

three sets of normal values for vascular resistance. They can be calculated in hybrid resistance units (mm Hg/L/min), multiplied by 80 and reported as absolute resistance units (dynes/sec/cm^5), or divided by cardiac index and reported as an index (Table 14-3).

Elevated systemic vascular resistance can be caused by anything that causes vasoconstriction: cold, inadequate perfusion; hypertension; or drugs that vasoconstrict, such as norepinephrine (Levophed), methoxamine (Vasoxyl), or epinephrine (Adrenalin). Warming a hypothermic patient to normal temperature or administering vasodilators such as nitroprusside, phentolamine (Regitine), or chlorpromazine (Thorazine) *decreases SVR.*

PVR is increased by constriction, obstruction (e.g., emboli), or compression of the pulmonary vasculature or by backpressure from the left heart. Hypoxemia, acidosis, and release of histamine from an allergic response also cause vasoconstriction with an increase in PVR. Over time, increased PVR causes changes in the pulmonary vasculature, resulting in pulmonary hypertension and eventually cor pulmonale (Table 14-4).

> **SIMPLY STATED**
> Cardiac output may decrease by one third before a significant drop in arterial blood pressure occurs. Because systemic arterial pressure is the product of SVR and cardiac output, reflex vasoconstriction may increase SVR and maintain a normal or increased blood pressure despite the decreasing cardiac output. The patient may suddenly "crash" when compensatory vasoconstriction is maximized and vasoconstriction can no longer maintain an adequate blood pressure.

Contractility

The third primary factor determining cardiac output is contractility, which is a measure of myocardial contraction strength. The strength of a cardiac contraction is modified by two major influences:

Table 14-3   Normal Values and Formulas for Vascular Resistances

Variable	Normal Range*	Formula
Pulmonary vascular resistance	<2 units 110-250 dynes/sec/cm^5	PVR = (MPAP − PCWP)/CO PVR = (MPAP − PCWP)/CO × 80[†]
Pulmonary vascular resistance index	225-315 dynes/sec/cm^5/m^2	PVRI = (MPAP − PCWP)/CI × 80[†]
Systemic vascular resistance	15-20 units 900-1400 dynes/sec/cm^5	SVR = (MAP − CVP)/CO SVR = (MAP − CVP)/CO × 80[‡]
Systemic vascular resistance index	1970-2400 dynes/sec/cm^5/m^2	SVRI = (MAP − CVP)/CI × 80[‡]

*Normal values for adults. Sources vary in normal values reported, but values are within the same general ranges.
[†]Conversion factors of 79.92 and 79.96 may also be used.[28,29]
Data from Shoemaker WC: Monitoring of the critically ill patient. In Shoemaker WC and others: *Textbook of critical care medicine*, ed 2, Philadelphia, 1989, WB Saunders; Pollard E, Seliger E: *An implementation of bedside physiological calculations*, Waltham, Mass, 1985, Hewlett-Packard; and Daily EK, Schroeder JS: *Techniques in bedside hemodynamic monitoring*, ed 4, St. Louis, 1989, Mosby.

Table 14-4	Causes of Pulmonary Hypertension and Cor Pulmonale
Mechanisms	**Related Disorders**
Loss of pulmonary vasculature and tissue (blockage, compression, destruction)	Primary pulmonary hypertension, multiple pulmonary emboli, pulmonary thrombosis Malignant metastasis, collagen-vascular diseases Inflammatory and fibrosing disease of the lung (diffuse interstitial pneumonia, sarcoidosis, the pneumonconioses)
Pulmonary vasoconstriction resulting from hypoxia and acidosis	COPD (emphysema, bronchitis, asthma) Neuromuscular disorders (e.g., myasthenia gravis, Guillain-Barré syndrome, poliomyelitis) Extreme obesity (pickwickian syndrome) Thoracic spine and chest wall deformities
Increased pulmonary venous pressure	Mitral valve stenosis, left atrial embolus or tumor, rheumatic heart disease Idiopathic veno-occlusive disease
Increased pulmonary blood flow (left-to-right shunt)	Ventricular septal defect, patent ductus arteriosus
Increased blood viscosity	Polycythemia

Modified from Margulies DM, Thaler MS: *The physician's book of lists*, New York, 1983, Churchill Livingstone.

- Change in the initial muscle length caused by stretch of the cardiac muscle (preload)
- Change in contractility or inotropic state of the heart at any given amount of muscle stretch

For all practical purposes, contractility can be thought of as a change in the force and speed of shortening of the heart muscle that is independent of changes in preload or afterload. Referring back to Figure 14-3, an increase in contractility is shown to be associated with an increase in cardiac output, despite no change in the preload. Conversely, heart failure is usually accompanied by decreased contractility with a downward shift of the ventricular function curve and a lowering of cardiac output for a given preload.

Factors Related to Contractility

Myocardial contractility is related to the following factors:
- Sympathetic nerve stimulation
- Inotropic drugs
- Physiologic depressants
- Damage to the heart
- Coronary blood flow

Sympathetic nerve stimulation

Sympathetic nerve stimulation with release of norepinephrine and other circulating catecholamines results in an increase in the strength and the rate of cardiac contraction: the fight-or-flight response. Conversely, inhibiting the sympathetic nervous system with a drug or by total spinal anesthesia depresses contractility. Parasympathetic stimulation (vagal stimulation) also decreases contractility.

Inotropic drugs

Inotropic drugs are medications that affect the strength of contraction. A drug with a positive inotropic effect increases the force and velocity of contraction and myocardial oxygen consumption. Positive inotropic drugs include calcium, digitalis, epinephrine, norepinephrine, dopamine, dobutamine, amrinone, isoproterenol, and caffeine. If a positive inotropic drug is used to drive the heart when there is inadequate preload, myocardial oxygen supply and demand can become increasingly mismatched and even result in myocardial infarction. Therefore it is necessary to maximize preload before "driving" the heart with these drugs.

Drugs with a negative inotropic effect decrease the strength of contraction but may also decrease the myocardial oxygen demand. Negative inotropic drugs include beta blockers, barbiturates, and many antiarrhythmic agents, such as procainamide and quinidine. In a patient with angina resulting from myocardial ischemia, negative inotropic agents such as beta blockers may be used to enhance the relationship of myocardial oxygen supply to demand.

Physiologic depressants

Physiologic depressants include hypoxia, hypercapnia, and acidosis. Decreased extravascular calcium and elevated potassium and sodium levels can severely depress contractility and cause the heart to become flaccid. An excess of calcium ions has the opposite effect, causing the heart to go into spastic contraction. Low potassium and sodium levels are associated with cardiac fibrillation. Conduction disturbances and arrhythmia from any cause can decrease cardiac performance.

Damage to the heart

Damage to the myocardium, valves, or conduction system reduces the pumping ability of the heart. Loss of ventricular substance results in decreased contractility because of the reduced effectiveness of muscle contraction, as in cardiomyopathy, myocardial ischemia, and myocarditis. The muscle in the area of a myocardial infarction may have no contraction or, over time, may even balloon out and develop into a ventricular aneurysm.

Chronic increase in the workload of the heart over time will result in enlargement of the chambers and hypertrophy of the muscle.

Coronary blood flow

The flow of blood through the myocardium is influenced by myocardial oxygen demand. When myocardial oxygen demand is increased, coronary blood flow increases. This autoregulation of coronary blood occurs within a MAP range of 60 to 180 mm Hg. Coronary blood flow continues throughout the cardiac cycle but is depressed during systole and increased during diastole. When MAP or diastolic pressure falls, perfusion of the coronary sinus may be compromised, resulting in decreased myocardial oxygen delivery and a subsequent fall in contractility.

Normal *coronary perfusion pressure (CPP)* is 60 to 80 mm Hg and is calculated as follows:

$$CPP = Diastolic\ BP - PCWP$$

> **SIMPLY STATED**
> **Factors Affecting Contractility**
> Decreased contractility generally is caused by loss of contractile muscle mass resulting from injury, disease, dysrhythmias, drugs, or poor perfusion.
> Increased contractility can be caused by sympathetic nerve stimulation or inotropic drugs.

Variables Used to Assess Contractility

Unfortunately, it is not possible to directly conclude that the cause of low cardiac output is decreased contractility. In addition, there is no absolute hemodynamic measure of contractility.

Stroke volume is a good indicator of ventricular performance and is directly related to the degree of myocardial fiber shortening and circumferential ventricular size. Other variables used to describe ventricular performance and pumping efficiency include *ejection fraction, cardiac work, stroke work*, and their indices, which were described earlier in this chapter. These calculations are used to describe the work the heart can do and thereby imply its contractile ability.

Rate-pressure product is a simplified approach to evaluating cardiac work. It is obtained by multiplying the easily obtained variables of HR and systolic blood pressure, based on the well-established fact that increases in HR and blood pressure result in increases in myocardial oxygen demand. Values

greater than 12,000 are thought to indicate increased myocardial work and increased oxygen demand.

Echocardiography and radionuclide cardiac imaging, discussed later in this chapter, can provide visual assessment of ventricular volumes and function. Transthoracic electrical bioimpedance, a noninvasive method of measuring cardiac performance variables, can also be used to assess the ventricular contractile state.

> **SIMPLY STATED**
> Cardiac output is determined by a complex set of interrelated physiologic variables, including the volume of blood in the heart (preload), the downstream resistance to ejecting blood from the heart (afterload), the contractility and compliance of the heart muscle, and the metabolic requirements of the body. A single measurement of cardiac output represents the interaction of all the variables. Cardiac output reflects not only heart function but also the response of the circulatory system to acute and chronic disease and the effect of therapeutic interventions (see Table 14-5).

METHODS OF MEASURING CARDIAC OUTPUT

The indicator-dilution method using thermodilution, the estimated Fick method, echocardiography, transthoracic bioimpedance, and radionuclide imaging are the most common techniques for measurement of cardiac output in critical care units.

Invasive Methods

Thermodilution Cardiac Output

Thermodilution cardiac output measurement requires the placement of a thermodilution pulmonary artery catheter and the appropriate thermodilution cardiac computer for the type of catheter used. The indicator measured for this technique is change in blood temperature. Sterile dextrose in water or normal saline solution at least 2° C colder than blood temperature is injected into the proximal port (right atrium) of the pulmonary artery line. The temperature change (cooling, sometimes called *heat loss*) is detected by a thermistor bead located just behind the balloon of the catheter, which is positioned in the pulmonary artery (Figure 14-6). A temperature-time curve is recorded by the computer. Thermodilution output measurements can be repeated as often as every 60 seconds because the blood rewarms in one pass through the system and there is no recirculation, as with optical dyes.

Acceptable variations in thermodilution injection technique

Accurate thermodilution results can be achieved using iced, refrigerated, or room-temperature injectant in most patients.[4-6]

Table 14-5	Conditions Associated With Alteration in Hemodynamic Measurements Used to Evaluate Low Cardiac Output		
Normal Hemodynamics	Altered Hemodynamics	Conditions	Usual Correction
Preload			

Right heart
  CVP and RAP =
  2-6 mm Hg or
  4-12 cm H$_2$O
Left heart
  LAP, PCWP, PADP =
  6-15 mm Hg
  EDV = 120-180 mL/beat
Urine output 30 mL/hr
	Low pressure or EDV
	↓CVP, ↓PCWP, and
	  ↓ urine output
		1. Inadequate vascular volume.
		2. ↓SVR (vasodilation) from drugs, spinal anesthetic, fever, sepsis.
		3. SVR may ↑ (vasoconstriction) to maintain MAP and CO if significant hypovolemia has developed.
			1. Volume expansion: intravenous solutions, blood, albumin.
			2. Stop vasodilators; volume expansion, vasoconstriction.
			3. Volume expansion; if SVR does not ↓, vasodilation and additional volume may be needed.

	High pressure or EDV = poor pump/too much volume		

	1. ↑CVP or PCWP	1. a. Cardiac failure.
		   b. Cardiac tamponade.
			1. a. Inotropic drugs, diuretics.
			   b. Volume expansion and isoproterenol until correction of tamponade.

	2. ↓CVP and ↑PCWP	2. Left heart failure, intraoperative myocardial infarction, left heart valve malfunction.	2. Inotropic drugs, vasodilate to ↓ SVR, surgical correction.

	3. ↑CVP and ↓PCWP	3. a. Right heart failure/valve malfunction.
		   b. Chronic pulmonary disease.
		   c. Pulmonary embolism.
			3. a. Inotropic drugs, surgical correction.
			   b. ↓PVR, watch for hypovolemia with low PCWP.
			   c. Heparin, inotropic drugs, vasopressors, surgical correction.

Afterload			

SVR = < 20 units or
  900-1400
  dyne/sec/cm^5
Urine output:
  Adult ≈ 30 mL/hr
  Pediatric ≥ 1 mL/kg/hr
Extremities warm
Capillary refill < 3 sec
	1. ↑SVR, ↓CVP and PCWP	1. Vasoconstriction: body's natural response to maintain perfusion to vital organs when BP drops; ↓ temperature.	1. Volume expansion; warm to normal temperature, watch for hypovolemia with vasodilation from warming.

	2. ↑SVR and ↑PCWP	2. ↑SVR is compensation for failing pump; if uncorrected, will proceed to downward cycle of cardiac failure to cardiogenic shock.	2. Vasodilators, diuretics, inotropic drugs.
	3. ↓SVR	3. Vasodilation: spinal anesthetic, ↑ temperature, vasovagal response, sepsis.	3. Stop vasodilators/diuretics; consider volume expansion; inotropic drugs, possible vasoconstrictors.
Contractility			

Cl = 2.5-4.0 L/min/m^2
SV = 60-130 mL
SVI = 30-50 mL/m^2
RVSWI = 8.8 ±
  0.9 g/min/m^2
LVSWI = 56 ±
  6 g/min/m^2
	Causes of decreased contractility:
	1. ↓ Volume.
			1. Volume expansion; in some failing hearts, PCWP must be kept at 15 mm Hg or higher to maintain contractility.

BP, Blood pressures; *CPP*, cerebral perfusion pressure; *CVP*, central venous pressure; *LAP*, left atrial pressure; *PADP*, pulmonary artery diastolic pressure; *RAP*, right atrial pressure; *SVR*, systemic vascular resistance. For other abbreviations, see text.

Continued

Table 14-5	Conditions Associated With Alteration in Hemodynamic Measurements Used to Evaluate Low Cardiac Output—cont'd		
Normal Hemodynamics	Altered Hemodynamics	Conditions	Usual Correction
Contractility—cont'd			
MAP = 80-100 mm Hg Diastolic BP = 60-80 mm Hg CPP = 60-80 mm Hg *See Table 14-2 for formulas.*	2. Inadequate coronary perfusion/heart muscle.	2. Inadequate diastolic pressure; coronary stenosis, occlusion; myocardial ischemia, infarction; ventricular aneurysm, congenital defects, surgery.	2. Maintain MAP > 60 mm Hg, diastolic pressure > 50 mm Hg (watch for drop in diastolic pressure with vasodilators). Angioplasty, surgery. Inotropic drugs when volume is adequate (driving heart when volume is low could lead to myocardial infarction). Low-dose inotropic support may be used continuously for 24-48 hr after surgery to support a weak myocardium.
	3. HR > 110 beats/min. HR < 60 beats/min.		3. ↓ rate: ensure adequate volume; β blockers, calcium antagonists. ↑ rate: atropine; rarely, isoproterenol. Pacemaker (CO may ↓ if loss of atrial kick).
	4. Arrhythmia.	4. ↓ K$^+$, Ca^{2+}, O$_2$. Drug-induced. Other.	4. Replace K$^+$, Ca^{2+}, maintain adequate Pao$_2$. Withdraw/change medication. Treat with antiarrhythmics, cardioversion, pacemaker.
	5. Negative inotropic drugs. β blockers (propranolol), antiarrhythmics, barbiturates.		5. ↓ or discontinue medication; inotropic drugs as needed.
	6. ↑ SVR (heart must work harder to pump against vasoconstriction).		6. Vasodilators with volume expansion if necessary; inotropic drugs.
	7. ↓ Po$_2$, pH, K$^+$, Na$^+$, Ca^{2+}, ↑ Pco$_2$, K$^+$, Na$^+$.		7. Correct oxygenation electrolytes, acid-base balance.

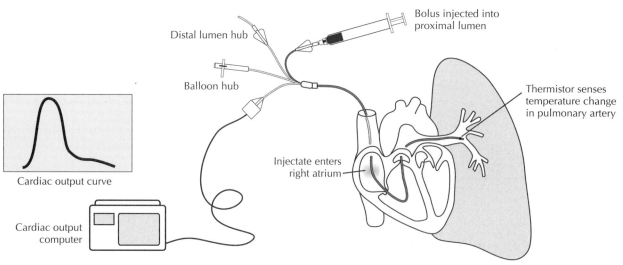

Distal lumen hub

Bolus injected into proximal lumen

Balloon hub

Thermistor senses temperature change in pulmonary artery

Injectate enters right atrium

Cardiac output curve

Cardiac output computer

Figure 14-6 Thermodilution cardiac output measurement.

Injection can be via the proximal injectant lumen, proximal infusion lumen, right atrial port, venous infusion port, or the side port of the introducer catheter.[7-9] An average of multiple determinations with *injections equally spaced throughout the respiratory cycle* has been shown to provide the best estimate of mean cardiac output.[10] Manual injection at end-exhalation may not accurately reflect the average cardiac output, especially in mechanically ventilated patients.[10] Use of an injection gun and a connecting system that measures the injectant temperature as it enters the catheter produces more consistent thermodilution cardiac output readings.

Accuracy and reproducibility of results for both methods depend on extremely careful attention to detail and technique. Indicators must be measured precisely and injected as a bolus in less than 3 seconds. Computers must be calibrated, carefully maintained by biomedical engineers, and balanced before each measurement. Catheters must be properly located and patent, and tips must be away from the wall of the vessel. The cardiac monitor should be watched during cardiac output measurements because arrhythmia may change the cardiac output. When a significant arrhythmia does occur, the cardiac output should be recorded separately (not averaged into the set) and noted to occur with the identified arrhythmia. Then another output measurement is obtained, averaged into the set, and recorded as cardiac output without the presence of arrhythmia.

Fick Cardiac Output

The *Fick method of cardiac output* measurement is based on Adolph Fick's principle that the cardiac output of the heart can be calculated if the oxygen uptake ($\dot{V}o_2$) is measured and the amount of oxygen in each volume of arterial blood (Cao_2) and mixed venous blood ($C\bar{v}o_2$) is known. Thus the cardiac output can be calculated as follows:

$$CO\,(L/min) = \frac{O_2 \text{ absorbed by the lungs (mL/min)}}{\text{Arteriovenous } O_2 \text{ difference (mL/L)}}$$

or

$$CO = \frac{\dot{V}o_2}{Cao_2 - C\bar{v}o_2}$$

Accurate calculation of a Fick cardiac output reading requires the collection of inspired and expired gases as well as arterial and mixed venous blood samples while the patient is in a steady state. This method is usually considered the gold standard against which other forms of cardiac output measurement are validated, but it is rarely used in the ICU. However, by using a normal or expected value of oxygen consumption and measuring the arteriovenous oxygen difference, an estimated Fick cardiac output reading can be obtained in the ICU setting. Three steps are required:

1. *Calculate the expected oxygen consumption* ($\dot{V}o_2$). The normal range of oxygen consumption is 120 to 160 mL/min/m^2, with an average of 125 mL/min/m^2. For a patient with a body surface area of 2 m^2, oxygen consumption would be calculated as follows:

$$\dot{V}o_2 = 125 \text{ mL/min/m}^2 \times 2 \text{ m}^2 = 250 \text{ mL/min}$$

2. *Calculate the arterial and mixed venous oxygen contents and arteriovenous oxygen difference.* The following example is calculated for a hemoglobin of 14 g/100 mL, an arterial oxygen saturation (Sao_2) of 90%, and a mixed venous oxygen saturation ($S\bar{v}o_2$) of 60%.

Arteriovenous oxygen difference, sometimes referred to verbally as the "a − v O_2 difference," is the difference between arterial and venous oxygen contents. The normal range for arteriovenous oxygen difference is 3.0 to 5.5 vol%. The *lower* the $C(a - \bar{v})o_2$, the smaller the amount of oxygen removed per 100 mL of blood passing through the capillaries. Low values are seen when the following occurs:

- Well-oxygenated blood moves rapidly through the capillaries (high cardiac output)
- Cells extract less oxygen (septic shock)
- Oxygen is not released from hemoglobin (left-sided shift in the oxyhemoglobin dissociation curve)

Higher $C(a - v)o_2$ values indicate more oxygen was removed, as when the following occurs:

- Blood flow is slow (low cardiac output) *or*
- Tissue extraction of oxygen is high (increased oxygen consumption)

3. *Calculate the cardiac output. Remember to convert the mL/min/vol% to L/min:*

$$CO\,(L/min) = \frac{\dot{V}o_2}{C(a-v)O_2} = \frac{250 \text{ mL/min}}{5.628 \text{ vol\%}}$$
$$= 44.8 \text{ mL/min/vol\%}$$
$$= 44.8 \times 10 = 4480 \text{ mL/min} = 4.48 \text{ L/min}$$

Estimating cardiac output

When patients do not have arterial or pulmonary artery lines in place, the following additional assumptions may be applied to obtain an estimated cardiac output; however, the chance of error is increased with each assumption used.

- Arterial oxygen saturation is 95%.
- Central venous blood is used for the blood sample rather than obtaining a true mixed venous sample from the pulmonary artery line.

The level of arteriovenous oxygen difference is inversely proportional to CI in the patient with a stable oxygen consumption as follows:

$C(a - \bar{v})o_2$ (vol%)		Cardiac Index (L/min/m^2)
> 6	≅	< 2
> 5	≅	< 3
4	≅	3
> 3	≅	< 4
< 3	≅	> 5

Continuous Cardiac Output Monitoring

Other invasive methods used successfully for continuous measurement of cardiac output include electromagnetic flow probes placed around the aorta, miniature ultrasound probes attached to the adventitia of the ascending aorta, arterial pulse contour analysis, and transtracheal, transesophageal, and intravascular ultrasound. Modifications to the pulmonary artery catheter using fiberoptics, rapid-response thermistors, Doppler ultrasound, electrode bands for measuring impedance, and electrodes for intracardiac electrocardiography (ECG) have made it possible to monitor cardiac output, $S\bar{v}o_2$, right ventricular ejection fraction,[11-13] and other indices of right ventricular function at the bedside.[14] Methods for continuous cardiac output monitoring that have developed from this catheter technology include intracardiac impedance, "injectless" cold thermodilution, continuous thermodilution, and continuous $S\bar{v}o_2$ monitoring. Their correlation with standard cardiac output methods is being evaluated.[15-16]

Continuous $S\bar{v}o_2$ monitoring

Continuous $S\bar{v}o_2$ monitoring has been suggested as an alternative to intermittent, serial cardiac output measurements. Based on the Fick equation, if total body oxygen consumption, hemoglobin, and Sao_2 remain constant, a change in cardiac output should be reflected by a parallel change in $S\bar{v}o_2$. Although significant correlation between cardiac output and $S\bar{v}o_2$ has been shown in critically ill patients who are in a steady state, $S\bar{v}o_2$ has not been found to be predictive of cardiac index in postoperative cardiac surgery patients or mixed populations of critically ill patients.[17,18]

Pulse contour cardiac output monitoring

The pulse contour method is an analysis of an arterial pressure waveform by an analog computer. It requires simultaneous measurement of the arterial pressure and cardiac output by another method such as thermodilution, or the Fick method to obtain a baseline cardiac output reading. Thereafter a continuous cardiac output reading may be obtained via the arterial catheter used for arterial blood pressure monitoring if the patient does not have a change in peripheral vascular resistance. This technique has been shown to have moderate correlation with bolus thermodilution before and after cardiopulmonary bypass.[19]

Transtracheal, transesophageal, and intravascular ultrasound

Doppler ultrasonic transducers positioned on tubes or catheters measure the velocity of blood flow and the vessel diameter from which volumetric blood flow in liters per minute can be calculated. These transducers have been used in different body locations to obtain cardiac output measurements.

The *transesophageal* transducer is positioned in the esophagus at the level of the fifth and sixth vertebrae (approximately 35 cm from the mouth) and pointed posteriorly to assess descending aortic blood flow. Signals can be obtained every 2 to 10 minutes. Transesophageal probes have been left in place for up to 4 days without significant complications.[20]

Transtracheal Doppler ultrasound[21] is accomplished via a transducer attached to the end of an endotracheal tube so that it can be in continuous contact with the tracheal wall. Because these devices look at flow in the descending aorta, which does not contain total cardiac output, they cannot provide an actual cardiac output measurement. However, they can provide measures of flow—including flow time, peak velocity, and stroke distance—that correlate with SV. One-time calibration using transcutaneous Doppler ultrasound cardiac output measurements has been used in an attempt to find a proportionality factor that could be used to convert the flow measurements to actual cardiac output measurement. This technique has not proved to be reliable. However, these devices may find more use in situations where it is important to identify hemodynamic changes but where it is not necessary to know the actual cardiac output.

Continuous *intravenous Doppler ultrasound* cardiac output measurements[22] are obtained via a transducer mounted on the distal section of a pulmonary artery catheter and positioned in the main pulmonary artery proximal to the bifurcation. Cardiac outputs obtained by this method have a moderate correlation ($r = 0.73$) to bolus thermodilution.[23]

Continuous thermodilution cardiac output

Two methods for obtaining continuous cardiac output measurements using the thermodilution method are being used. They have the advantage of *not* requiring a calibration cardiac output measurement by another standard cardiac output technique.

"Injectless" cold thermodilution uses a balloon on the proximal section of a pulmonary artery catheter. Iced solution is automatically injected into the balloon and withdrawn at intervals. The distal temperature changes are analyzed as they would be for a bolus thermodilution measurement. The practicality of using this automatic iced injector at the patient's bedside may be a limiting factor to the use of this technique.

Another continuous thermodilution technique measures volumetric flow using a specialized thermal filament located near the proximal injectant port of the pulmonary artery catheter. The filament, usually situated in the right ventricle, adds small amounts of heat to the blood in a specific, repetitive, on-off pattern that the computer can recognize as unique to the catheter and not caused by other physiologic or environmental events. These pulses serve as the indicator, which is then sensed by the distal thermistor in the same way the injectant would be sensed using the standard bolus thermodilution technique. Computer analysis produces a curve much like the standard thermodilution curve and the cardiac output. Measurements are the average of data collected over the previous 3 to 5 minutes and are updated on the screen every 30 seconds. Heat production is minimal because the blood temperature sensed by the distal thermistor typically is less than 0.05° C.

Noninvasive Methods

Noninvasive methods for measuring cardiac performance include transthoracic electrical bioimpedance, echocardiography, radionuclide cardiac imaging, estimates of cardiac index from pulse pressure, and partial carbon dioxide rebreathing.

Continuous Measurement of Cardiac Performance Using Transthoracic Electrical Bioimpedance

Transthoracic electrical bioimpedance provides continuous, real-time, noninvasive measurement of variables that describe global blood flow, left ventricular performance, pumping efficiency, and volume status. Because blood is the most electrically conductive substance in the body and the thorax can act like a transducer, the electrical conductivity in the thorax can be translated into blood flow data. Eight ECG-type electrodes, two on each side of the neck and two on each side of the chest, form the interface between the patient and the computer terminal. Digitally displayed variables include cardiac output, SV, HR, ejection velocity, ejection time, and thoracic fluid index. Additional variables include end-diastolic volume, peak flow, index of contractility, acceleration index, ejection ratio, and systolic time ratio.

This technique is promising because continuous real-time hemodynamic data can be obtained noninvasively. However, difficulty in obtaining accurate measurements in patients with sepsis, intracardiac shunts, cardiac arrhythmia, and hypertension and has limited widespread clinical use.[24,25]

Periodic Noninvasive Measurement of Cardiac Performance

Echocardiography

Echocardiography[26] provides a noninvasive method of obtaining periodic data on cardiac performance. The use of *Doppler color flow*[27] mapping with *two-dimensional* and *M-mode echocardiography* allows assessment of global ventricular function, including left ventricular volume, ejection fraction, fractional shortening, and circumferential fiber shortening. Additionally, echocardiography can be used to describe intracardiac blood flow and the origin of intracardiac shunts, diagnose pathologic lesions in and around the heart and great vessels, evaluate regional wall motion and its relationship to coronary artery insufficiency and myocardial infarction, and suggest the possibility of rejection in the infant with a transplanted heart. Although echocardiography does not provide continuous assessment of cardiac function, the portability of the current machines allows quality studies to be performed at the patient's bedside in the ICU. However, bandages, obesity, inability to turn or maintain a desired position, and air trapping in the lungs (as occurs with emphysematous patients) may make it difficult to obtain an adequate study using transthoracic imaging.

When a quality image cannot be obtained using a chest transducer, *transesophageal imaging* can be performed. Esophageal imaging provides especially good images of the chambers and the mitral valve because the transducer is positioned immediately behind the left ventricle or left atrium.

Radionuclide cardiac imaging

Radionuclide cardiac imaging[26] techniques can be used to provide periodic information about cardiac performance. Thallium-201 can be injected and myocardial perfusion scanning can be done with a gamma camera or single-photon emission computed tomography. Areas of decreased perfusion or scars pick up a reduced amount of thallium, creating "cold" spots on the image. Radionuclide angiography can be done by two techniques: *first pass* and *gated blood pool* (multiple gated acquisition). Technetium-99m is the radioisotope injected in both cases. The images obtained permit visualization of wall motion and calculation of ejection fraction.

Pulse pressure

Pulse pressure (the difference between the systolic and diastolic arterial pressure) can be used as a rough estimate of stroke index (1 mm Hg = 1 mL/m^2) because SV is the major determinant of pulse pressure. This estimate does not take into account the effects of peripheral vascular resistance on cardiac output but may have some value for obtaining cardiac output trends when hemodynamics are changing rapidly and it is not possible to obtain cardiac outputs by any other method.

Partial CO_2 rebreathing

Partial CO_2 rebreathing is a method of cardiac output monitoring based on a modification of the Fick principle. This "indirect Fick" method uses the Fick method applied to carbon dioxide produced by the body and eliminated through gas exchange by the lungs.

> **SIMPLY STATED**
> Each cardiac output measurement technique provides an estimate of cardiac output at a point in time—the time the measurement was obtained. Each method has advantages, disadvantages, and a margin of error. Accurate measurement depends on proper technique. As with all monitoring, the trend of multiple measurements over time, and correlation with the patient's clinical status, is vital to forming safe and accurate clinical decisions.

REVIEW QUESTIONS

1. Given a stroke volume of 62 mL and a heart rate of 88/min, what is the cardiac output?
   a. 5.5 L/min
   b. 6.2 L/min
   c. 7.0 L/min
   d. 11.0 L/min

2. What is the normal range for cardiac output in an adult?
   a. 2-4 L/min
   b. 4-8 L/min
   c. 6-10 L/min
   d. 10-13 L/min

3. T F Sympathetic nervous stimulation can cause the cardiac output to increase significantly.

4. T F Organs with lower metabolic requirements need more oxygen to function optimally.

5. Which of the following is true regarding the distribution of blood flow and venous return?
   a. 30% of the total blood volume is in the venous system.
   b. Blood is shunted to vital organs during cardiac failure.
   c. Circulatory function and pressures can be maintained with a loss of 40% of the blood volume.
   d. All of the above.

6. What is the normal range for cardiac index?
   a. $0.2-1.3$ L/min/m^2
   b. $1.5-2.6$ L/min/m^2
   c. $2.5-4.0$ L/min/m^2
   d. $4-8$ L/min/m^2

7. Which of the following correlates best with the oxygen requirements of the heart?
   a. Stroke volume
   b. Ejection fraction
   c. End diastolic volume
   d. Cardiac work

8. T F An ejection fraction of 32% would result in a severe reduction in exercise tolerance.

9. The amount of precontraction stretch applied to the ventricles is a definition of which of the following?
   a. Preload
   b. Afterload
   c. Contractility
   d. Ejection fraction

10. Preload of the left ventricle is assessed by which of the following parameters?
    a. Arterial diastolic blood pressure
    b. Mean arterial pressure
    c. Central venous pressure
    d. Pulmonary capillary wedge pressure

11. Which of the following would cause the measurement of preload to be reduced?
    a. Increased ventricular compliance
    b. Increased venous return
    c. Cardiac tamponade
    d. All of the above

12. T F Ventricular function curves are used to determine an optimal pressure/volume relationship to maintain adequate preload.

13. Which of the following is a possible hemodynamic effect of using mechanical ventilation?
    a. Reduced preload
    b. Reduced cardiac output
    c. Increased pulmonary vascular resistance
    d. All of the above

14. Which of the following would increase left ventricular afterload?
    a. Pulmonic valve stenosis
    b. Decreased blood viscosity
    c. Positive end-expiratory pressure
    d. None of the above

15. T F Systemic vascular resistance is a measure of right ventricular afterload.

16. Which of the following would increase pulmonary vascular resistance?
    a. Hypoxemia
    b. Acidosis
    c. Pulmonary emboli
    d. All of the above

17. Which of the following is true regarding cardiac contractility?
    a. It cannot be measured directly.
    b. It is increased by beta-blocking drugs.
    c. It is increased by hypercapnia.
    d. It is increased by parasympathetic neural stimulation.

18. Which of the following invasive cardiac output techniques requires the measurement of inhaled and exhaled gas concentrations?
    a. Thermodilution
    b. Fick
    c. Pulse contour
    d. Transtracheal Doppler

19. Which of the following invasive cardiac output techniques requires the placement of a pulmonary artery catheter?
    a. Thermodilution
    b. Fick
    c. Pulse contour
    d. All of the above

20. Which of the following is a noninvasive technique for determining cardiac performance?
    a. Echocardiography
    b. Transthoracic electrical bioimpedance
    c. Radionuclide cardiac imaging
    d. All of the above

REFERENCES

1. Shoemaker WC and others: *Textbook of critical care*, ed 4, Philadelphia, 2000, WB Saunders.
2. Guyton AC: *Textbook of medical physiology*, ed 7, Philadelphia, 1986, WB Saunders.
3. Guyton AC: *Human physiology and mechanisms of disease*, ed 4, Philadelphia, 1987, WB Saunders.
4. Price P, Fowlow B: Thermodilution cardiac output determinations: a comparison of iced and refrigerated injectate temperatures in patients after cardiac surgery, *Heart Lung* 22:266, 1993.
5. Pesola GR, Ayala B, Plante L: Room-temperature thermodilution cardiac output: proximal injectate lumen vs proximal infusion lumen, *Am J Crit Care* 2:132, 1993.
6. Pesola GR, Carlon GC: Room temperature thermodilution cardiac output: central venous vs right ventricular port, *Crit Care Med* 19:563, 1992.
7. Medley RS, DeLapp TD, Fisher DG: Comparability of the thermodilution cardiac output method: proximal injectate versus proximal infusion lumens, *Heart Lung* 21:12, 1992.
8. Hunn D and others: Thermodilution cardiac output values obtained by using a centrally placed introducer sheath and right atrial port of a pulmonary artery catheter, *Crit Care Med* 18:438, 1990.
9. Vicari M, Ogle V: Comparison of thermodilution cardiac output measurements by injection of the proximal lumen versus side port of the Swan-Ganz catheter, *Heart Lung* 14:126, 1985.
10. Thrush DN, Varlotta D: Thermodilution cardiac output: comparison between automated and manual injection of indicator, *J Cardiothorac Vasc Anesth* 6:17, 1992.
11. Rafferty T and others: Thermodilution right ventricular ejection fraction measurement reproducibility study in patients undergoing coronary artery bypass graft surgery, *Crit Care Med* 20:1524, 1992.
12. Dorman G and others: Use of a combined right ventricular ejection fraction-oximetry catheter system for coronary bypass surgery, *Crit Care Med* 20:1650, 1992.
13. Diebel L and others: End-diastolic volume: a better indicator of preload in the critically ill, *Arch Surg* 127:817, 1992.
14. Guerroero JE and others: Right ventricular systolic time intervals determined by means of a pulmonary artery catheter, *Crit Care Med* 20:1529, 1992.
15. Albert NM, Spear BT, Hammel J: Agreement and clinical utility of 2 techniques for measuring cardiac output in patients with low cardiac output, *Am J Crit Care* 8:464, 1999.
16. Burchell SA and others: Evaluation of a continuous cardiac output and mixed venous oxygen saturation catheter in critically ill surgical patients, *Crit Care Med* 25:388, 1997.
17. Vaughn S, Puri VK: Cardiac output changes and continuous mixed venous oxygen saturation measurement in the critically ill, *Crit Care Med* 16:496, 1988.
18. Sommers MS and others: Mixed venous oxygen saturation and oxygen partial pressure as predictors of cardiac index after coronary artery bypass grafting, *Heart Lung* 22:112, 1993.
19. Gratz I and others: Continuous noninvasive cardiac output as estimated from the pulse contour curve, *J Clin Monit* 8:20, 1992.
20. Valtier B and others: Noninvasive monitoring of cardiac output in critically ill patients using transesophageal Doppler, *Am J Respir Crit Care Med* 158:77, 1998.
21. Abrams JH, Weber RF, Holeman KD: Continuous cardiac output determinations using transtracheal Doppler: initial results in humans, *Anesthesiology* 7:11, 1989.
22. Allard MW, Robinson LM, Leone BJ: *The continuous determination of cardiac output using a flow directed Doppler pulmonary artery catheter* [abstract], presented at Society of Cardiovascular Anesthesiologists 12th Annual Meeting, Orlando, Fla, May 13-16, 1990, 207.
23. Segal J and others: *Instantaneous and continuous cardiac output using a Doppler pulmonary artery catheter*, Mountain View, Calif, 1989, Cardiometrics.
24. Yakimets J, Jensen L: Evaluation of impedance cardiography: comparison of NCCOM3-R7 with Fick and thermodilution methods, *Heart-Lung* 24:194, 1995.
25. Atallah MM, Demain AD: Cardiac output measurement: lack of agreement between thermodilution and thoracic electric bioimpedance in two clinical settings, *J Clin Anesth* 7:182, 1995.
26. Clements FM, deBruijn NP: Noninvasive cardiac monitoring, *Crit Care Clin* 4:435, 1988.
27. Trindale PT and others: Automatic cardiac output measurement (ACOM): clinical applications of a new noninvasive tool, *Int J Card Imaging* 14:147, 1998.
28. Shoemaker WC: Monitoring of the critically ill patient. In Shoemaker WC and others: *Textbook of critical care medicine*, ed 2, Philadelphia, 1989, WB Saunders.
29. Pollard E, Seliger E: *An implementation of bedside physiological calculations*, Waltham, Mass, 1985, Hewlett-Packard.
30. Guyton AC: *Human physiology and mechanisms of disease*, ed 4, Philadelphia, 1987, WB Saunders.

BIBLIOGRAPHY

Baum GL and others: *Textbook of pulmonary diseases*, ed 6, vols I and II, Philadelphia, 1998, Lippincott-Raven.
Bernstein DP: Noninvasive cardiac output measurement. In Shoemaker WC and others: *Textbook of critical care*, ed 4, Philadelphia, 1999, WB Saunders.
Biondi JW, Schulman DS, Matthay RA: Effects of mechanical ventilation on right and left ventricular function, *Clin Chest Med* 9:55, 1988.
Braunwald E: Assessment of cardiac function. In Braunwald E, editor: *Heart disease*, ed 3, Philadelphia, 1996, WB Saunders.
Braunwald E and others: Mechanisms of cardiac contraction and relaxation. In Braunwald E, editor: *Heart disease*, ed 4, Philadelphia, 1996, WB Saunders.

Daily EK, Schroeder JS: *Techniques in bedside hemodynamic monitoring*, ed 4, St Louis, 1989, Mosby.

Darovic GO: *Hemodynamic monitoring: invasive and noninvasive clinical application*, Philadelphia, 1995, WB Saunders.

Fishman AP and others: *Fishman's pulmonary disease and disorders*, ed 3, vols I and II, New York, 1998, McGraw-Hill.

Gillman PA: Continuous measurement of cardiac output: a milestone in hemodynamic monitoring, *Am J Nurs* 199:55, 1992.

Kacmarek RM, Hess D, Stoller JK: *Monitoring in respiratory care*, St Louis, 1993, Mosby.

Marini JJ: Monitoring during mechanical ventilation, *Clin Chest Med* 9:73, 1988.

Pinsky MR: The influence of positive-pressure ventilation on cardiovascular function in the critically ill, *Crit Care Clin* 1:699, 1985.

Robotham JL, Peters J, Takata M: Cardiorespiratory interactions. In Bone RC and others, editors: *Pulmonary and critical care medicine*, ed 2, St Louis, 1994, Mosby.

Rubin LJ: Pulmonary hypertension and cor pulmonale. In Bone RC and others, editors: *Pulmonary and critical care medicine*, ed 2, St Louis, 1994, Mosby.

Wood SE, Osguthorpe S: Cardiac output determination, *AACN Clin Issues Crit Care Nurs* 4:81, 1993.

15

Robert L. Wilkins
James R. Dexter

Assessment of Hemodynamic Pressures

LEARNING OBJECTIVES

Upon completion of this chapter, the reader should be able to accomplish the following:

1. Recognize the following regarding arterial cannulation:
   a. Indications for placing an A line
   b. Catheter description and common insertion sites
   c. Procedure for placement of the catheter
   d. Interpretation of arterial pressure waveforms
   e. Pressures measured and their interpretation
   f. Potential complications
2. Recognize the following regarding central venous pressure (CVP) monitoring:
   a. Indications for placing a CVP catheter
   b. Catheter description and insertion sites
   c. Procedure for placement of the catheter
   d. Interpretation of the CVP waveform
   e. Interpretation of pressures measured
   f. Relationship of CVP to left and right ventricular function
   g. Potential complications
3. Recognize the following regarding pulmonary artery (PA) pressure monitoring:
   a. Indications for placing a PA catheter
   b. Catheter description and insertion sites
   c. Procedure for placement of the catheter
   d. Interpretation of PA waveforms
   e. Interpretation of pressures measured
   f. Relationship between PA diastolic pressure and pulmonary capillary wedge pressure (PCWP)
   g. Techniques for obtaining an accurate PCWP reading
   h. Relationship between transmural pressure and PCWP
   i. Effect of positive end-expiratory pressure on PCWP measurements
   j. Potential complications of using the PA catheter

CHAPTER OUTLINE

Arterial Pressure Monitoring
Indications for Arterial Pressure Monitoring
Arterial Pressure Catheters and Insertion Sites
Procedure for Inserting an Arterial Pressure Line
Arterial Pressure Waveforms
Interpretation of Arterial Pressure Measurements
Complications of Continuous Arterial Pressure Monitoring

Central Venous Pressure Monitoring
Indications for Central Venous Pressure Monitoring
Central Venous Pressure Catheters and Insertion Sites
Procedure for Inserting a Central Venous Pressure Line
Central Venous and Atrial Pressure Waveforms
Methods of Measuring Central Venous Pressure
Interpretation of Central Venous Pressure Measurements
Complications of Central Venous Pressure Monitoring

Pulmonary Artery Pressure Monitoring
Indications for Pulmonary Artery Pressure Monitoring
Balloon Flotation Catheters and Insertion Sites
Placement of the Pulmonary Artery Catheter
Interpretation of Pulmonary Artery Pressures
Complications of Pulmonary Artery Catheters

KEY TERMS
central venous pressure (CVP)
mean arterial pressure (MAP)
pulmonary artery occlusion pressure
pulmonary capillary wedge pressure
pulse pressure
transmural pressure

Susan Jones Krider, RN, MS, contributed this chapter in the previous edition.

CHAPTER OVERVIEW

Hemodynamic monitoring can play an important role in the assessment and treatment of critically ill patients. It is performed to evaluate intravascular fluid volume by measuring central venous pressure (CVP) and pulmonary artery wedge pressure (PAWP); cardiac function by measuring cardiac output and cardiac index; and vascular function by measuring systemic and pulmonary vascular resistance. It can also suggest pericardial tamponade or stricture by measuring CVP, PAWP, right ventricular pressure, and PA pressure. Ideally, the information will be easily obtained, continuously available, and reliable, and the process of obtaining the information will not harm the patient.

Invasive hemodynamic monitoring is needed because clinical assessment (e.g., evaluating jugular venous distension, heart sounds) alone may not accurately predict hemodynamics in some patients. Before a catheter is placed in a patient, however, clinicians must consider the risk-benefit ratio of invasive monitoring. The risk of using invasive hemodynamic monitoring catheters is reduced when properly trained clinicians insert and maintain the system. The complications associated with placing a catheter in a major blood vessel are detailed later in this chapter.

Bedside monitors acquire and calculate physiologic data in real time and often transfer the data automatically to computers for trend analysis. But monitors do not always "tell the truth." Therefore, optimal invasive monitoring requires not only knowledge of the potential complications and appropriate clinical application of the acquired data but also understanding and control of the factors that alter the validity of the numbers. Therapeutic decision-making based on the numbers alone is never adequate and can be dangerous.

This chapter provides an introduction to the hemodynamic pressures most often monitored invasively in critically ill patients: arterial pressure, CVP, and PA pressures (Box 15-1). Indications and complications of invasive monitoring, normal and abnormal pressure waveforms, and clinical applications are discussed.

Table 15-1 summarizes the normal values and the most commonly used abbreviations for the pressures that are discussed. Although intracardiac pressures are essentially the same in adults and children, heart rate and blood pressure vary significantly by age. Table 15-2 lists normal heart rates and blood pressures for children from infancy through 16 years. Remember that "normals" are obtained from studies on healthy people and may be neither normal nor desirable for a specific patient. Nevertheless, normal values are useful as reference ranges in the intensive care unit (ICU).

> **SIMPLY STATED**
> Monitors do not always "tell the truth." Therapeutic decision-making based on numbers alone is never appropriate and can be dangerous, even deadly.

BOX 15-1   The Heart as Two Pumps: An Overview of Hemodynamic Pressure Relationships

When discussing hemodynamic parameters it is necessary to think of the heart as two separate pumps. The right heart receives blood from the venous system (venous return) and pumps blood to the pulmonary system. The left heart receives blood from the pulmonary system and pumps blood to the systemic circulation. In normal states, both hearts pump at the same time and move the same amount of blood.

Both atria are filling chambers for the ventricles. Their pressures are approximately equal and they have the same waveform. When the AV valves open (tricuspid and mitral), the pressures in the atrium and ventricle are equal; therefore atrial pressure usually reflects the ventricle's filling pressure (end-diastolic pressure).

Both ventricles pump blood into an arterial tree and create two waveforms: ventricular and arterial. Their waveforms have the same shape characteristics but their pressures are significantly different. The right heart pumps to a low-resistance circuit, the lungs, and thus produces a lower pressure. The left heart pumps to a high-pressure circuit, the body, so it has to produce a high pressure.

Alterations in blood flow and resistance to flow are reflected backward through the cardiopulmonary circuit as pressure changes. Pulmonary hypertension causes pressure to increase in the right heart and eventually the venous system.

$\uparrow$ Lung pressure $\rightarrow$ $\uparrow$ PAP $\rightarrow$ $\uparrow$ CVP $\rightarrow$ $\uparrow$ Venous congestion

A failing left ventricle will cause blood to "dam up" in the left heart, then the lungs, and eventually alters the entire circuit.

$\uparrow$ LAP $\rightarrow$ $\uparrow$ PCWP $\uparrow$ $\rightarrow$ PAP $\rightarrow$ $\uparrow$ CVP $\rightarrow$ $\uparrow$ Venous congestion

The following simple diagram illustrates the dynamic relationship between the two hearts, and shows where pressures are measured. Marking a patient's pressure changes helps clarify where there is and is not a problem (e.g., $\uparrow$ PCWP with normal PAP and CVP indicates a left heart problem that has not altered the lungs or right heart).

Pressures:	CVP			PAP	PCWP	LAP				Arterial BP	
Venous system		RA	RV		Lungs	LA		LV	Aorta	Arterial circulation	
Blood flow $\rightarrow$						$\leftarrow$ Alterations in resistance and flow are reflected backward					

CVP, Central venous pressure; *LAP*, left atrial pressure; *PCWP*, pulmonary capillary wedge pressure; *PAP*, pulmonary artery pressure; *BP*, blood pressure. *RA*, right atrium; *RV*, right ventricle; *LA*, left atrium; *LV*, left ventricle; vertical bars indicate heart valves. (Requests for reprints of the AHA Reports on Human Blood Pressure Determination by Sphygmomanometry should be sent to the Office of Scientific Affairs, American Heart Association, 7272 Greenville Avenue, Dallas, TX 75231-4596.)

Table 15-1	Normal Hemodynamic Pressure Values	
Pressure	Abbreviation	Normal Value
Arterial pressure	BP	120/80 mm Hg (90/60 in teenage girls)
Mean arterial pressure	MAP	80-100 mm Hg
Central venous pressure	CVP	< 6 mm Hg; < 12 cm H_2O
Right atrial pressure	RAP	2-6 mm Hg (mean pressure)
Right ventricular pressure	RVP	20-30/0-5 mm Hg
Right ventricular end-diastolic pressure	RVEDP	2-6 mm Hg
Pulmonary artery pressure	PAP	20-30/6-15 mm Hg
Mean pulmonary artery pressure	MPAP or $\overline{PAP}$	10-20 mm Hg
Pulmonary capillary wedge pressure	PCWP, $\overline{PCWP}$, PAOP, PWP	4-12 mm Hg
Left atrial pressure	LAP	4-12 mm Hg (mean pressure)
Left ventricular pressure	LVP	100-140/0-5 mm Hg
Left ventricular end-diastolic pressure	LVEDP	5-12 mm Hg

From Daily EK, Schroeder JS: *Hemodynamic waveforms: exercises in identification and analysis.* St Louis, 1983, Mosby.

Table 15-2	Normal Heart Rates and Blood Pressures in Children		
		Heart Rate*	
Age	Blood Pressure Average for Males (Girls 5% lower)	Average	Range
Neonate	75/50	140	100-190
1-6 mo	80/50	145	110-190
6-12 mo	90/65	140	110-180
1-2 yr	95/65	125	100-160
2-6 yr	100/60	100	65-130
6-12 yr	110/60	80	55-110
12-16 yr	110/65	75	55-100
	Range: ±20%		

Data from Rubenstein JS, Hageman JR: Monitoring of critically ill infants and children. *Crit Care Clin* 4:621, 1988.
*Heart rates rounded to nearest 5.

ARTERIAL PRESSURE MONITORING

Indications for Arterial Pressure Monitoring

The attending physician may place (or request) an arterial catheter into a patient with significant hemodynamic instability or a patient who will require frequent arterial blood draws. Patients with severe hypotension (shock), severe hypertension, or unstable respiratory failure are likely candidates to have continuous arterial pressure monitoring. Patients in need of medications that affect blood pressure (e.g., vasodilators or inotropic agents) may benefit from arterial pressure monitoring.

Arterial Pressure Catheters and Insertion Sites

Two arterial pressure catheter sizes are in common use, and selection is determined by the planned insertion site. The smaller catheter is ideal for use in the radial and other small arteries but is not adequate for femoral or other large arteries. The larger of the two catheters is much better for large arteries. The arterial catheter walls are relatively thin and stiff compared with central venous catheters (described below).

The catheter is usually placed in the radial, ulnar, brachial, axillary, or femoral artery. The radial artery is preferred because this site is readily accessible and usually has adequate collateral circulation. The radial artery site is easy to monitor and provides a stable site for blood withdrawal. The femoral artery provides pressure measurements that are less affected by peripheral vasoconstriction, but significant leakage of blood into the surrounding tissue can occur without detection.

Procedure for Inserting an Arterial Pressure Line

The "Seldinger" technique is used for most arterial catheter insertions. The technique involves using a needle to penetrate the artery, and a soft-tipped guidewire is then threaded through the needle into the artery. Next, the needle is removed, leaving the guidewire in place. Finally, the arterial catheter is advanced over the guidewire into position and the guidewire is removed, leaving the catheter in place. The relatively stiff walls of the arterial catheter allow advancement of the catheter over the guidewire without first inserting stiff dilators. The catheter is then sutured in place for security.

Options for placement of radial artery catheters range from using an intravenous catheter loaded on its insertion needle to using prepackaged arterial line kits that have the catheter preloaded on an introducer needle, with a guidewire loaded in the needle to provide easy access. Kits for femoral line placement commonly include the introducer needle, guidewire, and catheter as separate elements that are used in sequence.

Arterial Pressure Waveforms

An arterial waveform should have a clear upstroke on the left, with a dicrotic notch representing aortic valve closure on the downstroke to the right (Figure 15-1). If the dicrotic notch is not visible, the pressure tracing is dampened and probably is inaccurate, and the numbers are lower than the patient's actual pressure. The dicrotic notch disappears in some patients when the systolic pressure drops below 50 or 60 mm Hg.

Arterial pressure waves take on many different configurations in patients in the ICU (Figure 15-2). The left side of the pressure wave may become straight and even pointed on the top when there is an increase in circulating catecholamines that causes an increased inotropic response. A tall, narrow pressure wave is also seen in patients with a stiff aorta (arteriosclerotic vascular disease that is often accompanied by calcium visible in the aorta on chest x-ray). In these patients, the diastolic pressure may also fall, producing an exaggerated tall and narrow complex. Increases in heart rate and vascular resistance increase diastolic pressure. On the other hand, vasodilation that decreases vascular resistance can cause the diastolic pressure to drop. Because approximately 70% of coronary artery perfusion occurs during the diastolic phase, coronary artery perfusion may be compromised if the diastolic pressure falls below 50 mm Hg.

Respiratory Variation in the Arterial Pressure Waveform

Respiratory variation in the arterial pressure waveform normally goes unnoticed because arterial pressure is so high relative to the magnitude of usual respiratory pressure changes. The sensitivity of the monitor usually is set so that the screen covers a pressure range of 0 to 300 mm Hg, making changes of 10 mm Hg barely visible. When respiratory variation in the arterial pressure waveform is seen, the possibility of cardiac tamponade or other causes of paradoxical pulse must be considered (see Chapter 4). Increases in arterial pressure during inspiration (reverse pulsus paradoxus) are seen after heart surgery and in patients with left ventricular failure who are mechanically ventilated with positive end-expiratory pressure (PEEP). Dysrhythmias and pulsus alternans also cause variations in the height and shapes of the waveforms.

Interpretation of Arterial Pressure Measurements

Normal arterial pressure in the adult is approximately 120/80 mm Hg and increases gradually with age. Systolic pressures greater than 160 and diastolic pressures greater than 90 are considered hypertensive. A pressure below 90/60 mm Hg is known as hypotension in the adult patient.

Although arterial pressure is one of the most frequently monitored vital signs, it reflects only the general circulatory status. Pressure is the product of flow and resistance. Because

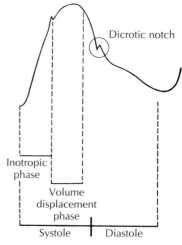

Figure 15-1 Arterial pressure waveform. Increase of circulating catecholamines can cause the inotropic phase to become steeper and form a point that may be higher than in the volume displacement phase. The circle marks the dicrotic notch that results from closure of the aortic valve. If the dicrotic notch cannot be visualized and the patient's systolic pressure is greater than 50 mm Hg, it can be assumed that the plumbing system is dampened.

neurovascular compensatory mechanisms can maintain blood pressure by vasoconstriction while flow is decreasing, low blood pressure is a late sign of deficits in blood volume or cardiac function. Earlier evidence of decreased blood volume or cardiac output are cold, clammy extremities caused by catecholamine-mediated peripheral vasoconstriction.

Arterial pressure decreases:
- With hypovolemia from fluid or blood loss (most commonly, bleeding)
- During cardiac failure and shock (most commonly, heart attack)
- With vasodilation (most commonly, sepsis)

Diastolic pressure must be watched carefully during the administration of vasodilators such as sodium nitroprusside, which may reduce diastolic pressure more rapidly than systolic or mean pressure. Because the coronary arteries receive most of their blood flow during diastole, diastolic pressure less than 50 mm Hg and mean pressure less than 60 mm Hg in an adult may result in compromised coronary perfusion.

Arterial pressure increases with the following:
- Improvement in circulatory volume and function
- Sympathetic stimulation (e.g., fear, medications)
- Vasoconstriction
- Administration of vasopressors

Administration of inotropic agents may or may not increase blood pressure. If a positive inotropic drug stimulates the heart under conditions of inadequate myocardial oxygenation or hypovolemia, the pressure may fall. Additionally, if the inotropic agent also causes vasodilation (e.g., isoproterenol [Isuprel]), the pressure may stay the same or fall as the medication is increased. In addition to systolic and diastolic blood pressure, arterial pressure monitoring allows assessment of pulse and mean arterial pressure.

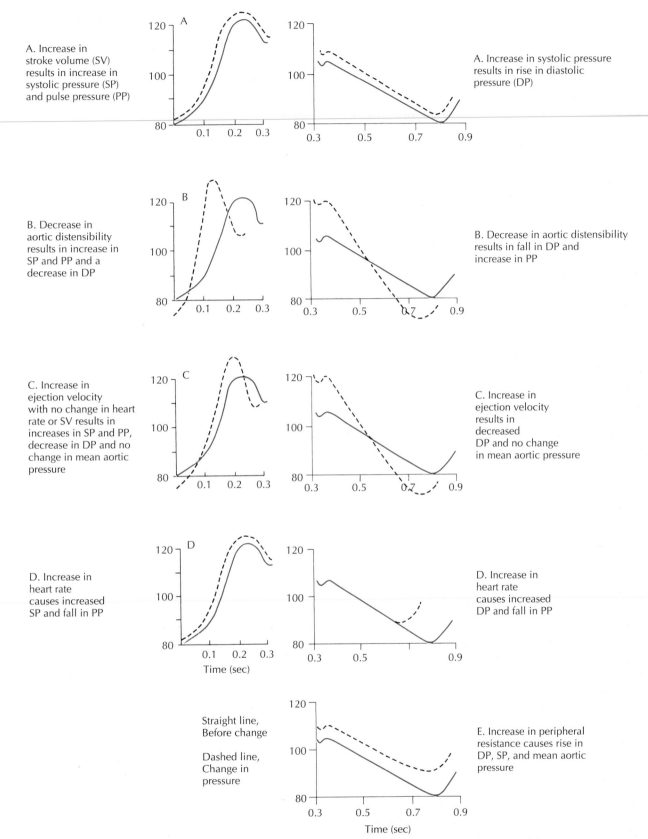

A. Increase in stroke volume (SV) results in increase in systolic pressure (SP) and pulse pressure (PP)

A. Increase in systolic pressure results in rise in diastolic pressure (DP)

B. Decrease in aortic distensibility results in increase in SP and PP and a decrease in DP

B. Decrease in aortic distensibility results in fall in DP and increase in PP

C. Increase in ejection velocity with no change in heart rate or SV results in increases in SP and PP, decrease in DP and no change in mean aortic pressure

C. Increase in ejection velocity results in decreased DP and no change in mean aortic pressure

D. Increase in heart rate causes increased SP and fall in PP

D. Increase in heart rate causes increased DP and fall in PP

Time (sec)

Straight line, Before change

Dashed line, Change in pressure

E. Increase in peripheral resistance causes rise in DP, SP, and mean aortic pressure

Time (sec)

Figure 15-2 Determinants of aortic pressures. Diagrams indicate general tendencies when other factors are held constant. *DP,* Diastolic pressure; *PP,* pulse pressure; *SP,* systolic pressure; *SV,* stroke volume. (Modified from Smith JJ, Kampine JP: *Circulatory physiology: the essentials.* Baltimore, 1980, Williams & Wilkins.)

The pulse pressure is the difference between the systolic and diastolic pressure. Normal pulse pressure is 30 to 40 mm Hg and is a reflection of stroke volume by the left ventricle and arterial system compliance. A decreasing pulse pressure is a sign of low stroke volume. An increasing stroke volume in a patient receiving fluid therapy is consistent with improved preload.

> **SIMPLY STATED**
> A pulse pressure < 30 mm Hg indicates a low stroke volume by the left ventricle. If the pulse pressure increases with fluid therapy, the patient was probably hypovolemic.

Mean arterial pressure (MAP) is an average of pressures pushing blood through the systemic circulation; therefore, it is the more important of the arterial pressures and an indicator of tissue perfusion. Normal MAP is considered to be 80 to 100 mm Hg. MAP is not an arithmetic average of systolic and diastolic pressures because the cardiac cycle spends about twice as long in diastole as in systole when the heart rate is in the normal range (50 to 100 beats per minute). Most monitors have a selector switch that computes MAP and displays it digitally. MAP can be estimated mathematically by either of the following formulas when it cannot be obtained from the monitor.

$$MAP = 1/3 \text{ Pulse pressure} + \text{Diastolic pressure}$$

or

$$MAP = \frac{\text{Systolic pressure} + (\text{Diastolic pressure} \times 2)}{3}$$

Circulation to the vital organs (i.e., kidneys, coronary arteries) may be compromised when MAP falls below 60 mm Hg. The patient may need fluid therapy or medications to increase left ventricular contractility (inotropics) or to increase vascular resistance in such cases. Elevated MAP is associated with increased risk of stroke and heart failure. Vasodilators or negative inotropic medications may be needed in such cases.

MAP is used in calculating derived hemodynamic variables such as systemic vascular resistance, left ventricular stroke work, and cardiac work (see Chapter 14).

Complications of Continuous Arterial Pressure Monitoring

Ischemia

Ischemia resulting from embolism, thrombus, or arterial spasm is the major complication of direct arterial monitoring. It is evidenced by pallor distal to the insertion site and usually is accompanied by pain and paresthesias. Ischemia can proceed to tissue necrosis if the catheter is not repositioned or removed. Thrombosis is prevented by irrigation with diluted heparinized solution. Bolus irrigation is done in very small amounts because flushing the line can result in retrograde flow and cerebral embolization.

Hemorrhage

Hemorrhage is possible if the line becomes disconnected or a stopcock is left open; therefore, the tubing should be kept on top of the bed sheets, where it can be observed. Blood flow through an 18-gauge catheter is sufficient to allow a 500-mL blood loss per minute, and exsanguination can occur. Bleeding and hematoma at the insertion site can also occur, especially if the catheter was placed through a needle. Sites should be assessed regularly while the catheter is in place and after removal of the catheter.

Infection

As with all invasive lines, the presence of an arterial catheter increases the risk of infection. The incidence of infection increases over time and is directly related to care of the lines and transducers; frequency of dressing, tubing, and solution change; to-and-fro motion of the catheter; and altered host defenses. Fever in any patient with invasive lines must trigger questions about the necessity of the lines and their role as cause of the infection process.

> **SIMPLY STATED**
> All invasive hemodynamic monitoring lines are a potential source of infection, bleeding, hematoma, embolus, thrombus, and impaired circulation. Fever in any patient with invasive lines must trigger questions about the necessity of the lines and their role in an infectious process.

CENTRAL VENOUS PRESSURE MONITORING

Central venous pressure (CVP) is the pressure of the blood in the right atrium or vena cava, where the blood is returned to the heart from the venous system. Because the tricuspid valve is opened between the right atrium and ventricle during diastole (ventricular filling), right atrial pressure or CVP also represents the end-diastolic pressure in the right ventricle (RVEDP) and reflects preload for the right ventricle. To obtain a CVP measurement, a venous catheter is placed in a major vein (see insertion discussion below).

Indications for Central Venous Pressure Monitoring

CVP monitoring is indicated to assess the circulating blood volume (adequacy of cardiac filling) or the degree of venous return or to evaluate right ventricular function. Patients who have had major surgery or blood loss due to trauma and those suspected of severe dehydration may benefit from placement of a CVP catheter to guide fluid replacement therapy. Patients with either cardiogenic or noncardiogenic pulmonary edema also need CVP monitoring to guide fluid therapy. In addition, the venous catheter is useful to evaluate the patient suspected of having damage to the right ventricle from myocardial infarction. Once the catheter is in place, the line can be used for rapid infusion of fluids or medications and to obtain blood samples for measurement of routine laboratory studies (e.g., complete blood counts and electrolytes).

Central Venous Pressure Catheters and Insertion Sites

The most common central venous catheters are 7-French, 3-lumen catheters with one distal port and two ports 3 to 4 cm from the distal end of the catheter (Figure 15-3). The multiple-lumen catheter allows infusion of blood and various medications and solutions through different ports and permits aspiration of blood samples or injections for cardiac output measurements without interrupting the infusion of medication. Catheters with walls that are impregnated with antibiotic are less commonly associated with infection than standard catheters. A less commonly used central venous catheter is 12-French and has two lumens solely for dialysis access. It can be placed in addition to a standard central venous line and is not used for medication delivery, pressure monitoring, or medication delivery.

Common sites for introduction of central venous catheters include subclavian, internal jugular, and femoral veins (Figure 15-4). Advantages of the subclavian approach are that it results in a much more stable catheter after placement. Disadvantages of the subclavian approach are that it is technically more difficult because the vein is harder to find and the catheter guidewire does not follow the subclavian vein as easily as it turns to form the superior vena cava. The subclavian vein is close to the subclavian artery, which is easily punctured, and the mediastinum can hold a fair amount of blood without external evidence of blood loss. The pleural surface is not far below the vein, so pneumothorax is not a rare complication of the procedure.

The internal jugular approach is easier; there is nearly a straight shot for the guidewire to reach the superior vena cava, there is less risk for pneumothorax, and hematomas are easier to see and control. Disadvantages of the internal jugular approach are that the catheter is much less stable after placement and is subject to kinking, breakage, and accidental removal.

Femoral central venous catheters are the easiest to place and have the least risk for complications, but they provide less reliable hemodynamic information because the catheter tip is far from the right atrium and pressure waveforms are often dampened. Most ICU patients must remain supine in bed so that the femoral catheter does not get kinked by the patient sitting up. Diarrhea makes the catheter somewhat harder to keep clean. A chest x-ray should be performed after subclavian or internal jugular central venous line insertion to ensure placement before use and to rule out pneumothorax.

Procedure for Inserting a Central Venous Pressure Line

Central venous line kits commonly include a hard-walled needle for venous penetration, a stiff plastic dilator, and a guidewire coiled in a plastic sheath with a "J" tip to prevent venous wall penetration. The J tip is held straight by a small

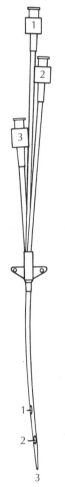

Figure 15-3 Triple-lumen central venous pressure catheter designed for placement through the internal or external jugular vein. The tip ends in the right atrium. The catheter does not have a balloon; air is never injected into ports.

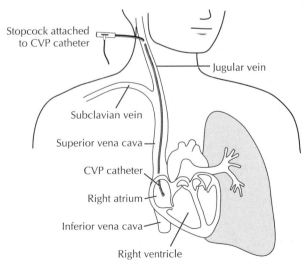

Figure 15-4 Central venous pressure (*CVP*) catheter inserted through the jugular vein with the tip positioned in the right atrium.

separate sheath to accommodate entry into the hub of the insertion needle.

The technique is nearly identical for subclavian, internal jugular, and femoral line insertions. The subclavian vein is entered from an insertion site at the edge of the distal third of the clavicle. The internal jugular can be entered from the head of the clavicle or a site behind the brachial artery. The femoral vein is most easily entered just medial to the femoral artery in the groin. The only difference in technique among these sites is that the head of the patient's bed is lowered for the subclavian and internal jugular insertions. This increases the size of the vein, making it easier to penetrate and thread the guidewire. This also decreases the risk of inadvertent air embolism. The head of the bed is elevated for the same reasons during placement of the femoral catheter.

The lumens of the CVP catheter are flushed with heparinized saline and the cap is removed from the lumen with the distal port. The guidewire is inserted and threaded and the needle withdrawn. A dilator is inserted over the guidewire and removed, and the distal port of the CVP catheter is threaded onto the guidewire. It is advanced to a depth that should leave the tip in the superior vena cava. The guidewire is then removed, the hub replaced, the port flushed

with heparinized saline, and the catheter is then stitched in place for security.

Central Venous and Atrial Pressure Waveforms

CVP waveforms reflect pressure changes in the right atrium. This is equivalent to the PAWP waveform, which approximates left atrial pressures. Both CVP and PAWP waveforms have three waves for each cardiac cycle: a, c, v (Figure 15-5).

The a wave results from atrial contraction and occurs during ventricular diastole. When there is no atrial contraction (atrial fibrillation), there is no a wave. Conversely, when the atrium contracts against a closed valve, as occurs during atrioventricular (AV) dissociation or with some junctional or ventricular pacemaker rhythms, large a waves called *cannon waves* occur. The downslope of the a wave (x descent) results from the decrease in atrial pressure as the blood moves into the ventricle and ends with the closure of the tricuspid valve (tricuspid on right, mitral on left).

The c wave occurs at the completion of AV valve closure. It represents the movement or bulging of the AV valve back toward the atrium during ventricular contraction.

The v wave results from atrial filling while the AV valve is closed during ventricular systole. The downslope of the v wave

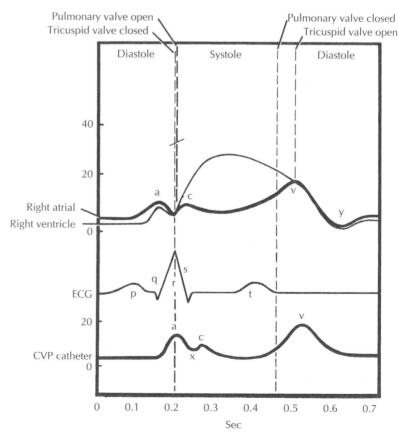

Figure 15-5 Central venous pressure *(CVP)* and right atrial pressure traces with a, c, and v waves shown in relation to the electrocardiogram *(ECG)* and ventricular pressure waves. When traces are recorded from long catheters, especially pulmonary artery catheters, there is usually a time delay in visualizing the pressure waveform so that the *a* wave coincides with the QRS complex rather than preceding it slightly, as occurs with the right atrial pressure trace. *a*, atrial contraction; *b*, closure of the AV valve; *v*, ventricular contraction.

(y descent) occurs when the tricuspid and mitral valves open and the ventricle begins to fill with blood. When an AV valve does not close all the way (incompetent or leaky valve), some of the blood is ejected backward into the atrium during systole (tricuspid regurgitation), creating exaggerated v waves and an elevated CVP measurement.

Respiratory Variations in the Central Venous Pressure Waveform

Respiratory-induced pressure changes are normal on CVP waveforms. If no respiratory artifact is seen on the trace and the patient is not holding his/her breath, the pressure must be assumed to be inaccurate. The most likely cause would be a kink or air in the tubing, a stopcock turned in the wrong direction, or a small clot or kink in the catheter. Rarely, when a hypovolemic patient is breathing spontaneously with a small tidal volume, no respiratory artifact or a, c, and v waves will be seen. If the patient is asked to take a deep breath, the waveform should fall below baseline as intrathoracic pressure falls with inspiration. The catheter and tubing should still be checked carefully for air and other causes of dampened pressure traces.

CVP decreases with spontaneous inspiration and increases with mechanical ventilation. When a patient is receiving intermittent mandatory ventilation, the pressure decreases with the spontaneous breaths. When the patient triggers a mechanical breath, the pressure decreases and then immediately rises above baseline levels when the ventilator breath is initiated.

The patient who is awake and alert can be asked to suspend breathing for several cardiac cycles until a mean venous pressure without respiratory artifact can be obtained. When the patient cannot assist and is not on PEEP, the ventilator can be disconnected for several cardiac cycles to obtain a pressure reading. When a patient is mechanically ventilated with PEEP, the pressures should be recorded on paper and the average end-expiratory pressure over several respiratory cycles should be used for both CVP and PA pressure measurements. Routine measurements are taken without interrupting the PEEP. Unless these precautions are taken, numbers obtained from the monitor represent the extremes of the patient's respiratory efforts and not the "real" CVP.

SIMPLY STATED
If no respiratory variation is seen on a central venous pressure, left atrial pressure, PA pressure, or pulmonary wedge pressure trace, the pressure must be assumed to be inaccurate.

Methods of Measuring Central Venous Pressure

CVP can be obtained using a transducer system or a water manometer (Figure 15-6). The CVP measurement is reported in mm Hg when the transducer system is used and in cm H_2O

when the water manometer is used. The reading from the water manometer must be converted to mm Hg for use in hemodynamic calculations. This is accomplished by dividing the centimeters of water by 1.36 (1.36 cm H_2O equals 1 mm Hg). For example, for 8 cm H_2O,

$$\frac{8 \text{ cm } H_2O}{1.36} = 5.9 \text{ mm Hg}$$

The transducer provides a more accurate assessment of mean CVP or right atrial pressure and also allows observation of the CVP waveform (see waveform analysis below).

The advantage of the water manometer is that it is inexpensive, does not require electronic equipment, and easy to use. The manometer is filled with intravenous fluid to a point above the expected CVP measurement. With the patient in the supine position, the zero level of the manometer is placed at the patient's right atrial level, and the stopcock is turned so that the manometer is opened to the patient. The fluid level in the manometer should fall rapidly until the level of the patient's CVP is reached, and then it should oscillate with respiration. The CVP is ideally read at the end of expiration because spontaneous inspiration causes the pressure to fall and mechanical ventilation causes the pressure to rise.

The criteria for interpretation of CVP by a water manometer include the following:
- X-ray verification that the tip of the catheter is in central venous position (if the subclavian or internal jugular route is used)
- Free-flowing intravenous fluid
- Ability to easily aspirate a blood sample from the CVP catheter
- A rapidly falling water column when the pressure is obtained
- Small oscillations at the top of the water column indicating the changes in the CVP throughout a cardiac cycle
- Larger oscillations occurring with respiration

Unfortunately, comparison of water manometer methods with transducer methods has demonstrated that the water manometer readings usually overestimate transducer-determined mean right atrial pressure (CVP). This is because the water only falls to the highest pressure in each cardiac cycle and not to the mean pressure. Additionally, the location of the catheter tip cannot be verified because the individual waves (a and v) cannot be seen, and wide fluctuations of the water column do not occur even when the catheter is located in the right ventricle.

Interpretation of Central Venous Pressure Measurements (Box 15-2)

CVP is regulated by a balance between the ability of the heart to pump blood out of the right atrium and ventricle and the amount of blood being returned to the heart by the venous system (venous return). In general, any peripheral factor that decreases the amount of blood returning to the heart decreases

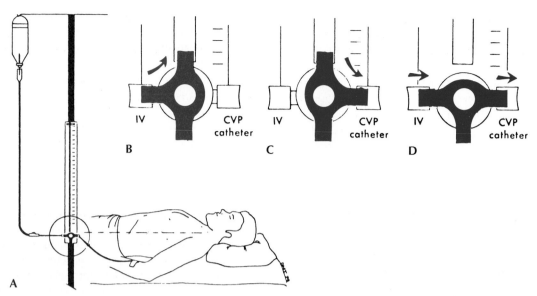

Figure 15-6 Procedure for measuring central venous pressure *(CVP)* with a manometer. **A**, Manometer and intravenous (IV) tubing in place. **B**, Stopcock turned so the manometer fills with fluid above the level of expected pressure. **C**, Stopcock turned so IV flow is off and fluid in manometer flows to the patient. Reading is obtained after fluid level stabilizes. **D**, Stopcock is turned to resume IV flow to the patient. (From Daily EK, Schroder JS: *Techniques in bedside hemodynamic monitoring*, ed 4. St Louis, 1989, Mosby.)

<table><tr><td>

BOX 15-2   Central Venous Pressure

CVP is pressure of the blood in the vena cava and right atrium and right ventricle during diastole when the tricuspid valve is open and unobstructed.
CVP measures right heart function and reflects:
• Preload and end-diastolic filling pressure
• Ability of the right heart to move blood through the lungs and left heart
CVP can reflect left-heart filling pressure in young patients with no hypertension, cardiac disease, or pulmonary disease.
CVP increases with:
• Increased venous return (volume)
• Increased intrathoracic pressure
• Decreased ability of the right heart to move blood
CVP decreases with:
• Decreased venous return (volume)
• Decreased intrathoracic pressure
• Increased ability of heart to move blood forward
Normal CVP:
• < 6 mm Hg by transducer
• < 12 cm H_2O by water manometer
If pressure is abnormally low or falling, think:
• Inadequate volume or volume loss
• Vasodilation (could be fever or medications)
• Plumbing or measurement problem
If pressure is abnormally high or climbing, think:
• Volume overload
• Heart compression (e.g., tamponade, pericarditis)
• Heart failure from pulmonary hypertension
• High intrathoracic or pulmonary pressure
• High ventilator pressures
• Intravenous infusion in line during pressure measurement
CVP can be used to monitor fluid challenges in adults and children.

</td><td>

CVP, and any factor that increases venous return increases CVP. When the pumping capacity of the right heart is increased, more blood is moved out of the right ventricle and CVP decreases. Conversely, decreased pumping ability of the heart results in an increase in CVP.

Elevations of CVP occur under the following conditions:
• Volume overload or fluids being given more rapidly than the heart can tolerate
• Increased intrathoracic pressure (CVP increases with positive-pressure breath or tension pneumothorax)
• Compression around the heart: constrictive pericarditis, cardiac tamponade
• Pulmonary hypertension (primary or secondary)
• Right ventricular failure (e.g., myocardial infarction, cardiomyopathy)
• Left heart failure severe enough to cause right heart failure
• Pulmonary valvular stenosis
• Tricuspid valvular stenosis or regurgitation
• Pulmonary embolism
• Increased large vessel tone throughout the body, resulting in venoconstriction
• Arteriolar vasodilation that increases the blood supply to the venous system
• Infusion of solution into the CVP line (especially by infusion pumps)
Causes of decreased CVP include the following:
• Vasodilation (by drug or increase in body temperature)
• Inadequate circulating blood volume (hypovolemia) caused by dehydration; actual blood loss; or large amounts of gastrointestinal loss, wound drainage, perspiration, urine output (diuresis), insensible losses (high temperature, low humidity), and losses to the interstitial space (edema, third-spacing)

</td></tr></table>

- Spontaneous inspiration
- Placement of the transducer or zero level of the water manometer above the patient's right atrial level (Box 15-3)
- Air bubbles or leaks in the pressure line

When a patient is hypovolemic but has pulmonary hypertension with decreased right ventricular function, the CVP reflects the elevated pressure from the loss of ventricular function and does not fall to levels that would be expected with hypovolemia.

> ## SIMPLY STATED
>
> CVP rises as the efficiency of the right heart to move blood through the lungs decreases. When the CVP is elevated and accurately measured while pulmonary pressures are normal or low, the cause of the problem resides in the right heart (e.g., right ventricular infarction or right heart valvular disease). If both CVP and PA pressure are elevated while the left-sided filling pressures are normal, the problem probably resides in the lung.

Central Venous Pressure as a Reflection of Left Ventricular Function

Can CVP be used to estimate left ventricular filling pressures and performance? Yes, under some circumstances. In patients with an ejection fraction greater than 0.50 (50% of the left ventricular end-diastolic volume) and no cardiopulmonary disease, excellent correlation has been found between central venous, left atrial, and pulmonary wedge pressures.

CVP is a reasonable option for management of intraoperative, postoperative, or volume replacement in young patients

---

> **BOX 15-3** | **Understanding the Effects of Transducer Position on Hemodynamic Pressures**
>
> Next time you are in the ICU, try this experiment. Look at a patient's pressure, then remove the transducer from its rack and raise it about a foot above the patient. The approximately 22–mm Hg drop in displayed pressure is caused by movement of the transducer, not a change in the patient's pressure. Next, lower the transducer to about a foot below the patient. The displayed pressure will increase by about 44 mm Hg (or, 22 mm Hg higher than the pressure when the transducer was in the rack).
>
> The following example shows the steps used to calculate the exact effect of an improperly positioned transducer on the pressure reading.
>
> | | |
> |---|---|
> | 1 inch | = 2.54 cm |
> | 1 ft (12 × 2.54) | = 30.48 cm |
> | 1 mm Hg | = 1.36 cm H_2O |
> | 30.48/1.36 | = 22.41 mm Hg |

---

with no history of heart disease or hypertension. However, in patients with valvular heart disease or coronary artery disease and in critically ill patients, CVP may not correlate well with left-heart filling pressures.

In a patient with pulmonary disease, the left heart pressures remain normal or may even be decreased, whereas the PA pressure and therefore right heart pressures are significantly elevated. Therefore, a patient with pulmonary hypertensive disease may benefit from monitoring of both the left and right heart pressures.

> ## SIMPLY STATED
>
> Patients with hypertensive pulmonary disease have increased pulmonary vascular pressures and CVPs resulting from the pulmonary disease process; therefore, CVP is not a good reflection of volume status. It is necessary to look more directly at left-heart filling pressure to determine whether the patient's volume status is adequate.

Complications of Central Venous Pressure Monitoring

Complications of using a CVP catheter can occur during placement or during its use over time. Placement of the catheter can cause problems such as bleeding or pneumothorax. Bleeding is often minimal since the venous system is under low pressure. Bleeding is more likely if the patient is taking heparin or has low platelet counts. It can also be severe if the subclavian artery is accidentally penetrated. Pneumothorax is uncommon but can occur if the catheter punctures the pleural lining. The most common complication associated with use of the catheter over time is infection. A less common complication is development of thrombus around the catheter. Accidental opening of the central venous line stopcock could allow air to enter the vein and result in an air embolus.

PULMONARY ARTERY PRESSURE MONITORING

The development of the pulmonary artery (PA) catheter by Drs. Swan and Ganz in the late 1960s[1] began a new era in assessment of left ventricular and hemodynamic performance. Placement of a flow-directed PA catheter into the patient's PA allows assessment of the filling pressures of the left side of the heart. Before the PA catheter was developed, the filling pressures for the left side of the heart were not known but estimated using the CVP measurement. As mentioned before, many critically ill patients have factors present that prevent a direct correlation of CVP and left-heart filling pressures. Thus the PA catheter can allow better assessment of the left side of the heart and provides numerous hemodynamic values. These values allow assessment of the following (Box 15-4):

BOX 15-4	Interpreting Pulmonary Artery Pressure

PA pressure is the product of the volume ejected by the right ventricle and resistance of flow through the pulmonary vasculature.

PA pressure measures right-heart function and reflects:
- Preload and end-diastolic filling pressure
- Ability of the right heart to move blood through the lungs and left heart

PA pressure can reflect left-heart filling pressure in young patients with no hypertension, cardiac disease, or pulmonary disease.

PA pressure increases with:
- Increased venous return (volume)
- Increased intrathoracic pressure
- Increased pulmonary vascular resistance

PA pressure decreases with:
- Decreased venous return (volume)
- Decreased intrathoracic pressure
- Decreased pulmonary vascular resistance

Normal PA pressure:
- Systolic 20 to 30 mm Hg
- Diastolic 6 to 15 mm Hg*
- Mean 10 to 20 mm Hg

If pressure is abnormally low or falling, think:
- Inadequate volume, volume loss
- Vasodilation (could be fever or medications)
- Plumbing or measurement problem

If pressure is abnormally high or climbing, think:
- Increased pulmonary vascular resistance
- Constriction, obstruction, compression of pulmonary vasculature (e.g., ↑ intrathoracic pressure, pulmonary hypertension, cardiac tamponade)
- Backpressure from high left-heart pressures
- Volume overload
- Technical problem or not reading at end-expiration

Pulmonary diastolic pressure can be used instead of wedge pressure if the diastolic is higher than the wedge and if none of the following is present:
- Tachyarrhythmia
- Vasoconstriction, increased pulmonary resistance
- Pulmonary emboli
- Fluctuating pulmonary vascular resistance

*Normal pulmonary artery diastolic pressure is 2 mm Hg higher than wedge pressure.

- Left ventricular preload via measurement of pulmonary artery diastolic pressure (PADP) and pulmonary capillary wedge pressure (PCWP)
- Pulmonary vascular resistance via measurement of PA mean systolic pressures and PCWPs; systemic vascular resistance via monitoring systemic arterial mean pressure and PA end-diastolic pressure
- Cardiac output
- Arteriovenous oxygen difference ($C[a - \bar{v}]O_2$) and left to right shunt based on increases in venous SaO_2 from CVP port and PA port

- Patient's response to therapy with vasoactive agents, fluid, and ventilation with PEEP
- Intermittent or continuous monitoring of mixed venous blood oxygenation status[2]

Indications for Pulmonary Artery Pressure Monitoring

Insertion of the PA catheter represents increased risk as compared to the CVP catheter. The additional risk is present because of the need for the catheter to pass through the right side of the heart and into the PA. The procedure may cause dysrhythmias or other serious complications (see discussion below). As a result, the PA catheter must be inserted only in those patients in whom the anticipated benefit outweighs the potential risks. Information defining risks and benefits has been accumulating over the past 20 years and has led to substantial changes in frequency of use in ICUs. More recent information suggests little improvement in mortality when information from PA catheters is used to manage critically ill patients. This information has decreased the use of PA catheters over the past several years.

Recent research has tried to identify the potential benefits of using a PA catheter in selected critically ill patients. Numerous studies have found that the measurements resulting from catheter-derived values do affect clinical decision-making and suggest the PA catheter is useful.[3,4] More recent and larger studies have not found benefits from the use of the PA catheter–derived values in terms of increased patient survival or shorter ICU/hospital stay in groups of patients previously thought to benefit from PA catheter placement.[5-7] Additional research is currently being done to identify which patients will benefit most from the use of PA catheters; however, the debate will probably continue for some time. Currently, there is no specific diagnosis or group of patients in which PA catheter placement is an absolute indication. Rather, the decision to place a PA catheter is individualized on a case-by-case basis. Common factors to consider include:
- Experience of the attending physician
- Availability of proper equipment and personnel to insert and maintain the catheter
- Diagnosis of the patient
- Cardiac history of the patient
- Pulmonary history of the patient

The common situations in which PA catheter monitoring is considered include:
- Diagnosis and treatment of patients with severe cardiogenic pulmonary edema, especially if the patient has unstable angina, has ventricular pathology, or does not respond to initial therapy
- Diagnosis and treatment of patients with severe acute respiratory distress syndrome (ARDS) who are hemodynamically unstable
- Monitoring of a patient who has had major thoracic surgery (e.g., coronary bypass surgery) with a recent history of myocardial infarction or poor ventricular function
- Diagnosis and treatment of patients in cardiogenic or septic shock

Balloon Flotation Catheters and Insertion Sites

PA catheters, also called Swan-Ganz catheters, are made of radiopaque polyvinylchloride and are approximately 110 cm long and marked in 10-cm increments. The balloon at the tip of the catheter is used both to float the catheter into position and to obtain wedge pressure measurements. The catheter is also called a *balloon-tipped, flow-directed* catheter (Figure 15-7). The size, configuration, and thermodilution computer

requirements vary according to manufacturer and specific application. Four- and five-French catheters with two or three lumens are available for use in children. Seven-french three-lumen catheters (plus an air channel for the balloon) are most commonly used for adults.

The distal lumen terminates at the tip of the catheter and is used for measuring PA pressures, aspirating mixed venous blood samples, and injecting medications. Some companies also provide a fiberoptic filament to the tip of the catheter that is used for monitoring $S\bar{v}O_2$.

The balloon lumen exits inside of the balloon just behind the tip of the catheter. This lumen is used only to inflate the balloon with air or carbon dioxide. Most balloons hold approximately 1.5 mL of air when fully inflated. The balloon is fully inflated during insertion to help the catheter float into the PA and to help prevent premature ventricular contractions when the catheter is passed through the right ventricle. Once the

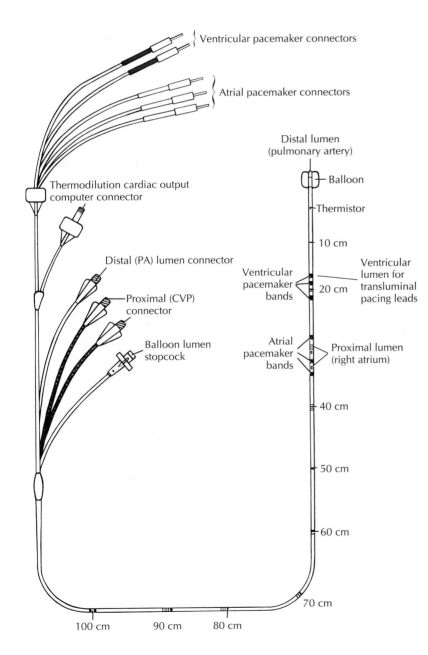

Figure 15-7 Idealized pulmonary artery *(PA)* catheter showing many of the features available on PA catheters; no catheters have all the features shown. Distal lumen opens into the PA. Fiberoptic filaments used for $S\bar{v}O_2$ monitoring (see Figure 13-12) and the balloon are also located at the tip. The thermistor bead is located 1.5 inches from the tip and is connected by a wire through the catheter to the connector for the thermodilution cardiac output computer. The proximal lumen located 30 cm back from the tip opens into the right atrium. Catheters are available for ventricular, atrial, or atrioventricular sequential pacing using either pacemaker bands positioned on the catheter or pacing leads, which are passed through the lumen. Ventricular bands or lumens are located 20 cm from the tip; atrial, 30 cm from the tip. *CVP*, Central venous pressure.

catheter is in place, only the amount of air necessary to obtain a wedge pressure reading is placed in the balloon.

The proximal lumen ends approximately 30 cm back from the tip of the catheter and rests in the right atrium when the catheter is properly placed. The proximal port is used for aspirating blood samples, measuring CVP, injecting drugs, and injecting the thermal bolus used for thermal dilution cardiac output measurements (see Chapter 14). Some catheters have two lumens ending in the right atrium: one for routine infusion of drugs or continuous pressure monitoring, the other for infusion of thermodilution materials and other periodic injections.

Thermodilution cardiac output catheters have a thermistor bead located approximately 1.5 inches from the tip of the catheter. The thermistor senses temperature changes in the blood and is used for obtaining body core temperature as well as thermodilution cardiac output measurements.

PA catheters are available with bands for atrial, ventricular, or AV sequential cardiac pacing. The pacemaker bands must stay in contact with the wall of the atrium or ventricle to work effectively. Another type of PA pacing catheter has a ventricular lumen 20 cm back from the tip in addition to the proximal (atrial) lumen. Specially designed pacing leads can be passed through the lumen and positioned more securely against the wall of the chamber. The pacer leads are then connected directly to the pacemaker. If cardiac pacing is not required, the lumen can be used for infusions and blood sampling.

The insertion sites for the PA catheter are the same as those for the CVP catheter. The subclavian and internal jugular are the most popular veins used in the ICU.

Placement of the Pulmonary Artery Catheter

The catheter can be positioned using fluoroscopy but is more often floated into place using pressure waveforms to indicate the catheter's position. The distal lumen of the catheter is connected to a transducer-monitor system; both the distal and proximal lumens are flushed until they are free of air bubbles, and then the catheter is placed through an introducer. The clinician placing the catheter usually inflates the balloon on the tip of the catheter when it reaches the superior vena cava or the right atrium. The inflated balloon allows the catheter to "float" through the right side of the heart and into the PA. The clinician observes the pressure waves generated by the pressure sensor in the tip of the catheter as it passes through the various anatomic structures (e.g., right atrium, right ventricle, PA). In this way, the clinician placing the catheter can know when the tip passes into the PA and is near the wedge position. The wedge position occurs when the balloon reaches a site in a pulmonary capillary that is too small to allow further advancement of the catheter. The waveforms generated by the catheter as it is inserted are briefly discussed below according to anatomic site.

Right Atrium

When the tip of the catheter reaches the great vessels, a CVP waveform appears on the monitor (Figure 15-8). The balloon is fully inflated while the catheter is still in the superior vena cava or atrium. This encourages the catheter to follow blood flow into the right ventricle and then into the PA and decreases the

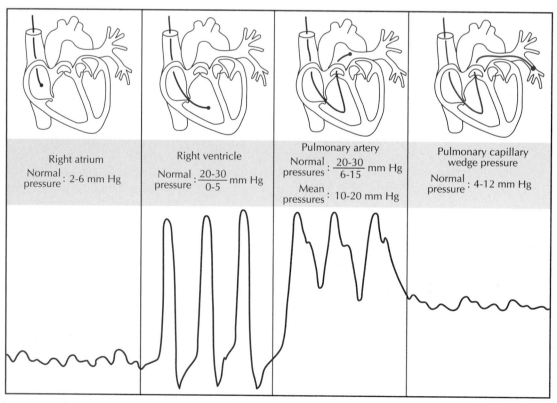

Right atrium	Right ventricle	Pulmonary artery	Pulmonary capillary wedge pressure
Normal pressure: 2-6 mm Hg	Normal pressure: $\frac{20\text{-}30}{0\text{-}5}$ mm Hg	Normal pressures: $\frac{20\text{-}30}{6\text{-}15}$ mm Hg Mean pressures: 10-20 mm Hg	Normal pressure: 4-12 mm Hg

Figure 15-8 Schematic of waveforms and normal pressures visualized as the pulmonary artery catheter is floated into position.

risk of premature ventricular contractions occurring while the catheter is in the ventricle.

Right Ventricle

A rapid increase in the height of the pressure waveform is seen when the catheter passes through the tricuspid valve into the right ventricle. This almost always provides a landmark in catheter insertion. Exceptions are patients with severe tricuspid regurgitation that produces marked pressure waves in the superior vena cava or patients with right heart dysfunction and very little generated pressure wave in the right ventricle. The right ventricular waveform is easily distinguished from the PA waveform because the right side of the waveform (downstroke) drops straight down to near zero as the ventricle relaxes during diastole. As soon as the ventricle relaxes, the tricuspid valve opens and blood begins to flow into the ventricle, causing the pressure wave to increase gradually. End-diastolic pressure occurs just before the upstroke created by ventricular isovolumetric contraction (see Figure 15-8).

The catheter is supposed to float easily from the right ventricle into the PA; however, achieving catheter placement in the PA can take from minutes to more than an hour. Difficult insertions are caused by a large, dysfunctional right ventricle, tricuspid regurgitation, and pulmonary hypertension with pulmonary valve incompetence. Placement is often most difficult in patients who would most benefit from the catheter-derived values. Under these circumstances, it is often necessary to position the catheter visually using fluoroscopy.

In most adults, catheters inserted through the subclavian or jugular vein are positioned in the PA when approximately 50 cm of catheter is inserted into the patient. When more than that amount has been inserted and no pulmonary waveform is obtained, it is generally assumed that the catheter is curling in the atrium or ventricle or is going down the inferior vena cava. The balloon is deflated and the catheter is withdrawn until the tip is in the atrium. The balloon is then reinflated and the catheter is reinserted. PA catheter insertion via femoral insertion site is much more difficult than via insertion sites that traverse the superior vena cava. Fluoroscopy should be planned at the onset of femoral PA catheter placements rather than as a last resort.

Pulmonary Artery

Entry into the PA is recognized by a change in the diastolic portion of the waveform. The PA maintains pressure throughout the cardiac cycle so that the baseline pressure usually increases to 8 to 15 mm Hg over right ventricular diastolic pressures. The PA waveform is a miniature of the peripheral arterial waveform, with a dicrotic notch and a gradual diastolic runoff that does not drop to zero.

Wedge Position

When the catheter wedges in a smaller branch of the PA, the forward flow of the pulmonary arterial blood is occluded. With pulsatile arterial blood flow stopped, the tip of the catheter "sees" the backpressure from the pulmonary venous system and left atrium and the waveform takes on the appearance of an atrial pressure waveform with a, c, and v waves (see Figure 15-8; Figure 15-9). The PA waveform should return when the balloon is deflated. Adjustments in catheter placement are often needed to keep the catheter tip in position to easily wedge but to avoid a permanently wedged position. Care should be taken to inflate

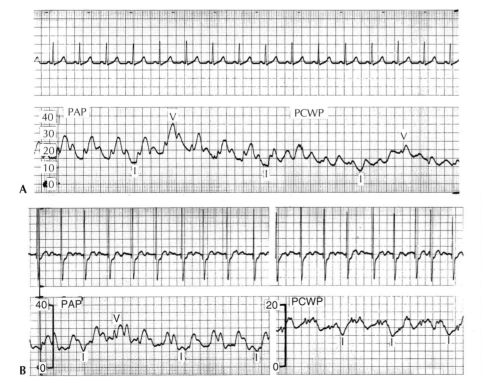

Figure 15-9 Pulmonary artery pressure *(PAP)* trace converting to wedge pressure. **A,** Patient is on intermittent mandatory ventilation of 12 and positive end-expiratory pressure of 5 cm H$_2$O. Note respiratory swing in pressure wave. Heart rate, 98 beats/min, normal sinus rhythm; PAP, 27/15 mm Hg; wedge pressure *(PCWP)*, 13 mm Hg. **B,** Note difference in appearance of waveforms in patient with atrial fibrillation. Heart rate, 87 to 102; PAP, 23/14 mm Hg; PCWP, 13 mm Hg. *I,* Spontaneous inspiration; *V,* intermittent ventilator breath.

the balloon only enough to provide a wedge reading because overdistension of the PA could cause rupture of the artery, which could be fatal.

Interpretation of Pulmonary Artery Pressures

As seen in the discussion above, the PA catheter provides numerous measurements including PA systolic, PA diastolic, and wedge pressure. Interpretation of each is discussed below.

Pulmonary Artery Systolic Pressure

PA systolic pressure is the highest pressure created when the right ventricle ejects blood through the pulmonary valve and into the PA and lungs. Like systemic arterial pressure, PA pressure is a product of the volume of blood ejected by the ventricle and the resistance of the pulmonary circulation. Normal PA systolic pressure is 20 to 30 mm Hg.

PA pressures decrease when the volume of blood ejected by the right ventricle decreases or when the pulmonary vasculature relaxes or dilates (decreased pulmonary vascular resistance).

PA pressures increase when pulmonary blood flow increases or when pulmonary vascular resistance increases. The right ventricle pumps increased amounts of blood into the lungs with volume overload or when it receives excess blood from left-to-right intracardiac shunts (e.g., atrial or ventricular septal defects or patent ductus arteriosus).

Resistance to pulmonary flow (increased pulmonary vascular resistance) can be caused by constriction, obstruction, or compression of the pulmonary vasculature or by backpressure from the left heart. Examples of conditions that can cause increased pulmonary vascular resistance include:

- Pulmonary emboli
- Acute or chronic lung disease that causes pulmonary vasoconstriction in response to hypoxia
- Cardiac tamponade or increased intrathoracic pressure compressing the vasculature and impeding forward flow
- Left heart failure and mitral valve regurgitation causing backpressure from the left heart into the lungs

Pulmonary arterial pressures average about 22/8 mm Hg, with a mean pressure of about 13 mm Hg. However, with pulmonary disease, it is not uncommon for the systolic pressure to exceed 45 mm Hg and the mean pulmonary pressure to exceed 35 mm Hg. Advanced pulmonary hypertension can result in pressures approaching systemic artery pressures. Such severe pulmonary hypertension can depress right ventricular function, which in turn decreases right ventricular output. With less blood moving forward, left ventricular preload is decreased, and subsequently left ventricular stroke volume and systemic oxygen transport may also decrease.

Pulmonary Artery Diastolic Pressure

PADP is normally 8 to 15 mm Hg and under normal conditions reflects pulmonary venous, left atrial, and left ventricular end-diastolic pressure (the mitral valve is open during diastole). Additionally, pulmonary capillary resistance and impedance to flow normally are minimal. Therefore, in the absence of severe pulmonary vascular changes, marked tachycardia, pulmonary embolism, and mitral valve stenosis or regurgitation, PADP can be used to monitor left ventricular filling pressure. Unfortunately, such ideal conditions are uncommon in the ICU and PADP is often unreliable as a measure of left ventricular filling pressure.

Normally, PADP is approximately 2 mm Hg higher than wedge pressure, but elevated pulmonary vascular resistance increases the gradient. In fact, a PADP-PCWP gradient that is greater than 5 mm Hg is characteristic of ARDS, sepsis, excessive PEEP, or other conditions that increase pulmonary vascular resistance. In contrast, pulmonary hypertension caused by left ventricular failure is characterized by a normal PADP-PCWP gradient (<5 mm Hg). With heart rates greater than 120 beats/min, the time for diastolic runoff is shortened and diastolic pressure increases and the gradient increases.

SIMPLY STATED

PADP may reflect filling pressures of the left ventricle if the mitral valve of the patient is normal and the pulmonary vascular resistance is normal. In most ICU patients, however, these conditions are not present.

Wedge Pressure

Normal pulmonary capillary wedge pressure (PCWP) is 4 to 12 mm Hg. Wedge pressure is lower than mean PA pressure and is usually about 2 mm Hg lower than PADP. These normal pressure relationships are easier to remember by keeping in mind that blood flows from higher pressure to lower pressure. Wedge pressure is also called pulmonary artery occlusion pressure (PAOP).

The PCWP reading is used to monitor left ventricular filling during diastole. Under normal conditions (e.g., healthy heart) the filling pressure correlates well with the volume of blood filling the ventricle (preload). When the heart is not healthy and a stiff left ventricle is present, the filling pressures increase and the filling volume does not. As a result, the PCWP reading must be interpreted in light of the patient's medical history.

Optimal PCWP values for any one patient depend on the condition of the left ventricle. In the normal heart, optimal stroke volume is obtained with a PCWP of 10 to 12 mm Hg. In the patient with left ventricular hypertrophy, a PCWP of 18 mm Hg or higher may be needed to optimize stroke volume. Thus, optimal PCWP varies from patient to patient and is identified by construction of left ventricular function curves for each patient. The function curves are created by measuring the stroke volume at various PCWP readings. This allows determination of the pressure readings that result in the best cardiac output. PCWP readings above or below this range cause the stroke volume to decrease.

PCWP readings increase for a variety of reasons. Left ventricular failure is a common cause. The lack of forward flow out of the left ventricle causes the left ventricle to dilate and blood to back up into the pulmonary circulation, resulting in an elevated PCWP. In some cases, the PCWP is markedly elevated, indicating overstretching of the left ventricle. This overstretching of the left ventricle causes the stroke volume to decrease and adds to the problem. Diuretics are usually needed, along with other therapy to reduce the PCWP and optimize left ventricular function.

PCWP also increases with mitral valve regurgitation and when the pulmonary venous circulation is obstructed with a tumor. The elevated PCWP does not correlate well with filling volume of the left ventricle in such cases. Box 15-5 summarizes situations in which wedge pressure overestimates left-heart filling pressure.

The most common cause of a decreased PCWP is hypovolemia. This is common after major surgery or trauma in which blood loss is significant. Severe dehydration can also lead to reduced PCWP readings.

SIMPLY STATED

The most common cause of an elevated PCWP is left ventricular failure.

BOX 15-5   Recognizing When Wedge Pressure Overestimates Left Ventricular Filling Catheter Tip in Zone I or II During PEEP or CPAP

PADP < PCWP

Smooth trace: no a or v waves

With changes in PEEP:
- PCWP increase > 50% of PEEP increase
- PCWP decrease > 50% of PEEP reduction

With catheter wedged:
- Inability to withdraw blood
- Mixed venous blood rather than "arterialized" blood
- Catheter tip above left atrial level on lateral chest film

Physiologic Conditions
- Pulmonary venous obstruction/compression (e.g., lung or mediastinal tumors, left atrial myxoma)
- Mitral valve stenosis or occlusion
- Mitral valve insufficiency: large v waves
- Decreased left ventricular compliance
- Inotropic drugs, hypertension
- Acute cardiac dilation
- Myocardial ischemia, hypertrophy, injury, infarction, infiltrate
- Pericardial disease or tamponade
- Increased intrathoracic pressure:
- PEEP or CPAP > 10 cm H_2O

Technical Problems
- Overinflation
- Incomplete wedge
- Catheter fling
- Underdampened trace
- Occluded catheter tip: clot, vessel wall, embolism
- Transducer below left atrial level
- Not end-expiratory reading
- Tubing or patient movement
- Cough or Valsalva maneuver during wedge

Obtaining an accurate wedge pressure

The accuracy of the wedge pressure reading is related to numerous factors including technical issues and position of the catheter within the chest. Table 15-3 summarizes the criteria used to ensure that the pressure measured is really wedge pressure.

The technical aspects of setting up a pressure monitoring system include calibrating the monitor and transducer, positioning the transducer and patient, verifying and maximizing frequency response and dampening characteristics, and recording the pressures at end-expiration. Attention to proper management of the technical steps is vital to obtaining accurate PA and wedge pressure measurements.

Another key point related to obtaining an accurate PCWP reading is the position of the catheter tip in relation to the heart. For wedge pressure to reflect pulmonary venous and therefore left atrial pressure, blood flow must be uninterrupted between the catheter tip and the left heart. This condition exists only in what West[8] has called zone III, an area of the lung where both pulmonary arterial and venous pressures exceed alveolar pressure.

As depicted in Figure 15-10, zone I theoretically has no blood flow because alveolar pressure exceeds both pulmonary venous pressure and MAP. In zone II, alveolar pressure exceeds venous pressure but is less than MAP. Because breathing (inspiration and expiration) and PA pressure (systolic and diastolic) are phasic, flow is intermittent. Hence, a catheter located in zone II measures pulmonary arterial pressure with the balloon deflated but reflects alveolar pressure when it is wedged.

The lung zones are not anatomically fixed zones but rather are functional, gravity-dependent zones, which are altered by position, blood flow, blood pressure, and ventilatory status (PEEP, continuous positive airway pressure (CPAP), air trapping). Zone II conditions dominate in supine patients. However, because the catheters are flow directed, they tend to advance to areas of continuous blood flow. Nevertheless, the location of the catheter tip at or below left atrial level should be verified by a lateral chest film.

To measure left heart pressure accurately, the catheter tip must be in zone III. When intravascular volume decreases (diuresis, hypovolemia, hemorrhage) or alveolar pressure increases (PEEP), zone III areas can convert to zone I or II. Catheters located at or below the left atrial level are less likely to be affected by these changes. Characteristics of non-zone III catheters are listed in Box 15-5.

Alterations in ventilatory patterns cause fluctuations in intrapleural pressure. End-expiration minimizes the influence of the pressure swings for both spontaneous and mechanical ventilation, provided the patient is not exhaling against positive pressure. Ideally, the pressure will be recorded from a calibrated paper trace that also records the ventilatory pattern so that the end-expiratory pressures are clearly identified over several respiratory cycles.

Wedging the balloon

Ideally, the catheter ends up in a portion of the PA that is at or below left atrial level, where a wedge trace with very clear a and

Table 15-3   Criteria for Wedge Pressure That Represents Left Heart Filling Pressure

Criteria	Characteristics
Distinct and valid pulmonary artery pressure trace before inflation	Frequency response not overdamped or underdamped. Transducer calibrated at left atrial level. Patient supine, head of bed ≤ 45 degrees.
Catheter tip in zone III	At or below left atrial level with lateral x-ray film.
PADP > PCWP	If PAPD < PCWP, consider non-zone III, tachycardia > 120 beats/min, and increased pulmonary vascular resistance.
Distinct PCWP trace immediately on wedge	*a* and *c* waves clearly visible. Elevated *v* waves suggest mitral regurgitation; may also be seen with MI and mitral stenosis.
Free flow with catheter wedged	No overinflation (climbing wave). Easy withdrawal of blood. Nondamped trace.
Change in PCWP < ½ change in airway pressure	Applies to both increase and decrease of PEEP or CPAP.
Aspiration of "arterialized" blood from distal port while catheter is wedged	$Pwo_2 - Pao_2 \geq 19$ mm Hg $Paco_2 - Pwco_2 \geq 11$ mm Hg $pHw - pHa \geq 0.08$
Pressure reading using the a wave at end-expiration	Obtain from paper if IMV or labored breathing. If monitor has algorithm to find end-expiration and if digital and paper recording agree: • Use systolic pressure for spontaneous breathing • Use diastolic pressure for continuous mechanical ventilation

PCWP, Pulmonary capillary wedge pressure; *PADP,* pulmonary artery diastolic pressure; *MI,* myocardial infarction; *PEEP,* positive end-expiratory pressure; *CPAP,* continuous positive airway pressure; Pwo_2, wedge pressure, oxygen; Pao_2, arterial oxygen tension; $Paco_2$, arterial carbon dioxide tension; $Pwco_2$, wedge pressure, carbon dioxide; *pHw,* wedge pH; *pHa,* arterial pH; *IMV,* intermittent mandatory ventilation.

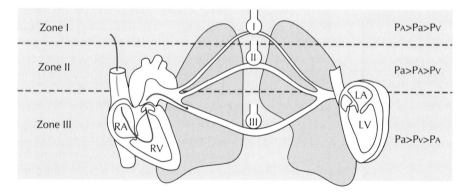

Figure 15-10 Pulmonary artery catheter wedged in zone III, where both pulmonary arterial pressures are greater than alveolar pressure, resulting in uninterrupted blood flow to the left heart and a wedge pressure that reflects pulmonary venous and left-heart pressures. Relationship of pressures is shown at the right. See text for explanation of West's zones I, II, and III. *LA,* Left atrium; *LV,* left ventricle; *PA,* alveolar pressure; *Pa,* pulmonary arterial pressure; *Pv,* pulmonary venous pressure; *RA,* right atrium; *RV,* right ventricle.

v waves is obtained using 0.8 to 1.5 mL of air. Locating the catheter tip in a slightly larger segment of the artery reduces the risk associated with catheter migration and decreases the likelihood of overinflation and eccentric balloon inflation. Subsequently, the balloon should be inflated with the minimum amount of air necessary to obtain a clear wedge reading. Placing too much air in the balloon (overwedging) results in a pressure waveform without clearly distinguishable a and v waves that gradually climbs upward across the screen. Rarely, overwedging may produce a waveform that gradually declines, without clearly distinguishable a and v waves.

The balloon should be left inflated only long enough to obtain the wedge trace; however, it must be remembered that it may take 5 to 20 seconds for equilibration of the left heart and

pulmonary pressures after balloon inflation. Integrity of the balloon is extended if it is permitted to empty on its own rather than by aspiration. Deflation of the balloon is confirmed by a clear PA trace.

The wedge position is verified first by the waveform. Before balloon inflation, the PA trace should be very clear, with systolic, dicrotic notch, and diastolic segments. On inflation, the waveform should immediately convert to a clear atrial pressure trace with no systolic segment or dicrotic notch. On balloon deflation, the waveform should convert immediately to a crisp PA trace.

It is possible to obtain a partial wedge, in which the systolic pressure is high enough to push blood around the inflated balloon but the artery is occluded during diastole. The trace is recognized by a systolic wave that converts to a wedge trace during diastole: half PA trace and half wedge trace. This waveform produces a pressure that is higher than true wedge pressure.

Wedge pressure readings normally are about 2 mm Hg lower than pulmonary diastolic pressure readings because blood flows from high pressure to low pressure. If the wedge pressure were higher, blood would be flowing backward. In fact, that does occur with mitral valve regurgitation, in which the valve does not close completely during systole and blood is ejected backward into the left atrium. This problem can be indicated by giant v waves, which are more than 10 mm Hg higher than the a waves. Recording the waveform on paper and using the a wave (atrial systole) at the end of expiration results in a more consistent and accurate reflection of left ventricular end-diastolic volume.

Relationship between transmural pressure and wedge pressure

Transmural pressure is the net distending pressure within the ventricle. It provides a true estimation of left ventricular end-diastolic filling because the effect of pressure around the heart is considered. Transmural pressure cannot be measured directly but is calculated by subtracting the pressure around the heart from the measured filling pressure in the heart.

Wedge pressure is used to estimate left ventricular filling pressure inside the heart. Intrapleural or esophageal pressure is used to approximate the pressure pushing on the heart from the outside.

During spontaneous breathing, intrapleural pressure is nearly zero at end-expiration. Therefore, as shown in the example that follows, end-diastolic pressure and transmural pressure are approximately equal and wedge pressure is a good estimator of left ventricular filling pressure in the patient during normal spontaneous breathing. However, positive-pressure ventilation, labored respiratory effort, coughing, and the Valsalva maneuver cause large swings in the intrapleural pressure. These pressure fluctuations can cause wedge pressure to overestimate or underestimate left ventricular filling pressure. The following example shows how a wedge pressure (PCWP) of 12 mm Hg can occur with very different transmural pressures. Remember that left ventricular filling pressure (PCWP) minus pressure around the heart (pleural pressure) equals pressure distending the left ventricle (transmural pressure).

	PCWP	–	Pleural pressure	=	Transmural pressure
Spontaneous breathing	12	–	0	=	12 mm Hg
20 cm PEEP	12	–	10	=	2 mm Hg
Partial airway obstruction	12	–	−10	=	22 mm Hg

The relationship between wedge and transmural pressures must be kept in mind in interpreting the numbers. The example "20 cm PEEP" shows how transmission of positive pleural pressure can cause the wedge pressure reading on the monitor or on paper to appear normal (12 mm Hg) while, in fact, the patient is really hypovolemic, with a transmural pressure of 2 mm Hg.

The example "partial airway obstruction" shows how filling pressure can appear to be normal (12 mm Hg) when the true filling pressure would be high (22 mm Hg).

Clinically, PEEP levels less than 10 cm H_2O have a limited effect on intrapleural pressure. However, when PEEP exceeds 15 cm H_2O, the effect of PEEP on transmural pressure is uncertain and is altered by lung compliance and changing venous return. As lung compliance decreases, (the lung gets stiffer), a smaller amount of the positive pressure is passed to the pleural space. This has led to the practice of estimating the effect of PEEP on wedge pressure by converting PEEP to millimeters of mercury (1.36 cm H_2O = 1 mm Hg) and subtracting part of PEEP from wedge pressure as follows:

- Compliant lungs: subtract ½ of PEEP from PCWP
- Noncompliant lungs: subtract ¼ of PEEP from PCWP

The effects of PEEP on transmural pressure also can be assessed by measuring pleural pressure. In practice, esophageal pressure is measured with a fluid-filled tube while the patient is in the lateral decubitus position. The esophageal pressure, which is essentially the same as pleural pressure, is then subtracted from the wedge pressure.

Removing the patient from PEEP while the wedge pressures are obtained has been suggested. However, this maneuver alters the pressure gradient for venous return to the thorax and may result in sudden "autotransfusion." In addition, sudden removal of PEEP has been reported to cause deterioration in gas exchange that is not readily corrected. In patients with left ventricular dysfunction, removal from mechanical ventilation with PEEP may be associated with increased PA pressure, hypoxemia, and deterioration in cardiac function. Removal of patients from mechanical ventilation with PEEP to obtain pressure readings is not recommended.

Complications of Pulmonary Artery Catheterization

PA catheterization has been associated with multiple complications. During cannulation of a central vein, it is possible for pneumothorax, hydrothorax, hemothorax, air embolism, and damage to the vein, nearby arteries, or nerves to occur. Movement of the catheter inside the heart can trigger bundle-branch block and supraventricular or ventricular dysrhythmia. Hypoxemia, acidosis, hypokalemia, hypocalcemia, and hypomagnesemia increase the likelihood of dysrhythmia. In addition, perforation of the heart or PA is possible.

The PA catheter, like all other invasive lines, is a source of embolus, thrombus, bleeding, hematoma, site infection, and sepsis. The constant movement of the catheter with heartbeat, breathing, and patient movement can result in catheter migration. It should be remembered that a balloon left inflated or a catheter that migrates into wedge position acts like a pulmonary embolus.

Pulmonary infarction and even PA rupture can result from overfilling the balloon while obtaining a wedge pressure as well as from catheter migration. Pulmonary infarction should be suspected and assessed whenever a patient with a pulmonary catheter coughs up blood-tinged sputum. An overfilled balloon can rupture, causing possible fragment or air embolism.

Catheter movement and catheter removal can trigger dysrhythmia as well as looping of the catheter in the ventricle, with possible knotting and valve damage. Lidocaine and emergency resuscitation equipment should be immediately available at both insertion and removal. Blood gases and serum electrolytes should be optimized to decrease the risk of dysrhythmia. Catheter resistance during removal is not normal and is an indication for obtaining a chest x-ray to assess the cause.

REVIEW QUESTIONS

1. T F Continuous measurement of blood pressure can be performed via arterial cannulation.

2. Which of the following patients is least likely to need placement of an indwelling arterial cannula?
   a. Patient in septic shock
   b. Patient in cardiogenic shock
   c. Patient with ARDS
   d. Patient with pneumonia

3. Which of the following is not a site used for arterial cannulation?
   a. Ulnar artery
   b. Radial artery
   c. Femoral artery
   d. Carotid artery

4. The dicrotic notch on the arterial pressure waveform represents which of the following?
   a. Pulmonic valve closure
   b. Aortic valve closure
   c. Tricuspid valve closure
   d. Mitral valve closure

5. T F The presence of a dicrotic notch in the arterial pressure waveform indicates an accurate pressure measurement.

6. T F Respiratory variation in the arterial pressure waveform may indicate cardiac tamponade.

7. Which of the following will cause the arterial pressure to decrease?
   a. Vasodilators
   b. Cardiac failure
   c. Hypovolemia
   d. All the above

8. Which of the following is true about MAP?
   a. It is normally 80 to 100 mm Hg.
   b. It is the arithmetic average of the systolic and diastolic pressures.

c. Organ perfusion will be reduced if MAP is less than 80 mm Hg.
   d. All of the above

9. Which of the following are possible complications of arterial cannulation?
   a. Infection
   b. Arterial spasm
   c. Thromboembolism
   d. All of the above

10. CVP is a reflection of which of the following?
   a. Right ventricular preload
   b. Right atrial pressure
   c. Right ventricular end-diastolic pressure
   d. All of the above

11. T F A CVP catheter can be used to administer intravascular drugs.

12. Which of the following is true about the CVP catheter?
   a. It is commonly inserted via the subclavian vein.
   b. The catheter can have multiple lumens.
   c. A balloon is located on the distal end.
   d. a and b only

13. The c wave of a CVP waveform represents which of the following?
   a. Atrial contraction
   b. Ventricular contraction
   c. Right atrial filling
   d. None of the above

14. T F Respiratory variation in the CVP waveform is an abnormal finding.

15. Which of the following is the correct method of measuring CVP in a patient receiving mechanical ventilation with PEEP?
   a. At end-inspiration on the ventilator
   b. At end-inspiration off the ventilator
   c. At end-exhalation on the ventilator
   d. At end-exhalation off the ventilator

16. T F In certain situations, CVP can be a good indicator of left ventricular function.

17. What is the normal value for CVP?
   a. Less than 6 mm Hg
   b. 6 to 8 mm Hg
   c. 8 to 12 mm Hg
   d. 12 to 18 mm Hg

18. Which of the following would cause the CVP to increase?
   a. Vasodilator therapy
   b. Spontaneous inspiration

c. Fluid overload
d. Air in the pressure-sensing line

19. Pulmonary artery pressure monitoring can be accomplished via the use of which of the following?
a. Pulmonary artery catheter
b. Swan-Ganz catheter
c. Balloon-tipped flow-directed catheter
d. All of the above

20. What size catheter typically is used for adults to monitor pulmonary artery pressures?
a. 4 to 5 French
b. 5 to 8 French
c. 8 to 10 French
d. 10 to 15 French

21. T   F   The distal lumen of the PA catheter is used to measure PCWP.

22. What is the approximate amount of air required to fill the balloon on a PA catheter?
a. 0.5 mL
b. 1.0 mL
c. 1.5 mL
d. 2.0 mL

23. During insertion of the PA catheter, when is the balloon inflated?
a. Immediately after the catheter is inserted into the venous site
b. When the catheter enters the right atrium
c. When the catheter enters the right ventricle
d. When the catheter enters the left atrium

24. What would be considered a normal value for PA pressure?
a. 15/4 mm Hg
b. 18/10 mm Hg
c. 25/10 mm Hg
d. 36/22 mm Hg

25. Which of the following would increase PA pressure?
a. Severe hypoxemia
b. Thromboembolism
c. Acidosis
d. All of the above

26. Which of the following statements is true about pulmonary capillary wedge pressure?
a. It is normally 4 to 12 mm Hg.
b. It is normally higher than PADP.
c. It reflects left ventricular afterload.
d. All of the above

27. T   F   A pulmonary diastolic pressure of 14 mm Hg and a wedge pressure of 12 mm Hg indicate zone III catheter placement.

28. Which of the following could cause PCWP to be artificially elevated?
a. PEEP or CPAP greater than 10 cm H_2O
b. Mitral valve stenosis
c. Reduced left ventricular compliance
d. All of the above

29. Your patient has a PA catheter in place and suddenly starts coughing up bloody sputum. What is the most likely cause of this?
a. Pneumothorax
b. Pulmonary infarction
c. Mitral valve stenosis
d. Myocardial infarction

30. What complication is most likely to occur during removal of the PA catheter?
a. Pneumothorax
b. Pulmonary infarction
c. Pulmonary embolism
d. Dysrhythmias

REFERENCES

1. Swan HJC and others: Catheterization of the heart in man with use of a flow-directed balloon-tipped catheter. *N Engl J Med* 283:447, 1970.
2. Cariou A and others: Continuous cardiac output and mixed venous oxygen saturation monitoring. *J Crit Care* 13:198, 1998.
3. Mimoz O and others: Pulmonary artery catheterization in critically ill patients: a prospective analysis of outcome changes associated with catheter-prompted changes in therapy. *Crit Care Med* 22:573-579, 1994.
4. Staudinger T: Diagnostic validity of pulmonary artery catheterization for residents at an ICU. *J Trauma* 44:902-906, 1998.
5. Sandham JD and others: A randomized, controlled trial of the use of pulmonary artery catheters in high-risk surgical patients. *N Engl J Med* 348:5-14, 2003.
6. Tuman KJ and others: Effect of pulmonary artery catheterization on outcome in patients undergoing coronary artery surgery. *Anesthesiology* 70:199-206, 1989.
7. Ramsey SD and others: Clinical and economic effects of pulmonary artery catheterization in nonemergent coronary artery bypass graft surgery. *J Cardiothorac Vasc Anesth* 14:113-118, 2000.
8. West JB: *Respiratory physiology: the essentials,* ed 5. Baltimore, 1995, Williams & Wilkins.

BIBLIOGRAPHY

Baum GL and others: *Textbook of pulmonary diseases,* ed 6, vols I and II. Philadelphia, 1998, Lippincott-Raven.

Civetta JM, Taylor RW, Kirby RR: *Critical care,* ed 3, Philadelphia, 1997, Lippincott-Raven.

Daily EK, Schroeder JS: *Techniques in bedside hemodynamic monitoring,* ed 5. St Louis, 1994, Mosby.

Dantzker DR, Scharf SM: *Cardiopulmonary critical care,* ed 3. Philadelphia, 1998, WB Saunders.

Darovic GO: *Handbook of hemodynamic monitoring,* ed 2. Philadelphia, 2004, WB Saunders.

Fishman AP and others: *Fishman's pulmonary disease and disorders,* ed 3, vols I and II. New York, 1998, McGraw-Hill.

Ilazinski MF: *Manual of pediatric critical care.* St Louis, 1999, Mosby.

Kinney MR and others: *AACN clinical reference for critical care nursing,* ed 4. St Louis, 1998, Mosby.

Lieberman K: Beyond the basics: monitoring with a pulmonary artery (Swan-Ganz) catheter. *J Emerg Nurs* 24:218, 1998.

Lynn-McHale DJ: Obtaining a pulmonary artery wedge pressure. *Crit Care Nurse* 17:94, 1997.

Schwartz GR, editor: *Principles and practice of emergency medicine,* ed 4. Baltimore, 1999, Williams & Wilkins.

Sheehy SB and others: *Manual of clinical trauma care: the first hour.* St Louis, 1999, Mosby.

Shoemaker WC and others: *Textbook of critical care,* ed 4. Philadelphia, 1995, WB Saunders.

C H A P T E R

16

Richard L. Sheldon
Judy L. Marcello

Flexible Fiberoptic Bronchoscopy

LEARNING OBJECTIVES

Upon completion of this chapter, the reader should be able to accomplish the following:

1. Define the basic terms used in endoscopy.
2. Identify basic technical data about flexible fiberoptic bronchoscopes as they relate to:
   a. Their size relative to the patients being examined
   b. The airway generations that can be examined
   c. The accessory equipment needed: light sources, biopsy forceps, brushes, needles, laser probes, and specialty forceps
3. List or identify the five most common indications for bronchoscopy and identify which indications are diagnostic applications and which are therapeutic applications.
4. Identify the uses of bronchoalveolar lavage, brushings (both sterile and nonsterile), and needle biopsies.
5. List the complications of flexible bronchoscopy and understand the relative risks involved in the procedure.
6. List the contraindications to performing a bronchoscopy.
7. List the essential equipment needed in order to perform a bronchoscopy safely.
8. Describe how to prepare a patient, step-by-step, for an outpatient bronchoscopy, including
   a. Explaining the procedure
   b. Instructing the patient on what to do and what not to do in the 6 hours before the procedure
   c. Obtaining informed consent
   d. Nebulizing lidocaine (Xylocaine)
   e. Starting an intravenous port for medication
   f. Preparing the nostril for insertion of the bronchoscope
   g. Preparing the suction device and the in-line trap
   h. Administration of "conscious sedation" medications
   i. Safety
   j. Handling specimens obtained during the procedure
   k. Monitoring the patient during and after the procedure
   l. Discharge criteria
   m. Sending the specimens to the laboratory
   n. Charting

CHAPTER OUTLINE

Characteristics and Capabilities of the Bronchoscope
Indications for Bronchoscopy
   Masses
   Hemoptysis
   Pneumonia
   Interstitial Lung Diseases
   Foreign Bodies
Complications
Outpatient Flexible Bronchoscopy
   The Role of the Respiratory Therapist

KEY TERMS

bronchoscopes   conscious sedation
bronchoscopy   endoscopy

CHAPTER OVERVIEW

The field of endoscopy* originated in the early twentieth century when Henry Plummer introduced rigid open-tube bronchoscopes to the Mayo Clinic in 1904. These early scopes were straight pieces of open pipe, beveled on the end to prevent tearing the trachea while being forced into the anesthetized patient with his/her head tipped back as far as possible. A simple light shining down the tube allowed limited viewing of the trachea and perhaps the mainstem bronchi. Although these rigid devices provided a limited view

---

Endoscopy is a general term used to describe procedures that look into the body's tubes and cavities. To extend the term to more specific parts of the body (e.g., the bronchi), the term *bronchoscopy* is used. Examining the esophagus is *esophagoscopy*; examining the colon is *colonoscopy*. Because the esophagus and the colon are part of the gastrointestinal tract, these examinations are performed with a *gastroscope*.

333

of the larger airways, they also allowed suctioning of large volumes of blood in the patient who was hemorrhaging from the lung. At the same time, ventilation could be provided to ensure better patient outcome. These early scopes have been replaced by more sophisticated instruments with lights at the tips and valves to allow general anesthesia, oxygenation, and biopsy.

The first application of flexible fiberoptics to the field of endoscopy was in 1957, when the technology was initially applied to gastroscopes. As experience grew and the techniques improved, it was only a matter of time before flexible fiberoptic technology was applied to the airways. In 1969 Shigeto Akeda of Japan brought to the Mayo Clinic the first bronchoscopes, which incorporated fiberoptics into a flexible tube suitable in size and length to enter the trachea and visualize the lower airway. The flexible fiberoptic bronchoscope has greatly improved our ability to perform lung pathology research and to apply high-quality diagnosis and treatment to patients with pulmonary disorders.

Respiratory therapists (RTs) become knowledgeable about flexible fiberoptic bronchoscopes because they often maintain the scopes and the accessory equipment. The RT has become indispensable in helping the physician perform the procedure in hospitals and outpatient clinics.

SIMPLY STATED

Endoscopy is a field of medicine that uses instruments to look into different parts of the body to diagnose various diseases and explain certain conditions. Bronchoscopy is the process of visualizing the airways below the larynx with a bronchoscope.

CHARACTERISTICS AND CAPABILITIES OF THE BRONCHOSCOPE

Currently, several companies manufacture excellent flexible fiberoptic bronchoscopes (bronchofibroscopes). The available scopes serve a wide range of applications, from small-diameter scopes used for viewing the airways of infants and children to larger-diameter scopes with suction channels used to remove large amounts of thick secretions from patients on ventilators in the intensive care unit. A small color television camera can be attached to the eyepiece of the scope. Images from these cameras can be recorded or used in teaching.

The standard flexible bronchoscope has an external diameter of 5.3 mm and a total length of 605 mm (Figure 16-1). It can pass easily down the trachea (first-order bronchus) and into the right or left mainstem bronchus and can enter most fourth-order bronchi and one third of all fifth-order bronchi (Figure 16-2). Visualization of half of the lung's sixth-order bronchi is possible.[1] Ultrathin scopes with a 2.7-mm external diameter and 0.8-mm biopsy channels will pass down 3.5-mm or larger endotracheal tubes, making it easier to study and perform biopsies on intubated infants and children.[2]

SIMPLY STATED

The standard adult bronchoscope is an instrument about 3 feet long and 0.5 inches thick, with hand controls for directing the tip and an eyepiece on the end. There are two ports near the hand controls: one for suctioning and the other for inserting biopsy tools and flushing fluids into distal airways.

The amount of tip angulation, which makes the scope directional, is crucial to the scope's utility and ability to visualize hard-to-reach but important airways. Scope tips can bend from the axial plane 130 degrees in one direction and 160 degrees in the other. The scope loses flexibility at the tip over time and with use; correcting this problem is expensive.

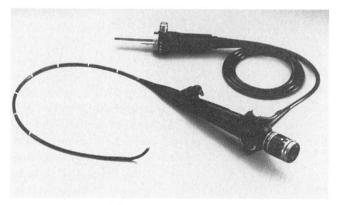

Figure 16-1 Standard flexible fiberoptic bronchoscope. The attachment for a light source is seen at the top of the photo. (Courtesy Olympus America Inc, Melville, NY.)

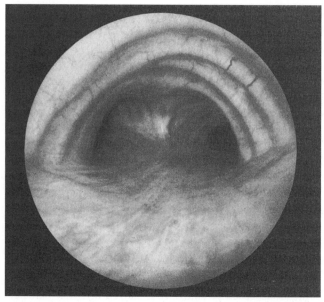

Figure 16-2 Normal main carina showing right and left mainstem bronchi.

Light sources for these scopes are critical. Light sources range in size from small portable boxes into which the scopes can be plugged (for performing bronchoscopy at bedside or in a clinic setting) to larger units that are less portable. These larger units deliver light at varied intensities, in different wavelengths, and in pulses for photography or other specialized jobs. The larger units can also blow air across the tip of the scope in order to maintain clean optics.

Biopsy devices can be passed down the scope and greatly extend the scope's use. The devices include biting and grasping forceps, brushes (shielded and unshielded), sheathed needles, and sampling catheters. The biting forceps come in various types (biting cusps with smooth edges or serrated edges). Smooth-cusped flexible forceps can be used if the physician needs to obtain a piece of lung parenchyma during the procedure. If a large, dense (tough) lesion is seen in the larger airways, a serrated forceps capable of cutting tissue is preferred. Positive findings (recognition of the specific type of abnormal tissue) in these large lesions using cutting forceps is almost 100%.[3] Because these forceps are metallic, they are easily visualized by a fluoroscope in radiology and thus can be visually directed using real-time fluoroscopy for direct biopsy of a small lesion.

A hollow needle fixed to a long, small-lumen plastic tube can be passed down the scope in order to perform biopsy on lesions under the mucosa and to obtain cells from coin lesions in the periphery of the lung. Positive yields (obtaining legitimate tissue samples) from submucosal lesions are less than for large cancers growing in the larger airways, but they can be as high as 87% if the biopsy is performed carefully.[4]

> **SIMPLY STATED**
> The bigger the lung tumor and the closer to the hilar area it is growing inside a large airway, the easier it is to make a tissue (adenocarcinoma, squamous cell, small cell, or large cell) diagnosis. If the cancer is outside an airway and in the periphery of the lung, it is less likely that flexible bronchoscopy will be able to get adequate tissue to make a diagnosis.

Unshielded brushes are used to harvest cells from tumor masses, both located centrally and in the periphery. The double-shielded sterile brush is used to gather microbiologically important material in order to diagnose infections in the lung. Because the bronchoscope is passed into the lung by way of the nose or the mouth, the entire scope immediately becomes contaminated with the patient's upper-tract bacterial mix (normal flora). Thus *unshielded* sampling badly misrepresents what is happening in the lower lung. Sterile double-shielded brushes are passed through the entire length of the scope until the bronchoscopist sees that the tip is well in view into the airway of concern. The wire brush is then advanced out of its wax-plugged and sterile inner sheath. The miniscule piece of sterile wax covering the end of the catheter to ensure sterility is pushed into the airway. This wax is inconsequential to the patient and is coughed out or melts and is included in the patient's mucus.

The sampling is done by gently brushing the airway. The wire is then drawn back into its sheath and pulled from the bronchoscope. The wire tip is cut off with sterile scissors and placed in a sterile container with pyrogen-free sterile normal saline.

> **SIMPLY STATED**
> Because the mouth harbors bacteria, shielded brushes must be used to get uncontaminated material from the area of the lung where pneumonias are located to accurately determine which organism is causing the pneumonia. When the offending organism is determined, the appropriate antibiotic can be selected.

Occasionally, patients accidentally inhale various objects. The list is amazing: everything from smooth, oblong objects such as peanuts, which are invisible to the roentgenogram and can go deep into the small airways, to irregular sharp-edged objects such as dentures and teeth, which can be seen on the roentgenogram. Grasping forceps and snares can be used with the bronchoscope to retrieve foreign objects (Figures 16-3 and 16-4). Grasping forceps are available with rubber tips for needle and nail removal; basket types are used for removal of marbles, seeds, and nuts; "pelican" types are used for food particles; and W-shaped forceps are used for the removal of coins.

Lasers can be used to obliterate tumors obstructing large airways. Flexible quartz monofilaments pass through the bronchoscope and conduct a laser beam to the end of the scope. The bronchoscopist can direct the red "aiming dot" with precision, step on the foot pedal to activate the laser beam, and send a pulsed beam of tissue-vaporizing laser energy into the tumor. Safety is a major issue here. Lasers are more likely to ignite airway fires if the oxygen concentration is high. Thus the F_{IO_2} should be kept below 0.30 whenever possible. Also, the laser beam can badly injure a retina if accidentally activated bursts hit an unprotected eye. A misdirected burst of laser energy can also penetrate the bronchial wall, puncture a large vessel, and cause massive and usually fatal pulmonary hemorrhage.

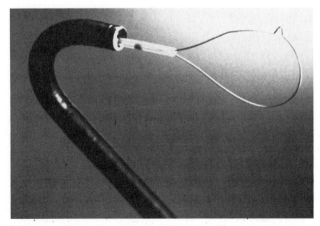

Figure 16-3 Electrosurgical snare. (Courtesy Olympus America Inc, Melville, NY.)

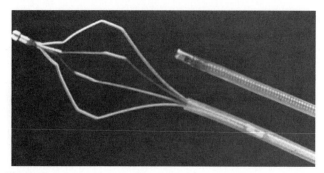

Figure 16-4 Retrieval snare. (Courtesy Olympus America Inc, Melville, NY.)

Other specialty catheters available for use through a bronchoscope include suture cutters, magnetic extractors, and injector catheters used to direct medications into an area of the lung. Coagulation electrodes and hot biopsy forceps are also available.

SIMPLY STATED

Laser treatment through a bronchoscope is usually reserved for patients in whom lung cancer has obstructed a large airway. Such patients are at high risk and should be operated on in the hospital's operating room.

INDICATIONS FOR BRONCHOSCOPY

There are two basic categories of indications for flexible fiberoptic bronchoscopy: *diagnostic* and *therapeutic* (Box 16-1).[5] The flexible fiberoptic bronchoscope is used most often for diagnostic purposes, with therapeutic indications being less common.

Masses

The most common indication for flexible bronchoscopy is to diagnose the cause of an abnormality seen on a chest roentgenogram. These abnormalities include infiltrates of any size or location, atelectasis, or mass lesions. These lesions are particularly troublesome if they have appeared on the chest radiograph recently and the patient has a significant smoking history. Bronchoscopy may be indicated in the patient with a normal chest radiograph if he/she has symptoms of a larger-airway lesion (e.g., persistent unexplained cough and stridor), especially if his/her smoking history is significant.

Coin lesions that occur in the lung periphery cannot be seen through a flexible bronchoscope. Fluoroscopy is used to aim the tip of the bronchoscope directly at the lesion. The biopsy forceps can be advanced to allow the bronchoscopist to bump the lesion with the forceps. Once the tip of the forceps is near the lesion, pieces are snipped off and sent for analysis. When coin lesions are assessed via bronchoscopy without the use of fluoroscopy, diagnostic yield is low. When fluoroscopy is used, yield is reported to be up to 67%.[6]

BOX 16-1   Indications for Flexible Bronchoscopy

Abnormal chest roentgenogram
   New or persistent shadow suggesting neoplasia
   Slowly resolving pneumonia
   Persistent atelectasis
   Unexplained and persistent pleural effusion
   Unexplained and persistent paralysis of a hemidiaphragm
   Interstitial fibrosis
Hemoptysis
Pneumonia
   Identification of causative organism
   Immunocompromised patients
Therapeutic
   Atelectasis (to remove mucus plugs and secretions)
   Laser excision of obstructing neoplasms
   Removal of foreign bodies
   Lung lavage in alveolar proteinosis
Unexplained and persistent cough or wheeze (stridor)
Tracheal disease (posttracheostomy)
Intensive care unit uses
   Difficult intubations
   Suctioning while patient is on a ventilator
Miscellaneous
   Unexplained hoarseness
   Brachytherapy (installing small radioactive "seeds" directly into tumor masses)
   Evaluation for possible upper airway burns and swelling in burn patients
   Bronchography
   Research (bronchoalveolar lavage)

Another application for flexible bronchoscopy in the setting of lung tumors is to examine the patient with a normal chest roentgenogram but sputum cytologies positive for carcinoma. Flexible bronchoscopy can be used occasionally for staging patients already diagnosed with carcinoma of the lung, but this process is better accomplished through mediastinoscopy.

SIMPLY STATED

Cancers starting in parts of the body other than the lung have different ways of metastasizing to the lung.

Hemoptysis

Usually, the patient with hemoptysis coughs up small amounts of blood and then stops. Occasionally, massive hemoptysis (> 200 mL/24 hr) occurs, and it signals the need for bronchoscopy in most cases. Whenever massive bleeding occurs, the patient should be examined with a large-bore rigid bronchoscope (Figures 16-5 and 16-6). This type of scope allows better removal of the blood while maintaining ventilation. After the

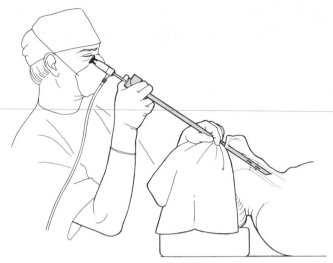

Figure 16-5 Placement of a rigid bronchoscope in the trachea of an anesthetized patient. (From Stradling P: *Diagnostic bronchoscopy,* ed 6, New York, 1991, Churchill Livingstone.)

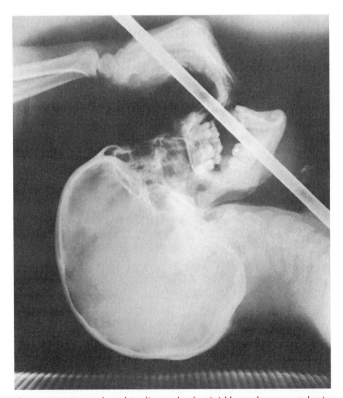

Figure 16-6 Lateral neck radiograph of a rigid bronchoscope tube in place. (From Stradling P: *Diagnostic bronchoscopy,* ed 6, New York, 1991, Churchill Livingstone.)

patient has been free of active bleeding for 1 or 2 days, he/she should be evaluated again with a flexible bronchoscope, especially if the patient smokes or the chest roentgenogram is abnormal.

Bronchitis is the most common cause of episodic hemoptysis in smokers. Most patients with hemoptysis caused by lung cancer have an abnormal chest roentgenogram.[7] In this setting, flexible bronchoscopy is definitely indicated.

Pneumonia

One of the most important clinical situations in which the flexible bronchoscope can be useful is in identifying the causative organism in difficult-to-diagnose pneumonia. This is particularly true if the patient is immunocompromised.[8] In such patients, the bronchoscope is passed to the infiltrated part of the lung and the tip of the scope is usually wedged into a fourth-order bronchus. Four or five 20- to 30-mL aliquots of pyrogen-free normal saline are flushed through the scope's inner channel to distend the distal bronchioles and flood the alveoli, thereby washing free samples of the offending microorganisms. A little more than half of the bronchoalveolar lavage (BAL) fluid is suctioned back into a collection chamber. This fluid is rich in microorganisms that are rarely found in sputum (e.g., *Mycobacterium tuberculosis, Pneumocystis carinii,* and fungal pathogens).[9] This fluid is sent to the laboratory for analysis (see Chapter 6).

For patients on ventilators who are receiving ineffective antibiotics, the diagnosis of persistent and potentially lethal pneumonias is a serious problem. Here the double-sheathed sterile brush is needed to determine which organism is the infective agent and which organism has merely colonized the lower respiratory tract. Even with careful attention to technique, if the patient is receiving antibiotics, the results of sterile brushing directly into an infiltrate may be misleading.[10]

Interstitial Lung Diseases

Several diseases infiltrate the lung in such a way as to give a roentgenographic pattern called *interstitial.* These diseases (e.g., idiopathic interstitial pneumonitis, sarcoidosis, pulmonary alveolar proteinosis, some of the collagen vascular diseases [rheumatoid arthritis, scleroderma], and certain cancers such as lymphoma and alveolar cell carcinoma) present as interstitial lung disease. Because of the difficulty of diagnosing these diseases, a piece of lung tissue must be examined under the microscope. The two options available to obtain lung tissue are open-lung biopsy (requiring general anesthesia, opening the chest in an operating room, and allowing postoperative time in the hospital) or flexible bronchoscopy.[11]

The flexible fiberoptic bronchoscope can be used to reach to the periphery of the lung and remove a small piece of lung for submission to the pathologist. A considerable amount of crush artifact is usually associated with these transbronchial biopsy (TBB) samples. In most cases, however, there is sufficient lung parenchyma to stain, examine, and provide a diagnosis. TBB samples are usually collected under fluoroscopic guidance in order to ensure accurate sampling because bleeding and pneumothorax are serious concerns.

BAL is useful in the diagnosis of some interstitial lung diseases (Table 16-1).[12] This technique requires close cooperation between the bronchoscopist and the assistant in order to distend terminal bronchioles and alveolar spaces rapidly with pyrogen-free normal saline and then collect this cell-rich fluid without contamination or loss.[12]

Table 16-1   Interstitial Lung Diseases and Fiberoptic Bronchoscopy

Disease	Technique	Findings
Sarcoidosis	TBB	Noncaseating granulomas
	BAL	Altered T-lymphocyte helper/suppressor ratio
Pulmonary alveolar proteinosis	TBB	PAS stain and alveolar exudates
Lymphangitic spread of cancer	TBB	Tumor cells in interstitial areas
Alveolar cell center	TBB	Tumor cells in alveolar space
Idiopathic interstitial fibrosis	BAL	Increased PMNs
Collagen vascular diseases	BAL	Increased PMNs
Pneumoconiosis	BAL	Increased PMNs
Bronchiolitis obliterans	BAL	Increased PMNs
Amiodarone toxicity	BAL	Lipid-laden macrophages
Goodpasture's syndrome	BAL	Hemosiderin-laden macrophages
Eosinophilic pneumonia	BAL	High eosinophil concentration
Hypersensitivity pneumonitis	BAL	Altered T-lymphocyte helper/suppressor ratio

TBB, Transbronchial biopsy; *BAL*, bronchoalveolar lavage; *PAS*, periodic acid-Schiff's stain; *PMN*, polymorphonuclear cells (neutrophils).

SIMPLY STATED

Interstitial lung diseases may necessitate several methods to obtain diagnostic material through a flexible bronchoscope, TBB, or BAL.

Foreign Bodies

If a large foreign body has been inhaled into the airway, a large-bore rigid bronchoscope inserted during general anesthesia is most useful to remove the object. Sometimes the object inhaled is small and passes beyond the reach of a rigid scope. In these cases the flexible fiberoptic bronchoscope is used. Regardless of the type of scope used, control of the airway is of the greatest concern. If the object is dislodged, it can move to a new location where obstruction of the airway can endanger the patient.

Of special concern is the ability to apply suction while removing foreign bodies. Prolonged suctioning while performing bronchoscopy may significantly reduce the inspired air, thereby creating a risk of intraoperative atelectasis and hypoxemia. Careful attention to suctioning technique and grasping of the foreign body in order to not damage the airway requires concentration by the medical staff.

COMPLICATIONS

Few complications are associated with fiberoptic bronchoscopy (Box 16-2). When they do occur, they are most often associated with medications used in the procedure, not the procedure itself. Overall mortality from flexible bronchoscopy is less than 0.01%. A careful preprocedure history and physical will identify

BOX 16-2   Complications of Flexible Bronchoscopy

Premedication
  Respiratory failure
  Hypotension
  Hyperexcitement
Local anesthesia
  Laryngospasm
  Bronchospasm
  Seizures
  Cardiopulmonary arrest
  Methemoglobinemia
Bronchoscopy
  Bronchospasm or laryngospasm
  Hypoxemia
  Cardiac arrhythmias
  Aspiration
During biopsy
  Pneumothorax
  Bleeding
  Loss of biopsy tip
Postprocedure
  Persistent bleeding
  Fever
  Pneumonia

Adapted from Fulkerson WJ: Current concepts: Fiberoptic bronchoscopy, *N Engl J Med* 311:511, 1984.

high-risk patients, and laboratory evaluation (prothrombin time, partial thromboplastin time, bleeding times, and platelet counts) looking for clotting abnormalities will alert the bronchoscopist that biopsy may be risky.

Bleeding and pneumothorax are potential complications associated with bronchoscopy. The risk of both problems can be reduced with careful attention to detail and technique. The risk of significant hemoptysis is greater in patients in whom a tissue biopsy has been obtained.

After bronchoscopy, patients may develop a transient low-grade fever. It occurs in about 5% of bronchoscopy patients, usually starting 6 to 8 hours after the procedure but lasting only 12 to 24 hours.[13] The exact cause of the fever is unknown but is not believed to be a sign of a new infection.

The longer the procedure goes on, the greater the risk of hypoxemia and hypercapnia. When these conditions occur, arrhythmias become more likely.[14] However, because the patient has received a large dose of lidocaine (Xylocaine), this will stabilize the myocardium and help prevent certain ventricular arrhythmias. Thus a considerable decay in oxygenation and ventilation may occur before arrhythmias are seen.

> **SIMPLY STATED**
> Flexible fiberoptic bronchoscopy is safe. Careful patient selection and attention to detail during and after the bronchoscopy make the risk/benefit ratio excellent for this procedure.

OUTPATIENT FLEXIBLE BRONCHOSCOPY

With the increasing demand for more cost-effective ways to render care, the outpatient clinic has been shown to be a safe and inexpensive site for routine flexible bronchoscopy.

The outpatient bronchoscopy room should be equipped with adequate suction capability, electrocardiograph, oxygen source, and a defibrillator with appropriate drugs, should cardiopulmonary resuscitation be needed. Specifically, Narcan and flumazenil (direct antagonists to opiates and midazolam, respectively) should be immediately available.

A complete history and physical examination are performed to assess the patient and the appropriateness of the bronchoscopy. Box 16-3 lists contraindications to performing the bronchoscopy in the outpatient setting.

> **SIMPLY STATED**
> There are specific contraindications to performing flexible bronchoscopy in the outpatient setting as opposed to the hospital. Because there is less support in an outpatient clinic if complications occur, these guidelines must be applied carefully to patient selection to ensure patient safety.

The Role of the Respiratory Therapist

Appropriate preparation of the patient for bronchoscopy is crucial to the success of the procedure. The preparation should start at home so that when the patient arrives at the outpatient

> **BOX 16-3 Contraindications for Outpatient Flexible Bronchoscopy**
>
> Recent myocardial infarction
> Lack of patient cooperation
> Unstable severe asthma
> Severe hypoxia
> Severe hypercapnia
> Bleeding disorders
> Potentially lethal cardiac arrhythmias
> Lung abscess
> Renal failure
> Immunosuppression
> Obstruction of the superior vena cava

facility, he/she has been fasting for 6 hours and is accompanied by a driver.

Before the procedure can be performed, an informed consent must be obtained from the patient (or closest relative if the patient is heavily sedated or comatose). The patient must understand the reason for the bronchoscopy (diagnostic or therapeutic) and other alternatives available to obtain similar results. The patient must understand the potential risks and complications of both the procedure and the anesthesia to be used. He/she must also be aware of what to expect after the procedure.

The patient is encouraged to ask questions about the bronchoscopy before signing the consent form. The bronchoscopist should already have explained the procedure in detail and should be available to answer any new questions. Risks and benefits are again discussed. Issues such as the patient's inability to speak during the procedure, supplemental oxygen, and "antigagging" medicines are covered. The concept of intravenous (IV) "conscious sedation" using Fentanyl and Versed is explained to the patient, and possible medication allergies are reviewed again. The effects and side effects of these two drugs must be explained. After all issues are covered to the patient's satisfaction, the consent is signed and witnessed.

The patient is then informed of the process necessary for adequate preparation. It is explained to the patient that, during the procedure, the RT will monitor and record the patient's vital signs, including blood pressure, heart rate, respiratory rate, temperature, and initial room air SpO_2. Cardiac status and pulse oximetry are monitored continuously while supplemental oxygenation via nasal cannula is supplied at a rate adequate to keep the patient in a safe range of oxygenation during all phases of the bronchoscopy.

> **SIMPLY STATED**
> Patient preparation should include answering all the patient's questions. The RT usually has this responsibility and must understand all aspects of the procedure.

The patient is now placed in a Fowler's position and given a medicated nebulizer treatment (unpressurized aerosol) containing 5 mL 4% topical Xylocaine over a 20-minute period. While the Xylocaine aerosol is being administered, an IV needle is inserted, usually in an antecubital vein, with a 23-gauge by ¾-inch butterfly or 24-gauge by ¾-inch angiocatheter. The IV line is connected to a heparin lock, then flushed with heparin and secured in place. This IV is the site for infusing the sedating drugs and is maintained for the duration of the procedure. A continuous saline infusion is not needed.

Upon completion of the medicated nebulizer treatment, the patient's most patent nostril is numbed with 3 mL 4% topical Xylocaine and 3 mL 2% viscous Xylocaine. The patient should be warned that this may be uncomfortable until the Xylocaine takes effect. Nasal oxygen is now supplied to the patient via nasal cannula.

The assistant now hooks up suction. Suction through the bronchoscope is critical to keep the airway clear of mucus and blood and to help keep the bronchoscope lens clear. The suction is connected to a sterile 80-mL specimen trap, which must be secured so it will not tip and thereby lose the washing from the patient's airway. Several of these traps are needed. Because the first one is usually contaminated with mouth flora, it is usually discarded, along with its contents. If heavy bleeding occurs during biopsy, the trap may become clogged with blood and thus inappropriate for cytologic analysis or cultures. It too is discarded.

The final stage of preparation is to administer IV Fentanyl and Versed to achieve conscious sedation. Administration of these medications can be repeated during the procedure if the patient has pain (Fentanyl or Demerol or Morphine) or is too restless (Versed). Total dosage of Versed should not exceed 10 mg. In certain patients, such as older adults and comatose patients, the dosage is greatly reduced or the drugs are eliminated completely. Often, the patient's recollection of the actual bronchoscopy is minimal when Versed is used. As soon as the patient relaxes and appears to be asleep, the bronchoscopy can begin.

Safety protocols require that the bronchoscopist and respiratory therapist wear a gown, mask, goggles, and gloves during the procedure.

The RT now assists the bronchoscopist directly. Several tasks must be done rapidly: handing the bronchoscopist more medication to instill in the airway, operating brushes and forceps, and processing the samples collected (Figure 16-7).

> **SIMPLY STATED**
> *Conscious sedation* is a term used to denote a state of anesthesia in which the patient is in a "twilight zone" for approximately 15 to 30 minutes. The medications used to achieve this state are given intravenously and can be reversed in seconds by specific antagonists, also given intravenously.

Samples are often obtained rapidly, so the RT must have an organized working surface with easily accessible supplies. Four medication cups should be available:

- One cup containing 3 mL 4% topical Xylocaine to be used if needed above the vocal cords
- One cup containing 6 mL 2% topical Xylocaine to be used if needed below the vocal cords
- One cup containing 15 mL 0.9% NaCl for irrigation (a larger container may be necessary if BAL is needed)
- One cup containing a 1:19 solution of epinephrine (1 mL 1:1000 epinephrine diluted with 19 mL 0.9% NaCl).

A labeled syringe is placed with each medication cup to match each medication. Two 5-mL syringes are placed next to the Xylocaine cups and two 10-mL syringes next to the NaCl and epinephrine cups.

It is important that when the syringes with Xylocaine are handed to the bronchoscopist during the procedure, they con-

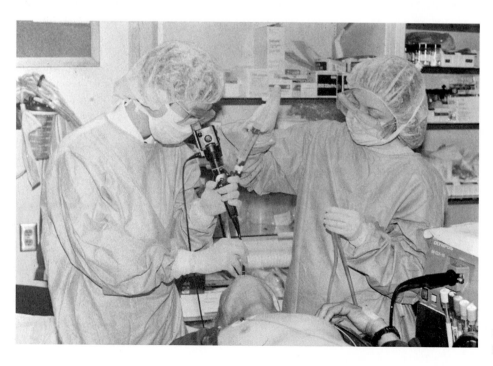

Figure 16-7 Typical outpatient setup for performing flexible bronchoscopy.

tain a known amount of Xylocaine, with plenty of air in the syringe barrel. This allows the bronchoscopist to push the Xylocaine all the way down the approximately 2 feet of the scope's channel. Because it is possible to administer an overdose of Xylocaine, having a small amount (1 mL) in each syringe helps limit the Xylocaine given. It is impossible to know how much Xylocaine the patient receives as a total dosage because the frequent suctioning during the procedure removes Xylocaine before it is absorbed. Nevertheless, it is important to keep the total dosage of Xylocaine below 300 mg. Seizures are the most common sign of acute Xylocaine overdose.

In addition to these cups, there should be four sets of frosted slides placed back to back and labeled legibly with the patient's name, history number, physician number (if applicable), and date. Two slide bottles with 90% alcohol and one biopsy specimen bottle containing 10% formalin should be available.

A 80-mL mucus specimen trap is placed in-line between the suction source and the bronchoscope. Standard biopsy forceps, a brush holder loaded with a disposable wire brush, and an aspiration needle accompanied by a 20-mL syringe filled with 5 mL 0.9% NaCl should be available, depending on the specimens the bronchoscopist needs to collect.

In order to obtain a lung brushing, the bronchoscopist gently brushes the abnormal-appearing area, then withdraws the brush from the scope. The therapist rubs the brush lightly on the frosted side of a slide, making a smear approximately the size of a dime. This slide is then placed in the slide bottle containing 90% alcohol. This procedure should take no longer than 10 seconds. Brushings rarely cause bleeding, so they are done before biopsy is performed with forceps or needle aspiration.

The bronchoscopist places lung biopsy tissues into a labeled specimen bottle filled with formalin. Usually four to six samples are obtained. It is often necessary for the assistant to tease the small piece of tissue out of the biopsy cusps with a needle. The assistant is often asked whether the specimen is lung tissue or useless blood clot or mucus. If bleeding occurs, the prepared epinephrine wash may be needed.

Obtaining a needle aspiration sample requires the bronchoscopist to place two or three drops of specimen on the frosted side of a slide. The therapist then places a second slide, frosted side down, on top of the original slide containing the specimen and slowly slides it across this slide. Both slides should be placed into a slide bottle containing 90% alcohol. This procedure is repeated with each new specimen collected.

BAL, if needed, is performed with repeated instillations of 10 to 20 mL 0.9% NaCl. The instillations are followed by suctioning into an 80-mL mucus specimen trap.

SIMPLY STATED
After patient safety, collection of samples and their careful management is the most important job of the assistant.

Upon completion of the bronchoscopy, the patient is monitored closely while recovering. Vital signs including blood pressure, heart rate, respiratory rate, and SpO_2 are recorded every 10 to 15 minutes. The physician must be notified of significant changes in any of these parameters. It is essential to recognize signs of increased discomfort, bleeding, or respiratory distress. The IV site should be examined periodically for signs of infiltration or blockage until its discontinuation.

Once the patient is alert and oriented, usually within an hour of procedure's completion, the patient is given a small sip of water to see whether his/her gag reflex and sensation in the throat have returned to normal. If these parameters are normal, the IV is removed and a final set of vital signs is obtained. The following criteria should be met before discharge:
- The patient is alert and oriented.
- Gag reflex is present.
- Sensation in the throat has returned to normal.
- Vital signs are stable.
- No bleeding is present.

Now is a good time for the bronchoscopist to explain the findings to the patient and to tell the patient that he/she may cough up small amounts of blood for up to 24 hours after the procedure. Larger amounts of blood, sudden shortness of breath, pain, or fever should prompt a call to the clinic. Arrangements are made for a return visit in 5 to 7 days to review the findings from the patient's specimens and to make recommendations.

The patient can then be disconnected from all monitors and assisted in dressing. A wheelchair should be available to transport the patient out to his/her attendant. It is imperative to remind the patient not to drive for several hours. The patient and attendant are reminded that if any unusual bleeding, shortness of breath, fever, or pain occurs, they are to call the clinic immediately.

All specimens must be handled appropriately for transport to the laboratory. Biopsies, brushings, needle aspirations, and lung washings should be labeled with the patient's name, history number, physician number, date, and site of origin. Necessary pathology or laboratory slips should also contain similar data, including what tests should be performed.

Finally, any additional charting should be completed, signed by the bronchoscopist, and filed in the patient's chart. The bronchoscopist must also make his/her own notes of the entire procedure, including indications, medications given, specimens collected, tests requested on the specimens, any intraoperative complications, and postoperative impression.

SIMPLY STATED
The 1-hour period after the bronchoscopy is completed is a busy time for the assistant. He/she is cleaning equipment, labeling samples, charting, and repeatedly assessing the patient's recovery from the procedure.

REVIEW QUESTIONS

1. What is the maximum depth that the standard adult bronchoscope can visualize in most patients?
   a. Third-level bronchi
   b. Fourth-level bronchi
   c. Fifth-level bronchi
   d. Sixth-level bronchi

2. What are double-shielded brushes used for during bronchoscopy?
   a. To clean the fiberoptics
   b. To obtain microbiologic samples
   c. To assist in cleaning the smaller airways of mucus plugs
   d. To assist in diagnosing malignancies

3. For what purpose are lasers used during bronchoscopy?
   a. To obliterate obstructing tumors
   b. To stop excessive bleeding
   c. To open mucus-plugged airways
   d. To improve visualization of smaller airways

4. What is the most common indication for the use of a bronchoscope?
   a. To retrieve inhaled foreign objects
   b. To obtain microbiologic samples
   c. To help diagnose abnormalities seen on chest x-ray
   d. To treat hemoptysis

5. For what condition is the rigid bronchoscope most likely to be used?
   a. Pneumonia
   b. Massive hemoptysis
   c. Tumors
   d. Interstitial lung disease

6. What complications associated with bronchoscopy are most common?
   a. Those associated with medications used in the procedure
   b. Pneumothorax
   c. Secondary infection
   d. Excessive bleeding

7. Why is the patient undergoing bronchoscopy who develops hypoxemia less likely to demonstrate arrhythmias?
   a. Use of sedative medications
   b. Use of Xylocaine before the procedure
   c. Lack of heart problems in most patients undergoing bronchoscopy
   d. Vagal stimulation from the scope

8. The respiratory therapist assisting the pulmonologist during a bronchoscopy should have medication cups of Xylocaine, normal saline, and _____ ready before beginning the procedure.

   a. Acetylcysteine (Mucomyst)
   b. Epinephrine
   c. Sterile water
   d. Versed

9. What is the most common sign of Xylocaine overdose during bronchoscopy?
   a. Tachycardia
   b. Bradycardia
   c. Seizures
   d. Apnea

10. Which of the following criteria is least important before discharge of the patient after bronchoscopy?
    a. Gag reflex present
    b. Stable vital signs
    c. No bleeding present
    d. Ability to swallow without pain

REFERENCES

1. Pulmonary Special Center of Research Grant No. HL-15063-02 from the National Heart and Lung Institute: Maximal extent of visualization of bronchial tree by flexible fiberoptic bronchoscopy, *Am Rev Respir Dis* 110:88, 1974.
2. Tanaka M and others: Assessment of an ultrathin bronchoscope that allows cytodiagnosis of small airways, *Chest* 106(5):1443, 1994.
3. Shure D, Astarita RW: Bronchoscopic carcinoma presenting as an endobronchial mass, *Chest* 83(6):865, 1983.
4. Shure D, Fedullio PF: Transbronchial needle aspiration in the diagnosis of submucosal and peribronchial bronchogenic carcinoma, *Chest* 88(1):49, 1985.
5. American Thoracic Society, Medical Section of the American Lung Association: Guidelines for fiberoptic bronchoscopy in adults, *Am Rev Respir Dis* 136(4):1066, 1987.
6. Cortese DA, McDougall JC: Biopsy and brushing of peripheral lung cancer with fluoroscopic guidance, *Chest* 75(2):141, 1979.
7. Weaver LJG, Soliday N, Cugell DW: Selection of patients with hemoptysis for fiberoptic bronchoscopy, *Chest* 76(1):7, 1979.
8. Jain P, Saundr S, Meli Y: Role of flexible fiberoptic bronchoscopy in immunocompromised patients with lung infiltrates, *Chest* 125:712-722, 2004.
9. Pisani RJ, Wright AJ: Clinical utility of BAL in immunocompromised hosts (review), *Mayo Clin Proc* 67(3):221, 1992.
10. Meduri GU and others: Management of bacterial pneumonia in ventilated patients: protected bronchial lavage as a diagnostic tool, *Chest* 101(2):500, 1992.
11. Depaso WJ, Winterbauer RH: Interstitial lung disease (review), *Dis Mon* 37(2):61, 1991.

12. Studdy PR and others: Bronchoalveolar lavage in the diagnosis of diffuse pulmonary shadowing, *Br J Dis Chest* 78(1):46, 1984.
13. Um SW and others: Prospective analysis of clinical characteristics and risk factors of post bronchoscopy fever, *Chest* 125:945, 2004.
14. Katz AS, Michelson EL, Stawicki J: Cardiac arrhythmias: frequency during fiberoptic bronchoscopy and correlation with hypoxemia, *Arch Intern Med* 141:603, 1984.

BIBLIOGRAPHY

Poe RH, Israel RH: Flexible fiberoptic bronchoscopy in 1998, *Respir Care* 43:811, 1998.
Stradling P: *Diagnostic bronchoscopy: a teaching manual,* ed 6, Edinburgh, 1991, Churchill Livingstone.

C H A P T E R

17

James A. Peters
Cheryl D. Thomas-Peters

Nutritional Assessment of Patients with Respiratory Disease

LEARNING OBJECTIVES

Upon completion of this chapter, the reader should be able to accomplish the following:

1. Recognize how nutrition and respiration are interrelated.
2. Recognize the functional importance of oxygen in nutrition.
3. Identify the nutritional significance of measuring oxygen uptake.
4. Identify the value of determining the basal metabolic rate and basal energy expenditure.
5. Recognize how starvation affects the following:
   a. Body weight
   b. Muscle mass (diaphragm and other respiratory musculature)
   c. Forced vital capacity, forced expiratory volume in 1 second, and diffusing capacity of the lung for carbon dioxide
   d. Surfactant production
6. Recognize how some respiratory treatment modalities may inhibit the nutritional status of patients.
7. Identify the by-products of anaerobic (without oxygen) metabolism.
8. Identify oxygen's importance in terms of adenosine triphosphate production.
9. Recognize how fat, carbohydrate, and protein metabolism affect the respiratory quotient.
10. Recognize the daily nutritional requirements for carbohydrate, protein, and fat.
11. Identify the protein requirements for normal and severely catabolic patients.
12. Recognize the significance of measuring nitrogen balance.
13. Recognize the problems associated with a low-protein diet.
14. Recognize the advantages and disadvantages of a high-carbohydrate diet in regard to the pulmonary system.
15. Identify the importance of vitamins and minerals in respiratory function.
16. Recognize the methods available for meeting nutritional requirements and their advantages and disadvantages.
17. Recognize the methods for assessing nutritional status.
18. Identify the role of the respiratory therapist in nutritional assessment in relation to inspection, auscultation, and laboratory findings.

CHAPTER OUTLINE

Interdependence of Respiration and Nutrition
   Nutritional Depletion and Respiration
   Therapeutic Interactions of Respiration and Nutrition
Respiratory System and Nutritional Needs
   Neurologic Component
   Respiratory Muscle Component
   Cardiovascular Component
   Gas Exchange Component (Lungs)
Metabolism
Nutritional Requirements
   Carbohydrate
   Protein
   Fat
   Vitamins, Minerals, Phytochemicals, and Other Nutrients
   Fluids and Electrolytes
Methods of Meeting Nutritional Requirements
Nutritional Assessment
   Data Gathering and Interpretation
   Role of Respiratory Therapists in Nutritional Assessment

KEY TERMS

adenosine triphosphate (ATP)
anabolism
anemia
basal energy expenditure (BEE)
body mass index (BMI)
basal metabolic rate (BMR)
cachectic
catabolism
creatine phosphate
creatinine
creatinine-height index (CHI)

direct calorimetry
gluconeogenesis
glycolysis
ideal body weight
indirect calorimetry
kilocalories (kcal)
lactic acid
metabolic cart
metabolism
nitric oxide (NO)
nitrogen balance
oncotic pressure
oxygen uptake
parenteral

protein energy
   malnutrition
respiratory quotient (RQ)
resting energy expenditure
   (REE)

serum albumin
serum transferrin
skinfold measurement
total parenteral nutrition
   (TPN)

CHAPTER OVERVIEW

The nutritional needs of patients with lung disease have emerged as a major factor influencing acute and long-term outcomes. The energy to breathe and allow the body to function, as well as to provide for purposeful body movements, comes from food. The quantity and quality of the food affect the efficiency of the metabolic process and influence the amount of oxygen needed and the amount of carbon dioxide exhaled. The nutrients in food can enhance or harm the immune function of the lung and thereby affect the patient's susceptibility to infection and ability to deal with environmental stress. The ability to assess and understand the role of nutrition in respiratory medicine is important for today's respiratory therapist (RT).

INTERDEPENDENCE OF RESPIRATION AND NUTRITION

Respiration and nutrition are interdependent (Figure 17-1). Air and food share common pathways during ingestion and then separate only briefly during "digestion," with air going to the lungs and food to the stomach. Oxygen and nutrients soon blend together in the blood and are distributed to the tissues of the body. The use of food for energy at the cellular level requires oxygen to support a controlled combustion process that produces energy molecules of adenosine triphosphate (ATP), which are used in all of the body processes (Figure 17-2).

Body heat is a result of a combustion process called metabolism. This metabolic fire requires fuel, and the fuel is food. For combustion to occur, oxygen must be present, and this is why we breathe. Unless oxygen is delivered to the cells, the food eaten cannot be used. Nutrition and respiration are truly interdependent. Clearly, breathing and oxygen can be considered part of nutrition.

Titrating the proper amount of oxygen and eliminating carbon dioxide (the metabolic "smoke" of the combustion process) is the job of the respiratory system, coupled closely with the cardiovascular system. The respiratory system must be sensitive to the metabolic needs of the whole body. This process requires an integration of several organ systems. The respiratory system consists of neurologic components, cardiovascular components, respiratory muscles, and lungs (Figure 17-3).

The metabolic rates of the tissues dictate the amount of oxygen needing to be picked up in the lungs. Oxygen uptake ($\dot{V}_{O_2}$) is a respiratory factor that can be measured in the laboratory or at the bedside. Nutritionally speaking, it is this measure

that indicates the patient's energy requirement. If $\dot{V}_{O_2}$ is measured while a person is in a resting, nonstressed state, the basal metabolic rate (BMR) or basal energy expenditure (BEE) can be calculated. The BEE is the measure obtained when a person is at absolute rest with no physical movement. The term resting energy expenditure (REE) is used when a person is simply resting. REE is most commonly reported and is often equal to BEE, but is often a little higher than BEE. The Harris-Benedict equation is commonly used for estimating BEE.[1] This regression equation was derived from normal subjects and therefore may not always apply to acutely ill and stressed patients in a critical care setting. To account for energy expenditures of daily living, this equation is adjusted upward by 15% to 20%. Other correction factors are applied for various metabolic conditions.

1. Basal energy expenditure (BEE) equation

$$\text{Men: BEE} = 66 + (13.7 \times W) + (5 \times H) - (6.8 \times A)$$
$$\text{Women: BEE} = 655 + (9.6 \times W) + (1.7 \times H) - (4.7 \times A)$$

where

   W = Weight in kilograms
   H = Height in centimeters
   A = Age in years

2. Percent energy multipliers of BEE for specific therapeutic goals

Type of Therapy	Kilocalories Required (per 24 hr)
Parenteral anabolic*	1.75 × BEE
Oral anabolic	1.50 × BEE
Oral maintenance	1.20 × BEE

Anabolic means to "build up"

Because calculating the BEE is only an estimate, it is preferable to measure the actual metabolic rate in order to know the patient's true energy needs. This eliminates some of the guesswork, especially for treating critically ill or metabolically challenged patients.

There are two ways to determine one's energy use: direct and indirect calorimetry. Energy production generates heat and heat is measured in calories. Direct calorimetry directly measures the heat given off by the body in a carefully designed room. This is not practical in clinical settings. Indirect calorimetry is the method of choice used clinically. Indirect calorimetry measures respiratory parameters ($\dot{V}_{O_2}$ and $\dot{V}_{CO_2}$) to determine the energy consumed by the body. Since oxygen is not stored in the body, measuring oxygen uptake ($\dot{V}_{O_2}$) correlates directly with energy (ATP) creation and use. Metabolism (REE) then can be measured by oxygen consumption and is directly related to the energy (calories) used. Since energy measurements by indirect calorimetry are respiratory measurements, RTs are best qualified to perform these measures in clinical settings. There is a place on the nutritional support team for RTs who are trained in indirect calorimetry measurements.

Indirect calorimetry measurements are now performed using a metabolic cart. A metabolic cart is a computer-controlled unit composed of oxygen and carbon dioxide gas analyzers and flow transducers. The cart automatically measures patients' air

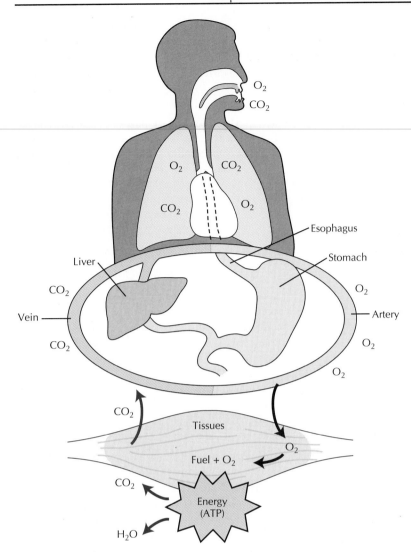

Figure 17-1 Nutrition and breathing are interrelated. Food and air share common ports of entry into the body, separate briefly before entering the lungs or stomach, and then travel together in the circulation. At the tissue level, food energy is released in the presence of oxygen. Final nutrient-air interaction results in production of adenosine triphosphate *(ATP)*, carbon dioxide, and water.

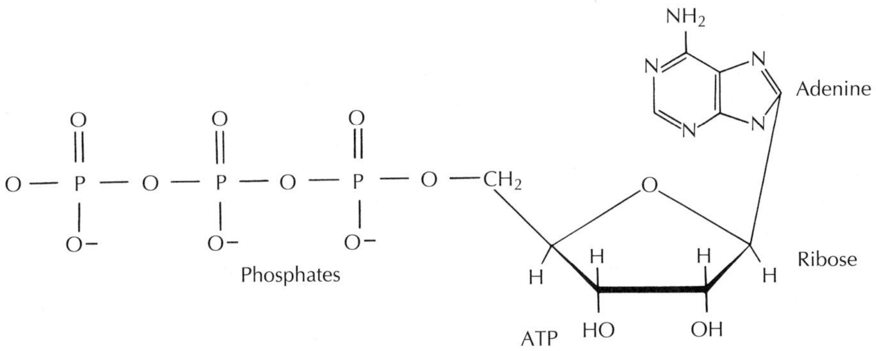

Figure 17-2 Functions of adenosine triphosphate *(ATP)* are as follows: muscle contraction and relaxation, active transport of substances across membranes, substrate for cyclic adenosine monophosphate, energy for synthesis of various chemical compounds, and energy storage.

flow and expiratory volumes, applies correction factors, and prints out and graphs the results. Having an understanding of this procedure will help the RT better understand what is automatically done by a metabolic cart. Following is a summary of the traditional energy measurement procedure.

1. Collect expired gas in a bag or Tissot spirometer for several minutes.
2. Analyze for carbon dioxide and oxygen (or oxygen and nitrogen).
3. Measure the volume of the gas collected in the bag.

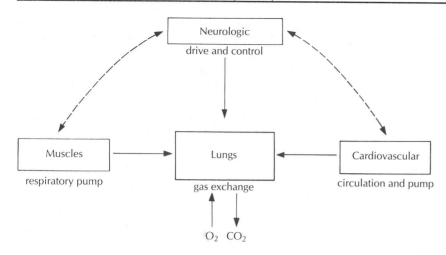

Figure 17-3 Block diagram illustrating components of the respiratory system. The neurologic component drives and controls respiration at the lungs via the respiratory muscles. It also affects the cardiovascular system by altering heart function and circulatory resistance. All components are necessary to achieve respiration. Nutritional quality and quantity directly affect the functioning of each system.

4. Calculate:
   a. If oxygen and carbon dioxide are measured:

$$\dot{V}_{O_2STPD} = \left[\frac{\dot{V}_{E\,ATPS} \times \left(P_B - H_2O\right) \times 21.55}{\text{collection time} \times (273 + temp°C)} \right]$$

$$\times \frac{1 - F_{EO_2} - F_{ECO_2} - \left(\dfrac{P_{H_2O}}{P_B}\right)}{\dfrac{1 - F_{IO_2}}{F_{IO_2}}} - F_{EO_2}$$

$$\text{Note:} \left(\frac{273°K \times 60\ sec}{760\ mm\ Hg} \right) = 21.55$$

If gas is analyzed with desiccant in line, then

$$\frac{P_{H_2O}}{P_B} = 0$$

where

$\dot{V}_{O_2STPD}$ = Oxygen uptake, standard conditions
$\dot{V}_{E\,ATPS}$ = Minute volume; ambient temperature and pressure, saturated
P_B = Barometric pressure
F_{EO_2} = Fraction of expired oxygen
F_{ECO_2} = Fraction of expired carbon dioxide
P_{H_2O} = Water vapor pressure
F_{IO_2} = Fraction of inspired oxygen

   b. $\dot{V}_{CO_2} = \dot{V}_{E\,STPD} \times \left(F_{ECO_2} - 0.0003\right)$

where $\dot{V}_{CO_2}$ = Carbon dioxide production

   c. $RQ = \left(\dfrac{\dot{V}_{CO_2}}{\dot{V}_{O_2}} \right)$

where RQ = Respiratory quotient

   d. If only oxygen and nitrogen are measured,

$$\dot{V}_{O_2} = \dot{V}_E \times \left(\frac{F_{EN_2}}{F_{IN_2}} \right) \times F_{IO_2} - \left(\dot{V}_E \times F_{EO_2} \right)$$

where

F_{EN_2} = Fraction of expired nitrogen
F_{IN_2} = Fraction of inspired nitrogen

For patients confined to a hospital bed, portable equipment is used. For patients who are not intubated and whose condition does not allow them to cooperate with the procedure using a nose clip and mouthpiece, a special hood or tent apparatus becomes necessary. The RT's interactions with the nutritional support team for metabolic measurements are most helpful because respiratory therapy departments are usually equipped and therapists are trained for such measurements.

In nutrition, energy is quantified in terms of kilocalories (kcal); 1 kcal is the amount of energy it takes to raise the temperature of 1 kg of water 1° C. (Although kilocalories have been used most frequently in clinical nutrition, the kilojoule [kJ] is often used in research, since kJ is the international unit for energy. To convert kilocalories to kilojoules, multiply kcal × 4.184. For approximately every 5 kcal burned, 1 L of oxygen is used by the tissues. Therefore if a patient's $\dot{V}_{O_2}$ is measured as 300 mL oxygen/min, then 300 mL oxygen × 60 minutes × 24 hours equals 432 L of oxygen required per day. And 5 kcal × 432 L oxygen/day equals 2160 kcal/day that should be given to the patient. If less than this amount of energy is given, the patient must use body energy stores, which are often depleted in chronically ill patients. The Weir or Lusk equation is used for more precise conversion of $\dot{V}_{O_2}$ to kilocalories.[2,3]

The Weir equation is as follows:

$$\text{kcal/min} = 3.94 \times \dot{V}_{O_2} + 1.11 \times \dot{V}_{CO_2}$$
$$BEE = \text{kcal/min} \times 1440\ \text{min (per day)}$$

Nutritional Depletion and Respiration

A patient who is not ingesting food enterally (through the gastrointestinal tract) probably will be placed on intravenous (IV) therapy. An IV solution of 5% dextrose running at 3 L/day will provide the patient with only 600 kcal/day (0.05 × 3000 mL × 3.41 kcal/g glucose). (Note: Glucose, when given in hydrated form [IV D5/W, etc.], yields 3.41 kcal/g; otherwise the yield is about 4 kcal/g of carbohydrate.) This is far from sufficient to meet a person's energy needs, much less protein, vitamin, and mineral needs.

Blood sugar levels are maintained from liver glycogen (carbohydrate) stores between meals and during fasting. The liver's glycogen stores come from the carbohydrates (starches and sugars) that are eaten in the diet. However, liver glycogen will be depleted within 12 to 16 hours unless sufficient carbohydrate is ingested again. When the liver glycogen is depleted, the body obtains sugar by converting protein (amino acids) to sugar. This process is called gluconeogenesis (*gluco* meaning "glucose sugar"; *neo* meaning "new"; and *genesis* meaning "to create"). The protein used for gluconeogenesis is obtained from functional proteins (muscles and enzyme systems) because protein is never stored like fat in the body. Protein in the body is always a part of structural or functional tissue, organ, enzyme, or other biochemical action molecules, or is in an "amino acid pool" in circulation while waiting to be incorporated into body systems. Therefore in patients who have a consistently poor nutritional intake, protein must be used for more and more of the body's energy needs. This leads to a loss of functional tissue. Skeletal muscle tissue, including the diaphragm and other respiratory muscles, lose muscle mass, with a resultant decrease in endurance and strength. The depletion of protein from the body is reflected in lowered blood albumin levels. In starvation or semistarvation states, respiratory muscle strength can diminish, producing a decrease in forced vital capacity (FVC) and forced expiratory volume in 1 second (FEV_1). Also occurring in starvation is a decrease in carbon monoxide diffusing capacity (DL_{CO}). The decline in FEV_1 also correlates with a decreased creatinine-height index, indicative of loss of muscle mass. Because our immune antibodies are composed of proteins, persistent low calorie and protein intake will also compromise the immune system, thereby limiting the body's ability to fight pneumonia or other infections.

If the calorie intake is less than needed, there will be a decrease in weight, as is commonly seen in patients with chronic obstructive pulmonary disease (COPD). Patients with emphysema are more commonly underweight than those with chronic bronchitis. Emphysema produces a catabolic state that usually results in weight loss, even when a normal quantity of food is consumed.

Measures of REE are consistently higher in malnourished emphysemic patients.[4] This increased REE leads to nutritional depletion and eventually malnutrition. Malnutrition can exacerbate symptoms of COPD by decreasing respiratory muscle strength and exercise tolerance, and can compromise immune function leading to increased respiratory infections.[5] Respiratory muscles develop into a hypermetabolic state, and this is a contributing factor in the elevated REE.[6] In addition, insufficient absorption of some nutrients may lead to muscle wasting and malnutrition. Short-term supplementation of the usual diet with additional protein (branched-chain amino-acid–enriched enteral formula) has resulted in improved body weight and respiratory muscle strength in patients with COPD.[7]

If an increased amount of food is consumed, weight can begin to normalize, but emphysematous patients are not comfortable eating larger quantities of foods. In one study it was necessary to increase intake above 140% of the BMR before they could improve the nutritional status of COPD patients.[8] If not continuously encouraged to do so, patients typically return to eating their normal amount, which is insufficient to maintain a normal weight.[9] Patients with chronic protein energy malnutrition (PEM; also known as protein-calorie malnutrition [PCM]) also experience higher morbidity and mortality. With loss of body protein, there is a subsequent loss not only of muscle and various enzyme systems, but also of immunoglobulins (IgA, IgG, and IgM). Thus susceptibility to respiratory infections is increased because of decreased immunocompetence.

Therapeutic Interactions of Respiration and Nutrition

Nutritional repletion in respiratory patients is often hindered by some of the necessary therapeutic actions. Bronchodilators may produce nausea; oxygen by nasal cannula disturbs the sense of smell and therefore taste, since 70% of the taste of food is contributed from the sense of smell. Medications the patients are taking may also interact with nutrients and render them less available for absorption or even inhibit specific metabolic enzymes. An intubated patient really complicates the process of eating. Furthermore, because large meals may hamper function in an already less-functional diaphragm, frequent small meals may be necessary, requiring greater effort in food preparation. Eating more frequently is also shown to burn more calories than fewer, larger meals eaten each day. These factors, along with shortness of breath, increased work of breathing, and a greater prevalence of peptic ulcers, increase the risk of malnutrition. Being knowledgeable about these facts can help the patient to improve both nutritional status and respiratory function.

The respiratory response to the body's need for oxygen and carbon dioxide elimination is usually regulated by the carbon dioxide produced ($\dot{V}CO_2$). At the oxygen sensor level, increased hydrogen ion (H^+) concentration in addition to carbon dioxide drives ventilation; this occurs when the amount of oxygen present is insufficient with respect to metabolic need, resulting in lactic acidosis. Oxygen levels, when low enough, become an important stimulus for breathing. In addition, a semistarved state can decrease hypoxic drive, rendering a patient less sensitive to the need for more oxygen.[10,11] This compromises a patient even further.

Oxygen uptake and carbon dioxide excretion are as much a part of nutrition as are eating and the elimination of food byproducts via the gastrointestinal tract and kidneys. Usually respiration is not thought of in this way because of the abundance of air and the minimal effort involved in its continuous "ingestion" (breathing). However, patients with respiratory disease often find themselves needing higher levels of the "nutrient" oxygen or assistance in getting rid of the metabolic waste, carbon dioxide. Under these conditions, breathing becomes a more conscious and deliberate effort. In critical care patients, both feeding and breathing often require continuous assistance. Just

---

SIMPLY STATED

Chronic nutritional depletion eventually weakens the muscles of breathing and can contribute to the onset of respiratory failure, especially in patients with chronic lung disease.

as patients require intubation when the ventilatory status is compromised sufficiently, they may require nasogastric (NG) or enteral tubes or parenteral (outside of the gastrointestinal tract) intravenous (IV) feeding. Matching a patient's energy and nutritional needs with ventilatory needs can become a challenge. Meeting this challenge translates into better survival for the patient.

RESPIRATORY SYSTEM AND NUTRITIONAL NEEDS

For optimal ventilatory function, proper nutrition is needed for all components of the respiratory system (see Figure 17-3).

Neurologic Component

The neurologic component drives and controls ventilation. The higher the $\dot{V}CO_2$ level, the greater the blood carbon dioxide concentration and therefore the greater the stimulus to the chemoreceptors. $\dot{V}CO_2$ is increased in the body by metabolism, buffering of fixed acids, or both. This in turn increases the electrical activity in the respiratory centers of the central nervous system (CNS), resulting in increased minute ventilation. The nervous system's fundamental requirement is for glucose. The energy derived from glucose is used to maintain an electrical charge across the nerve cell membrane, allowing for depolarization (action potential) and subsequent repolarization. The neurotransmitters at the synaptic ends are amino acids themselves or derivatives of them, and their presence is necessary for the relay of information from one neuron to another and from nerve to muscle. Apparently the sensitivity of the respiratory centers (either peripheral or central chemoreceptors) is affected by the amount and quality of protein ingested. The respiratory response to carbon dioxide or low levels of oxygen is increased with high protein intake.[12] However, too much protein may make some patients too sensitive to gas partial pressure changes, thus increasing the work of breathing. Giving the optimal amount of protein is the task of the nutritional support team.

Respiratory Muscle Component

The respiratory muscles make up the pump that drives the lungs. They receive the final stimulus from the CNS and produce the appropriate breathing rate and tidal volume as dictated by the CNS and local feedback pathways. The muscles require energy for contraction and relaxation. This energy is derived from blood glucose, free fatty acids from fat stores, and muscle glycogen. The muscle glycogen stores are the most readily available source of energy for the muscles; however, the amount of glycogen stored depends on the level of carbohydrate in the diet as well as the exercise history of the muscle. A muscle that has been exercised has a greater ability to store glycogen (muscle carbohydrate) after a meal than eating without having exercised first. In any case, for the body to store muscle glycogen, there must be an adequate amount of carbohydrate in the diet. The diaphragm, being the main muscle of respiration, needs adequate glycogen stores to be able to meet the metabolic demand of breathing.

Cardiovascular Component

The heart and the circulatory system are vital for pumping the blood through the lungs and throughout the body carrying both nutrients and oxygen to all the tissues. The requirements of the cardiovascular system for food energy for the heart muscle are similar to those of the respiratory muscles.

Protein is needed for maintaining and building up the heart muscle and other structural components of tissue. Protein is also a part of buffering actions, clotting factors in the blood, and transport of lipids and iron. Oncotic pressure in the blood is maintained primarily via albumin, the major blood protein produced by the liver. *Arginine,* one of the amino acids that make up proteins in the body, is the main contributor of nitrogen for the crucial vasodilating molecule nitric oxide (NO). NO plays the key role in relaxing the smooth muscles around the artery walls, resulting in vasodilation and thereby regulating blood flow throughout the body. NO is also involved in some end processes of the immune system. Arginine is found in highest concentrations in plant-based proteins.

Carbohydrate is the major fuel for heart muscle. Carbohydrate metabolism is also the source of *2,3-diphosphoglycerate (2,3-DPG)* that facilitates oxygen release in the tissue. Blood sugar levels come primarily from dietary carbohydrate and release of stored liver glycogen between meals. Regulation of blood sugar (glucose) is key to normal metabolic function.

Fat is an important component of all cell membranes and is a part of packaging of molecules that are produced by cells. Fat is also a source of fuel for heart muscle, especially when blood glucose levels or muscle glycogen runs low. *Essential fatty acids* are the backbone of prostaglandins and help regulate blood lipid levels, blood glucose levels, and blood pressure. The fat in nuts also appears to have anti-arrhythmic properties.

Vitamins and minerals are needed for maintenance of the metabolic pathways and integrity of cell membranes and antioxidant activity of cells. They are major players of all body enzyme and metabolic systems. Iron is a major mineral that is a structural part of the heme of the hemoglobin and is where oxygen attaches and is carried by the blood.

Water is the major constituent of the blood and body cells. Sufficient water intake is necessary for proper circulation, clearing of waste from the body, and maintenance blood pressure. What is eaten or drunk has a vital effect on the cardiovascular system.

Gas Exchange Component (Lungs)

The lungs, which introduce air from the atmosphere into the circulatory system, require a delicate balance of various systems to achieve efficient gas exchange. Alveolar ventilation must be matched with alveolar circulation to allow the efficient transfer of gases between blood and air. To prevent alveolar collapse, surfactant is needed to lessen the surface-active forces that promote collapse of the lung. Starvation leads to decreased surfactant synthesis as well as emphysematous changes in the lung.[13,14] Humidity and mucociliary performance in the lung require adequate hydration. Smooth muscle function, macrophage activity, and secretion of immunoglobulins (e.g., IgA) into mucus all depend on good nutrition.

METABOLISM

Because basic requirements for both oxygen and nutrients are determined by the cellular metabolic rate, an understanding of metabolism is essential for both respiratory and nutritional assessment.

Metabolism is the body's way of transferring energy from food to the body's energy currency molecules: adenosine triphosphate (ATP). The metabolic process can be divided into two pathways: those that break molecules down as energy is released (catabolism) and those that build up new molecules (anabolism) to be used in a structural or a functional role. The catabolic pathways produce ATP, which is used in the anabolic pathways for growth and maintenance of the organism or simply for the organism's movement in the environment. Therefore energy is the fundamental need of the body. If sufficient food is eaten, the body can maintain its equilibrium and satisfy the demands placed on it by changes in the environment. However, if too little food is ingested, the body must rely on energy previously stored. If the stored energy—fat and carbohydrate (glycogen)—is not sufficient, the body will break down protein to produce ATP. As mentioned previously, this condition is undesirable because the protein comes from functioning tissue and therefore lessens the functional capability of the organism.

If too much food energy is taken in, the body must use some of its energy to convert the excess carbohydrate or protein so it can store the excess in the form of fat. As the level of body fat increases, the metabolic cost of moving and breathing increases along with the risk of various diseases. Again the functional capability of the organism is decreased.

A basic understanding of the metabolic pathways is essential when planning nutritional and ventilatory support. Figure 17-4 illustrates schematically the major energy-producing pathways used by almost every cell of the body. The reader is encouraged to refer to biochemistry or physiology texts for a more complete discussion of metabolism.

The metabolic process can be viewed as having four major phases (see Figure 17-4). The first is the digestive phase, in which the food materials are broken down to the basic components: fat (fatty acids), carbohydrates (sugars), and protein (amino acids). The food components are then absorbed from the gastrointestinal tract into the blood, where they eventually travel to every cell in the body.

The second phase involves the catabolism of the food components within the cell down to a common molecule, acetylcoenzyme A (acetyl CoA). A small amount of the food energy is used directly to produce a few ATP molecules or transferred to molecular energy shuttles (energy intermediates) in this phase,

but acetyl CoA still contains the bulk of the food energy. It is also possible for the metabolic pathways in this phase to go in the opposite direction, from acetyl CoA to form the basic food components again. However, molecules move in this anabolic direction only when the cell has plenty of energy currency (ATP) available. Also note that anaerobic metabolism (energy—ATP—being formed without the presence of oxygen) can occur only in this second phase of metabolism, in the pathway labeled glycolysis. In anaerobic metabolism, pyruvate produces lactate (lactic acid) rather than acetyl CoA. The greater the energy production without sufficient oxygen, the more lactic acid produced. This can result in *lactic acidosis*. If this occurs, the acid must be buffered with bicarbonate (HCO_3), and carbon dioxide is produced in the process. This requires increased minute ventilation to eliminate the carbon dioxide generated.

Whereas the phases just described have different pathways for each of the food components, the third phase uses the same *tricarboxylic acid (TCA)* pathway (also called the Krebs or citric acid cycle), regardless of the origin of the acetyl CoA. The rest of the food energy is removed in the TCA phase, again transferring the energy to molecular energy shuttles. It is here that most of the energy-depleted carbon "skeletons" are discarded as carbon dioxide. For the TCA cycle to be active, the energy shuttles *nicotinamide adenine dinucleotide (NAD)* and *flavoprotein adenine dinucleotide (FAD)* must be able to unload their energy-rich hydrogen and electrons into the respiratory transport chain (oxidative phosphorylation). This requires the presence of oxygen. Without it, the TCA cycle grinds to a halt.

The fourth phase is the final destination of the molecular energy shuttles, where they "dump" their energy-rich loads of hydrogen and electrons into the oxidative phosphorylation system, where ATP molecules are mass produced. This is also the final destination of the oxygen that was inhaled. Here the energy is extracted from the hydrogen and electrons; in the energy-depleted form, the hydrogen and electrons combine with oxygen to form water.

It is in the metabolic pathways just outlined where the body's oxygen is used and carbon dioxide is produced. The oxygen used can be measured and is expressed as the oxygen uptake per minute ($\dot{V}O_2$). The measured carbon dioxide produced per minute is expressed as the $\dot{V}CO_2$. The ratio of $\dot{V}CO_2$ to $\dot{V}O_2$ is the respiratory quotient (RQ). The RQ is determined simply by the amount of fat, carbohydrate, or protein one has eaten or is metabolizing. Pure fat metabolism has an RQ of 0.7, protein has a value of 0.85, and carbohydrate has a value of 1.0. A mixture of the three different types of foods used for energy at the same time results in an RQ of around 0.8. (This is the R value used most often in the alveolar air equation.)

NUTRITIONAL REQUIREMENTS

The basic nutritional requirements include carbohydrate, protein, fat, vitamins, minerals, and water. In light of the present

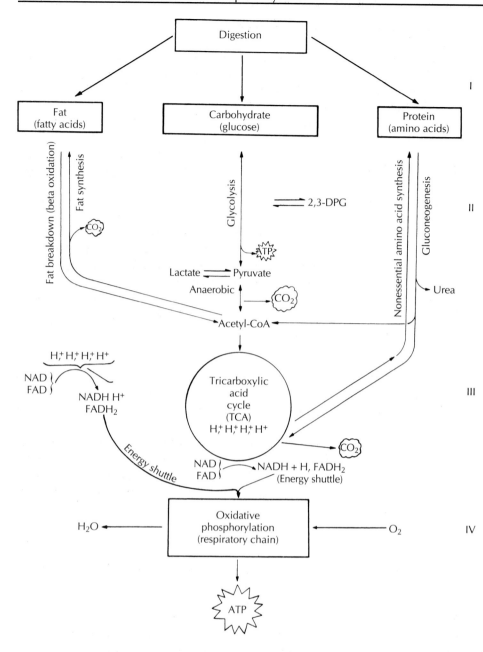

Figure 17-4 Four major phases of metabolism are schematically illustrated. **Phase I,** Digestion and nutrient absorption of fat, carbohydrate, and protein. **Phase II,** Breakdown of fatty acids, glucose, and amino acids to acetyl-CoA, which either can go on to synthesize (directly or indirectly) fat, carbohydrate, or amino acids, as need be, or can have more energy extracted from it in phases III and IV. **Phase III,** Tricarboxylic acid cycle, where most of the body's CO2 is produced and where most of the molecular energy shuttles (nicotinamide adenine dinucleotide [NAD], flavoprotein adenosine dinucleotide [FAD]) receive their energy supply in the form of hydrogen atoms. Shuttles transport energy to the respiratory chain. **Phase IV,** Inner mitochondrial membrane where oxidative phosphorylation (production of adenosine triphosphate [ATP] in the presence of oxygen) occurs. Oxygen is the final acceptor of the now energy-depleted electrons and hydrogen ions. *2,3-DPG,* 2,3-Diphosphoglycerate; *FADH,* flavoprotein adenine dinucleotide dehydrogenase; *NADH,* nicotine adenine dinucleotide dehydrogenase.

discussion, it would not be wrong to include oxygen as a nutrient because food is of no value unless oxygen is present, although traditionally it is not included in discussions of nutritional requirements. Carbohydrate, protein, and fat provide the energy the body needs as well as the basic chemical skeletons on which structural and functional body systems are built. Vitamins, being part of coenzymes, work along with enzymes in various metabolic pathways and allow specific reactions to occur. Minerals often are elements of specific molecules, such as hemoglobin, cytochromes, and thyroxin. Water is the medium in which the various chemical reactions take place within cells. It is also responsible for the fluidity of the blood, which allows blood to circulate.

The optimal amount of each of the nutritional elements has not been determined precisely, especially for those required in trace amounts. There is agreement that a minimum nutrient level should be high enough so that deficiency symptoms can-

not be detected and low enough to prevent toxicity. Within this range there is much discussion as to what is the right amount because nutritional requirements can vary from person to person. Greater or lesser amounts of specific nutrients may be needed because of genetically induced enzyme defects, various disease states, varying amounts of energy expenditure, and various drug-nutrient interactions. Because of the complexity of nurturing the body, a careful nutritional assessment by a nutritional support team, composed of at least a physician and dietitian, is essential. A clinical pharmacologist, for diets that are given parenterally, and an RT, for assessing $\dot{V}o_2$ and $\dot{V}co_2$, are important additions to the team.

Carbohydrate

The food component that should compose the largest amount of the dietary intake is carbohydrate. Carbohydrate can be broadly classified as complex or simple. The complex carbohydrates are starches (sugar molecules linked together in long branching chains) and are readily found in a variety of foods, the best sources being grains, vegetables, and fruits. Foods high in complex carbohydrates usually contain the vitamins required in the metabolic pathways for catabolism. In addition, these foods provide water, fiber, protein, and chemical components that inhibit disease processes. Simple carbohydrates are free sugars and, of the natural foods, are found in the largest amounts in fruits. However, the majority of sugar consumed comes from processed, refined foods. Ingestion of simple carbohydrates should be held to a minimum because their nutritional value is quite low but their metabolic demand is quite high (i.e., they travel down the glucose metabolic pathway or go to fat synthesis, but do not "pay any taxes" in the form of vitamins or minerals for the maintenance of the metabolic machinery). They can provide a quick form of energy, but when ingested alone they can stimulate an exaggerated insulin response because of their rapid absorption from the intestinal tract. Complex carbohydrates tend not to trigger this response because they have to be broken down to free sugars—which takes time—before they are absorbed. Various complex carbohydrate foods differ from one another in their effects on blood sugar levels.

Carbohydrate has often been contrasted with fat. Because the $\dot{V}CO_2$ with fat metabolism is lower than that with carbohydrate, it has been suggested by some that minimizing the dietary intake of carbohydrate is to the advantage of the patient with respiratory disease. A patient's response to carbohydrate should be evaluated so that adverse effects can be avoided. It appears, however, that when high levels of carbohydrate are given enterally to patients with COPD who retain carbon dioxide, elevated arterial carbon dioxide tension ($PaCO_2$) levels do not always occur.[15-18] In fact, there are even some advantages. A load of ingested carbohydrate can elevate the arterial blood oxygen level (PaO_2) by a modest amount of 7 to 9 mm Hg.[15,19] This is of definite benefit to patients with low oxygen saturations. When the oxygen saturation is low, small increases in PaO_2 can produce significant increases in oxygen content. In addition, a high-carbohydrate diet can significantly increase endurance[20] and allow a given amount of work to be performed with less oxygen than with low-carbohydrate diets.[21] The low-$\dot{V}CO_2$ advantages of a high-fat diet may be offset in some patients by the increased oxygen requirement for a given work rate. The major problem that has arisen with carbohydrate intake in patients with respiratory disorders occurs when glucose has been given in excess. The increased $\dot{V}CO_2$ (a result of both the high RQ of glucose metabolism and its conversion to fat) has induced respiratory difficulty in patients being weaned from mechanical ventilators.[22-24] This has been observed primarily when glucose has been administered by the parenteral (IV) route.

Clearly the problem with glucose lies not in its use, but in its abuse. It is recommended that with the use of parenteral nutrition in critically ill patients, fat should be infused along with the glucose. The infused fat not only helps provide energy but inhibits the fat synthesis pathway, thereby preventing excessive carbon dioxide production.

Despite the advantages of carbohydrates, diets must be individualized for each patient. Patients with more severe COPD often do better with a higher fat content in the diet and less carbohydrate because there is less CO_2 production. But this does not lessen the importance of carbohydrates. Various carbohydrate and dietary fat percentages should be tried until the best combination is found for each patient. This point is stressed because there is a tendency to simply put patients with COPD on a high-fat diet without determining how much carbohydrate they can handle before their condition becomes compromised. Generally, carbohydrates should make up about 55% to 60% of the caloric intake of enterally fed patients. Follow-up assessment of patients by a registered dietitian familiar with COPD allows proper dietary adjustments.

Protein

Protein should make up 12% to 15% of the caloric intake. The recommended dietary allowance (RDA) of protein for a healthy person has been set at 0.8 g/kg of body weight each day. Thus a 70-kg person should obtain about 56 g of protein each day. Typically a person who ingests an adequate number of calories each day, from a variety of foods, will get sufficient protein. Following are two methods for estimating protein needs in healthy or sick people.

Caloric-nitrogen ratio
   150:1 for the average hospitalized patient
   100:1 for extreme hypermetabolism
   450:1 for renal insufficiency (without dialysis)
   300:1 for the normal healthy adult
Grams of protein per kilogram of body weight
   0.8 g/kg for the normal healthy adult
   1.2 to 1.5 g/kg for the average hospitalized patient
   2.0 to 2.5 g/kg for severe catabolic problems

Nitrogen values are often referred to in discussion of protein requirements because nitrogen is only found in the amino acids that make up proteins. So measuring nitrogen, which is a simple laboratory measure, is the easiest way to measure protein intake or excretion. *Amino acids* make up all the proteins. Amino acids contain an acid group, COOH, and an amino group, NH_2. The amino group is the nitrogen-containing portion of the amino acid. Specific laboratory methods are used to measure nitrogen in the blood (blood urea nitrogen [BUN]) or in the urine (urinary urea nitrogen [UUN]). Because every 100 g of proteins contains 6.25 g of nitrogen, grams of nitrogen can readily be converted to grams of protein by multiplying by 6.25. Conversely, to find how much nitrogen there is in a given amount of protein, in grams, one simply divides by 6.25 (or the appropriate factor for the specific protein).

When considering adequacy of protein intake, both quantity and quality of the protein must be considered. The quality

---

> **SIMPLY STATED**
> Excessive glucose intake leads to an increase in CO_2 production, and the respiratory system must work harder to rid the body of this extra CO_2.

of a protein is determined by the amount of essential amino acids it contains. *Essential amino acids* cannot be synthesized by the body in sufficient quantities to meet body needs—or cannot be synthesized at all. Of the 20 amino acids, 9 are considered essential for the healthy adult: histidine, isoleucine, leucine, lysine, methionine, phenylalanine, threonine, tryptophan, and valine. By definition, the greater the number of essential amino acids contained in a protein, the higher its quality. However, in clinical nutrition, we are finding that simply being high in the essential amino acids does not equate with being the best protein. The ratio of various key amino acids is emerging as an important factor in nutritional health. Soy protein is considered a high-quality protein, along with milk or egg protein; however, with soy protein, we find an additional benefit of lower insulin stimulation and a lowering of cholesterol. With milk or egg protein, there is an opposite effect. Plant-based proteins lower many of the risk factors for many chronic diseases. Most of the plant proteins have lower essential amino acid profiles than do animal proteins, but instead of this being detrimental, it is being found that there is a health and longevity advantage.

As with anything else, the extremes of protein intake, either too little or too much, can have detrimental effects. Too little protein compromises the immune system, promotes edema and ascites, produces generalized wasting of muscle tissue, and retards growth and proper development in children. Too much protein, although not as harmful, increases the requirements for some other nutrients, notably calcium and water. In addition, there may be an increase in the work of breathing, as noted previously, and increased stress on the liver and kidneys (of concern mostly in patients with liver or renal insufficiency). The final consideration involves the body's acid-base balance. Protein is the major source of fixed acids that are ingested (fixed acids must be cleared by the kidney; volatile acids, like carbon dioxide, can be cleared by the lungs). Patients with COPD who are in a state of respiratory acidosis may experience more difficulty if an increased fixed acid load—large quantity of protein—is ingested. Protein from plant-based sources are more alkaline in nature. In fact, fruits and vegetables leave an alkaline residue in the body after metabolism and they help buffer the acids from the proteins. Without sufficient fruits and vegetables, more calcium must be pulled from the bones, forming calcium carbonate, which is then used to buffer the fixed acids from the proteins. So, for patients who have respiratory acidosis and are in need of more protein intake, their acid-base balance is better regulated by adding more plant-based foods in the diet.

To establish the optimal amount of protein, a patient needs the measurement of protein intake (nitrogen intake) and nitrogen excretion. A patient whose intake of nitrogen equals excretion of nitrogen is said to be in nitrogen balance. If more nitrogen is excreted than ingested, *negative* nitrogen balance exists. Conversely, *positive* nitrogen balance exists when the nitrogen intake is greater than the nitrogen excretion. Patients who are severely ill or who are simply not getting enough calories are often in negative nitrogen balance. This is undesirable because it indicates that body protein is being used for energy. Patients who are nutritionally depleted need to be in positive nitrogen balance to build up body tissues. In the well-nourished patient, the clinical goal is to maintain nitrogen balance.

> **SIMPLY STATED**
>
> A negative nitrogen balance is common in critically ill patients who are not able to eat and indicates that more nitrogen is excreted than ingested. Body protein stores are being consumed in such cases, and muscle wasting is occurring.

Fat

Dietary fat plays a number of important roles in the body. The fat-soluble vitamins—A, D, E, and K—are carried in fats and oils. These vitamins are involved in immunity, antioxidant activity, and blood clotting. Fat is energy dense and contains twice as many calories per gram weight as carbohydrate or protein. Because of this, fat is the best storage form for energy, and this is why the body stores excess calories in the form of fat in the adipose tissue. Fat is also the most efficient way to provide more calories to hospitalized patients when they are fluid restricted or cannot tolerate large volumes of food. Fat provides a feeling of fullness (satiety), improves palatability of food, and is digested more slowly than proteins and starches. There are two *essential fats*, linolenic (omega 3) and linoleic (omega 6), that the body must obtain from the diet. These fats are needed for modulation of inflammatory processes, nerve function, and other essential chemical activities.

Within the body, fat is involved in many different functions. Notably, fat is a component of all cell membranes, provides energy storage and organ protection, and is the major component of surfactant (dipalmitoyl lecithin). However, these tasks do not require much fat to be eaten. The typical American diet is composed of more than 30% of calories from fat. This is more than necessary. With excess dietary fat comes increased risk of heart disease, breast cancer, colon cancer, and lung cancer in women. Increased fat also decreases oxygenation of the tissues,[25,26] impairs pulmonary gas diffusion (DL_{CO}), and hinders capillary circulation by promoting the clumping of red blood cells.[27] However, these outcomes do not always occur because the effects seen depend on the amount of fat that is circulating, the rate of clearance of fat, and possibly the type of fat. As the fat content of the diet increases, there is a measurable decrease in $\dot{V}CO_2$. For many patients with COPD, this results in less dyspnea and improved function.[28-30]

> **SIMPLY STATED**
>
> Excessive fat intake can decrease tissue oxygenation. Strive for a balance between fat and carbohydrate intake so oxygenation is maximized and carbon dioxide production is minimized.

The main concern of nutritionists is to determine the optimal percentage of calories that should come from carbohydrate and protein. With that established, the remaining amount of calories required can come from fat.

With the quantity of fat determined, one must be concerned with the quality of fat. Fat can be either *saturated* (no double bonds present in the fatty acid chain) or unsaturated (some of the fatty acid carbons contain double bonds). Unsaturated fat is of two types: *polyunsaturated* (more than two double bonds in the fatty acid chain) and *monounsaturated* (only one double bond present). Most of the fat eaten should be mono-unsaturated type. Mono-unsaturated fat, found in olives, nuts, and avocados, has numerous health benefits. This type of fat lowers total and low-density cholesterol (LDL) with no adverse effect on the high-density lipoprotein cholesterol (HDL), thereby lowering risk for heart disease.[31,32] Mono-unsaturated fat also helps regulate both blood sugar and blood pressure. Olive oil or canola oil are the recommended choices. Despite all the information available about the advantages and disadvantages of given foods and optimal combinations of carbohydrate, fat, and protein, dietary patterns established early in life are difficult to change in later years. Patients should be encouraged to eat foods that provide good nutrition as well as not aggravate a compromised respiratory condition. However, some patients will not adapt to a change in diet, and in these cases any nutrition is better than no nutrition.

Vitamins, Minerals, Phytochemicals, and Other Nutrients

Vitamins can be classified into two main categories: water soluble and fat soluble. Water-soluble vitamins are those of the B group and vitamin C. The fat-soluble vitamins are A, D, E, and K. Vitamins are co-factors in the enzyme systems needed for various metabolic pathways and body processes. The minerals can be divided into either macronutrient elements or micronutrient (trace) elements. Minerals are used in all of the body chemical reactions and are part of numerous enzyme systems. It is just as important to supplement with minerals as it is with vitamins when there appears to be a deficient food intake.

For most people who eat a variety of foods each day, ingesting the recommended amounts of vitamins and minerals is not difficult. But when physiologic functioning has been altered by a disease process, an increased need for specific nutrients may arise. Vitamin and mineral supplementation will also be more necessary when there is a decreased consumption of food because of, for example, loss of appetite. The less eaten, the more difficulty there will be in obtaining all the different nutrients. Furthermore, various medications can interact with the absorption, function, or excretion of some nutrients, thereby altering the required amount. Studies show that in older people, supplementation with a basic vitamin and mineral results in fewer infections and more days of wellness each year.[33-35] However, not all studies confirm these findings.[36] The differing results might be due to different levels or combinations of supplementations. There appears to be a consistent finding that

higher levels of antioxidant levels in the blood correlate with improved lung function, but this may be more likely from the diet rather than the supplements.[37] Subjects with higher plasma beta-carotene are shown to have higher FVC levels.[38] Higher intakes of vitamin C or beta-carotene is protective for FEV_1 and FVC.[39] These observations are important for COPD patients, since it is found that there is a decrease in plasma antioxidants in people who smoke; this is not only associated with decreased lung function but greater mortality.[40-42] It has also been found that a deficiency of vitamins C and E are associated with more wheezing symptoms.[43] Higher levels of dietary intakes of antioxidants appear to be associated with higher skeletal muscular strength in elderly persons.[44] This relationship would apply to the respiratory muscles, which are skeletal muscles.

A few nutrients deserve special mention because of their importance in patients with lung disease. Iron's role in oxygen transport and use in hemoglobin and myoglobin and within the respiratory transport chain make it necessary to maintain iron at normal levels. It has also been found that anemia is associated with decreases in muscular strength.[45] Vitamin A promotes optimal functioning of mucous membranes and helps promote resistance to respiratory tract infections.[46] Vitamin A depletion induced by cigarette smoking has been associated with development of emphysema in rats.[47] *Carotene*, a vitamin A precursor, and vitamin C have been found to be associated with a decreased risk of certain types of lung cancers.[48,49] A number of studies show that the benefits from these nutrients are better realized from eating the fruits and vegetables that contain them than from simply supplementing the isolated vitamin. Vitamins E and C and selenium, which are antioxidants, appear to help lessen the effects of oxygen toxicity and ozone on lung tissue.[50-53]

Any chronically ill patient may have altered eating habits that are insufficient to meet nutrient requirements. The severity of nutritional depletion appears to be related to the severity of COPD despite an adequate caloric intake.[54] This may result in a need for supplementation of some or all of the vitamins and minerals.

Phytochemicals are plant components that make up plant colors and other active components of plants. Intake of plant phytochemicals, as would be obtained from eating whole plant foods, lowers risk for chronic diseases, including asthma.[55] Flavonoids and other phytochemicals, which are only found in plant foods—especially fruits, vegetables, and berries—have potent antioxidant tissue-protective effects that are vital to health and disease prevention. Diets need to ensure generous amounts of these types of foods.

COPD patients, as with other patients with chronic diseases, are often found to have an underlying inflammatory component. Skeletal muscle loss in COPD appears to be linked with systemic inflammation.[56] It is also known that the underlying problem with asthma is airway inflammation, which leads to bronchoconstriction. Dietary omega-3 polyunsaturated fatty acids, which are found in flax seeds and fish oils, have important antiinflammatory effects in the body and may benefit patients with lung disease.[57,58]

For further information, the reader is referred to any of the many nutrition texts.

Fluids and Electrolytes

Adequate fluid intake is extremely important for patients with respiratory disorders. Proper function of the lung's mucociliary clearance mechanism requires good hydration. Although the body is composed of about 60% water by weight, it is constantly losing water via urine, feces, sweat, breathing, and, in patients with respiratory problems, expectoration. This requires continual fluid replacement.[59,60]

Patients with respiratory problems often develop heart failure (right or left or eventually both), which complicates the fluid replacement process. The need for fluids must be carefully balanced with the need to restrict fluids because of the fluid retention resulting from the heart problem. In a patient who has a heart problem, both fluid and sodium intake must be monitored. Sodium levels determine how much water the body will retain; therefore, dietary sodium often must be limited.

Water is the best fluid to replace water. However, fruit or vegetable juices add some variety as well as some nutrition and more calories for those who need more caloric intake. Low-sodium juices can be obtained. Drinks containing caffeine promote bronchodilation to some extent because caffeine is in the same family as theophylline, both being xanthines.[61] But if a patient is using theophylline-type bronchodilators and is also a heavy user of drinks containing caffeine, there is a greater chance of side effects. Because the ingestion of alcohol has been correlated with decreased FVC and FEV_1,[62] bronchoconstriction,[63] impairment of lung defenses,[64] and increased likelihood of sleep apnea,[65] its use is contraindicated. Good nutrition for the respiratory system involves not only getting enough of that which is essential, but also avoiding that which is harmful.

Patients receiving IV fluids must have the input and output amounts monitored continually so that neither too much nor too little is given. Fluid overload often results in pulmonary congestion or edema, further complicating a poorly functioning lung.

In addition to serum sodium levels, potassium and chloride values should be checked. All of these electrolytes play an important role in acid-base balance and nerve function. Potassium also plays an important role in heart, muscle, and nerve function, as well as in stimulation of aldosterone secretion (along with angiotensin II) from the adrenal cortex.

One must not forget that fluid and sodium intake can occur with medication and normal saline nebulization. Nebulized fluid retention is most critical when dealing with small children and infants, especially when an ultrasonic nebulizer is used.

SIMPLY STATED

Excessive intake of sodium can lead to fluid retention, especially in the patient with heart failure.

METHODS OF MEETING NUTRITIONAL REQUIREMENTS

Nutritional requirements can only be met once the food has entered the body. This is obvious; however, it is not always achieved easily. Dietitians often work against such patient factors as loss of appetite, dyspnea that is increased with eating, inability to eat normal amounts of solid food, fluid restrictions, inability to take food by mouth, and a comatose state. Careful evaluation of a patient's nutritional needs, food preferences, educational and economic status, cooking facilities, and self-help level is necessary. All factors influence a patient's ability to reach the nutritional goals set.

The routes of nutritional administration can be either enteral or parenteral. The preferred route is enteral. If a patient is intubated and cannot take food by mouth, tube feeding is instituted via an NG tube. The last resort, when all other attempts at feeding are unsuccessful, is total parenteral nutrition (TPN). TPN is the feeding of patients by direct infusion of nutrients into either a peripheral or a central vein. There is a reluctance to feed patients by TPN because it is not as efficient as the enteral route, it is expensive, and there are increased risks of complications such as infection. However, because nutrition is so important, it is used. Nutritionally depleted or hypermetabolic patients should never go without nutritional support for more than a day.

Patients with emphysema are often underweight and need to gain, whereas those with chronic bronchitis are likely to be overweight and need to lose. Patients with COPD may find it uncomfortable to eat a large meal because a flattened diaphragm along with a full stomach makes it even more difficult to function. To avoid this problem, frequent small meals may be helpful. The goal for a patient with emphysema is a positive nitrogen balance and an increase in caloric intake because respiratory muscle function improves with an increase in weight (muscle mass). The goal for an overweight patient with bronchitis is maintenance of nitrogen balance with decreased caloric intake because respiratory muscle function improves with a loss of weight (fat).

Patients being assisted by continuous mechanical ventilation provide an additional nutritional challenge. Positive-pressure breathing can affect splanchnic (internal organs of the abdomen) circulation as well as increased resistance to portal blood flow to the liver, increased resistance to bile flow down the bile duct, and decreased blood flow to the kidneys. These effects are increased as the pressure is increased and are most pronounced with the use of continuous positive-airway pressure (CPAP) or positive end-expiratory pressure (PEEP). However, these effects may reach significance only for a minority of patients. Yet any alteration in blood flow in the gastrointestinal tract, liver, or kidneys can have an effect on the nutritional status of the patient, thus making it more difficult to meet his/her nutritional requirements.

NUTRITIONAL ASSESSMENT

The RT is not responsible for the nutritional assessment of the patient but should be familiar with the process and may actually participate in it. Because the RT and the nurse usually spend the most time with a patient, their observations are valuable. A complete nutritional assessment is performed by the dietitian, with some factors being assessed by other members of the nutritional support team. The components of nutritional assessment consist of medical and diet histories, anthropometric (weight and various body) measurements, biochemical evaluations, and immunologic evaluations. The areas to be assessed in determining the patient's nutritional profile are summarized in Box 17-1.

BOX 17-1   Areas Requiring Assessment to Determine Patient's Nutritional Profile

Physiological

Types of diseases present
Severity of illness
Metabolic stress of disease
Medications being used
Genetic deficiencies
Activity level
Resting metabolic rate
Food allergies
Present nutritional status
Anthropometric
Biochemical
Immunologic

Psychosocial

Mental state (mood, alertness)
Culture
Food preparation skills
Appetite
Learned eating behaviors/habits (food preferences)
Motivation
Habits: alcohol, smoking
Education
Income

Environmental

Mechanical hindrances to eating (continuous mechanical ventilation and tracheostomy)
Food availability
Temperature
Humidity

Measurement Indication

Skinfold thickness
Skinfold + arm circumference = arm, muscle circumference, muscle and fat area
Weight for height
Amount of body fat
Body protein reserves (an indicator of protein energy nutrition)
Body fat stores (an indicator of energy reserves)
Result of long-term nutritional status

Data Gathering and Interpretation

History

Following is a list of conditions to be sought in the medical history:
- Multiple surgical or nonsurgical trauma
- Fever
- Infection
- Burns
- Long bone fractures
- Hyperthyroidism
- Prolonged corticosteroid therapy

These conditions increase a patient's metabolic rate or caloric and other nutrient requirements. Such metabolic challenges pose a serious threat to the homeostatic maintenance of a marginally nourished patient with COPD. A patient with one of these conditions should be evaluated further with a metabolic rate assessment (BEE) using indirect calorimetry.

During the patient interview, information is sought in the following important areas:
- Occupation and usual daily activity
- Use of supplemental oxygen
- Usual energy and nutrient intake via 24-hour recall or food frequency pattern
- Special diet at home
- Food aversions, intolerances, and allergies
- Medications and nutritional supplements
- Mechanical feeding problems (e.g., chewing, swallowing)
- Changes in appetite
- Changes in food intake or food patterns
- Gastrointestinal problems (e.g., nausea, vomiting, heartburn)
- Elimination pattern and consistency of stool
- Maximum weight attained and how long ago it was attained
- Usual weight
- Alcohol intake
- Smoking or other tobacco habits

This information is usually obtained from the patient or family members during the initial workup.

Physical Examination

The physical examination often yields clues to the patient's nutritional status; however, many signs of nutritional deficiency can be missed by the inexperienced practitioner. Look at the health of the patient's hair and check for sparseness, dyspigmentation, or easy "pluckability." Does the patient's skin show areas of drying, cracking, or pigment change? Are there swollen parotid glands or an enlarged liver? Is there weight loss or muscle wasting, edema, mental apathy, or confusion? These are some of the signs of malnutrition. Of course, these signs are rather nonspecific and therefore only suggestive of malnutrition. When these signs are present in a patient, more sensitive and objective methods of assessment should be used to confirm or rule out compromised nutritional status.

Following is a summary of some basic anthropometric measurements and their nutritional assessment value.

The assessment most commonly used and easiest to perform during the physical examination involves weighing and measuring. Measurements of weight, height, and arm circumference require little effort or time yet give important information. Because height and weight can vary with the time of day and the amount of clothing or shoe heel height, the measurements should be performed in the same way each time and the pertinent information recorded so that serial measurements are meaningful. Bed scales can be used for weighing ventilator dependent patients. The weight of any ventilator tubing should be subtracted from the total. A weight loss of 5% of the usual body weight, or an unintentional weight loss of 10 lb or more, indicates increased nutritional risk. Although body weight has limited value in detecting malnutrition, low body weights correlate with poor medical outcomes. The clinical team should make certain that water retention is not masking a patient who is actually underweight and that water loss is not interpreted as nutritional depletion. If a fluctuation or change in weight of several pounds is observed during a 24-hour period, it is most likely caused by water retention or loss.

The body mass index (BMI) is the primary method for assessment of the appropriateness of weight for a given height. The BMI is determined by: weight (kg)/height (m^2). Figure 17-5 shows a look-up table for finding the BMI without having to calculate it. A BMI in the range of 20 to 25 is considered optimal. A BMI from 25 to 30 is considered overweight; 30 to 35 is stage 1 obesity; 35 to 40 is stage 2 obesity; and 40 to 45 is stage 3 obesity. As the BMI exceeds 27, the risk for weight-related problems begins to increase. BMIs that are below 19 are associated with malnutrition problems and increased pneumonia infections. BMI is shown to be significantly associated with FEV_1 and FEV_1/VC.[66] In COPD patients, the best survival outcomes are associated with those who have higher BMIs and in whom low BMI is an independent risk factor for dying.[66-68]

A quick estimate of ideal body weight can be determined from the following rule: allow 105 lb for the first 5 feet of height and 5 lb for each additional inch. This does not account for variations in frame size but is useful for rapid estimation as to appropriateness of a patient's weight. The ideal body weight can also be used for estimating a patient's anatomic dead space (1 mL/lb ideal body weight) or for determining a starting tidal volume for a ventilator-dependent patient (5 to 7 mL/lb ideal body weight). The term ideal body weight simply refers to the weight the patient probably *should* weigh.

Body weight is often divided into two types: fat weight and lean body weight (lean body weight = total weight − fat weight). The problem is never simply a weight problem. A patient weighs too much only when the percentage of total body weight made up of fat exceeds about 23% for males and 28% for females. A method for estimating the percent of body fat is the skinfold measurement.

Triceps skinfold thickness

Measurement of skinfold thickness with the use of calipers is a fairly simple procedure (proper technique is important) that yields data on the fat and protein reserves in the body. The triceps skinfold is the most common place of measurement; however, several other sites can be used, usually in addition to the triceps area. Skinfold thickness coupled with measurements of the upper arm circumference, arm muscle circumference, and arm muscle area provide accepted estimates of protein energy malnutrition. The arm fat area may also be calculated and, when used along with triceps skinfold measurements, improves the body fat weight estimate.[69] These measurements are all compared with standard normal values to assess the degree of malnutrition. As with other tests, the exact value obtained with any one measurement may not be as important as the trend seen with serial measurements. It is important to establish baseline data for a patient when first admitted. Then the first signs of malnutrition can be detected and appropriate treatment implemented before serious deficiency symptoms occur.

Other, more accurate methods for assessment of body fat include underwater weighing, body volume displacement, and electrical bioimpedance measurements.[70] Only the last has a role in the hospital setting.

Laboratory Biochemical Tests

Laboratory biochemical tests tend to reflect body changes more quickly and be more accurate than anthropometric tests. Table 17-1 summarizes their relative sensitivities to body nutritional change and suggests guidelines for interpretation.

Creatine phosphate is used in muscle as an energy reserve molecule. When there is an increased demand for ATP, creatine donates a phosphate to ADP, making ATP. The more muscle mass there is in the body, the more creatine there will be. Creatine is metabolized to creatinine, the form in which it is largely excreted. The clearance of creatinine from the blood by the kidneys is a good indicator of renal function. Measurement of 24-hour urinary excretion of creatinine correlates with the patient's lean body weight (muscle mass): the greater the muscle mass, the higher the urinary excretion of creatinine. When expressed in terms of height, a measure generally unaffected by malnutrition, urinary excretion of creatinine can be used as a general measure of malnutrition. The creatinine-height index (CHI) is a predictor of muscle mass but may not correlate well with arm muscle circumference, probably because of the many factors that govern the excretion of creatinine. In young females and older men, if the creatinine excretion is related to the total arm length, the ability to predict malnutrition is improved.

Levels of serum albumin, the major protein fraction of blood, correlate well with body protein reserves of muscle mass. The measurement of serum albumin levels provides a useful screening tool for detecting protein energy undernutrition. However, because the turnover of serum albumin is slow (half-life is 20 days), a change in nutritional status is not soon reflected by this measurement. The time lag of 1 to 2 weeks for the serum albumin level to show a change after a nutritional alteration has occurred is too long to effectively manage the nutrition of most critically ill patients.

Prealbumin—also called *thyroxin-binding prealbumin (TBPA)* because it carries about one third of the body's thyroxin

BMI Table for Determining Optimal Weight for Given Height

Height in Inches

↓	56	57	58	59	60	61	62	63	64	65	66	67	68	69	70	71	72	73	74	75	76
100	22	22	21	20	20	19	18	18	17	17	16	16	15	15	14	14	14	13	13	13	12
105	24	23	22	21	21	20	19	19	18	18	17	16	16	16	15	15	14	14	14	13	13
110	25	24	23	22	22	21	20	20	19	18	18	17	17	16	16	15	15	15	14	14	13
115	26	25	24	23	23	22	21	20	20	19	19	18	18	17	17	16	16	15	15	14	14
120	27	26	25	24	23	23	22	21	21	20	19	19	18	18	17	17	16	16	15	15	15
125	28	27	26	25	24	24	23	22	22	21	20	20	19	18	18	17	17	17	16	16	15
130	29	28	27	26	25	25	24	23	22	22	21	20	20	19	19	18	18	17	17	16	16
135	30	29	28	27	26	26	25	24	23	23	22	21	21	20	19	19	18	18	17	17	16
140	31	30	29	28	27	27	26	25	24	23	23	22	21	21	20	20	19	19	18	18	17
145	33	31	30	29	28	27	27	26	25	24	23	23	22	21	21	20	20	19	19	18	18
150	34	33	31	30	29	28	27	27	26	25	24	24	23	22	22	21	20	20	19	19	18
155	35	34	32	31	30	29	28	28	27	26	25	24	24	23	22	22	21	20	20	19	19
160	36	35	34	32	31	30	29	28	28	27	26	25	24	24	23	22	22	21	21	20	20
165	37	36	35	33	32	31	30	29	28	28	27	26	25	24	24	23	22	22	21	21	20
170	38	37	36	34	33	32	31	30	29	28	27	27	26	25	24	24	23	22	22	21	21
175	39	38	37	35	34	33	32	31	30	29	28	27	27	26	25	24	24	23	23	22	21
180	40	39	38	36	35	34	33	32	31	30	29	28	27	27	26	25	24	24	23	23	22
185	42	40	39	37	36	35	34	33	32	31	30	29	28	27	27	26	25	24	24	23	23
190	43	41	40	38	37	36	35	34	33	32	31	30	29	28	27	27	26	25	24	24	23
195	44	42	41	39	38	37	36	35	34	33	32	31	30	29	28	27	27	26	25	24	24
200	45	43	42	40	39	38	37	36	34	33	32	31	30	30	29	28	27	26	26	25	24
205	46	44	43	41	40	39	38	36	35	34	33	32	31	30	29	29	28	27	26	26	25
210	47	46	44	43	41	40	38	37	36	35	34	33	32	31	30	29	29	28	27	26	26
215	48	47	45	44	42	41	39	38	37	36	35	34	33	32	31	30	29	28	28	27	26
220	49	48	46	45	43	42	40	39	38	37	36	35	34	33	32	31	30	29	28	28	27
225	51	49	47	46	44	43	41	40	39	38	36	35	34	33	32	31	31	30	29	28	27
230	52	50	48	47	45	44	42	41	40	38	37	36	35	34	33	32	31	30	30	29	28
235	53	51	49	48	46	44	43	42	40	39	38	37	36	35	34	33	32	31	30	29	29
240	54	52	50	49	47	45	44	43	41	40	39	38	37	36	35	34	33	32	31	30	29
245	55	53	51	50	48	46	45	43	42	41	40	38	37	36	35	34	33	32	32	31	30
250	56	54	52	51	49	47	46	44	43	42	40	39	38	37	36	35	34	33	32	31	30
255	57	55	53	52	50	48	47	45	44	43	41	40	39	38	37	36	35	34	33	32	31
260	58	56	54	53	51	49	48	46	45	43	42	41	40	38	37	36	35	34	33	33	32
265	60	57	56	54	52	50	49	47	46	44	43	42	40	39	38	37	36	35	34	33	32
270	61	59	57	55	53	51	49	48	46	45	44	42	41	40	39	38	37	36	35	34	33
275	62	60	58	56	54	52	50	49	47	46	44	43	42	41	40	38	37	36	35	34	34
280	63	61	59	57	55	53	51	50	48	47	45	44	43	41	40	39	38	37	36	35	34

Weight in Pounds

Figure 17-5   The body mass index (BMI) is determined by aligning a patient's weight with their height. The BMI is found where the row of weight intersects the column of height. See text for more explanation. (Courtesy www.niddk.nih.gov.)

(thyroid hormone)—also carries *retinol-binding protein (RBP)*. These two proteins quickly reflect nutritional deprivation or refeeding treatment because of their short half-lives (TBPA, 2 days; RBP, 12 hours).[71] Either can be used for assessing nutritional repletion in critically ill patients because the response time for these values is 3 days or less.[72]

Serum transferrin, the protein that transports iron in the body, has a half-life of 4 to 8 days. However, because of its wide range of normal values and its unpredictable response to refeed-ing in depleted patients, it has limited clinical use in nutritional assessment. The *total iron-binding capacity (TIBC)* of transferrin may also be used. However, it may overestimate transferrin levels because iron can also bind to other proteins in the blood. Transferrin levels may be elevated during iron deficiency anemia, the second and third trimesters of pregnancy, estrogen therapy, or oral contraceptive use. Other hormones and disease states have a variable effect on serum transferrin levels and TIBC.

Table 17-1	Current Laboratory Biochemical Tests and Guidelines for Interpretation			
Measurement or Index	Deficient	Normal	Sensitivity	
Creatinine-height index (CHI) (%)	40	60	Poor	
Serum albumin level (g/dL)	2.5	3.5-5.0	Limited because of long half-life (20 days)	
Serum transferrin level (mg/dL)	100	200-400	Poor; unpredictable response to refeeding	
Total iron-binding capacity (TIBC) (mg/dL)	<250	250-350	Poor; increased in pregnancy, iron deficiency, oral contraceptive use; iron may bind to proteins other than serum transferrin	
Nitrogen balance	Negative balance	Equilibrium	Poor; nitrogen excretion often underestimated	
Thyroxin-binding prealbumin (TBPA) (mg/dL)	<10	10-20	Very good; half-life short (2 days)	
Retinol-binding protein (RBP) (μg/dL)	<3	3-6	Very good; half-life short (12 hr)	
Total lymphocyte count (cells/mm^3)	<1200	2000-3500	Limited; decreased in injury, chemotherapy, radiotherapy, surgery; increased in infection	
Differential count for lymphocytes (%)		20-45	Limited	
Skin antigen testing	Negative	Positive	Good	

Nitrogen balance measurements, using 24-hour urine specimens, are essential for protein assessment and are commonly performed in acute care settings. However, an underestimation of nitrogen excretion can occur in patients with burns, diarrhea, vomiting, or other nitrogen-losing conditions.[73] A commonly used clinical estimation is nitrogen balance = grams of nitrogen intake − (24-hour grams of urine urea nitrogen + 4 g).

Immunocompetence, or being dependent on globulin proteins (as mentioned previously), can also be used to help assess PEM. Total lymphocyte count (lymphocytes make the immunoglobulins) or their function can be measured. An easy test of their function (which requires them to have ample protein to make their antibodies) is to challenge them with skin antigen testing. Antigens used are those to which a patient is most likely to have been previously exposed. With these, a quick antigen-antibody reaction should be seen at the skin testing site, much like a positive tuberculin skin test reaction. However, if the patient is protein deficient, the skin test reaction will be greatly diminished or absent.[74] It should be noted that an iron deficiency can also diminish the response.[75]

As can be seen, no one test constitutes a perfect assessment of a patient's nutritional status. But with the appropriate use of selected anthropometric and biochemical measurements, along with astute observations by respiratory care practitioners, an adequate nutritional profile can be developed. Other sources should be consulted for further discussion of nutritional assessment.[76]

> **SIMPLY STATED**
> No single measurement can determine the patient's nutritional status. A combination of the history, physical examination, and laboratory tests is often needed to determine the patient's nutritional needs.

Role of Respiratory Therapists in Nutritional Assessment

The members of the health care team not involved in direct nutritional assessment, if alert to the information discussed so far, can contribute significantly to achieving good nutrition for patients with respiratory disorders. Signs or symptoms of potential nutritional problems should be sought during routine patient care.

In examining a patient with respiratory problems, the first step is to observe. Although malnutrition can never be diagnosed by simple inspection (except in extreme cases), much information can be learned by simply looking. During this time various differential diagnoses can be formulated, which subsequent findings will confirm or disprove.

Inspection Findings

One should note the effects of body mass on breathing efficiency. Cachectic (nutritionally depleted) patients have readily outlined bony structures with depression of the intercostal spaces. Accessory muscles of respiration are often visible in these patients. Because severe muscle wasting can decrease lung function in those *without* lung disease, malnourished patients with COPD have compounded breathing difficulties. Patients who are obese have difficulty breathing in direct proportion to their excess fat weight. Obesity imposes a restrictive condition on top of whatever lung condition already exists. Figure 17-6 illustrates the effects of excess fat weight on the mechanics of breathing. Note the increased energy that must be expended during inspiration. Pregnancy can produce similar interference with the mechanics of breathing.

> **SIMPLY STATED**
> Obesity hinders movement of the diaphragm and increases the work of breathing.

During inspection of the patient, the amount of effort that can be generated during coughing should be observed. Muscle weakness accompanies poor nutrition. Also, the viscosity of the sputum should be noted. This, along with jugular venous pressure (JVP) estimation, can give clues to fluid balance. Of course, in patients with right ventricular heart failure, the JVP will be elevated by factors other than simple fluid overload. In addition, a distended abdomen, as with ascites (fluid retention), may cause fluid balance as well as breathing problems. Edema of the extremities should also be noted; when present, it may require alterations in the patient's fluid and sodium intake.

Auscultation Findings

Coarse or fine crackles in the lung bases on auscultation can indicate either fluid overload or a loss of blood protein (oncotic pressure). Wheezing may be associated with some food intolerances or foods that contain yellow food coloring. As previously mentioned, alcohol can produce wheezing in some people. Aspirated food can also produce wheezing. The fine, late inspiratory crackles of atelectasis may result from decreased surfactant production resulting from malnutrition. Hearing the S_3 heart sound of congestive heart failure could suggest that fluid problems occur. An S_4 heart sound can be associated with severe anemia.

Laboratory Findings

Decreases in pulmonary function measures such as FVC or FEV_1 may indicate protein energy deficiency or severe malnutrition. Decreased FVC can also occur with excess fat weight because of fat's restrictive effects. Decreases in peak expiratory pressure (PEP) and peak inspiratory pressure (PIP) are also associated with poor nutrition. Altered lung compliance, as measured in the laboratory, or effective compliance, as measured when taking ventilator parameters, can result from fluid and serum albumin changes acutely or from chronic malnutrition.

Arterial blood gas (ABG) values can be altered with nutrition, as mentioned before. Increased $PaCO_2$ levels can result from excess parenteral infusion of glucose or simply from insufficient muscle energy to achieve adequate ventilation. The chemoreceptor set point can also be altered by changes in protein (amino acid) intake, thereby altering sensitivity to $PaCO_2$ levels. Oxygenation parameters (oxygen saturation, oxygen content, hemoglobin) are all affected by nutritional status. Anemias can result from deficiencies in iron, folic acid, or vitamin B_{12}. Some patients may not be able to tolerate high intakes of fat or lipid infusions because of the resulting lowered PaO_2.

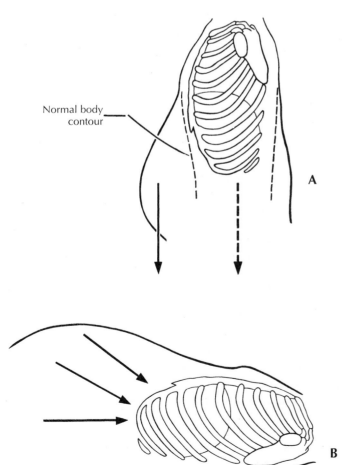

Normal body contour

A

B

Figure 17-6 Effects of obesity on mechanics of breathing. **A,** In normal-weight persons, the weight of viscera is borne by the pelvic area, and the net weight force is in the direction of the dotted arrow. However, in obese people, the net force of the weight *(solid arrow)* is not supported by the pelvic area, and weight pulls directly down on the ribs. This favors the expiratory phase, making inspiration more difficult. **B,** In the supine position, the weight of viscera pushes up on the diaphragm, again making inspiration difficult.

Changes in pH can indicate changes in dietary intake of potassium, sodium, or foods that leave an alkaline or acidic residue. Low PaO_2 levels, with subsequent lactate production, can lower pH as well. As alluded to earlier, any change in the $PaCO_2$ set point can alter acid-base balance.

The RT can become directly involved in the nutritional assessment of patients by measuring $\dot{V}O_2$ in determining energy needs. In addition, the eating environment and conditions that may affect the eating process should be assessed. An effort should be made to have clean equipment in the patient's room, to empty suction bottles, and to remove or hide sputum cups during mealtimes. A prerequisite to good nutrition is a good appetite, and a good appetite is hard to invoke unless the surroundings are pleasant. The RT can further assist by helping patients receive adequate oxygen therapy during and after meals and by scheduling breathing treatments to not interfere with mealtimes. Patients who are using oxygen masks should have an order for oxygen via cannula while eating. Attending to the oxygenation of the patient is of great nutritional importance. A decrease in oxygen saturation while eating can occur in patients with severe COPD.[77] A patient who is short of breath may not eat, and if the patient does eat, food metabolism may be compromised.

Rarely is a respiratory problem caused by nutrition alone; however, the RT will often see nutritional deficiencies complicating an existing lung problem. Being alert to the effect of nutrition on respiratory function may help stabilize the condition of a patient with lung disease that was previously deteriorating because of nutritional neglect.

REVIEW QUESTIONS

1. T F   Oxygen is required for the optimal production of ATP.

2. T F   Oxygen uptake ($\dot{V}O_2$) is a nutritional indicator of the patient's energy needs.

3. Which of the following is true about the basal energy expenditure?
   a. It requires a $\dot{V}O_2$ measurement in order to calculate.
   b. It gives an estimation of the patient's nutritional needs.
   c. If it is not met, use of body energy stores is required.
   d. All of the above.

4. Measuring the patient's energy expenditure using oxygen consumption is referred to as:
   a. Direct calorimetry.
   b. Indirect calorimetry.
   c. Simple calorimetry.
   d. Complex calorimetry.

5. Which of the following is a pulmonary effect of starvation?
   a. Increased DL_{CO}
   b. Increased FEV1

   c. Increased risk of pneumonia
   d. None of the above

6. Which of the following might hinder attempts at nutritional repletion in patients with respiratory disease?
   a. The use of bronchodilators
   b. Simple oxygen therapy
   c. Intubation
   d. All of the above

7. What element must be stored in sufficient quantities to meet the metabolic demands of the diaphragm?
   a. Arginine
   b. Glycogen
   c. 2,3-DPG
   d. Fat

8. Which of the following is true about anaerobic metabolism?
   a. It can cause a metabolic acidosis.
   b. It results in excess lactate production.
   c. It results in excess production of CO_2.
   d. All of the above.

9. What is the RQ value of a patient on a pure carbohydrate diet?
   a. 0.60
   b. 0.70
   c. 0.85
   d. 1.00

10. Which of the following should the majority of dietary intake be made up of ?
    a. Fat
    b. Carbohydrate
    c. Protein
    d. None of the above

11. Which of the following may be more difficult with a high-carbohydrate diet?
    a. Oxygenation
    b. Cellular gas exchange
    c. Oxygen transport
    d. Weaning from mechanical ventilation

12. What is nitrogen balance useful in determining?
    a. The adequacy of protein intake
    b. The adequacy of carbohydrate intake
    c. The need for vitamin supplementation
    d. Fluid and electrolyte balance

13. Which of the following is associated with a low-protein diet?
    a. Increased work of breathing
    b. Increased fixed acid load
    c. Immune compromise
    d. Increased stress on the kidneys

14. Which of the following is *not* associated with a high-fat diet?
    a. Increased risk of heart disease
    b. Decreased tissue oxygenation
    c. Decreased DL_{CO}
    d. Increased CO_2 production

15. What mineral plays a very important role in oxygen transport?
    a. Calcium
    b. Iron
    c. Zinc
    d. Magnesium

16. T F Total parenteral nutrition is the first choice for nutritional supplementation.

17. Which of the following is *not* associated with an increased metabolism?
    a. Severe burns
    b. Severe infection
    c. Trauma
    d. Hypothyroidism

18. Which of the following might indicate poor nutritional status?
    a. Body weight less than ideal
    b. Negative nitrogen balance
    c. Negative response to skin antigen testing
    d. All of the above

19. What test is most useful for screening the patient for protein malnutrition?
    a. Thyroxin-binding prealbumin
    b. Serum transferrin
    c. Creatinine-height index
    d. None of the above

20. T F Aiding a patient's nutritional status may be as simple as helping to relieve his/her dyspnea.

REFERENCES

1. Roza AM, Shizgal HM: The Harris Benedict equation reevaluated: resting energy requirements and the body cell mass, *Am J Clin Nutr* 40:168, 1984.
2. Wier JB, De V: New methods for calculating metabolic rate with special reference to protein metabolism, *J Physiol* 109:1, 1949.
3. Lusk G: *The elements of sciences of nutrition,* Philadelphia, 1928, WB Saunders.
4. Cohen RI and others: Body composition and resting energy expenditure in clinically stable, non-weight-losing patients with severe emphysema, *Chest* 124:1365, 2003.
5. Ezzell L and Jensen GL: Malnutrition in chronic obstructive pulmonary disease, *Am J Clin Nutr* 72:1415, 2000.
6. Jounieaux V, Mayeux I: Oxygen cost of breathing in patients with emphysema or chronic bronchitis in acute respiratory failure, *Am J Respir Crit Care Med* 152(6 Pt 1):2181, 1995.
7. Yoneda T and others: Clinical benefit of nutritional assessment and support in patients with chronic obstructive pulmonary disease, *Nippon Kyobu Shikkan Gakkai Zasshi* 34(suppl):79, 1996.
8. Thorsddottir I, Gunnarsdottir I: Energy intake must be increased among recently hospitalized patients with chronic obstructive pulmonary disease to improve nutritional status, *J Am Dietetic Assoc* 102:247, 2002.
9. Frey JG and others: Chronic obstructive pulmonary disease patients undergoing home oxygen therapy: a study of clinical parameters, nutritional status and ambulatory capacity, *Rev Mal Respir* 15(1):69, 1998.
10. Doekel RC and others: Clinical semi-starvation: depression of hypoxic ventilatory response, *N Engl J Med* 295:358, 1976.
11. Gorini M and others: Neural respiratory drive and neuromuscular coupling in patients with chronic obstructive pulmonary disease (COPD), *Chest* 98:1179, 1990.
12. Weissman C, Askanazi J: Nutrition and respiration, *Clin Consult Nutr* 2(Suppl):5, 1982.
13. Sahebjami H, Wirman JA: Emphysema-like changes in the lungs of starved rats, *Am Rev Respir Dis* 124:619, 1981.
14. Sahebjami H, Vassallo CL, Wirman JA: Lung mechanics and ultrastructure in prolonged starvation, *Am Rev Respir Dis* 117:77, 1978.
15. Gieseke T, Gurushanthaiah G, Glauser FL: Effects of carbohydrates on carbon dioxide excretion in patients with airway disease, *Chest* 71:55, 1977.
16. Prusaczyk WK and others: Differential effects of dietary carbohydrate on RPE at the lactate and ventilatory thresholds, *Med Sci Sports Exerc* 24:568, 1992.
17. Sue CY and others: Effect of altering the proportion of dietary fat and carbohydrate on exercise gas exchange in normal subjects, *Am Rev Respir Dis* 139:1430, 1989.
18. Talpers SS and others: Nutritionally associated increased carbon dioxide production. Excess total calories vs high proportion of carbohydrate calories, *Chest* 102:551, 1992.
19. Saltzman HA, Salzano JV: Effects of carbohydrate metabolism upon respiratory gas exchange in normal men, *J Appl Physiol* 30:228, 1971.
20. Hansen JE, Hartley H, Hogan RP: Arterial oxygen increase by high-carbohydrate diet at altitude, *J Appl Physiol* 33:441, 1972.
21. Astrand PO: Something old and something new . . . very new, *Nutr Today* 1968, p 9.
22. Askanazi J and others: Respiratory changes induced by the large glucose loads of total parenteral nutrition, *JAMA* 243:1444, 1980.
23. Efthimiou J and others: Effect of carbohydrate rich versus fat rich loads on gas exchange and walking performance in

patients with chronic obstructive lung disease, *Thorax* 47:451, 1992.

24. De Meo MT, Mobarhan S, Van De Graaff W: The hazards of hypercaloric nutritional support in respiratory disease, *Nutr Rev* 49:112, 1991.

25. Swank RL, Nakamura H: Oxygen availability in brain tissues after lipid meals, *Am J Physiol* 198:217, 1960.

26. Talbott GD, Frayser R: Hyperlipidemia, a cause of decreased oxygen saturation, *Nature* 200:684, 1963.

27. Williams AV, Higginbotham AC, Knisel MH: Increased blood cell agglutination following ingestion of fat, a factor contributing to cardiac ischemia, coronary insufficiency, and anginal pain, *Angiology* 8:29, 1957.

28. Angelillo VA and others: Effects of low and high carbohydrate feedings in ambulatory patients with chronic obstructive pulmonary disease and chronic hypercapnia, *Ann Intern Med* 103(6 Pt 1):883, 1985.

29. Kuo CD, Shiao GM, Lee JD: The effects of high-fat and high-carbohydrate diet loads on gas exchange and ventilation in COPD patients and normal subjects, *Chest* 104(1):189, 1993.

30. Frankfort JD and others: Effects of high- and low-carbohydrate meals on maximum exercise performance in chronic airflow obstruction, *Chest* 100(3):792, 1991.

31. Fraser G and others: A possible protective effect of nut consumption on risk of coronary heart disease: the Adventist health study, *Arch Intern Med* 152:1416, 1992.

32. Sabate J and others: Effects of walnuts on serum lipid levels and blood pressure in normal men, *N Engl J Med* 328:603, 1993.

33. Chandra RK: Effect of vitamin and race-element supplementation on immune responses and infection in elderly subjects, *Lancet* 340(8828):1124, 1992.

34. Jain AM: Influence of vitamins and trace-elements on the incidence of respiratory infection, *Nutr Res* 22:88, 2002.

35. Langkamp-Henken B and others: Nutritional formula enhanced immune function and reduced days of symptoms of upper respiratory tract infection in seniors, *J Am Geriatr Soc* 52:3, 2004.

36. Graat JM and others: Effect of daily vitamin E and multivitamin-mineral supplementation on acute respiratory tract infections in elderly persons: a randomized controlled trial, *JAMA* 288:715, 2002.

37. Chen R and others: Association of dietary antioxidants and waist circumference with pulmonary function and airway obstruction, *Am J Epidemiol* 153:157, 2001.

38. Grievink L and others: Plasma concentrations of the antioxidants beta-carotene and alpha-tocopherol in relation to lung function, *Eur J Clin Nutr* 53:813, 1999.

39. Grievink L and others: Dietary intake of antioxidant (pro)-vitamins, respiratory symptoms and pulmonary function: the MORGEN study, *Thorax* 53:166, 1998.

40. Dietrich M and others: Smoking and exposure to environmental tobacco smoke decrease some plasma antioxidants and increase gamma-tocopherol in vivo after adjustment for dietary antioxidant intakes, *Am J Clin Nutr* 77:160, 2003.

41. Lykkesfeldt J and others: Ascorbate is depleted by smoking and repleted by moderate supplementation: a study in male smokers and nonsmokers with matched dietary antioxidant intakes, *Am J Clin Nutr* 71:530, 2000.

42. Fletcher AE and others: Antioxidant vitamins and mortality in older persons: findings from the nutrition add-on study to the Medical Research Council Trial of Assessment and Management of Older People in the Community, *Am J Clin Nutr* 78:999, 2003.

43. Bodner C and others: Antioxidant intake and adult-onset wheeze: a case-control study Aberdeen WHEASE Study Group, *Eur Respir J* 13:22, 1999.

44. Cesari M and others: Antioxidants and physical performance in elderly persons: the Invecchiare in Chianti (InCHIANTI) study, *Am J Clin Nutr* 79:289, 2004.

45. Cesari M and others: Hemoglobin levels and skeletal muscle: results from the InCHIANTI study, *J Gerontol A Bio Sci Med Sci* 59:M249, 2004.

46. Goodman DS: Vitamin A and retinoids in health and disease, *N Engl J Med* 310:1023, 1984.

47. Li T and others: Vitamin A Depletion induced by cigarette smoke is associated with the development of emphysema in rats, *J Nutr* 133:2629, 2003.

48. Michaud DA and others: Intake of specific carotenoids and risk of lung cancer in 2 prospective US cohorts, *Am J Clin Nutr* 72:900, 2000.

49. Riboli E, Norat Teresa: Epidemiologic evidence of the protective effect of fruit and vegetables on cancer risk, *Am J Clin Nutr* 78(suppl):5598, 2003.

50. Kann HE Jr and others: Oxygen toxicity and vitamin E, *Aerospace Med* 35:840, 1964.

51. Cross CE and others: Enhanced lung toxicity of O_2: in selenium-deficient rats, *Res Commun Chem Pathol Pharmacol* 16:695, 1977.

52. Richard C and others: Vitamin E deficiency and lipoperoxidation during adult respiratory distress syndrome, *Crit Care Med* 18:4, 1990.

53. Frank L: Antioxidants, nutrition, and bronchopulmonary dysplasia, *Clin Perinatol* 19:541, 1992.

54. Fiaccadori E and others: Hypercapnic-hypoxemic chronic obstructive pulmonary disease (COPD): influence of severity of COPD on nutritional status, *Am J Clin Nutr* 48:680, 1988.

55. Knekt P and others: Flavonoid intake and risk of chronic diseases, *Am J Clin Nutr* 76:560, 2002.

56. Eid AA and others: Inflammatory response and body composition in chronic obstructive pulmonary disease, *Am J Respir Crit Care Med* 164:1414, 2001.

57. Freedman SD and others: Association of cystic fibrosis with abnormalities in fatty acid metabolism, *N Engl J Med* 350:560, 2004.

58. Schwartz J: Role of polyunsaturated fatty acids in lung disease, *Am J Clin Nutr* 71(suppl):393s, 2000.

59. Cavaliere F and others: Airway secretion electrolytes: reflection of water and salt states of the body, *Crit Care Med* 17:891, 1989.

60. Rubin BK and others: Respiratory mucus from asymptomatic smokers is better hydrated and more easily cleared by mucociliary action, *Am Rev Respir Dis* 145:545, 1992.

61. Becker AB and others: The bronchodilator effects and pharmacokinetics of caffeine in asthma, *N Engl J Med* 310:743, 1984.

62. Lebowitz MD: Respiratory symptoms and disease related to alcohol consumption, *Am Rev Respir Dis* 123:16, 1981.

63. Geppert EF, Boushey HA: Case report: an investigation of the mechanism of ethanol-induced bronchoconstriction, *Am Rev Respir Dis* 118:135, 1978.

64. Heinemann HO: Alcohol and the lung: a brief review, *Am J Med* 63:81, 1977.

65. Dolly FR, Block JA: Increased ventricular ectopy and sleep apnea following ethanol ingestion in COPD patients, *Chest* 83:469, 1983.

66. Chailleux E and others: Prognostic value of nutritional depletion in patients with COPD treated by long-term oxygen therapy: data from the ANTADIR observatory, *Chest* 123:1460, 2003.

67. Bartolome R and others: The body-mass index, airflow obstruction, dyspnea, and exercise capacity index in chronic obstructive pulmonary disease, *N Engl J Med* 350:1005, 2004.

68. Landbo C and others: Prognostic value of nutritional status in chronic obstructive pulmonary disease, *Am J Respir Crit Care Med* 160:1856, 1999.

69. Frisancho AR: New norms of upper limb fat and muscle areas for assessment of nutritional status, *Am J Clin Nutr* 34:2540, 1981.

70. Schols AM and others: Body composition by bioelectrical impedance analysis compared with deuterium dilution and skin-fold anthropometry in patients with chronic obstructive pulmonary disease, *Am J Clin Nutr* 53:421, 1991.

71. Gofferje H: Prealbumin and retinol-binding protein highly sensitive parameters for the nutritional state in respect to protein, *Med Lab* 5:38, 1979.

72. Shetty PS and others: Rapid turnover transport proteins: an index of subclinical protein-energy malnutrition, *Lancet* 2:230, 1979.

73. Blackburn GL and others: Nutritional and metabolic assessment of the hospitalized patient, *J Parenter Enteral Nutr* 1:11, 1977.

74. Vitale J: Impact of nutrition on immune function. In *Nutrition in disease series,* Columbus, Ohio, 1979, Ross Laboratories.

75. Strauss RG: Iron deficiency infections and immune function: a reassessment, *Am J Clin Nutr* 31:660, 1978.

76. Peters JA, Burke K, White D: Nutrition in the pulmonary patient. In Hodgkin JE, Zorn E, Connors G: *Pulmonary rehabilitation: guidelines to success,* Woburn, Mass, 1984, Butterworth.

77. Brown SE, Casciari RJ, Light RW: Arterial oxygen desaturation during eating in patients with severe chronic obstructive pulmonary disease (COPD) (abstract), *Chest* 3:346, 1979.

CHAPTER 18

Ralph Downey III
Ronald M. Perkin

Assessment of Sleep and Breathing

LEARNING OBJECTIVES

Upon completion of this chapter, the reader should be able to accomplish the following:

1. Identify the percentage of men believed to have problems related to sleep apnea.
2. Identify the characteristics of non–rapid eye movement and rapid eye movement sleep.
3. Identify the physiologic effect of the different types and stages of sleep on the cardiovascular and respiratory systems in the healthy adult.
4. Recognize a definition of obstructive, central, and mixed sleep apnea. Also recognize a definition of the related terms hypopnea and upper airway resistance syndrome.
5. Identify the criteria for mild, moderate, and severe sleep apnea.
6. Identify the factors believed to be responsible for the pathophysiology of obstructive sleep apnea.
7. Identify the clinical features of patients with obstructive sleep apnea (OSA).
8. Identify the metabolic and cardiac complications associated with OSA.
9. Recognize the symptoms and behavior problems associated with sleep apnea in children.
10. Identify the age at which the peak incidence of sudden infant death occurs.
11. Identify the parameters typically monitored during a polysomnogram.
12. Identify the purpose of the multiple sleep latency test and potential causes of abnormalities.

CHAPTER OUTLINE
Normal Sleep Stages
Non–Rapid Eye Movement Sleep
Rapid Eye Movement Sleep (Sleeping)
Sleep-Related Breathing Disorders
Definitions of Sleep-Disordered Breathing
Sleep-Disordered Breathing Severity

The Sleep-Disordered Breathing Continuum
Upper Airway Resistance Syndrome
Obstructive Sleep Apnea and Hypopnea
Children and Infants with Sleep-Disordered Breathing
Central Sleep Apnea in Children
Sudden Infant Death Syndrome and Apparent Life-Threatening Events
Assessment of Sleep-Related Breathing Disorders
Bedside Observations
Laboratory Assessment

KEY TERMS

apparent life-threatening events (ALTEs)
central apnea
delta sleep
hypopnea
micrognathia
multiple sleep latency test (MSLT)
non–rapid eye movement (NREM) sleep
obstructive sleep apnea (OSA)
polysomnogram (PSG)
rapid eye movement (REM) sleep
respiratory disturbance index (RDI)
retrognathia
sleep apnea
sleep continuity theory
sleep latency
sudden infant death syndrome (SIDS)
upper airway resistance syndrome (UARS)

CHAPTER OVERVIEW

For most people, sleep is a time to relax and recover from the day's efforts. For those with sleep disorders, however, sleep may not provide refreshment and recovery. In addition, when a sleep-related breathing disorder is present, sleep can precipitate life-threatening problems.

Sleep-related breathing problems occur in about 5% of adult men, with this figure being somewhat lower in women.[1] In adults over 60 years of age, the incidence of sleep-related breathing abnormalities increases significantly, with one report identifying a 37% incidence in this age group.[2]

Sleep disorders centers (SDCs) exist to evaluate and diagnose sleep-related breathing problems and a host of other sleep disorders. The recognition of sleep apnea problems and their clinical importance has led to a dramatic increase in the number of SDCs. Respiratory therapists (RTs) serve as technicians for the SDCs because of their expertise in breathing disorders. In this setting the RT may work as a sleep technician to evaluate patients with sleep disorders. In the hospital setting, RTs have many opportunities to observe patients with sleep disorders. In order to understand disturbed sleep, it is helpful to understand the basics of normal sleep.

NORMAL SLEEP STAGES

Everyone sleeps. Most humans sleep about 8 hours a night. Until recently, sleep was thought to be a homogeneous state of dormancy; however, sleep is a heterogeneous physiologic state

of activity. The normal sleeper progresses through a standard sequence of sleep during the night. Two basic types of sleep exist: non–rapid eye movement (NREM) and rapid eye movement (REM) sleep. The sleep stages of NREM and REM cycle every 60 to 90 minutes.

Non–Rapid Eye Movement Sleep

Sleep begins with NREM. NREM sleep has four different stages (Figure 18-1). Normal sleepers enter sleep stage 1 first. This stage is characterized by large eye rolls and low-amplitude waves on the electroencephalogram (EEG). During this transitional stage between sleep and wakefulness, the sleeper experiences drowsiness.

Within minutes after entering sleep stage 1, most sleepers progress to sleep stage 2. Sleep stage 2 is characterized by sleep spindles on the EEG recording (a quick burst of waveforms at 12 to 14 Hz), along with K complexes (large 75 μV waves) (see

Awake-low voltage-random, fast

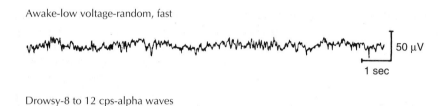

50 μV

1 sec

Drowsy-8 to 12 cps-alpha waves

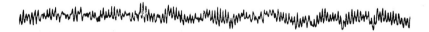

Stage 1-3 to 7 cps—theta waves

Theta waves

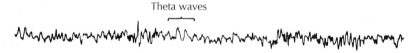

Stage 2-12 to 14 cps-sleep spindles and K complexes

Sleep spindle

K complex —

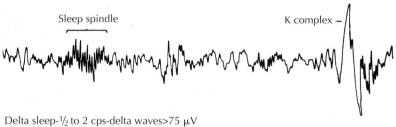

Delta sleep-½ to 2 cps-delta waves>75 μV

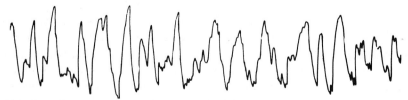

REM Sleep-low voltage-random, fast with sawtooth waves

Sawtooth waves   Sawtooth waves

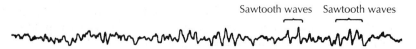

Figure 18-1 Human sleep stages. *REM,* Rapid eye movement. (From Hauri P: *The sleep disorders: current concepts,* ed 2, Kalamazoo, Mich, 1982, Upjohn.)

Figure 18-1). Sleep stage 2 is a deeper sleep state than sleep stage 1 and is the predominant stage of NREM sleep in adults. Approximately 10 to 20 minutes after entering sleep stage 2, the sleeper moves into sleep stages 3 and 4, which reflect increased depth of sleep. During sleep stages 3 and 4, commonly called *slow-wave sleep,* the sleeper may be difficult to rouse. Slow-wave sleep (also called delta sleep) is characterized by the presence of extremely high-amplitude waves (> 75 µV) (see Figure 18-1). The amount of time the sleeper stays in slow-wave sleep decreases with age and pathologic states.

Respiratory rate slows during NREM sleep.[3] The decrease in ventilation that results often causes a rise in arterial carbon dioxide pressure ($PaCO_2$) in the early stages of sleep. Also, during the beginning moments of sleep, respiration tends to be irregular in most persons.[3-5] However, once deeper stages of NREM sleep are reached, ventilation generally becomes rhythmic and continues to be so until the person wakens or enters REM sleep. Blood pressure decreases during NREM sleep about 5% to 10% during stages 1 and 2 and 8% to 14% in delta sleep.[6]

> ### SIMPLY STATED
> Breathing is regular during the deeper stages of NREM sleep, as compared with the lighter stages. Muscle tone is diminished during deeper stages of sleep.

Rapid Eye Movement Sleep (Dreaming)

REM begins in normal sleepers after 60 to 90 minutes of sleep. REM sleep is characterized by dreaming and by many profound physiologic changes (described later). Sleepers awakened from REM sleep almost always report dreaming, whereas those awakened from slow-wave sleep rarely report dreamlike experiences.

The normal sleeper experiences four or five REM episodes each night. REM episodes increase progressively in length and intensity throughout the night. The initial REM episode may last only 5 minutes, whereas the later episodes occurring toward morning may last 30 to 60 minutes. REM sleep accounts for about 20% to 25% of total sleep time over the human life span. Infants spend 55% to 80% of their time dreaming, and this drops off to adult amounts after about 6 months of life.

Because dreaming takes place in REM sleep, it may be regarded as a time of pleasure by the normal sleeper. However, for the sleeper with breathing difficulties, REM sleep may be a time of peril. During REM sleep, muscle tone, as measured by the electromyogram (EMG), is at a minimum. Thus during REM sleep, the sleeper is partially paralyzed. In addition, respiratory efforts are chaotic, even in healthy persons.[1,4] REM sleep, unlike slow-wave sleep, is associated with a diminished response to hypercapnia and hypoxemia.[5] This effect, coupled with a decrease in upper airway muscle tone, increases vulnerability to upper airway obstruction and hypoxemia during sleep. This is particularly true when respiration is compromised by

pulmonary disease or small upper airway dimensions (e.g., excessive upper airway tissue). Furthermore, the heart rate is variable during REM sleep, and cardiac arrhythmias are more common. Blood pressure often increases slightly over its NREM level.

Sleep amount is not the only factor predicting subsequent daytime performance and sleepiness. This is noted in sleep apnea patients. Sleep apnea patients may sleep more than 8 hours per night but are still profoundly sleepy in the daytime. Sleep continuity (the amount of continuous uninterrupted sleep between sleep arousals) is an important factor in determining the degree of daytime sleepiness.

Sleep continuity theory predicts that as sleep interruption increases, daytime alertness decreases.[7] Numerous studies have identified that sleepers who experience frequent arousals during the night have more sleepiness during the subsequent day.[7-11] Those who experience fewer interruptions during sleep are more alert and functional the following day. The amount of time in any sleep stage 1, 2, 3, 4 or REM does not predict performance or degree of sleepiness.

> ### SIMPLY STATED
> REM sleep is believed to be the time during which the sleeper experiences dreaming. The healthy sleeper experiences four or five REM episodes each night.

SLEEP-RELATED BREATHING DISORDERS

People with sleep disorders can exhibit a diverse spectrum of sleep difficulties, from sleeplessness (insomnia) to excessive daytime sleepiness. Sleep disorders may be present at birth but are much more common in adulthood and old age. The focus of this chapter is sleep-related breathing disorders (SDB). In this chapter the SDB continuum (primary snoring, upper airway resistance syndrome [UARS], and obstructive sleep apnea [OSA]),[12] will be discussed. In addition, central sleep apnea with a focus on sudden infant death syndrome and apparent life-threatening events (ALTE) will be described.

Definitions of Sleep-Disordered Breathing

Sleep apnea is defined as a cessation of airflow for at least 10 seconds, which occurs during sleep. Three types of apnea have been identified: *obstructive, central,* and *mixed.* Obstructive sleep apnea (OSA) is defined by an airflow reduction of > 70%, in the presence of respiratory effort. OSA is present when breathing is intermittently absent or significantly decreased during sleep despite persistent effort to breathe. Central sleep apnea (CSA) is defined as a 10-second or more period of apnea with no respiratory effort. Thus the drive to breathe is intermittently abnormal. Mixed apnea is present when patients have periods of both obstructive and central apnea during the same night of sleep.

A common term associated with OSA is hypopnea. Hypopnea is defined as a 30% reduction in airflow in the presence of a $\geq 4\%$ reduction in SaO_2 during sleep. Although airflow continues, the amount is markedly reduced and thus results in hypoxemia. Hypopneas also cause temporary arousals from sleep similar to obstructive apnea episodes.

In addition to apnea and hypopnea, ventilation during sleep can be disturbed by upper airway resistance syndrome (UARS). UARS occurs when there is increased negative intrathoracic pressure seen intermittently during breathing (increased work of breathing) with sleep but no significant oxygen desaturations. Such breathing difficulties often cause arousal from a deeper stage of sleep to a lighter stage. The patient who experiences these arousals may not remember them the next day because they do not become fully conscious in most cases. Thus the patient reports that his/her sleep was uneventful.

The exact type and severity of sleep-disordered breathing problems present in any patient is best determined in a sleep center using a polysomnogram (PSG). The PSG monitors multiple parameters during an all-night study of the patient's sleep. The PSG is described in detail later in this chapter.

An adult PSG is positive for sleep apnea if the respiratory disturbance index (RDI) is > 5 (the RDI is defined as the total of obstructive apneas, hypopneas, and central apneas per hour). In infants and children a PSG is considered abnormal if the RDI is > 1, if the oxygen saturation is < 92%, or if the end tidal CO_2 is > 53 mm Hg during episodes of apnea.[13,14]

Sleep-Disordered Breathing Severity

Sleep disorder specialists have not agreed on a single criterion of what constitutes mild, moderate, and severe sleep apnea. We do not attempt to divide the apnea indices into mild, moderate, and severe for children, since there are not enough data to support the diagnostic distinctions in this age group. In our SDC, we consider an RDI of 5-20 to be mild apnea, 20-40 to be moderate apnea, and greater than 40 to be severe apnea in adults. Although dividing groups in this way may provide an idea about the relative severity, many factors co-exist in these patients that may cause the clinician to consider one patient more severe than another. The most common co-factors are the level of excessive daytime sleepiness and the amount of changes in SaO_2 during the course of a PSG.

THE SLEEP-DISORDERED BREATHING CONTINUUM

Perhaps a helpful way to think about SDB is that the SDB syndromes lie on a continuum, which ranges from mild snoring to severe OSA (Figure 18-2). The SDB continuum can be helpful in understanding where a patient's particular SDB condition lies relative to another patient's SDB condition, or how a particular SDB condition changes with treatment or time. For example, inadequate treatment of severe OSA may leave the patient with UARS; therefore the patient is prone to the symptoms and clini-

cal consequences of UARS. This continuum is clinically helpful in SDB assessment. In this example, the UARS patient would then need further treatment to eliminate upper airway resistance and snoring so that symptoms are completely resolved.

Upper Airway Resistance Syndrome

As part of the SDB continuum, UARS patients have similar symptoms to those patients with snoring and OSA.[12,15] Patients with severe UARS have frequent sleep interruptions and PSG changes similar to those patients with OSA. One of the most important distinctions between UARS and OSA is that UARS patients do not become hypoxic during sleep, like their OSA counterparts. UARS patients have excessive daytime sleepiness (because of poor sleep continuity).

UARS patients often benefit from nasal continuous positive-airway pressure (CPAP), like snorers and OSA patients. Because of the similarities between UARS and OSA, but the increased complexity of making the UARS diagnosis, it is thought that UARS is underrecognized and undertreated.[15]

Obstructive Sleep Apnea and Hypopnea

OSA and hypopneas are the most common forms of SDB in adults. OSA is thought to occur because of an upper airway occlusion during sleep, and hypopnea is thought to be due to partial airway closure. OSA/hypopnea may be caused by several anatomic abnormalities, including micrognathia (small lower jaw), large tongue, large tonsils, retrognathia (underdevelopment of the mandible), or a deviated septum. Although the exact pathophysiological mechanism of OSA/hypopnea remains unclear, it is clear that the most common site of the obstruction is in the pharynx.

Pathophysiology

During sleep, the tissues in the upper airway relax to levels not seen during the waking state. As the airway becomes narrowed

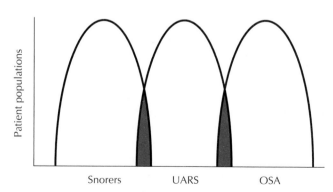

Figure 18-2 The continuum used to assess the patient with sleep-disordered breathing. The continuum ranges from primary snoring with no clinical signs and symptoms to obstructive sleep apnea *(OSA)* with severe clinical consequences. *UARS*, Upper airway resistance syndrome. (Modified from Downey R, Perkin RM, MacQuarrie J: *Sleep* 16:620, 1993.)

or occluded, there is an increased negative upper airway pressure. In response to the occlusion, the inspiratory muscles contract more forcefully and cause an increased negative intrathoracic pressure to overcome the obstruction. This is analogous to breathing through a wet paper straw. As you try to pull air through the straw, it closes more tightly.

Upper airway obstruction usually causes hypoxemia and sleep arousals. Muscle tone returns to the tissues in the upper airway with arousal, and the apnea is terminated. Normal ventilation resumes and the patient slowly drifts off to a deeper stage of sleep. The upper airway collapses again and the hypopnea/apnea returns. This sequence may recur throughout sleep and is usually worse when the patient is supine, in REM sleep, or when the upper airway tone is reduced by sleep deprivation, sedatives, or consumption of alcohol.

It has been shown that the predominant site of upper airway collapse in OSA is within the pharyngeal segments, between the tip of soft palate to the glottic inlet.[16] Examination of the OSA patient's airway may reveal enlarged tonsillar pillars, redundant soft palate tissue, macroglossia, and/or retrognathia. Such physical findings would lead to the conclusion that collapse of the upper airway during sleep is highly likely. This may be true, but the physical findings described are not always predictive of OSA on a PSG.[17]

Genetic factors may play a role in OSA. The diameter of the upper airway is smaller in some people with normal weight, and this tends to be inherited.[18] The role of compliance of the upper airway is also important. Patients with increased compliance of the upper airway are more prone to occlusion during sleep. Body habitus also plays a role in the incidence of OSA. The majority of patients who are seen in the SDC are overweight (60%-90% are at least 1 SD above normal weight); however, not all are. Therefore upper airway collapse in SDB depends on a number of complex interacting factors.[19,20]

Clinical Features of Obstructive Sleep Apnea

OSA patients suffer a number of consequences from their disorder (Box 18-1). Excessive daytime sleepiness (EDS) is experienced by many OSA patients and can be one of the most dangerous symptoms they develop. EDS is associated with impaired cognitive and psychomotor function. Drivers with untreated OSA are more likely to fall asleep while driving than are non-OSA drivers.[21] Drivers who fall asleep tend to be involved in more serious collisions.[22,23] However, most patients with sleep apnea do not have automobile crashes. Moreover, there are currently no reliable tests to decide who is safe or unsafe driving.

The typical history of a patient with OSA is an obese middle-aged man who snores loudly, is excessively sleepy, and is reported to stop his breathing at night. Snoring is almost always present in patients with OSA. When a patient's history is taken, the exclusion of other causes of poor sleep continuity (e.g., periodic limb movement disorder, depression, medical disorders, environmental interferences) is important. The three cardinal symptoms of sleep apnea can be remembered as an alliteration of three S's: Snoring (loud, habitual), Spousal apnea report or witnessed apneas by others, and Sleepiness (daytime, excessive).

BOX 18-1 Clinical Features of Obstructive Sleep Apnea

Snoring
Excessive daytime sleepiness
Morning headaches
Sleep fragmentation
Memory loss
Confusional awakenings
Personality changes
Impotence
Night sweats
Cardiac dysrhythmias
Pulmonary and systemic hypertension
Congestive heart failure
Enuresis

Other Symptoms

Non-restorative sleep
A choking sensation or gasping during the night
Morning headaches, probably because of hypercapnia during sleep
Insomnia
Restless sleep
Sore throat or dry throat upon waking in the morning
Cognitive deficits; memory and intellectual impairment
Decreased vigilance
Morning confusion
Personality and mood changes, including depression and anxiety
Sexual dysfunction, including impotence and decreased libido
Gastroesophageal reflux

SIMPLY STATED
Patients with OSA complain of excessive daytime sleepiness and loud snoring (observed by their bed partner).

Physical Examination

Airway features of OSA may include severe nasal obstruction, low-hanging soft palate, large uvula, enlarged tonsils/adenoids, macroglossia, and large neck circumference (collar size > 17.5 in). Systemic arterial hypertension (HTN) is present in approximately 50% of patients with OSA. Craniofacial abnormalities may be present, including malocclusion of jaws with anterior over jet of incisor teeth. Patients with obesity hypoventilation syndrome (and some patients with OSA) may have evidence of pulmonary HTN, right heart failure (e.g., JVD and pedal edema) and congestive heart failure (CHF). Some patients develop polycythemia because of intermittent hypoxemia at night caused by SDB.

Medical Characteristics of SDB Patients

One important risk factor for adult and childhood OSA is obesity,[24-26] and obesity is rapidly increasing in children.[24] An increase of one standard deviation (SD) in any measure of body composition is related to a three- to five-time increase in the risk of OSA.[25,26] Recently, a link between SDB in obese children and the presence of insulin resistance has been made.[27]

In a study of 62 obese children, researchers demonstrated a positive correlation between the degree of hyperinsulinemia and SDB severity. The RDI, glucose level, and measures of the degree of hypoxemia during sleep were associated with fasting insulin level.[28] Similar to the findings observed in obese children, studies of adult obese subjects with SDB found a higher degree of insulin resistance compared with weight-matched control subjects without SDB.[27-33] The importance of these observations stems from the belief that insulin resistance is the primary precursor of the metabolic syndrome, which includes a constellation of obesity, HTN, insulin resistance, and hyperinsulinemia[29]

Changes in the heart rate and cardiac dysrhythmias are more common in OSA patients. Bradycardia often occurs during the apneic period and is followed by tachycardia immediately after the apnea.[34] Premature ventricular contractions occur in approximately 20% of patients with OSA and are the most common dysrhythmia.[35] Asystole occurs in about 10% of cases and usually lasts for only a few seconds. HTN is common in OSA patients, as is poor HTN control[36-38] Once co-factors such as gender and BMI are accounted for, OSA patients are two times more likely to develop HTN than are nonapneic control patients. OSA patients are almost two times as likely to have a stroke versus non-OSA patients.[39]

CHF is associated with OSA and CSA. Correction of the CSA and OSA may lead to improvement in longevity in CHF patients. Mansfield and others[40] have examined the use of CPAP in OSA and heart failure. Patients were optimized on traditional medications for their CHF before entering the study. Patients were randomized into two groups: control or treatment. The treatment group received CPAP for 3 months while the control group only received lifestyle advice for 3 months. CPAP significantly improved cardiac function, sympathetic activity, and quality of life. Interestingly, this effect was not correlated with the patient's RDI. This study concluded that CPAP improves heart function, particularly the left ventricle's effectiveness, decreases sympathetic nervous system tone, and improves quality of life in OSA patients.

CHILDREN AND INFANTS WITH SLEEP-DISORDERED BREATHING

Snoring is a hallmark symptom of OSA in the child, as in the adult.[41-43] Pediatric SDB patients can be of any age or gender and may be overweight or have failure to thrive. In the infant, specific and numerous anomalies are linked with sleep apnea, more so than in the typical adult patient, making evaluation of pediatric sleep apnea more complex (Box 18-2). PSG features are also quite different in infants and children. Unfortunately, questionnaires cannot reliably predict OSA in the child.[41]

The SDB child may be either sleepy or hyperactive and have a variety of other problems, including developmental

---

BOX 18-2   Syndromes Commonly Associated with Sleep-Disordered Breathing in Children

Adenotonsillar hypertrophy
Craniofacial anomalies or abnormalities
Obesity
Neuromuscular disorders
Prader-Willi syndrome
Sickle cell disease
Mucopolysaccharidoses
Bronchopulmonary dysplasia
Chronic nasal obstruction
Laryngomalacia

Adapted from Gozal D: Sleep-disordered breathing and school performance in children, *Pediatrics* 102:616-620, 1998.

---

delay, poor school performance, aggressive behavior, and social withdrawal.[44,45] Although rare, brain damage, seizures, and coma can result from asphyxial brain damage.[45] Untreated OSA can have a negative influence on school performance and behavior. Gozal[46] found that first-graders who had an unusually high prevalence of snoring and nocturnal gas exchange abnormalities were poor achievers until their SDB was treated. After treatment, their academic scores significantly improved.

Inattentive and hyperactive behavior is highly prevalent among school-aged children and is often associated with a clinical psychiatric syndrome such as attention-deficit/hyperactivity disorder (ADHD).[47] In many instances, unrecognized medical conditions underlie the problematic behavior.[48] One such medical condition may be obstructive sleep-disordered breathing.[49] Clinical series from the SDCs report that inattentive and hyperactive behavior are common among children with OSA or UARS[50,51] and that treatment of either form of SDB is often associated with improved behavior and decreased need for medication.[47,51-53] These results underscore the importance of screening all children who have symptoms suggestive of ADHD for sleep problems. SDB may either play a causative role or exacerbate the clinical appearance of ADHD in a given child.[53]

Central Sleep Apnea in Children

Documented cases of CSA make up less than 10% of all cases of adult sleep apnea[54] but are more often seen in infants and young children.

Pathophysiology

CSA occurs when there is a cessation of airflow resulting from lack of movement of the diaphragm; thus CSA represents a loss of ventilatory drive or rhythmicity. During sleep, behavioral control of ventilation may be absent, placing ventilation under the control of the metabolic system. Ventilation is governed by afferent input from chemoreceptors and vagal intrapulmonary receptors during sleep. The development of sleep-induced apnea represents instability of these control mechanisms that maintain normal blood gas homeostasis. In addition, normally sleep depresses both hypoxic and hypercapnic ventilatory response.[55] In children, various factors may play a role in precipitating an episode of CSA, which may include cardiac, hematologic, infectious, metabolic, neurologic, gastrointestinal, or neuromuscular abnormalities.[44]

Clinical Features of Central Sleep Apnea

Many patients with CSA experience few daytime effects. The most significant difference between OSA and CSA patients is their body habitus. CSA patients often have a normal body habitus, whereas the OSA patient is often obese. Because most persons with sleep apnea have components of both OSA and CSA, many of the clinical features of each type are common to most SDB patients. The reason most sleepers have a mixed component of apnea is not known.

SUDDEN INFANT DEATH SYNDROME AND APPARENT LIFE-THREATENING EVENTS

Most people associate breathing problems in infants with sudden infant death syndrome (SIDS); however, SIDS is only one of the many potential sleep-related breathing disorders in children. SIDS, by definition, has no known cause. It is the leading cause of death in children under the age of 1 year. SIDS has a peak incidence between 2 and 4 months of age, and the majority of cases occur in the first 6 months of life.

Apparent life-threatening events (ALTEs) are events in which the infant appears to be dying because of apnea during sleep and may have associated skin color changes (pallor and cyanosis) and muscle tone changes. The number of infants in the United States who experience ALTEs is not known.

OSA may be a risk factor for ALTEs and SIDS.[56-60] The exact relationship between ALTEs and SIDS is not known. Data from a large-scale prospective study in Belgium, however, revealed that patients who had undergone PSG, and who later died of SIDS, had episodes of OSA, less movement time, and more regurgitation after feeding. CSA was not a significant predictor of SIDS in this study.[56] Other data suggest that supine sleep is safer than prone sleep in otherwise healthy infants.[61] Deaths have been reduced because of the promotion of infants sleeping on their backs. There has been a 15% to 20% decrease since the guidelines were written by the American Academy of Pediatrics.[61] The frequency of prone sleeping has thus decreased and the SIDS rate has decreased by more than 40%.[62,63]

Despite these encouraging statistics, SIDS remains the highest cause of infant death beyond the neonatal period, and there are still several potentially modifiable risk factors. Although some of these factors have been known for many years (e.g., maternal smoking), the importance of other hazards, such as soft bedding and covered airways, have been demonstrated only recently.[63]

ASSESSMENT OF SLEEP-RELATED BREATHING DISORDERS

Bedside Observations

Observation of the hospitalized patient during sleep may provide the opportunity to evaluate the patient's gross sleeping characteristics. The evaluator should identify whether the patient snores and should pay strict attention to whether the patient has pauses in respiration. If pauses are present, they should be timed. As part of this observation, the sleeping position, presence or absence of cyanosis, and breathing effort should be noted. If the patient is hospitalized for several days or nights, a series of observations may coalesce into a broad evaluation of the patient's sleeping pattern. A referral to a sleep center for the appropriate diagnosis is in order if the patient is noted to have pauses in breathing with sleep.

Laboratory Assessment

The primary tool used to evaluate patients with sleep-disordered breathing is the PSG. During the PSG, electroencephalogram (EEG) is used to determine sleep stages, arousals, and other abnormal EEG activity. Eye movements are measured using a two-channel electrooculogram (EOG). This is useful to detect the onset of REM sleep. Chin EMG recording is used to measure chin muscle activity. The EMG is particularly important in the identification of REM sleep, because in REM sleep there is a complete loss of chin activity on the EMG (Figure 18-3). The typical clinical PSG also includes a one-lead ECG to recognize arrhythmias associated with episodes of apnea and a leg EMG (electrodes placed over the anterior tibialis muscles of both legs) to determine whether the patient experiences leg movements during sleep.

To record respirations, electrodes are placed on the upper and lower chest or abdomen to detect movement in these regions, and a dual bead thermistor is used to detect oral and nasal airflow (Figure 18-4). Snoring microphones pick up noise in the throat and thus can be a good qualitative indication of the presence of snoring. Snoring typically has a recurrent pattern that is often easy to detect. Snoring is characterized by its volume (mild, moderate, or loud), its presence in different sleep positions (supine, prone, side), and its quality (wheezing, stridorous, cacophonous) by the technician.

End-tidal CO_2 or transcutaneous CO_2 is routinely monitored in infants and children. SpO_2, via pulse oximetry, is measured concomitantly during the PSG and can be directly correlated with the changes in respiration. For example, during apnea it is common for oxygen saturation to decrease (see Figure 18-4).

It is important to note that oximetry alone is insufficient to diagnose or exclude SDB. Some practitioners use oximetry as a "screening" test for sleep apnea. This is unfortunate because a negative oximetry (one that does not show recurrent SaO_2 changes) cannot exclude UARS. Moreover, it may delay care.

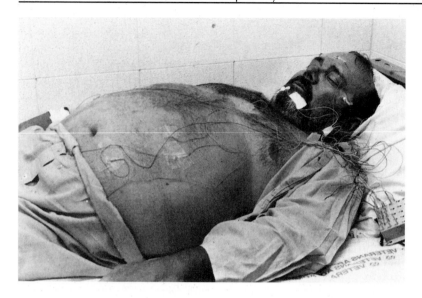

Figure 18-3 Patient with sleep apnea syndrome being monitored with electrodes to detect chest and abdominal movement. Electroencephalograph lead placement includes C3-A2, OZ-A1, and electrodes to detect eye movements. Chin electromyograph detects muscle tension.

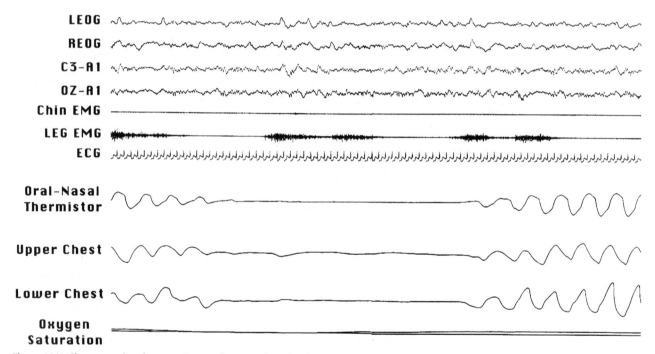

Figure 18-4 Sleep recording from a patient undergoing clinical polysomnography (sleep study):

Channel 1: left eye electrooculogram (*LEOG*)

Channel 2: right eye electrooculogram (*REOG*)

Channel 3: electroencephalogram (*EEG*): C3 placement referenced to A1

Channel 4: EEG: central channel (*CZ*) placement referenced to A1

Channel 5: chin electromyograph (*EMG*)

Channel 6: leg EMG

Channel 7: electrocardiogram (*ECG*)

Channel 8: nasal-oral thermistor (measures airflow through the mouth and nose)

Channel 9: upper chest movement

Channel 10: lower chest movement (abdomen)

Channel 11: oxygen saturation reading from oximeter.

Many SDCs, including ours, use a split night study protocol, where the first part of the PSG night is spent making the SDB diagnosis, and, if appropriate, the second half is spent titrating CPAP to correct SDB.

The American Academy of Sleep Medicine has guidelines written for PSG testing.[64] In the view of the panel of experts who have reviewed the existing data, the PSG is the gold standard for diagnosing patients suspected of having sleep apnea. Oximetry monitoring to screen for OSA and home testing are of limited use. A list of member centers that meet the highest professional standards set forth by sleep medicine practitioners can be found at www.AASM.org.

SIMPLY STATED

The gold standard for evaluating the patient thought to have OSA is the PSG.

Multiple Sleep Latency Testing

In the patient whose reported sleepiness seems out of proportion to his/her level of SDB, a multiple sleep latency test (MSLT) is recommended after an overnight PSG. Sleep latency is defined as the amount of time required for sleep onset after going to bed. Individuals with excessive daytime sleepiness will fall asleep quickly even during daytime naps repeated throughout the day.

The MSLT is the most reliable and valid test used to assess daytime sleepiness objectively. After sleeping the same amount of time at night in the SDC as they do at home, patients take a series of four or five naps, every 2 hours during hours they are normally awake. Before the MSLT, patients must be drug free for a period of about 2 weeks, especially from drugs that may affect sleep (particularly REM sleep). The sleep-wake schedule must be routine for at least 7 days before testing, and a nocturnal PSG must be performed the night before the MSLT to rule out other sleep disorders that may affect the test results.[65]

An MSLT is interpreted by measuring the average sleep latency for four or five daytime naps taken by the patient. It is normal to stay awake for more than 15 minutes during the daytime on the MSLT. At the other extreme, if someone falls asleep in less than 5 to 8 minutes on average, this is considered to be severe sleepiness.[66] This level of sleepiness is not specific to one sleep disorder but is often associated with OSA, UARS, narcolepsy, and sleep deprivation, among other sleep disorders.

SIMPLY STATED

The MSLT measures true daytime sleepiness. The patient who consistently falls asleep in less than 8 minutes during a daytime nap is suffering from a sleep disorder that needs immediate attention.

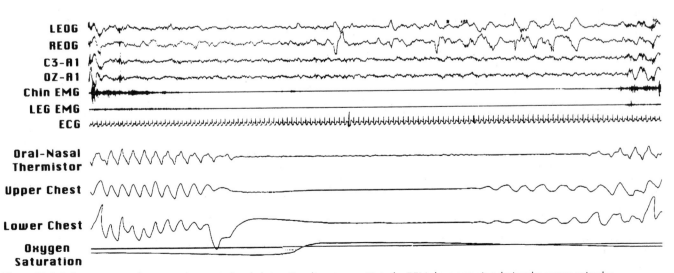

Figure 18-5 Polysomnogram demonstrating central and obstructive sleep apnea. Note the REM sleep occuring during the apnea episodes.

CASE STUDY 1

D.B. is a 40-year-old man who comes to his attending physician in the outpatient clinic with complaints of severe fatigue and daytime sleepiness. D.B. is accompanied by his wife, who states that her husband snores loudly throughout the night with occasional pauses in breathing followed by gasping for air. D.B.'s wife indicates that D.B. is a restless sleeper. D.B. smokes two packs of cigarettes per day and has been smoking for the past 22 years.

Physical examination:

D.B. is 68 in. tall and weighs 240 lb. Therefore, his body mass index (BMI) is 36.5. He appears lethargic but is oriented to time, place, and person. His vital signs at rest are: blood pressure, 140/85 mm Hg; respiratory rate, 26 breaths per minute; and heart rate, 110 beats per minute. D.B. has a short, thick neck with enlarged tonsils and a hypopharynx that is narrowed by excessive fatty tissue. D.B. is a mouth breather with nasal-sounding speech. His breath sounds are diminished bilaterally. A loud P_2 was noted during auscultation over the precordium.

Laboratory data:

A routine ECG revealed right axis deviation and was consistent with cor pulmonale. The complete blood count was normal except for polycythemia. A chest film revealed mild cardiomegaly. The patient was referred to the sleep center for a PSG. The PSG study revealed the following:

Obstructive and hypopnea index:	50
Central apnea index:	0
Minimum SaO_2:	75%
No. of desaturation events:	137
Arousals per hour of sleep:	50

Stage 1 sleep:	50% (normal = 1%-5%)
Stage 2 sleep:	25% (normal = 45%-55%)
Stage 3 and 4 sleep:	0% (normal = 0%-5%)
REM sleep:	20% (normal = 15%-25%)
Technician comments:	Loud snoring in all sleep positions: restlessness observed throughout the night.

Interpretation and Impression:

Severe OSA is present because the apnea index is greater than 40. Frequent arousals occur, which probably explains D.B.'s excessive daytime sleepiness. The frequent episodes of desaturation may be contributing to the cor pulmonale because the hypoxemia triggers significant increases in pulmonary vascular resistance. The distribution of sleep is abnormal and consistent with frequent nocturnal arousals. The patient is experiencing no delta sleep (stages 3 and 4), less than normal amounts of stage 2 sleep, and an increased amount of stage 1 sleep. Figure 18-5 provides a sample of the PSG demonstrating the obstructive apnea in this case.

Recommendations:

- CPAP trial with pressure titration during the course of follow-up PSG.
- Orthodontic appliance evaluation may be considered if CPAP is not tolerated. Ear, nose, and throat consultation for evaluation of the upper airway problems.
- Dietary consultation and endocrinology evaluation for obesity.
- Follow-up sleep study to evaluate effects of treatment, if indicated clinically.

REVIEW QUESTIONS

1. What percentage of men are thought to have a sleep-related breathing disorder?
   a. 1%
   b. 5%
   c. 7.5%
   d. 10%

2. What is the predominant stage of NREM sleep?
   a. Stage 1
   b. Stage 2
   c. Stage 3
   d. Stage 4

3. T F Breathing tends to be irregular during the early stages of NREM sleep.

4. T F Blood pressure tends to increase during the initial stages of sleep.

5. T F During REM sleep the sleeper is partially paralyzed.

6. T F Breathing is very regular during REM sleep in most sleepers.

7. Which of the following is the key concept related to the definition of central sleep apnea?

a. Intermittent absence of respiratory effort
b. Intermittent upper airway obstruction
c. Intermittent central airway obstruction
d. Intermittent reductions in tidal volume

8. Hypopneas are most closely linked to what type of SDB problem?
   a. Central apnea
   b. Obstructive apnea
   c. UARS
   d. All of the above

9. Which of the following is *not* believed to be responsible for the onset of obstructive sleep apnea?
   a. Relaxation of the upper airway muscles
   b. Tremendous increase in upper airway resistance
   c. More forceful contraction of the inspiratory muscles
   d. Significant decrease in static lung compliance

10. Which of the following clinical features is *not* typical for adult patients with obstructive sleep apnea?
    a. Excessive daytime sleepiness
    b. Inspiratory stridor during daytime examination
    c. Loud snoring during sleep
    d. Impaired cognitive function

11. What is the most common arrhythmia seen in OSA patients?
    a. Bradycardia
    b. PVCs
    c. Asystole
    d. First-degree block

12. Which of the following problems is/are seen in children with SDB?
    a. Excessive daytime sleepiness
    b. Hyperactivity
    c. Aggressive behavior
    d. All of the above

13. What is the peak age of onset for SIDS?
    a. Birth to 2 months
    b. 2 to 4 months
    c. 3 to 8 months
    d. 6 to 10 months

14. Which of the following parameters is *not* typically monitored during a polysomnogram?
    a. EEG
    b. ECG
    c. Leg EMG
    d. Minute volume

15. Which of the following tests is used to assess the degree of daytime sleepiness?
    a. Polysomnogram
    b. MSLT

c. Bonet's insomnia questionnaire
d. None of the above

REFERENCES

1. White DP: Disorders of breathing during sleep: introduction, epidemiology and incidence, *Semin Respir Med* 9:529, 1988.
2. Carskadon M, Dement W: Respiration during sleep in the aged human, *J Gerontol* 36:420, 1981.
3. Douglas NJ, White DP, Weil JV: Respiration during sleep in normal man, *Thorax* 37:840, 1982.
4. Kreiger J: Breathing during sleep in normal subjects, *Clin Chest Med* 6:577, 1985.
5. Naifeh KH, Kamiya J: The nature of respiratory changes associated with sleep onset, *Sleep* 4:49, 1981.
6. Shepard JW, Bradley TD: Hypertension, cardiac arrhythmias, myocardial infarction, and stroke in relation to obstructive sleep apnea, *Clin Chest Med* 13:437, 1992.
7. Bonnet MH: Effect of sleep disruption on sleep, performance, and mood, *Sleep* 8:11, 1985.
8. Downey III R, Bonnet MH: Performance during frequent sleep disruption, *Sleep* 10(4),354, 1987.
9. Bonnet MH: Performance and sleepiness as a function of frequency and placement of sleep disruption, *Psychophysiology* 23:263, 1986.
10. Bonnet MH: Performance and sleepiness following moderate sleep disruption and slow wave sleep deprivation, *Physiol Behav* 37:915, 1986.
11. Colt HG, Helmut H, Rich GB: Hypoxemia vs sleep fragmentation as cause of excessive daytime sleepiness in obstructive sleep apnea, *Chest* 100:1542, 1991.
12. Downey R III, Perkin RM, MacQuarrie J: Upper airway resistance syndrome: sick, symptomatic but underrecognized, *Sleep* 16:620, 1993.
13. Marcus CL and others: Normal polysomnographic values for children and adolescents, *Am Rev Respir Dis* 146:1235, 1992.
14. Uliel S and others: Normal polysomnographic respiratory values in children and adolescents. *Chest* 125(3):872, 2004.
15. Guilleminault C and others: Recognition of sleep-disordered breathing in children, *Pediatrics* 98:871, 1996.
16. Remmers JE and others: Pathogenesis of the upper airway occlusion during sleep. *J Appl Physiol* 44:931, 1978.
17. Downey III R, Lim R, and Wilms DJ: Predicting obstructive sleep apnea severity using waking laryngoscopy and the Muller maneuver. *Sleep Res* 19, 225. 1990
18. Smith PL, Schwartz AR: Biomechanics of the Upper Airway During Sleep. In Pack, AI (Ed): *Sleep Apnea: Pathogenesis, Diagnosis, and Treatment.* Marcel-Dekker, New York, 2002.
19. Younes, M.: Contributions of upper airway mechanics and control mechanisms to severity of obstructive apnea, *Am J Respir Crit Care Med* 168:645, 2003.

20. Dempsey JA and others: Sleep-induced respiratory instabilities. In Pack, AI (Ed): *Sleep Apnea: Pathogenesis, Diagnosis, and Treatment.* Marcel-Dekker, New York, 2002.

21. Findley LJ, Unverzagt ME, Suratt PM: Automobile accidents involving patients with obstructive sleep apnea, *Am Rev Respir Dis* 138:337, 1988.

22. Findley LJ, Weiss J, Jabour E: Serious automobile crashes caused by undetected sleep apnea, *Arch Intern Med* 151:1451, 1991.

23. Findley LJ, Levinson MP, Bonnie RJ: Driving performance and auto accidents in patients with sleep apnea, *Clin Chest Med* 13:427, 1992.

24. Strauss RS, Pollack HA: Epidemic increase in childhood overweight, 1986-1998. *JAMA* 286:284, 2001.

25. Young T and others: The occurrence of sleep-disordered breathing among middle-aged adults. *N Engl J Med* 328:1230, 1993.

26. Redline S and others: Risk factors for sleep-disordered breathing in children. Associations with obesity, race, and respiratory problems. *Am J Respir Crit Care Med* 159:1527, 1999.

27. De la Eva RC and others: Metabolic correlates with obstructive sleep apnea in obese subjects. *J Pediatr* 140:654, 2002.

28. Vgontzas AN and others: Sleep apnea and daytime sleepiness and fatigue: relation to visceral obesity, insulin resistance and hypercytokinemia. *J Clin Endocrinol Metab* 85(3):1151, 2000.

29. Liese AD, Mayer-Davis EJ, Haffner SM: Development of the multiple metabolic syndrome: an epidemiologic perspective. *Epidemiol Rev* 20:157, 1998.

30. Willi SM and others: The effects of high-protein, low-fat, ketogenic diet on adolescents with morbid obesity. *Pediatrics* 101:61, 1998.

31. Naresh M and others: Sleep-disordered breathing and insulin resistance in middle-aged and overweight men. *Am J Respir Crit Care Med* 165:677, 2002.

32. Mary SM and others: Obstructive sleep apnea is independently associated with insulin resistance. *Am J Respir Crit Care Med* 165:670, 2002.

33. Harsch IA and others: Continuous positive airway pressure treatment rapidly improves insulin sensitivity in patients with obstructive sleep apnea syndrome. *Am J Respir Crit Care Med* 169:156, 2004.

34. Zwillich CW and others: Bradycardia during sleep apnea: its characteristics and mechanisms, *Am Rev Respir Dis* 125:234, 1982.

35. Romaker AM, Ancoli-Israel S: The diagnosis of sleep-related breathing disorders, *Clin Chest Med* 8, 1987.

36. Grote L, Hedner J, Peter JH: Sleep-related breathing disorder is an independent risk factor for uncontrolled hypertension. *J Hypertens* 19:679, 2000.

37. Lavie P, Hoftstein V: Sleep apnea syndrome: a possible contributing factor to resistant hypertension. *Sleep* 24:721, 2001.

38. Logan AG and others: High prevalence of unrecognized sleep apnea in drug-resistant hypertension. *J Hypertens* 19(12):2271, 2001.

39. Moe T and others: Sleep disordered breathing and coronary artery disease: Long term prognosis. *Am J. Respir Crit Care Med* 164:1910, 2001.

40. Mansfield DR and others: Controlled trial of continuous positive airway pressure in obstructive sleep apnea and heart failure. *Am J Respir Crit Care Med* 169:361, 2004.

41. Brouillette R and others: A diagnostic approach to suspected obstructive sleep apnea in children, *J Pediatr* 105:10, 1984.

42. Carroll JL and others: Inability of clinical history to distinguish primary snoring from obstructive sleep apnea syndrome in children, *Chest* 108:610, 1995.

43. Nieminen P and others: Snoring children: factors predicting sleep apnea, *Acta Otolaryngol* S529:190, 1997.

44. Perkin RM, Downey R III, MacQuarrie J: Sleep disordered breathing in infants and children, *Respir Clin North Am* 5(3):395, 1999.

45. Brooks LJ: Sleep-disordered breathing in children, *Respir Care* 43:394, 1998.

46. Gozal D: Sleep-disordered breathing and school performance in children, *Pediatrics* 102:616, 1998.

47. Chervin RD and others: Inattention, hyperactivity, and symptoms of sleep-disordered breathing. *Pediatrics* 109:449, 2002.

48. Zametkin AJ, Ernst M: Problems in the management of attention-deficit-hyperactivity disorder. *N Engl J Med* 340:40, 1999.

49. Chervin RD. Attention-deficit-hyperactivity disorder (letter). *N Engl J Med* 340:1766, 1999.

50. Guilleminault C, Korobkin R, Winkle R: A review of 50 children with obstructive sleep apnea syndrome. *Lung* 159:275, 1981.

51. Guilleminault C and others: Children and nocturnal snoring-evaluation of the effects of sleep related respiratory resistive load and daytime functioning. *Eur J Pediatr* 139:165, 1982.

52. Ali NJ, Pitson D, Stradling JR: Sleep disordered breathing: effects of adenotonsillectomy on behavior and psychological functioning. *Eur J Pediatr* 155:56, 1996.

53. Owens JA and others: Parental and self-report of sleep in children with attention-deficit/hyperactivity disorder. *Arch Pediatr Adolesc Med* 154:549, 2000.

54. Guilleminault C, van den Hoed J, Mitler M: Clinical overview of the sleep apnea syndromes. In Guilleminault C, Dement W (eds): *Sleep apnea syndromes,* New York, 1978, Alan R Liss.

55. Onal E: Central sleep apnea. *Semin Respir Med* 9:547, 1988.

56. Kahn A and others: Sleep and cardiorespiratory characteristics of infant victims of sudden death: a prospective case-control study. *Sleep* 15:287, 1992.

57. Guilleminault C and others: Five cases of near-miss sudden infant death syndrome and development of obstructive sleep apnea syndrome, *Pediatrics* 73:71, 1984.

58. Guilleminault C and others: Upper airway resistance in infants at risk for sudden infant death syndrome. *J Pediatr* 122:881, 1993.

59. Tishler PV and others: The association of sudden unexpected infant death with obstructive sleep apnea. *Am J Respir Crit Care Med* 153:157, 1996.

60. McNamara F, Sullivan CE: Obstructive sleep apnea in infants: Relation to family history of sudden infant death syndrome, apparent life-threatening events, and obstructive sleep apnea. *J Pediatric* 136:318, 2000.

61. American Academy of Pediatrics Task Force on Infant Positioning and SIDS: Positioning and SIDS. *Pediatrics* 89:1120, 1992.

62. American Academy of Pediatrics: Positioning and sudden infant death syndrome (SIDS): update, *Pediatrics* 98:1216, 1996.

63. American Academy of Pediatrics Task Force on Infant Sleep Position and Sudden Infant Death Syndrome. Changing concepts of sudden infant death syndrome: Implications for infant sleeping environment and sleep position. *Pediatrics* 105:650-656, 2000.

64. American Sleep Disorders Association: Indications for Polysomnography Task Force: Practice parameters for the indications for polysomnography and related procedures. *Sleep* 20(6):406-422, 1997.

65. Association of Sleep Disorders Centers Task Force on Daytime Sleepiness, Carskadon MA, chairman: Guidelines for the multiple sleep latency test (MSLT): a standard measure of sleepiness, *Sleep* 9:519, 1986.

66. Aldrich MS, Chervin RD, Malow BA: Value of the multiple sleep latency test (MSLT) for the diagnosis of narcolepsy, *Sleep* 20(8):620, 1997.

BIBLIOGRAPHY

Guilleminault C, editor: *Sleeping and waking: indications and techniques,* Menlo Park, Calif, 1982, Addison-Wesley.

Kryger MH, Roth T, Dement WC: *Principles and practice of sleep medicine,* ed 3. Philadelphia, 2000, WB Saunders.

Downey R III, Wickramasinghe H. Sleep Apnea. Sharma S and others, editors. Available at www.Emedicine.com.

Hoffstein V. Apnea and snoring: State of the art and future directions. *Acta Otorhinolaryngol Belg* 56:205-236, 2002.

Assessment of the Home Care Patient

LEARNING OBJECTIVES

Upon completion of this chapter, the reader should be able to accomplish the following:

1. Identify the importance and benefits of respiratory home care.
2. Identify the type of patients who receive home respiratory care.
3. Recognize the key elements involved in home respiratory care assessment.
4. Recognize the role of the respiratory therapist in home care.
5. Identify the components involved in the initial home care evaluation.
6. Recognize the purpose and the procedure for developing a plan of care.
7. Identify helpful strategies to use during patient education in the home.
8. Recognize the purpose of follow-up care.

CHAPTER OUTLINE

Importance of Respiratory Home Care
The Home Care Patient
Hospital Versus Home Care Assessment
Qualifications of the Home Care Respiratory Therapist
Assessment and the Home Visit
  Initial Visit
  Plan of Care
  Patient Education and Training
  Follow-Up Care
  Equipment Maintenance
  Discharging the Patient

KEY TERMS

home care
home medical equipment (HME)

CHAPTER OVERVIEW

Home care continues to be a rapidly growing segment of patient care.[1] This is partially explained by the fact that chronic obstructive pulmonary disease (COPD) is ranked the fourth most common cause of death in the United States and the only major disease that is rising in prevalence and mortality.[2,3] Home care is considered an essential component of the short- and long-term treatment of the patient with COPD and other pulmonary diseases. In today's healthcare climate of cost controls and managed care, treating patients at home—the least expensive site of care—is the preferred method whenever possible. Although the patient's personal residence is still the primary site of care, group homes, assisted living facilities, and residential treatment facilities are other common sites for home care.

Respiratory home care is defined by the American Association for Respiratory Care as "those prescribed respiratory services provided in a patient's personal residence. Prescribed respiratory care services include, but are not limited to, patient assessment and monitoring, diagnostic and therapeutic modalities and services, disease management, and patient and caregiver education."[4] Increasing numbers of respiratory therapists (RTs) are employed as respiratory home care providers, primarily with home medical equipment (HME) companies. Many RTs find themselves without the necessary skills to practice respiratory home care proficiently. These skills include time management, communication and teaching skills, decision making, and the ability to perform all types of respiratory therapy modalities (and some nonrespiratory modalities). The most important skill at which the RT must be proficient is patient assessment. This chapter presents the many aspects of assessment used to evaluate the home care patient.

IMPORTANCE OF RESPIRATORY HOME CARE

Soaring costs for acute medical care and changes in third-party reimbursement have shifted the focus of care toward reducing the length of a patient's stay in an acute care facility and moving the patient more quickly along the healthcare continuum. As a result, procedures once performed only in an acute care facility, such as tracheostomy tube changes, aerosolized antibiotic treatments, and ventilator weaning, are now being done in the patient's home. The availability of such services and the personnel to perform them enables physicians to discharge their patients from the hospital earlier and many times to not admit them at all.

The major benefits of home care are obvious: It decreases overall expenditures for medical care while reducing the length and number of future hospitalizations. However, there are other benefits that are important in their own right. Home care enhances a patient's ability to independently manage his/her care. Staying at home improves the patient's quality of life. It allows technology-dependent patients to go home rather than being placed in a long-term care facility. In addition, with the number of people with chronic medical conditions estimated to rise from 105 million in the year 2000 to 167 million in 2050, home care will also provide RTs with many new opportunities.[5]

THE HOME CARE PATIENT

A wide array of patients can benefit from home care services. It is estimated that 44% of patients discharged from the hospital require ongoing medical care that cannot be performed by family. An estimated 20% of patients older than 65 years have functional and physical problems that impair their ability to perform essential activities of daily living.[6]

The home care RT primarily sees patients with some form of chronic lung disease. Emphysema, asthma, and chronic bronchitis are health problems the RT is likely to see daily. Sleep-disordered breathing, infant apnea, and other debilitating illnesses also are seen. Box 19-1 lists some of the most common disorders the home care RT encounters.

A patient with an acute exacerbation of his/her COPD may need short-term home care services designed to instruct and evaluate the patient on the use of home oxygen equipment, compressor nebulizer therapy, or a new medication schedule. Assessments should be performed to determine need, response

to therapy, and compliance and to identify emergent problems that could lead to a rebound hospitalization. Goals of care might be to assist the patient in becoming independent with his/her care: to self-administer nebulizer treatments as prescribed, to use and maintain the oxygen equipment as instructed, and to know when to call the oxygen provider. Once these goals are accomplished, the patient would be discharged from services.

Conversely, a patient requiring mechanical ventilation for life support requires home care services for as long as he/she remains at home. The technical nature of home ventilators and ancillary equipment necessitates frequent evaluation and maintenance to ensure proper function. Home ventilator users also require frequent physical assessment, again to determine compliance and response to therapy and to identify changes and emergent problems.

In the middle of the spectrum are patients who require limited home care services for days, weeks, or months for the treatment of infections, management of a tracheostomy or newly prescribed oxygen therapy, or stabilization on a program of noninvasive ventilation, for example. Home care services are terminated once the need no longer exists; however, the patient whose condition has changed or who has had a change in caregivers, environment, or equipment may need to have those services restarted.

SIMPLY STATED

The home care RT sees many types of patients and equipment, from technically simple to technically complex, very young to very old, with pulmonary and nonpulmonary diseases.

HOSPITAL VERSUS HOME CARE ASSESSMENT

The home care RT uses many of the methods of assessment used in the acute care setting. Many of the techniques of physical examination described in this book are used in home care (see Chapters 4 and 5). The major differences in assessment of the patient at home are the parameters evaluated and the types of diagnostic tools used. The primary tools used to conduct a home care patient assessment are very basic and may be considered rudimentary by the critical care practitioner. A stethoscope, sphygmomanometer, and oximeter are the most common devices used for physical assessment. Peak flowmeters and respirometers are used to assess basic pulmonary function on select patients, such as asthmatic and ventilator-assisted patients. End-tidal carbon dioxide monitors and portable diagnostic sleep-recording devices are used with increasing frequency, again for select patients. Oxygen analyzers, liter meters, and calibrated pressure gauges are used to monitor the function of home respiratory equipment.

It is important to understand the limitations of these portable assessment instruments. Most importantly, each

---

BOX 19-1   Disorders Commonly Encountered in Respiratory Home Care

- Chronic obstructive pulmonary disease
- Acute and chronic bronchitis, bronchiolitis
- Stable and unstable asthma
- Acute and resolving pneumonia
- Restrictive lung diseases
- Sleep-disordered breathing
- Acute upper respiratory infections
- Airway clearance problems
- Ventilatory insufficiency disorders
- Infant apnea, apnea of prematurity

parameter assessed must be taken as part of the whole, and the RT must understand that an abnormal reading may not be abnormal for a particular patient. For example, the heart rate of a patient with COPD may normally be 120 beats/min, or his/her respiratory rate may normally be 20 breaths/min. This is why it is so important to perform an initial assessment on each patient and establish baseline parameters.

The tools themselves have limitations. Blood pressure measurements usually are done using an aneroid sphygmomanometer and cuff. Blood pressure measurements can be inaccurate if performed improperly. Using a cuff that is too narrow or applying the cuff too tightly results in erroneously high readings. The RT should also take care not to press on the artery too hard with the head of the stethoscope, because this could result in erroneously high diastolic pressure readings.[7] Some patients use self-administered blood pressure units to monitor their blood pressure. Used correctly, these units are very accurate. However, it is fairly easy to use them incorrectly, which can give the patient inaccurate results. The RT should review the patient's technique and review the manufacturer's instructions to ensure that the equipment is being used properly. It is also useful to compare the patient's readings with those obtained using the RT's blood pressure cuff. It is important for the patient to take his/her blood pressure readings at the same time each day, using the same arm and sitting in the same position each time.

Peak flowmeters are also valuable when used properly. They are most commonly used to monitor patients whose disease has an asthmatic component, particularly children. Changes in peak flow readings are indicative of changes in airway reactivity and patency. Proper technique is essential to obtain accurate readings, and the patient should be instructed to use the peak flowmeter on waking in the morning before using a bronchodilator. Each patient should have his/her own peak flowmeter; there is variability between brands, as well as between flowmeters within brands, which could give inconsistent results.[8]

Pulse oximeters are used often in the home care setting but most often by the home care RT or home health nurse. It is considered medically unnecessary for most home care patients to have ongoing or continuous monitoring by pulse oximetry (and most insurance companies will not pay for oximeters for home use). If oximetry is indicated, the user should understand how to obtain an accurate reading and how to avoid inaccurate readings. For example, if the patient's hands are cold, the oximetry readings could be erroneously low. If the patient smokes, the readings could be erroneously high. Excessive movement, high levels of ambient light, or a low battery in the oximeter can also result in inaccurate readings. The user must understand these issues and be instructed to use the oximetry readings as part of a whole assessment; changes should not be made based on oximetry readings alone.[9]

Oxygen analyzers are used very commonly in home respiratory care, but like oximeters, they are not necessary for continuous monitoring in most cases. (Oxygen analyzers occasionally are used to monitor ventilator use in children, but even in these cases, they may not be medically necessary.) Oxygen analyzers are used most often to evaluate the function of oxygen equipment during servicing or troubleshooting. They must be calibrated according to the manufacturer's recommendations at least daily, and the RT must use care when carrying an oxygen analyzer in his/her car to avoid damaging it.

Arterial blood sampling and analysis can be performed in the home, often by mobile blood gas laboratories. Sputum and venous blood samples can be collected, and even electrocardiograms can be obtained in the home. The ability to collect such information allows the physician to determine and institute treatment, in many cases avoiding hospitalization. It is also much more convenient for the homebound patient; for example, it is much easier to get and transport a sputum specimen to an outpatient clinical laboratory or emergency department than to transport the patient there to have the sample taken.

RTs are not the only healthcare professionals seeing patients at home. Rather, the RT is most often part of a healthcare team that includes home health nurses; speech, physical, and occupational therapists; social workers; dietitians; home health aides; and lay caregivers. As a team, these people gather vital information about the patient that is used to develop a comprehensive care plan.

> **SIMPLY STATED**
>
> Continuous monitoring of parameters such as SpO_2 or FIO_2 usually is not considered medically necessary in the home care setting.

QUALIFICATIONS OF THE HOME CARE RESPIRATORY THERAPIST

The role of the RT in home care is to select, set up, and train the patient in the use of respiratory equipment and HME and to monitor and assess the patient for continued safe use of that equipment.[10] RTs who choose to perform home care must be highly competent, possess good critical thinking skills, and be extremely versatile. The job requires well-honed skills including the abilities to teach a patient to use a complex piece of equipment with confidence, evaluate a patient using the most basic tools in an uncontrolled environment, anticipate problems, and make good decisions about the patient's ongoing plan of care or service.[11]

Most RTs are employed by HME providers, although there are RTs who are employees of or consultants to home health agencies. (Home health agencies provide skilled nursing care.) Most HME companies rely on RTs who have previous hospital patient care experience and are well versed in all respiratory therapy modalities.

The RT often is the only skilled professional the HME company has on staff. Therefore home care RTs must be extremely versatile. The RT may be called on to set up and troubleshoot equipment that is never used by an RT in a hospital. For example, it is not uncommon for the RT to have to set up, maintain, and instruct a patient on the use of enteral feeding or intravenous pump equipment. The home care RT may also be asked to show a patient how to use a walker, wheelchair, or other durable medical equipment. Of course, the RT must be adequately trained before setting up equipment with which he/she is not familiar.

The home care RT must also have a good working knowledge of insurance reimbursement. The acute care RT seldom has to be concerned with how a procedure or supply is paid for or who pays for it. The acute care RT can administer oxygen therapy without worrying about whether a patient qualifies for coverage under his/her health insurance policy, and there usually is no limit to the number of suction catheters, ventilator circuits, or medication nebulizers a patient can use. However, the home care RT must understand the rules and guidelines for reimbursement.[12,13] The RT who understands reimbursement issues and can provide high-quality care within the dynamic and convoluted realm of health insurance is a great asset to the patient.

SIMPLY STATED

The home RT must be familiar with respiratory care procedures, as well as many nursing care procedures, nonrespiratory equipment, and reimbursement issues.

ASSESSMENT AND THE HOME VISIT

Assessment is one of the most important aspects of respiratory home care. The results of a thorough assessment affect all other aspects of the patient's care, such as the type of equipment required, instruction of the patient and other caregivers, whether ancillary services such as nursing are necessary, and the type of monitoring and follow-up the patient will need.

Most often, the RT sees a patient because a piece of respiratory equipment has been ordered from the HME provider. This referral can come from several sources: the physician's office, the hospital discharge planner, the insurance case manager, the home health nurse, and sometimes, the patient or his/her family. Box 19-2 lists the types of respiratory equipment for which an RT sees a home care patient.

Initial Visit

Once the referral is received, the RT schedules an initial home visit with the new patient. The purpose of this visit is to set up and teach the patient how to use the equipment that was prescribed. In some instances, the equipment has already been set up before the RT's arrival. Most HME providers use specially trained service technicians to deliver, set up, and train the patient in the use of certain types of respiratory equipment, such as home oxygen equipment. The RT then sees the patient, usually within 48 hours.

In either case, the RT uses the initial visit to perform a comprehensive evaluation of the patient. The results of this assess-

---

BOX 19-2   Respiratory Equipment Necessitating a Home Care Respiratory Therapist Visit

- Invasive and noninvasive ventilators
- Oxygen therapy equipment
- Compressor nebulizers
- Intermittent positive pressure breathing devices
- Bland aerosol therapy
- Continuous positive airway pressure and bilevel pressure devices
- Suction machines for oral, endotracheal, and intermittent gastric suction
- Mechanical airway clearance devices (percussors, flutter valves, exsufflation devices)
- Cardiorespiratory (apnea) monitors
- Portable sleep-recording devices
- Oximeters
- Airway adjuncts (tracheostomy tubes, laryngectomy tubes, transtracheal oxygen catheters)

---

ment affect all other aspects of the patient's home care program. It also establishes a baseline from which the patient is compared during subsequent visits. Box 19-3 highlights the elements of the comprehensive initial evaluation.

Medical History

During the first home visit, the RT interviews the patient and caregivers and then examines the patient. The patient interview is conducted to establish the patient's current medical status and symptom profile. Smoking status, pulmonary risk factors, and previous medical history (including surgeries and hospitalizations) should be determined. Any treatments or therapies the patient is undergoing should be identified. The RT should also ask the patient whether his/her immunization record for influenza and pneumococcal vaccines is current and identify any drug allergies the patient has. A medical history of the patient's family should also be obtained.

BOX 19-3   Key Elements of the Initial Evaluation

Patient	*Environment*
Past and current medical history	Cleanliness, safety hazards
Symptom profile	Smoke alarm, fire extinguisher
Medication review	Adequate electricity
Physical examination	Heating, cooling
Evaluation of functional limitations	Space for equipment, supplies
	Adequate cleaning facilities
Psychosocial evaluation	Telephone
Nutritional status	Emergency access
Caregiver evaluation	Equipment needs
Advance directives	

Medication Review

The RT reviews the patient's current medication regimen. This review identifies all prescription, over-the-counter, and herbal remedies the patient is taking. The RT evaluates the patient's level of understanding about how he/she should be taking medication and assesses compliance. It is helpful to ask the patient how he/she keeps track of medications and suggest the use of a medication scheduling pill holder for simplification, if needed. The RT should also ask to see the patient's technique for using metered-dose inhalers, dry powder inhalers, and medication nebulizers. If the RT determines that the patient is not using his/her medications as prescribed, the RT should inform the patient's physician. The RT can also recommend that the patient consult with a pharmacist for advice and clarification. A visit by the home health nurse may also be indicated to teach the patient to take his/her medications properly.

Nutritional Review

The patient's nutritional status is also evaluated, and the RT should inquire about any dietary restrictions (e.g., sodium, sugar, fat, calories). The RT should determine how many meals the patient eats per day; it is common for patients with pulmonary disease to eat poorly or decline food rather than suffer the dyspnea associated with its preparation and consumption. Such a patient would benefit from instruction in energy conservation techniques to help him/her prepare food and eat it. An important question to ask during the nutritional assessment is whether the patient leaves his/her oxygen cannula on during cooking and eating. It is common to discover that patients remove their oxygen cannula while cooking, because they are afraid of the danger of using oxygen around sources of heat. Many patients also remove their oxygen cannula during meals, often for cosmetic reasons. Identifying these issues would prompt problem solving by the RT and patient. For example, a visit by a home health dietitian could be suggested or the patient could be encouraged to use a local meal preparation and delivery service such as Meals on Wheels. Chore workers or personal attendants can be hired to assist the patient with meal preparation. A review of oxygen safety while cooking would also be appropriate. The RT can also reinforce any dietary recommendations that have already been made for the patient.

Physical Examination

During the initial home visit, a physical examination usually is performed. Age, height, weight, and general appearance are recorded. Vital signs, including blood pressure, pulse rate, respiratory rate and quality, and pulse oximetry, are taken. It is important to note that pulse oximetry can be done only on the order of the patient's physician. Many RTs have standing orders with their referring physicians that allow the RTs to perform oximetry on their patients. Auscultation; palpation of the chest; and observation for cyanosis, clubbing, and peripheral edema also are done. Examination techniques are standard, as seen in this and other texts.[7,14]

Some aspects of the physical examination may need to be altered to protect the patient's privacy. The home care therapist may be the only person in the room with the patient when the examination is being performed. Therefore it may be considered improper for the RT to ask the patient to disrobe for auscultation of the lungs. This is especially true when an RT examines a patient of the opposite sex. In such cases, auscultation must be performed over the patient's shirt or nightclothes, keeping in mind that extraneous sounds may occur when the patient's clothing rubs against the chest piece of the stethoscope. The RT will also encounter the patient who does not want to have his/her feet or legs examined for edema. Obtaining the patient's permission to perform the physical examination is essential to making the encounter comfortable for both the patient and the RT.

Part of the physical examination often includes some form of diagnostic testing. Peak flow, tidal volume, negative inspiratory force, and forced vital capacity are done on patients for whom such testing is appropriate. Observation of abnormal sputum may prompt a physician's order for sputum sample collection and analysis. End-tidal CO_2 breath sampling may be ordered for a patient with suspected ventilatory insufficiency.

HME providers that are accredited by the Joint Commission on Accreditation of Healthcare Organizations for clinical respiratory services can allow the RT to perform a patient's initial physical assessment without a physician's order; however, the RT can perform ongoing physical assessments of the patient only under written orders by the patient's physician.

Physical and Functional Limitations

Evaluation of physical and functional limitations is performed to identify any physical or functional problems that could reduce the patient's ability to care for himself/herself. The RT must look for physical deficits in eyesight, hearing, speech, strength, endurance, and mobility. The RT must also evaluate a patient's cognitive abilities. Any limitations could affect the patient's potential for self-care and limit his/her ability to safely manage any medical equipment that has been prescribed. If the patient has other people assisting in his/her care, consideration must be given to any functional or physical limitations those caregivers may have.

Several functional areas must be considered. The patient's ability to independently perform basic activities of daily living is assessed. Such activities include personal care, cooking, and independent or assisted mobility within the home. For example, the patient with COPD may appear unkempt because he/she cannot bathe and dress without severe shortness of breath. The patient may not use his/her portable oxygen tank because he/she does not have the hand strength to turn on the oxygen regulator. Perhaps he/she cannot walk from the living room to the bathroom without stopping or assistance or does not have enough strength to get up out of a chair. That same patient may have difficulty seeing the calibration markings on an oxygen tank or a medication eyedropper. The RT may even have had difficulty scheduling the initial visit because the patient could not hear the telephone ringing.

Cognitive function is also important to assess. A patient with short-term memory problems may have difficulty remembering the RT's instructions on how to fill up the portable oxygen tank. A patient who is depressed may not listen to instructions or may refuse the oxygen altogether. Cognitive impairment caused by stroke or even some types of medications can interfere with the patient's ability to use HME safely or without caregiver assistance. If there are caregivers, they will need evaluation to ensure that they have the cognitive abilities to manage the patient's care or equipment.

Psychosocial Evaluation

A psychosocial assessment should be performed during the initial visit. This assessment looks at the patient's self-image, outlook on his/her present and future situation, home status and support systems, and work history.[15] Home care patients can be anxious, embarrassed, angry, or depressed over their state of health and often feel that they are a burden to their families. They may have difficulty coping with being dependent on others for help with basic activities of daily living, particularly when this involves role reversal. For example, a male patient who has always had control and authority may have difficulty coping with losing that control and having to be assisted by his wife or being told what to do by healthcare workers. This patient may try to exert control by not complying with treatment regimens or refusing treatment altogether. The female patient with COPD who has always done all the cooking and cleaning may have difficulty allowing someone else to do it for her. She may continue to try to perform these duties, to the detriment of her health.

Patients with chronic lung disease often express feelings of hopelessness about their future. They may feel or may have been told that their condition is "terminal" and that there is no hope for improvement. Patients who have recently been prescribed oxygen often express the feeling that, because they need supplemental oxygen, they are dying. These patients may believe that there is no reason to continue treatment and basically give up. Many chronically ill patients isolate themselves because of the anxiety and embarrassment they feel about their declining health. Other patients deny their medical condition and ignore or refuse treatment.

Patients forced to retire because of declining health may become depressed at the loss of their role as breadwinner. They may be concerned about family finances; some patients are so concerned about finances that they refuse medications or equipment because they feel they cannot afford them. They feel that they have become a physical and financial burden on their families. Depression can lead to hostility toward caregivers, refusal of care or treatment, and verbal expression of suicidal thoughts. Anxiety can lead to medication abuse, increased shortness of breath, trouble sleeping, and other problems.

Caregivers in the home can also suffer from depression and anxiety. The COPD patient's spouse may have to quit work to care for the patient and may be concerned with financial problems while also having to worry about the patient's health. The asthmatic child's mother may overuse emergency services because of her fear of a life-threatening asthma attack. A wife

Questions to Ask Yourself
WHEN TRYING TO IDENTIFY PHYSICAL AND FUNCTIONAL LIMITATIONS IN PATIENTS AND CAREGIVERS

- Is the patient able to walk unaided or does he/she need a walker, cane, or other walking aid? Is the patient able to walk without significant shortness of breath? Is the patient able to climb a flight of stairs if the home has stairs? Does the patient have any weakness, arthritis, pain, swelling, or reduced range of motion in his/her feet, ankles, or legs?
- Does the patient have arthritis in his/her hands? Is the patient able to make a fist? Does the patient need assistance when performing an activity with his/her hands? Do the patient's hands shake? Does the patient have the strength to lift a portable oxygen tank or nebulizer?
- Does the patient have any hearing or vision problems? Can the patient read medication containers accurately? Is the patient able to read the gauges, flowmeters, or other indicators on the HME? Can the patient read the written instructions provided with his/her medications and equipment? Can the patient hear the alarms made by the equipment? Can the patient hear the telephone, doorbell, or normal speaking voices?
- Can the patient shower or bathe without assistance? Can the patient dress without assistance? Is the patient exhausted or short of breath after bathing or going to the toilet? Does the patient using oxygen need a higher flow rate during these activities?
- Is the patient able to make his/her own bed? Does the patient do his/her own cleaning and laundry?
- Is the patient able to prepare meals? Does the patient need assistance with food shopping? How many meals does the patient eat per day?
- Does the patient have difficulty remembering how to use any of the medical equipment? Does the patient remember which HME company has provided his/her equipment? Can the patient remember when his/her last bronchodilator treatment was? Can the patient remember how many times per day to take each of his/her medications?
- Do the patient's breathing problems limit his/her lifestyle in any way? Is the patient homebound?

Adapted from Dunne PJ, McInturff SL: The home visit. In Dunne PJ, McInturff SL: *Respiratory home care: The essentials,* Philadelphia, 1997, FA Davis.

may resent having to take care of her husband and believe that she has little choice in doing so.

Caregiver burnout is a common problem in the home. It is important that the RT look for signs of burnout, such as abuse and neglect. Box 19-4 lists some behavioral clues the RT should look for during this evaluation.

BOX 19-4	Signs and Symptoms of Psychosocial Problems in the Home

- Fear
- Shame
- Depression
- Evasive answers
- Embarrassment
- Social isolation
- Physical signs of abuse
- Demonstration of verbal abuse

The RT should notify the patient's physician of any psychosocial problems; a visit from a social worker may be indicated. The social worker can assist the patient and family with financial issues, caregiver burnout, and adjustment problems. The social worker can also assist the patient and family with decisions about advance directives if these have not been made.

Cultural, ethnic, and religious beliefs can also affect the patient's home care program. Language differences can make it difficult for the patient to convey or obtain information. The RT may need to locate an interpreter to translate; often there is a family member available who can perform this role. Many equipment user manuals are now written in several languages to help overcome this problem.

Some cultures encourage extended families to live together in a single dwelling. This can be advantageous, because it increases the number of potential caregivers and reduces the feeling of isolation suffered by some patients. It can be less of an advantage when care must be divided between the patient and other family members, particularly small children. Other patients may have religious beliefs that require an alteration in the home care program; for example, a patient may decline visits on days of worship or may decline treatment on religious grounds. A patient may request religious counsel as part of his/her healthcare team or request that prayers be said for him/her. The RT should always respect the patient's spiritual, as well as physical, needs.

Environmental Assessment

An environmental assessment is done to determine whether problems exist in the physical environment that would affect patient care. The home is inspected to identify health, fire, and safety hazards.[16] The home's walkways should be free of anything that could cause the patient to stumble; for example, throw rugs should be removed if the patient has gait problems or uses a walking aid. Halls and doorways should be wide enough for the patient to pass through, particularly when he/she uses a walker. Emergency exit routes must be identified and a plan for the quick removal of the patient should be developed and posted for all caregivers and emergency personnel.

Many older homes have electrical outlets that are not grounded properly. Patients often use multiplug adapters that are overloaded or in ill repair. Depending on the amount of medical equipment the patient needs, the home may not supply enough amperage on a circuit to power the equipment and the other appliances the patient wants to use. In extreme cases, some patients do not have electricity at all or "borrow" it from neighbors via extension cords. Inspection by a professional electrician may be needed to determine whether modifications are necessary to support the patient's equipment needs. In some cases, it may not be possible to place equipment safely in the home.

The home should be inspected for functioning smoke alarms and fire extinguishers.[16] There should be plenty of room for all equipment and supplies the patient will need; this is critical when oxygen is going to be used. Oxygen equipment must be placed at least 6 feet away from any heat sources and should not be placed on or near heater vents or in closets. Equipment powered by compressors, such as oxygen concentrators, nebulizers, and ventilators, must have enough free space around it to allow for adequate air intake and cooling. Other furniture may need to be removed to make space for hospital beds and other large equipment.

The home should have a working telephone. Touch-tone telephones with oversized numbers are available for patients with poor vision, and telephones with amplifiers or lights are helpful to patients with hearing deficits. Cordless telephones are ideal for patients who become short of breath trying to get to a ringing phone. Cordless phones also are handy to keep at the patient's bedside; this enables the caregiver to stay at the patient's side instead of having to leave the room to make a call, particularly in an emergency. However, cordless phones and other electronic devices should not be placed on or too close to equipment such as ventilators or apnea monitors because of the potential for electromagnetic interference, which can damage equipment and render it inoperable.

Patients with pulmonary impairment may not tolerate wide fluctuations in ambient temperature, so the home should be evaluated for its heating and cooling systems. Wood-burning stoves and fireplaces can aggravate lung problems, particularly asthma, as do stoves or heaters that are not vented. When inspecting the home of an asthmatic patient, the RT must be particularly careful to identify possible triggers such as old carpeting, pets, mold, and wood fires.[17]

SIMPLY STATED

An assessment of the physical environment should always be performed during the initial visit, even if a physical assessment of the patient is not going to be performed.

Equipment Needs

The nature of the patient's illness usually dictates the type of medical equipment needed. The environmental assessment indicates the suitability of that equipment and the adaptations or additions that may be necessary. The patient who lives in an older home with an inadequate electrical system may need a liquid oxygen system rather than an oxygen concentrator. A patient living in a large or two-story home may need to have oxygen equipment placed on both floors or at both ends of the house to prevent the use of more than 50 feet of oxygen tubing. Careful observation of where and how the equipment will be used is essential.

The patient using a home ventilator will likely need battery-powered equipment as backup if he/she lives in an area with frequent power outages. A patient who lives in a small mobile home may not have enough room for a hospital bed, and if that patient suffers from orthopnea, arthritis, or another need for frequent changes in body position, it is necessary to find other ways to elevate the head during sleep or to facilitate positioning.

If the functional assessment reveals that the patient has difficulty with personal care such as bathing or using the toilet, adaptive equipment may be indicated to make these activities less taxing and, more importantly, less hazardous. Bath seats and shower chairs allow the patient to sit down while bathing, and handheld shower attachments make cleaning much easier. Properly mounted grab bars and tub rails provide an added measure of safety. A home evaluation by a physical therapist is useful in ensuring that the patient's environment is properly equipped to allow the patient to function as independently and safely as possible.

> **SIMPLY STATED**
>
> A comprehensive initial evaluation will help the RT determine the most appropriate respiratory and home medical equipment for the patient.

Plan of Care

The objective of the comprehensive initial evaluation is to provide vital information the practitioner will use to develop an individualized plan of care or service. The plan of care or service is developed from problems identified during the initial evalua-

tion. Desired outcomes are established and processes are delineated to correct the problems and achieve those outcomes. Goals should be specific, measurable, attainable, realistic, and within a specified time frame.

The physician orders home care services for a patient because that patient has specific medical needs. The type of service the physician orders is the *plan of treatment.* This is essentially a prescription that includes the type of therapy, dosage, frequency, and method of administration, as well as any physical parameters the physician wants assessed, such as oxygen saturation or blood pressure. For example, the plan of treatment for the home oxygen patient might state, "Oxygen at 1 L/min via nasal cannula at rest and 2 L/min with activity via oxygen concentrator, with pulse oximetry spot check monthly and with change in shortness of breath." During the initial home visit, the RT assesses the patient as ordered, sets up and instructs the patient and caregivers in the use of the equipment, reviews the physician's prescription, and evaluates the patient's environment to determine whether the equipment is appropriate for the environment.

During the initial evaluation, the RT will also identify specific problems or needs the patient may have in regard to the prescribed treatment. For example, the patient may be unable to read the flowmeter on the oxygen concentrator, which is a problem because the flow is supposed to be changed from 1 L/min to 2 L/min with activity. Perhaps the patient is too weak to carry a portable oxygen cylinder. The patient may feel that the oxygen equipment is too embarrassing to wear in public, so he/she refuses to use the portable oxygen system outside the house. The patient's spouse may have short-term memory problems and cannot remember the instructions for cleaning the filters on the concentrator. Table 19-1 shows a sample plan of care or service for this home oxygen patient based on the physician's order for treatment.

Patient Education and Training

Part of the initial home visit is spent training the patient and caregivers in how to use the prescribed medical equipment and perform the related respiratory care procedures. Assessment is

Table 19-1	Sample Plan of Care or Service	
Problem	Goal	Action
Hypoxia by O_2 saturation	Patient will maintain saturation above 90%	Monitor O_2 saturation by pulse oximetry monthly and as needed
Patient cannot see flowmeter on concentrator	Patient will use O_2 at 1 L/min at rest and 2 L/min with activity	Instruct patient's family in how to change flow rate on concentrator as prescribed
Patient cannot carry portable oxygen tank	Patient will use portable oxygen as prescribed when away from house	Supply patient with smallest aluminum oxygen cylinder with oxygen-conserving device
Patient refuses to wear oxygen in public	Patient will wear oxygen as prescribed	Review health problems associated with hypoxia, provide patient with clear nasal cannula, encourage patient to carry portable cylinder in backpack or other carrying bag

the most important skill the RT must have, but the ability to teach runs a close second. Indeed, RTs have been shown to be uniquely effective in teaching patients.[18] The RT must be able to convey technical information in a simple and meaningful way and to verify that what was taught was also understood. Each person learns differently, and the RT must determine how each particular patient learns best. Some learn best by visualization or by reading. Others learn better by listening, and some learn best by doing.[19] The RT probably will use a combination of all three methods during training.

The patient should be taught to use the equipment or perform the procedure independently whenever possible. If the patient is unable to use the equipment or perform the procedure, he/she should still be involved in the training. It is important that the patient be confident that the caregivers understand and can adequately perform the necessary procedures.[20] Box 19-5 outlines some useful teaching strategies.

> **SIMPLY STATED**
> Patients should be trained to use equipment or perform procedures themselves whenever possible.

It may be necessary for the RT to return to the patient's home two or three times to continue the training sessions, particularly when there are several pieces of equipment to learn to use. It is common for patients and families to be overwhelmed during the RT's initial visit, especially if the patient was discharged from the hospital that day and other healthcare professionals are also trying to see the patient. Patients who are overwhelmed probably will not remember all the instructions the RT may give them. It is important for the RT to evaluate how much the patient has understood and provide additional training as necessary. The RT will factor this into the plan of care or service and use follow-up visits to provide the additional training and monitor the patient's and caregiver's ongoing performance. For example, the goal of the plan of care or service may be, "The patient will properly clean the inner cannula of the tra-

cheostomy tube daily and as needed within the next 30 days." Knowing that learning to clean an inner cannula is difficult, the RT might schedule home visits daily for the first week to train, retrain, and monitor the patient's progress on performing this task. As the patient becomes proficient, the RT would reduce the frequency of the home visits and would monitor the patient's technique during those visits. During a follow-up visit, the RT may notice that the patient has some redness and irritation at the stoma site, probably from not changing the drain sponges often enough. The RT will use this opportunity to review tracheostomy care, frequency of sponge changes, and prevention of stomal irritation.

Follow-Up Care

The plan of care or service should also include the RT's plan for follow-up care. Based on the issues identified during the initial evaluation and the desired outcomes, the patient may or may not need ongoing physical assessment and evaluation. This is usually a function of how ill or unstable the patient is or what type of equipment the patient is using. For example, the RT probably would not perform ongoing assessments on a patient using a compressor nebulizer, or if follow-up was indicated, it would be for a short duration. The RT may have found during the initial evaluation that the patient seemed to have difficulty remembering how to schedule his/her treatments, and a follow-up visit would be made. Once it is established that the patient is taking treatments as prescribed, he/she no longer needs follow-up.

A patient just discharged from the hospital with home oxygen who is still medically unstable may need frequent follow-up and assessment until his/her condition stabilizes. For example, the patient may need to be seen weekly for the first 2 weeks, then every other week for the next month, and then monthly after that. A very stable, long-term patient on oxygen may not need physical assessment at all, but rather will need ongoing equipment monitoring.

It is ideal to reassess the patient completely during each follow-up visit, particularly when the home visits are done less frequently. The RT often will identify something that has changed from the initial evaluation, and emergent problems often are found this way. It may be during a periodic visit to evaluate the oxygen equipment that the RT notices a change in the patient's shortness of breath or an increase in pedal edema. The RT may have found that the patient is using portable cylinders faster than expected or that the patient is not using as much oxygen as he/she should, as evidenced by the hour meter on the concentrator. The essence of the follow-up visit is that the RT will always find something that has changed about the patient, equipment, or environment and that the plan of care or service is continually evolving based on the goals that are met and new problems that are identified. Table 19-2 reviews physical changes that may be found during a follow-up visit and the actions the RT should take.

A growing trend in follow-up care is telemonitoring. This is usually done via telephone modem on equipment specially designed for remote monitoring. This equipment collects and

---

BOX 19-5   Helpful Strategies to Use During Patient Education and Training

- Reduce outside stimuli and ensure the learner's attention.
- Present only the necessary information.
- Use simple terms.
- Use demonstration equipment, videotapes, or audiotapes.
- Demonstrate the procedure exactly as it should be performed.
- Ask for a return demonstration.
- Have the learner practice several times.
- Limit the training session to 30 minutes when possible.
- Encourage the learner to ask questions.
- Leave printed instructions.
- Leave a 24-hour telephone number.

Table 19-2	Interpretation of Signs and Symptoms in the Home Care Patient	
Finding	Possible Cause	Action
Dyspnea, cyanosis	Malfunction of equipment, poor compliance with treatment, change in physical status	Check oxygen equipment, assess patient, review energy conservation techniques and pursed-lip breathing, contact physician
Wheezing	Bronchospasm, congestive heart failure, pulmonary infection	Examine patient, verify compliance with medication regimen, review medication nebulizer procedures, contact physician
Increased sputum or change in sputum color	Lung or airway infection	Assess patient, check temperature, check compliance with therapy and cleaning of equipment, contact physician
Pedal edema	Heart failure, fluid overload	Assess patient, verify function of oxygen equipment, check compliance with oxygen therapy, verify compliance with medication regimen
Poor appetite	Depression, dyspnea, fever	Assess patient, examine medication schedule, review energy conservation techniques, contact physician

stores data that can track usage and compliance and identify and categorize events such as breathing problems or heart arrhythmias. Some telemonitoring equipment also has video capabilities that allow the healthcare professional not only to interview the patient but also to monitor blood pressure, listen to the patient's lungs, inspect wounds, and perform other physical assessment tasks. Telemonitoring reduces the amount of time required to do a visit, because it eliminates the driving time involved, allowing the healthcare professional to see more patients in a day. Telemonitoring is not widely used yet, partly because of the expense involved in providing the equipment, which is not reimbursable.

Equipment Maintenance

An essential aspect of follow-up care is equipment maintenance. RTs assess the patient, caregivers, and environment, as well as various types of equipment for appropriateness and proper function.

Each manufacturer of medical equipment has specific guidelines for periodic preventive maintenance and servicing. For home ventilators, filters must be replaced, settings verified, and batteries checked. Home ventilators also must be replaced periodically for more extensive maintenance, usually after a specific number of hours. Oxygen equipment also needs routine monitoring and maintenance. Output concentration and flow rates of oxygen concentrators must be checked and external and internal filters replaced. Flow rates of liquid oxygen equipment must be checked routinely for accuracy, and rings and seals must be replaced periodically. An electrical safety check should be performed on all electrically powered equipment at least every 12 months.

The patient or caregiver is often responsible for performing some of the routine maintenance on home care equipment. The patient should be taught how to change external filters on oxygen concentrators, compressor nebulizers, ventilators, and con-

tinuous positive airway pressure (CPAP) equipment. He/she also should be taught how to clean and disinfect nebulizers, humidifiers, and tubing and how to properly dispose of tubing and cannulas that are not cleanable. The patient should also be taught routine troubleshooting procedures and how and when to contact the equipment provider for help and service.

Some types of home oxygen equipment include monitoring devices to assist with equipment maintenance. Oxygen concentrators can be equipped with oxygen concentration indicators (OCIs), which alert the user if the concentration output drops below a certain level. OCIs are helpful in ensuring that the patient is always receiving an adequate concentration of oxygen; for example, an oxygen concentrator without an OCI may still put out the prescribed flow of 2 L/min, but the concentration of that flow may be 80%, 75%, or even lower. The patient has no way to know that the inspired oxygen level is too low except that he/she may not feel as good.

Oxygen equipment providers can also monitor oxygen equipment in the patient's home by modem. Use patterns, tank contents, concentration, and flow rates can be monitored by computer. Equipment telemonitoring systems can help reduce the number of service calls an oxygen provider has to make to a patient's home and can identify equipment problems more rapidly. However, these systems are an additional expense to the provider and therefore have limited use.

RTs perform many routine maintenance procedures during their follow-up visits. This gives them the opportunity to check the patient's adherence to cleaning and maintenance schedules. The RT can monitor patient compliance by checking hour meters on equipment such as oxygen concentrators, ventilators, and CPAP machines. Any variances that are discovered should prompt a review of cleaning, maintenance, and the physician's prescription for treatment.

The RT should also evaluate the appropriateness of the equipment during the follow-up visits. A change in the patient's condition could mean that the equipment is no longer the best choice. For example, if a patient's oxygen needs to be increased, an oxygen concentrator with an "E" cylinder in a cart for portability may not allow the patient to leave the home for as long as necessary. Instead, a liquid oxygen stationary system and portable oxygen system would allow the patient to be away from home longer.

Discharging the Patient

Most home care patients are not followed by the RT indefinitely. The ultimate goal of respiratory home care is to provide the patient with the tools to manage his/her own care. These tools include the knowledge base, equipment, procedures, and self-monitoring capability.

The plan of care is established to work through the problems and issues found during the RT's home visits. As problems are identified, goals are set to achieve desired outcomes and correct the problems. For most patients, the goals are achieved and the patient becomes capable of self-monitoring. At this point, the patient is discharged from respiratory care services.

If the patient continues to use medical equipment such as oxygen, ventilators, and apnea monitors, he/she will at least continue to need service visits to monitor the function of that equipment. Those services may or may not be performed by the RT. Some HME providers use specially trained service technicians to make these service calls, and others use RTs to service life support equipment and service technicians to monitor oxygen and nebulizer equipment. These service technicians are trained to identify and report back any problems that might require a patient contact by the RT.

SUMMARY

As stated in the American Association for Respiratory Care's Position Statement on Home Respiratory Care Services, the RT, "by virtue of education, training, and competency testing, is the most competent healthcare professional to provide prescribed home respiratory care."[4] The home care RT has the ability to affect the quality of life of their patients every single day. The RT's exceptional skills in assessment, patient education, and decision making enhance the safety and well-being of patients who have the privilege of receiving their care at home.

REVIEW QUESTIONS

1. Which of the following is true about respiratory home care?
   a. Its use is increasing.
   b. It usually involves rudimentary forms of patient care and clinical expertise.
   c. The technology required for respiratory home care lags behind hospital-based therapy.
   d. It is performed mostly by on-the-job trainees.

2. T   F   The type of patients receiving home respiratory care varies widely.

3. Which of the following is the most important skill in respiratory home care?
   a. Treatment of physical disease
   b. Treatment of psychologic problems
   c. Patient assessment skills
   d. Management of physical and monetary resources

4. Which of the following would *not* be performed during a respiratory home care visit?
   a. Arterial blood gas sampling and analysis
   b. Mixed venous blood gas analysis
   c. Collection of sputum samples
   d. Sleep studies

5. T   F   The services of the home care RT usually are reimbursed by most insurance plans, including Medicare.

6. T   F   The RT often is the only healthcare professional caring for the patient with chronic lung disease in the home.

7. Which of the following is true about the initial home care evaluation?
   a. It may include diagnostic evaluation.
   b. It is performed by a physician.
   c. It involves evaluation of the patient only.
   d. a and c.

8. Which of the following is true about the patient's plan of care or service?
   a. It is based solely on the initial evaluation.
   b. It identifies issues and establishes goals for the patient.
   c. It is developed to establish equipment services only.
   d. All of the above.

9. Which of the following would be a part of the environmental assessment?
   a. Determining whether the person(s) with whom the patient lives is (are) willing to care for the patient
   b. Determining whether home care equipment is functioning properly
   c. Determining space requirements for ambulation and equipment
   d. a and c only

10. Which of the following is part of follow-up care?
    a. Reducing care to minimize cost
    b. Developing a treatment plan
    c. Assessing the patient's compliance with the therapy
    d. All of the above

11. Which of the following is *not* associated with loss of appetite in the home care patient?
    a. Depression
    b. Dyspnea
    c. Fever
    d. Hypertension

REFERENCES

1. Levine SA, Boal J, Boling PA: Clinician's corner: Home care, *JAMA* 290:9, 2003.

2. National Center for Health Statistics: FastStats: Deaths/mortality, Centers for Disease Control, October 2003. Available at www.cdc.gov/nchs/fastats/deaths.htm.

3. Mannino DM: Chronic obstructive pulmonary disease: Definition and epidemiology, *Respir Care* 48:12, 2003.

4. American Association for Respiratory Care Position Statement: *Home respiratory care services,* Dallas, 2000, AARC.

5. Dunne PJ, McInturff SL: The rationale for respiratory home care. In Dunne PJ, McInturff SL, editors: *Respiratory home care: The essentials,* Philadelphia, 1998, FA Davis.

6. American Medical Association: *Medical management of the home care patient: Guidelines for physicians,* ed 2, Chicago, AMA, 1998.

7. Krider SJ: Vital signs. In Wilkins RL, Krider SJ, Sheldon RL, editors: *Clinical assessment in respiratory care,* ed 5, St Louis, 2005, Mosby.

8. Second Expert Panel on the Management of Asthma: Component 1: Measures of assessment and monitoring. In *Highlights of the expert panel report 2: Guidelines for the diagnosis and management of asthma,* Pub No 97-4051A, Bethesda, MD, 1997, National Institutes of Health.

9. McInturff SL, O'Donohue WJ: Respiratory care in the home and alternate sites. In Burton GG, Hodgkin JE, Ward JJ, editors: *Respiratory care: A guide to clinical practice,* ed 4, Philadelphia, 1997, JB Lippincott.

10. Spratt G, Petty TL: Partnering for optimal respiratory home care: Physicians working with respiratory therapists to optimally meet respiratory home care needs, *Respir Care* 46:5, 2001.

11. Mishoe SC: Critical thinking in respiratory care practice: A qualitative research study, *Respir Care* 48:5, 2003.

12. Smith R: The home care game, *J Respir Care Pract* 11(6):47, 1998.

13. Miller LS, Dunne PJ: Reimbursement. In Dunne PJ, McInturff SL, editors: *Respiratory home care: The essentials,* Philadelphia, 1998, FA Davis.

14. Bates B: The physical examination of an adult. In Bates B, Bickley LS, Hoekelman RA, editors: *A pocket guide to physical examination and history taking,* ed 2, Philadelphia, 1995, JB Lippincott.

15. Bates B: Clinical thinking and the patient's record. In Bates B, Bickley LS, Hoekelman RA, editors: *A pocket guide to physical examination and history taking,* ed 2, Philadelphia, 1995, JB Lippincott.

16. Consumer Product Safety Commission: *Safety for older consumers home safety checklist,* CPSC Document #701, Washington, DC. Available at www.cpsc.gov/cpscpub/pubs/701.html.

17. Second Expert Panel on the Management of Asthma: Component 2: Control of factors contributing to asthma severity. In *Highlights of the expert panel report 2: Guidelines for the diagnosis and management of asthma,* Pub No 97-4051A, Bethesda, MD, 1997, National Institutes of Health.

18. Stoller JK: Are respiratory therapists effective? Assessing the evidence, *Respir Care* 46:1, 2001.

19. Fuchs CP: A practical model for teaching clinical decision-making, *AARC Times* 20(8):40, 1996.

20. Pulmonary Rehabilitation Focus Group: Clinical practice guideline: Providing patient and caregiver training, *Respir Care* 41(7):658, 1996.

Documentation of the Patient Assessment

CHAPTER OVERVIEW

This chapter reviews why so much time and energy is spent documenting patient care. Sometimes the paperwork is so time consuming that it seems counterproductive because it reduces time that could be spent with the patient; however, documentation of the care provided and the patient's response is essential to the entire process of healthcare. This chapter reviews the medical-legal aspects of patient care documentation, with emphasis on the Joint Commission on Accreditation of Healthcare Organizations (JCAHO) requirements. Several different charting methods are presented. The reader of this chapter will appreciate how good documentation is essential from a legal perspective and, more importantly, how it provides better communication among members of the healthcare team and ultimately improves patient care.

GENERAL PURPOSES OF DOCUMENTATION

Once you have completed your bedside patient assessment, talked to other members of the healthcare team, taken notes, reviewed the information in the medical record, and discussed the information with the patient's physician, it's time to record your own assessment and plan into the medical record. The very process of collecting the data involves the mental process called *critical thinking.* The critical thinking process requires many skills, including interpretation, analysis, evaluation, inference, explanation, and self-regulation.[1] The really difficult part is over, and now all you have to do is describe, very briefly, your thoughts and findings in a concise and professional manner. Because you are using a medical-legal document, you need to understand some fundamental principles before writing in the patient's medical record.

The reasons for creating a record of the patient's interactions with any health service organization (HSO) include the following:

- To serve as a legal record. The medical record is more than just a collection of data; it is a legal document.

- To collect evidence in support of the patient's complaints. When the clinical facts about the patient's condition are collected, the correct diagnosis can be confirmed and the patient's clinical progress can be better documented.

- To provide communication between members of the healthcare team. The clinical notes, reports, flow sheets, vital signs, and test results enable the physician and other members of the team to document that the patient has received high-quality care according to each profession's standards of care or hospital policies. Each discipline has unique perspectives to bring to the discussion of a patient's care plan.

- To support appropriate reimbursement. The hospital is a business that must collect revenues; therefore, the medical record is also a financial document. The medical record must clearly show the nature of the patient's needs in the form of the diagnosis. Medicare and many insurance systems reimburse the hospital based on the patient's diagnosis.

- To support operation of the HSO and its allocation of internal resources and to provide documentation of compliance with JCAHO and state standards of care. This type of documentation provides data for legally mandated reports to state and federal agencies. These reviews of the medical records and related financial records, as well as the subsequent reports from those reviews, are used to show the hospital's board of supervisors and administration that the business is functioning as it should.

- To serve as an educational tool. Every healthcare professional must learn how to use the medical record correctly. At first the medical record is very intimidating, but with time it becomes more familiar. The initial problem is often just finding the information you need. The medical record provides documentation of the clinical manifestations and course of the disease process and the patient's responses to interventions. For this reason, even the experienced healthcare worker can learn from a good medical record. By reviewing a patient's record, you can learn both what has worked and what has not on this particular patient. Furthermore, by reviewing large numbers of patient medical records, we learn how to more accurately describe each patient's condition and determine how to better treat patients with specific diseases. Most human research is based on or related to medical records. Extracting data from medical records is a complex process that requires skill and diligence.

As noted, the patient's medical record is subject to review by different professionals for several reasons. By far the most common and compelling reason to scrutinize a patient's record, or the HSO's handling of medical records in general, is to improve the quality of medical care.

SIMPLY STATED

A retrospective review of patient charts can provide students and other clinicians with the opportunity to see how patients with a certain problem were diagnosed, what treatment was given, and how the patients responded to that treatment.

JOINT COMMISSION ON ACCREDITATION OF HEALTHCARE ORGANIZATIONS AND LEGAL ASPECTS OF THE MEDICAL RECORD

JCAHO reviews all HSOs in order to improve the quality of patient care. If any healthcare organization fails to comply with JCAHO standards, JCAHO will revoke its accreditation. This means that the organization can no longer receive federal money in the form of Medicare payments. Soon thereafter (probably a matter of a few days), most states will cease Medicaid payments, and most, if not all, private insurance companies will stop allowing admissions to or treatment by that facility. Furthermore, each state's health department will start an on-site inspection and probably revoke that organization's license to do business. JCAHO has revoked accreditation of hospitals and skilled nursing facilities in the past.

JCAHO inspectors look for documentation of high-quality patient care. The stated goal of the Management of Information section of the JCAHO Comprehensive Accreditation Manual for Hospitals (CAMH) "...is to support decision making to improve patient outcomes, improve healthcare documentation, assure patient safety, and improve performance in patient care, treatment, and services, governance, management and support processes."[2] This section of the manual details some of the expectations and standards that apply to the documentation of assessments and routine charting. JCAHO specifies in detail what must be included in patient documentation. How each organization accomplishes these tasks is left up to that facility. The on-site JCAHO survey team members have a scoring system to evaluate the effectiveness of the organization's compliance with these requirements, and this includes reviewing many medical records to confirm compliance. The survey team members may also provide examples from other organizations to demonstrate compliance with the letter and spirit of the regulation. JCAHO survey team members often emphasize that they are there to help the HSO, not to punish individuals or the organization.

The following are JCAHO statements from the 2004 manual about required medical record elements.[2] Although there have been some changes in the format of the manual, and in the accreditation process itself, most all of the underlying expectations have remained constant.

- IM.2.10 Information privacy and confidentiality are maintained.
- IM.2.20 Information security, including data integrity, is maintained.

    These first two standards are directed toward guarding the patient's rights to privacy (the individual's right to limit the disclosure of personal information) and confidentiality (the safekeeping of data/information so as to restrict access to individuals who have need, reason, and permission of such access).[2] These standards are consistent with both state and federal laws and regulations. Violations of these expectations, or related laws and regulations, can result in legal action resulting in fines for the institution, and/or even closure of the facility, plus civil and/or criminal prosecution of the offender(s) (depending on the details of the incident) that could result in personal fines in the hundreds of thousands of dollars, loss of job(s), loss of professional licenses, and in the worse cases even jail time. The federal law known as the "Health Insurance Portability and Accountability Act of 1996," or HIPAA, details the legal expectations and professional standards regarding the transmission (verbal, written, electronic, etc.) of patient information. These professional standards can be simply summarized by saying that what you learn about a patient is on a "need to know" basis, and you are not to share that information outside of that professional "need to know" context. Generally, we need to refer almost all questions coming from relatives and friends to the other professional team members, such as the nurse, social worker, and naturally, the physician. These issues become complex at times, particularly when we are dealing with a culturally diverse environment.

- IM.4.10 The information management system provides information for use in decision-making.

    This standard gets into the expectation of organization of the medical record, in that it needs to be accessible, accurately recorded, complete, and organized for efficient retrieval of needed information.[2]

- IM.6.10 The hospital has a complete and accurate medical record for every patient assessed or treated. (This standard includes the following topics.)
  - Only authorized individuals make entries in the medical record.
  - Standardized formats are used for documenting all care, treatment, and services provided to patients. (Each hospital has the authority to establish its own standardized formats.)
  - Every medical record entry is dated, the author identified, and when necessary according to law or regulation and the hospital policy, the record is authenticated (for paper-based records, counter-signatures are entered for purposes of authentication after transcription or verbal orders are dated when required by law, regulation, and/or hospital policy).

- The medical record contains sufficient information to identify the patient; support the diagnosis/condition; justify the care, treatment, and service; document the course and results of care, treatment, and service; and promote continuity of care among providers (this expectation is linked to PC.4.10, see below).
- The hospital (and/or department) has a policy and procedure on the timely entry of all significant information into the patient's medical record.

- IM.6.20 Records contain patient-specific information, as appropriate, to the care, treatment, and services provided. (This expectation includes the following.)
  - Documentation and findings of assessments
  - Reason(s) for admission or care, treatment, and services
  - The goals of treatment and the treatment plan
  - Progress notes made by authorized individuals
  - All reassessments and plan of care revisions, when indicated
  - Relevant observations
  - The response to care, treatment, and services provided

- M.6.50 Designated qualified personnel accept and transcribe verbal orders from authorized individuals.

    Communication problems during the giving and taking of verbal orders have resulted in serious patient complications and even death. This alarming problem has caused JCAHO to include in the National Patient Safety Goals the expectation that all verbal orders are to be read back to the person giving the order. This must occur to verify the complete and correct order is being recorded and acted upon. The person who gave the order, within a specified time frame, must authenticate all verbal orders. Because of errors or problems in communications regarding verbal orders, there is a general movement in the healthcare industry away from accepting verbal orders.

    Guidelines regarding the authority to accept verbal orders are outlined in most states' respiratory care practice acts. The general rule is that respiratory therapists (RTs) can take (receive) orders for only those treatments or services that they directly provide, which therefore excludes drugs that we do not directly administer. We can, however, take orders for routine labs, chest x-rays, and standardized multidisciplinary protocols that are related to our practice. The expectation is still the same, although the text of the 2004 CAMH no longer includes the following statement: "Respiratory Care services are provided to patients consistent with a written prescription by the patient's physician and are documented in the patient's medical record." All orders (written and verbal) must be dated, identifying the names of the individuals who gave and received the order. Under certain circumstances, two persons should be present to take a verbal order or be on the phone line, and then one of these persons needs to repeat the order back to the physician before recording and carrying out the order. Both persons that heard the verbal directive should cosign the order in the medical record. The medical record must also indicate who implemented the order and what time the order was carried out.

- PC.4.10 Development of a plan of care, treatment, and services is individualized and appropriate to the patient's needs, strengths, limitations, and goals.

   This also means that respiratory therapy staff members should integrate the information from various assessments (such as both the physician and nurse evaluations) of the patient to identify and assign priorities to the patient's care needs. Then we should base our care decisions on the identified patient needs and care priorities. Attention should be paid to treating symptoms, such as dyspnea, and using accepted professional standards of practice, such as the American Association for Respiratory Care (AARC) clinical practice guidelines.

- PC.2.20 The hospital defines in writing the data and information gathered during assessment and reassessment. (Most often, the department's policies and procedures detail this expectation.)

- PC.3.230 Diagnostic testing necessary for determining the patient's healthcare needs is performed.

- PC.2.120 The hospital defines, in writing, the time frame(s) for conducting the initial assessment(s).

- PC.2 pr.150 Patients are reassessed as needed.

   The preceding means that there should be reassessments at regular intervals in the course of care to determine a patient's response to care. Furthermore, any significant change in a patient's condition should result in a reassessment, and the results or observations should be communicated to the other healthcare team members as appropriate.

These professional expectations are scrutinized carefully when the patient or his/her family believes that the patient did not receive high-quality care or, more specifically, when it is believed that there has been some form of negligence.

SIMPLY STATED

JCAHO standards for documentation provide direction to all clinicians about what should be charted, how often, and to what level of detail. Without such standards, documentation would vary so much between healthcare facilities that patient records would be of little value.

Negligence is defined as an instance of failure to use reasonable amount of care ("ordinary prudence") that results in injury or damages to another. Negligence has been committed when someone (who becomes the defendant) has failed to live up to a required duty of care owed to another person (the plaintiff). Generally, the legal definition of negligence requires the presence of the following four conditions:

- The defendant owed a duty of care to the plaintiff.
- The defendant breached that duty.
- The plaintiff suffered a legally recognizable injury.
- The defendant's breach of duty of care caused the plaintiff's injury.

As an RT, you have a duty of care to your patients. The scope of your duty to a patient (and family) is outlined by your professional standards (e.g., the AARC clinical practice guidelines, your state's respiratory care practice act and business and professional laws, the position statements of your state's society, and the JCAHO standards). Your scope of practice is further defined, or limited by, your job description in your place of employment. Staying within your job description, the limits of your state's practice act, and the professional expectations keeps you professionally safe.

Concerns regarding ethical situations or clinical conflicts between disciplines should not be entered into the patient's medical record. Issues such as these need to be referred to the institutions' quality management department or, as needed, to the risk management department, through the proper channels. Every healthcare organization is required by JCAHO to have a performance improvement process that ensures that patient safety issues can be brought up in a "no fault" manner, and that every employee is instructed on how to report or access this process.

The absence of information or the lack of documented recognition of specific problems could constitute malpractice. There is a legal term *res ipsa loquitur*, which means, "the thing speaks for itself." Simply put, if it was not charted, it was not done. For example, if it were not recognized that a patient on a ventilator had severe chronic obstructive pulmonary disease (COPD) and was at very high risk for auto–PEEP, and the patient suffered injury or death, this could turn into a legal problem (though this example is not likely). However, if:

- Clinical notes show that auto-PEEP was being monitored with every ventilator parameter;
- There was documentation of communication between the RT, physician, and nurse about the auto-PEEP problem; and
- Bronchodilator therapy was started and ventilator changes were made, both in an attempt to decrease auto-PEEP,

then the presumption should be that due care was taken and the patient's death was not caused by neglect or malpractice in this regard.

The medical record must accurately convey the course and results of the patient care provided. Therefore, the accurate recording of the date, time, and place of events is essential. Late entries into the medical record are often a necessary but undesirable event. The standard calls for all information to be entered into the medical record in a timely manner. But what is timely? In one case (*Joseph Brant Memorial Hospital v. Koziol* [1978]), a nurse did not chart her observations for 7 hours on a postoperative patient who then died during her shift. The delay in charting was interpreted by the court as having not made the observations. Vital signs and parameters should be charted immediately. Late entries of clinical notes or descriptions should be clearly marked as late entries and show the time entered and the time or period covered in the note.

TYPES OF MEDICAL RECORDS

The different kinds of entries into the medical record depend on the purpose of that entry. The major types that are most familiar to the RT are treatment records, flowcharts or parameter sheets, and test results.

Treatment records are concerned with a single event at a specific time. The treatment record shows when, how, and with what drugs or equipment a treatment was given and the patient's response to this therapeutic intervention. The treatment record can contain patient-subjective information of the response to the treatment, but the majority of the treatment record is objective information. This type of documentation should include the following:

- Date and time of test or treatment
- Type of test or treatment
- Drugs and their dosages, if used
- Result, or response to treatment, including adverse reactions
- Goals, objectives, or end-point criteria for the treatment

Flowcharts or parameter sheets have similar requirements for dates, times, changes in equipment settings, and, most importantly, the patient's responses to the therapeutic intervention. Flowcharting and parameter charting have become increasingly important in the sophisticated environment of the intensive care unit (ICU). This type of documentation is designed to show that the healthcare worker looked for and responded to adverse events or trends or responded to opportunities to reduce invasive procedures and medications. The need to record accurate ventilator and monitor alarm settings is often overlooked by busy healthcare workers. If a patient were to die from a massive tension pneumothorax after hours of high peak pressures with an inappropriately set high peak pressure alarm, a strong case might be made for malpractice.

Tests are mostly objective observations of clinical laboratory results (e.g., arterial blood gas [ABG] or electrolytes) or physiologic responses to clinical challenges (e.g., fluid challenges or PEEP curves). Because tests are seen as integral to the clinical course of the patient's care, the date and time of the test and its subsequent reporting to the physician are very important.

Treatment records, parameter sheets, and test result forms typically do not pose a problem for most clinicians, but some find documentation of patient assessments to be a challenge. Assessment notes, medical histories, and clinical notes are extremely important in conveying information and documenting that due care has been taken. These types of documentation demonstrate the efforts to collect all of the information about the patient and determine his/her medical needs.

ORGANIZING PATIENT INFORMATION

There is no single best way to record medical information, especially patient assessments. The problem you face clinically is to organize the patient information and your assessment in a logical, professional presentation.

The most popular method of documenting patient assessments is the SOAP (subjective, objective, assessment, and plan) charting method. We will start with the SOAP format to demonstrate how to document a patient assessment because this format is an excellent teaching tool.

Step 1: Data Collection

As one astute physician has pointed out, "Data collection has been likened to picking flowers rather than mowing a lawn" (author unknown). For novices, a great deal of time and effort goes into collecting and organizing data without knowing its relevance. Novices do this because they do not know which information is valuable and which is not. As practitioners become more expert, they spend less time and effort in the collection of data because they know which data are clinically meaningful. The collection and organization of relevant data to make correct decisions is complex. The goal of data collection is to come to an accurate conclusion about the patient's conditions and needs. To do so, it is necessary to start with proper bedside examination techniques. Sloppy examination methods lead to invalid data and inaccurate conclusions.

The first two steps of this system call for subjective and objective data collection (the *S* and *O* of *SOAP*). Subjective information is what the patient can tell you about how he/she feels. According to experts, obtaining a good medical history from the patient can give you a 70% chance of correctly identifying a patient's problem before doing a single test. It is also evidence of the patient's level of consciousness. If the patient is comatose, that is all the subjective information you can gather; any additional information must be objective. Other people's observations can be included in this section because they may be able to fill in some of the following questions. Remember, when you use another person's report about a subjective issue, it is always hearsay. Hearsay information can be entered into the SOAP only if you document who was the source of the information.

The major questions to answer in the subjective section include the following:

- What is the patient's chief complaint?
- How does the patient feel at the time of the assessment?
- Can the patient contribute any information that affects his/her diagnosis or treatment plan?
- What is the patient's level of consciousness?

The *O* in *SOAP* stands for objective. This is everything you see, hear, feel, smell, and learn from tests and procedures. This part of the data collection can include the following:

- Vital signs
- Physical examination of the head and neck, abdomen, and extremities for physical evidence of respiratory problems
- Physical examination of the thorax (heart and lungs) by inspection, palpation, percussion, and auscultation (see Chapter 5)
- Review of clinical laboratory studies (see Chapter 6)
- Review of ABGs (see Chapter 7)
- Review of pulmonary function test (see Chapter 8)
- Review of chest radiographs, computed tomograms, and magnetic resonance images (see Chapter 9)
- Review of electrocardiograms (ECGs) (see Chapter 10)
- Review of ICU hemodynamic data and cardiac outputs (see Chapters 14 and 15)
- Review of respiratory mechanics monitoring (see Chapter 13)

Step 2: Assessment

Your assessment of the patient's data involves critical thinking, going through clinical and scientific reasoning processes, and forming a hypothesis about the nature and cause of the patient's problems. You use this hypothesis to form a "problem list," which helps you focus on the patient's problems. We will use a patient case to illustrate how to develop a problem list (Case Study 1). See Box 20-1.

Problems can also fit into additional categories:

- Current versus potential problems. Potential problems include events or outcomes that you want to prevent, such as volume trauma, esophageal-tracheal fistulas, or reduced cardiac outputs from excessive mechanical ventilation.

BOX 20-1   Assessment and the Development of a Problem List

How do you organize and report the information in Case Study 1 so that you can quickly identify the patient's problems? All of this information can be used as the subjective and objective information of the SOAP. You can start with almost any sign or symptom you want; just make sure you use all the information you have. As you review each piece of information, ask yourself the following questions:

- Are the data normal or abnormal? (As a corollary, are the data normal in an abnormal setting?) As an example, a $PaCO_2$ of 40 mm Hg is textbook normal, but if it is associated with a minute ventilation of 15 L/min, the patient has a severe dead space disease process. In this case, a $PaCO_2$ of 32 mm Hg is not normal for a patient with dyspnea, and the PaO_2 is abnormal.
- If the findings are abnormal, are they mildly, moderately, or severely out of the norm? In this case, the acid-base and carbon dioxide levels are mildly out of line with normal ABG values, but the 53 mm Hg PaO_2 is moderately reduced.
- Is this an acute or chronic problem for the patient? Does the patient have an acute episode superimposed on a chronic problem? For example, in this case the hypoxemia may be a worsening of a chronic problem. More data are needed for further evaluation.
- Are any of these signs and symptoms related to each other? In this case, the patient is complaining of pain in his right elbow, but this sign probably is not related to his primary cardiopulmonary disease process. However, his inspiratory crackles and the leg pain have a high probability of being related to his cardiopulmonary disease process.
- Do the data indicate that there is something you can do about the patient's condition? Obviously, you can do something about the oxygenation problem, but you may not be able to administer the needed intravenous drugs because your scope of practice limits what you can and cannot give the patient.

CASE STUDY 1

You are called to the emergency room to help a patient who is complaining of shortness of breath and to give him a bronchodilator treatment. On arrival, you find a 65-year-old, moderately obese man sitting upright on the examination table in a single-patient examination room. You observe that his respiratory rate is about 20 breaths/min, with pursed-lip breathing and slight cyanosis around the lips, and he is unable to say more than a few words per breath. He is complaining of right elbow pain. His cardiac rate is 126 and irregular. On auscultation, you hear crackles in both lung bases. He reports a nonproductive cough for the last 2 days, with increasing shortness of breath (SOB), an inability to lie down flat, and increasing leg pain. You notice that he is

unable to tie his shoes because his feet are so swollen and that his legs are very red, shiny, and painful to the touch. His current peak expiratory flow (PEF) is 50% of predicted. A room air ABG was done before your arrival: pH, 7.47; $PaCO_2$, 32 mm Hg; PaO_2, 53 mm Hg; HCO_3, 23 mEq; B.E., O; SaO_2, 89%. No chest x-ray has been done.

You give the ordered bronchodilator treatment with O_2, but the patient reports no subjective relief. No changes in vital signs are noted. His color does improve a little during the treatment (O_2 at 6 L/min), and his breath sounds are unchanged. His cough is nonproductive, and there is no measurable change in the peak flow after treatment.

- Respiratory versus nonrespiratory problems. The nonrespiratory problems that RTs are interested in include cerebral blood flow, infections, ascites, and causes of metabolic acidosis. You need to know enough about these and similar topics to identify how "nonrespiratory" problems result in cardiopulmonary signs and symptoms.

Another guiding principle is this: "Do not confuse the cause or diagnosis with the patient problem." For example, the cause is smoking, the diagnosis is heart and lung disease, and the patient problem is chronic hypoxemia.

RTs do not diagnose; we objectively identify patient problems or define and describe signs and symptoms. This may be a subtle difference at times, but it is a necessary distinction for medical-legal reasons. If we stick to our areas of expertise, we will always be on safe medical-legal ground.

We can define the problems we identify using the following five major types:

- Airway management: from the nose and mouth down to the terminal respiratory bronchiole. This includes any problem that can be treated with artificial airways, pulmonary hygiene, cough assisting, suctioning, postural drainage, and in some circumstances even PEEP.
- Ventilation: the act of ventilating the patient's lungs. Acute and chronic hypoventilation problems fall into this area.
- Oxygenation: the process of delivering oxygen down to the cellular level. This includes cardiac output as a component of delivered oxygenation (Do_2).
- The work of breathing (WOB): the mechanics of both spontaneous and artificial ventilation of the lungs. Most of our treatments have a direct or indirect positive effect on WOB; for instance, oxygen therapy reduces the amount of cardiopulmonary work the patient has to do to maintain a certain amount of ventilation or Pao_2. We can measure the mechanical WOB in joules per breath or joules per minute, but measuring the oxygen cost of breathing is too difficult to perform clinically.
- Signs of acute cardiopulmonary problems that do not have a respiratory cause: a good example is diabetic ketoacidosis with Kussmaul's breathing, wherein the pulmonary manifestation is relieved with the administration of insulin.

From this perspective, you can see that RTs focus on a fairly narrow scope of practice. Furthermore, this short problem list is clearly integrated into our full range of therapeutic interventions, from life support and emergency issues to daily supportive therapies such as simple oxygen therapy.

Documenting the problem in the medical record helps to prioritize patient needs and improve communication between the different disciplines. This method of linking the data with problem identification is a crucial learning step and cannot be stressed enough. If you document the relationships between the data and the identified problem, other members of the health-care team can follow your logic (Box 20-2).

SIMPLY STATED

The assessment part of the SOAP record is not used by RTs to diagnose the patient's problem but rather to formulate a list of the patient's cardiopulmonary problems in order of severity.

Step 3: The Plan

Now that you have listed the patient's problems, what are you going to do about each of them? Each patient problem should indicate an intervention and therapeutic objective. For instance, in our case study, the hypoxemia should be treated with oxygen. The amount of oxygen and the therapeutic objective must be negotiated with the physician. The physician order becomes the plan (e.g., "Oxygen at 2 L/min via nasal cannula; titrate to keep SpO_2 at 92% or greater").

Consulting with the physician for patient orders is very important. As you repeatedly demonstrate effective data collection, problem identification, and appropriate therapeutic suggestions and communicate effectively with the physician, you build a professional relationship based on trust. This trust (or lack thereof) between the physician and therapist contributes to the reputation of your department and profession.

Two things are evident in the case from the information you gathered:

- The patient is acutely ill and requires interventions that may necessitate admission to the hospital for further investigation.
- This may not be primarily a respiratory problem, and further information is needed to identify the underlying cause of the patient's symptoms.

A good medical plan must include a goal against which one can measure. Factors to consider when establishing or evaluating an objective include the following:

1. The purpose of the treatment. By stating a goal for the treatment or therapy, the RT is meeting the expectations of the ordering physician and the needs of the patient. Every RT should know how to judge the effectiveness of the therapies he/she is administering and be able to guide both physicians and nurses in understanding the rationale for these goals.
2. Responsiveness of the patient. If the therapy is administered correctly, the patient should respond in a predictable fashion. Assuming that the treatment was

BOX 20-2	Problem List for Case Study 1 Patient

1. Hypoxemia: Pao_2, 56 mm Hg; Sao_2, 89%; cyanosis of the lips
2. SOB: pursed-lip breathing and tachypnea
3. Crackles in both bases
4. Unresponsiveness to bronchodilators: PF 50% pre- and post-Rx
5. Edema of the lower extremities
6. Tachycardia with irregular beats

BOX 20-3	The Plan (Physician Orders) for Case Study 1 Patient

1. Oxygen via nasal cannula at 2 L/min; titrate to keep SpO_2 90% to 92%; ABG to follow
2. Morning ABG, plus prn if condition worsens; SpO_2 q4hr
3. Complete blood cell count (CBC), creatine phosphokinase (CPK), electrolytes
4. Chest x-ray (CXR)
5. ECG
6. Four puffs Atrovent qid
7. Four puffs Proventil, prn for SOB
8. Lasix 50 mg bid, monitor intake and output of fluids (I&Os)

done correctly, if the patient does not meet the therapeutic goal, there are two basic possibilities:

A. The patient problem was not identified correctly and the patient has a different problem.

B. The patient is a lot sicker than you thought. A good example would be status asthmaticus, which by definition is asthma that does not respond to conventional treatment.

3. Objectives are critical for knowing when to make decisions or perform further interventions. When ordered to give a beta-2-adrenergic bronchodilator to improve the SOB, it might be wise to evaluate the patient's responsiveness by comparing the current PEF against his/her prior PEF.

4. Objectives can be used as end-point criteria for the termination of the therapy. For example, if a patient reaches a PaO_2 of 110 mm Hg on 1 L/min nasal cannula, it is probably time to discontinue the oxygen.

There can be a number of barriers to correctly setting up patient plans:

- Inadequate data collection to make correct decisions (most common)
- Failure to recognize patient problems
- False assumptions about relationships between the data and the identified problem
- Confusing the disease with the problem, or confusion of the cause with the problem; this barrier leads to ineffective intervention (Box 20-3)

The physician has continued the assessment by including additional tests (information collection) to assess cardiac signs and symptoms (e.g., ECG, CXR, CPK, and heart sounds) and to confirm or eliminate additional diagnoses. The physician has recognized that there is a high probability that there is a cardiac problem. As an RT, you cannot state that there is a cardiac problem; that is a diagnosis and is out of your scope of practice. You can correctly relate the signs of a cardiac problem (e.g., tachycardia, irregular heart beats, and edema of the lower extremities) and the signs of cellulitis.

Step 4: Implementation of the Plan

The next step is to actually give the treatment or perform the test. During the administration of bedside treatment, you still

have to use critical thinking skills to ensure that you are performing the procedure or test correctly. Furthermore, you need to keep in mind the technical aspects of equipment operation necessary for safe and effective care.

As you are doing the treatment or test, continue to collect data so you can move on to the next step of evaluating the effectiveness of the plan.

Step 5: Evaluation of the Results of the Plan and Implementation

An important question to ask is whether you correctly identified the problem. To answer this, it is necessary to go through another few questions:

- Was there any evidence of adverse effects?
- Did you see the response that you expected, given your knowledge of the patient and the technology used?

By actively seeking answers to these and similar questions, and then acting on the observed results, you are returning to the data collection, assessment, plan, and implementation steps outlined earlier. This cycling through the steps of the respiratory (scientific) process is essential for good patient care.

SIMPLY STATED

Clinicians who blindly follow physician orders are doing a disservice to their patients. The competent caregiver is constantly evaluating the effects of therapy and documenting the results in the patient's medical record. It may be necessary to call the attending physician if serious adverse effects occur or if the patient requires a change in therapy.

CHARTING METHODS

Most currently used charting systems are based on some variation of the problem-oriented medical record. All of the following charting systems require a clear outline of the patient's problems and corresponding physician orders or professional care plans to address those problems. Patient assessments can be written either on profession-specific forms or in the multidisciplinary progress notes, depending on the hospital standards. Three popular formats for writing progress notes are described in this section. Your hospital will state which of the following methods is acceptable.

Subjective, Objective, Assessment, and Plan Charting

As noted earlier, SOAP is one of the most popular documentation methods, in part because it is believed to be the best presentation of the patient's conditions and clearly shows how the physician or healthcare worker arrives at his/her professional conclusions.

Assessment, Plan, Implementation, and Evaluation Charting

A primary goal of the assessment, plan, implementation, and evaluation (APIE) method is to condense the data-collection statements and emphasize evaluation of the effectiveness of the interventions.

Problem, Intervention, and Plan Charting

At the other extreme from the detailed presentation of SOAP charting is the minimalist approach: problem, implementation, and plan (PIP) charting. PIP charting is based on the assumption that the data collection has already been done in the medical record and that the subjective and objective information gathering of SOAP charting is redundant. Some people dislike this method because they like to see the evi-

dence and logic leading to the assessment and resulting order. However, the PIP method works well for the experienced clinician who is pressed for time, wants to meet charting requirements, and needs to be brief. Under the "Problem" section, the patient's problem is stated simply, often with reference to the evidence that brought the author to this conclusion. Next is the "Intervention" section, which describes what is going to be done for the patient. This is often identical with the physician orders or standards of care for the services being provided. The "Plan" section shows how the intervention will be assessed or carried out, depending on the intervention.

Comparison of Charting Methods

The following patient scenario will be used to illustrate these different charting styles.

 CASE STUDY 2

The head nurse calls you to the medical floor on the night shift because a patient has awakened short of breath. You find a 65-year-old man sitting upright in his bed, leaning forward on the night stand. He is pursed-lipped and using accessory muscles to breathe, with a prolonged expiratory phase, at a rate of 16 to 18 per minute. In the dim light of his semiprivate room it is hard to see his color, but his skin is warm and moist over his upper torso and his chest has an increased anteroposterior diameter. His SpO_2 is 86% on room air. On auscultation, you hear crackles in the right base and expiratory low-pitched wheezing in the upper lung fields bilaterally. Breath sounds in the left lung base are very diminished. He has expectorated at least 10 cc of thick greenish-yellow sputum; no blood is seen. By palpation his pulse is rapid and occasionally irregular. He was admitted 6 hours earlier for a knee fracture incurred during a fall that afternoon. When interviewed, he relates that he has COPD but hasn't been receiving any treatment for it for the last 6 months. When he was taking medications it was only one metered dose inhaler (MD), four puffs in early morning and afternoon, but he doesn't remember the name of the medication. The physician has been paged, but it is 1:00 AM. You and the nurse agree to do the following:

1. Start oxygen therapy at 2 L/min via nasal cannula.
2. Repeat SpO_2 after O_2 therapy.
3. Get an ECG, stat.
4. Page the physician again and call the nursing and respiratory supervisors.

Immediately after completing these interventions and telling your supervisor what you have done, you sit down to chart your assessment and what has transpired.

SOAP Format Example

Date: 1/30/04
Time: 0130

S. *"I can't breathe," "I'm not on any inhalers at this time," "I have COPD."*

O. *Patient is very SOB, skin is warm and moist. Using accessory muscles, pursed-lip breathing, and long expiratory phase. Expectorated 10 cc of thick yellow and greenish sputum. Crackles in right base, left base diminished, low-pitched wheezing throughout. SpO_2 on room air 86%.*

A. *1. Signs and symptoms of respiratory distress and hypoxemia.*
   2. Retained secretions, possible bronchospasm.

P. *1. Call physician and appropriate supervisors: done.*
   2. Start on 2 L/min nasal cannula: done.
   3. Repeat SpO_2: done at 0155 = 89%.
   4. ECG: done at 0145.
   5. Request orders for above, stat ABG, and bronchodilator therapy, sputum culture and sensitivity.

APIE Format Example

Date: 1/30/04
Time: 0130

A. *1. Signs and symptoms of respiratory distress and hypoxemia.*
   2. Retained secretions, possible bronchospasm.

P. *1. Call physician and hospital supervisors.*
   2. Start on 2 L/min nasal cannula.
   3. Repeat SpO_2.
   4. ECG.
   5. Request orders for above, stat ABG, and bronchodilator therapy, and sputum C&S.

I. *1. Calls made.*
   2. Started on 2 L/min nasal cannula.
   3. ECG done.

E. *At 0210: Patient's SOB decreased but not totally reversed; SpO_2 89% on O_2.*

CASE STUDY 2– Cont'd

PIP Format Example

Date: 1/30/04
Time: 0130

P.   1. *Signs and symptoms of respiratory distress and hypoxemia.*
     2. *Retained secretions, possible bronchospasm.*
I.   1. *Call physician and hospital supervisors: done.*

   2. *Start on 2 L/min nasal cannula: done and Spo_2 89% at 0155.*
   3. *ECG: done at 0145.*
P. 1. *Continue O_2 therapy and monitor patient's level of SOB and Spo_2.*
   2. *Request orders for above, stat ABG, and bronchodilator therapy.*

CASE STUDY 3

You are just starting your morning shift in the adult ICU, and you have been assigned a 22-year-old woman with a history of acute asthma. The shift report to you is that she has been on q1hr bronchodilator therapy with 1 mL albuterol in 5 mL normal saline for 18 hours; concurrently she has been receiving 55% FIO_2 Ventimask, with a "prn ABG for SOB" order and with a continuous pulse oximeter and ECG. She has been alert and cooperative, and her SOB had diminished through the night shift. Her admission ABG on 55% FIO_2 was pH 7.46, Paco_2 30, Pao_2 70, HCO_3 22, BE-1, Sao_2 94%, Hgb 12.0, HbCO 0.7%.

When you arrive in the ICU, you note a slightly sleepy but easily aroused cooperative young adult. Her Spo_2 is reading 94% on 55% FIO_2, heart rate is 126 beats/min, and respiratory rate is 20 breaths/min without accessory muscle use. Auscultation reveals that she has bilateral inspiratory and expiratory wheezing. Her chest x-ray report states that there is hyperinflation noted bilaterally, with patchy infiltrates and atelectasis the right lung base. Her radial pulses are strong and unaffected by her respiratory pattern. Her stat morning electrolyte levels are all within normal limits; her CBC shows elevated eosinophilia but otherwise is within normal limits. You start her treatment at 0700 and finish at 0715; vital signs and breath sounds are unchanged through the treatment. You finish your charting and go to your next patient.

At 0745 the nurse calls you and asks you to come see the same asthmatic patient. You immediately recognize that her ECG rate and respiratory rate have increased in the last 30 minutes, and her accessory muscle use has increased. She is becoming restless, pulling her Ventimask off and complaining of increasing SOB. You cannot hear any breath sounds over her right lower lobe. With the nurse helping hold the patient's arm steady, you draw an arterial sample. Her Spo_2 is now 89% on the Ventimask when she keeps it on. Before you go to analyze the ABG, you put her on a partial rebreather mask per physician orders. Her ABG is pH 7.26, Paco_2 52 mm Hg, Pao_2 50 mm Hg, HCO_3 22, BE-5, Sao_2 87%, Hgb 12.0. On your return, the patient's physician is at the bedside, and she tells you the patient is going to be intubated and placed on a ventilator. The anesthetist is called to intubate as you go to get the ventilator. The patient is successfully intubated and placed on the ventilator per physician initial orders. Before you start an in-line bronchodilator treatment, you note and report that her auto-PEEP is 12 cm H_2O at a respiratory rate of 14 breaths/min with an inspiratory/expiratory (I/E) ratio of 1:3.5. After the in-line treatment, the breath sounds, peak pressures, and auto-PEEP are all unchanged, but the Spo_2 has improved to 95%.

According to hospital policy, you now have to write an assessment in the medical record.

SOAP Format Example

Date: 1/31/99
Time: 0850

S.   *"I can't breathe!" "Help me!"*

O.   *Increasing SOB, despite q1hr bronchodilator treatments; increasing Paco_2 to 52 mm Hg with falling pH, Pao_2 decreasing to 50 mm Hg concurrently, right lung sounds much more diminished than at start of shift. Patient was intubated and placed on a ventilator. Initial settings: respiratory rate of 14 breaths/min with an I/E ratio of 1:3.5; VT at 0.7 L, FIO_2 70%; Spo_2 95%. Auto-PEEP is 12 cm H_2O initially on ventilator.*

A.   1. *Acute hypercapnia, respiratory acidosis.*
     2. *Hypoxemia despite oxygen therapy.*
     3. *Increased work of breathing with profound SOB.*
     4. *Greatly diminished breath sounds in right lower lobe area.*
P.   1. *Intubate and place on ventilator: done.*
     2. *Increase FIO_2: done.*
     3. *Repeat ABGs: pending.*
     4. *Continue bronchodilator therapy in-line, q1hr: started.*
     5. *Monitor sedation needs and effectiveness.*
     6. *Monitor auto-PEEP.*
     7. *Check tube placement on CXR.*
     8. *Adjust the ventilator settings, post-ABG, to new settings per physician orders.*

CASE STUDY 3— Cont'd

APIE Format Example

Date: 1/31/99
Time: 0850

  A. *1. Acute hypercapnia and respiratory acidosis.*
     2. Hypoxemia despite oxygen therapy.
     3. Increased work of breathing with profound SOB.
     4. Greatly diminished breath sounds in right lower lobe area.
  P. *1. Intubate and place on ventilator.*
     2. Increase FIO_2.
     3. Repeat ABGs.
     4. Continue bronchodilator therapy in-line q1hr.
     5. Monitor sedation needs and effectiveness.
     6. Monitor auto-PEEP.
     7. Check tube placement and CXR.
     8. Adjust the ventilator settings, post ABG, to new settings per physician orders.
  I. *1. Intubated and placed on ventilator with the following settings: respiratory rate of 14 breaths/min, with an I/E ratio of 1:2.5; V_T at 0.7 L, FIO_2 70%.*
     2. Increased FIO_2; done.
     3. Continue bronchodilator therapy in-line q1hr: done.
     4. Monitor auto-PEEP.

  E. *1. Patient is resting on ventilator, sedated.*
     2. ABG: pending.
     3. SpO_2 is 95% currently.
     4. Breath sounds unchanged.

PIP Format Example

Date: 1/31/99
Time: 0850

  P. *1. Acute hypercapnia and respiratory acidosis.*
     2. Hypoxemia despite oxygen therapy
     3. Increased work of breathing with profound SOB.
     4. Greatly diminished breath sounds in right lower lobe area.
  I. *1. Intubated and placed on ventilator.*
     2. Increased FIO_2.
     3. Repeat ABGs: pending.
     4. Continue bronchodilator therapy in-line q1hr: done.
  P. *1. Monitor sedation needs and effectiveness.*
     2. Monitor auto-PEEP.
     3. Check tube placement and CXR.
     4. Adjust the ventilator settings, post-ABG, to new settings per physician orders.

SUMMARY

The role of the RT in the documentation of the patient assessment is well defined. He/she must be able to not only assess the patient's condition accurately, but also document the findings in the patient's medical record using a prescribed format that meets JCAHO and legal requirements. The documentation of patient assessments serves a variety of purposes that are important to the business of the healthcare organization. A variety of documentation formats are available, each of which has its own advantages. Regardless of the method chosen, each recording in the patient chart must be accurate, concise, and available to other clinicians for review. High-quality documentation after each patient encounter promotes improved communication within the healthcare organization and promotes improved patient outcomes.

REVIEW QUESTIONS

1. T   F   The patient's medical record is a financial document.

2. T   F   The patient's medical record is a legal document.

3. Which of the following organizations influence what needs to be documented in a patient's medical record?
    a. Joint Commission on Accreditation of Healthcare Organizations
    b. Medicare

    c. Financial intermediaries
    d. All of the above

4. What is the primary goal of the Joint Commission on Accreditation of Healthcare Organizations?
    a. Monitor financial reimbursement of hospitals
    b. Review healthcare organizations to improve the quality of healthcare
    c. Provide healthcare workers with a safe work environment
    d. Monitor the ethical practice of medicine at healthcare organizations

5. Which of the following statements is most appropriate for the RT in the assessment section of the SOAP documentation?
    a. Onset of asthma
    b. Viral pneumonia
    c. Hypoxemia on room air
    d. Diabetic ketoacidosis

6. T   F   The patient's medical record can serve as an educational tool for students.

7. Your medical-legal duties to the patient are outlined by:
    a. JCAHO standards.
    b. AARC code of ethics as respiratory care practitioners.
    c. Your state's Respiratory Care Board's practice act.
    d. Your job description and employer's policies and procedures.
    e. All of the above.

8. All of the following are examples of "objective" data, *except:*
   a. Laboratory results.
   b. Observation of a patient's sleep apnea.
   c. The patient's report of the amount of sputum he/she produces daily.
   d. The physician's interpretation of the patient's ECG.

9. What does the letter "I" stand for in the APIE method of documentation?
   a. Implementation
   b. Impact
   c. Inconsistencies
   d. None of the above

10. Which method of documentation is probably best for a clinician pressed for time?
    a. SOAP
    b. APIE
    c. PIP
    d. APIA

REFERENCES

1. Wood KJ: *Critical thinking: cases in respiratory care,* Philadelphia, 1998, FA Davis.
2. *Comprehensive accreditation manual for hospitals,* Chicago, 2004, Joint Commission on Accreditation of Healthcare Organizations.

BIBLIOGRAPHY

Maher VF: Legal aspects of clinical care. In Dantzker DR, MacIntyre NR, Bakow ED: *Comprehensive respiratory care,* Philadelphia, 1995, WB Saunders, pp 1182-1190.

Meeham MJ: Legal aspects of therapist driven protocols: do therapist driven protocols place therapists in a legally compromising position? *Respir Care Clin North Am* 2(1):133, 1996.

North SD, Serkes PC: Improving documentation of initial nursing assessment, *Nursing Management* 27(4):30, 1996.

Roach WH: Legal review: incentives for completing medical records—the legal risks, *Topics in Health Records Management* 10(3):78, 1990.

Thomas JP: *Healthcare records: a practical legal guide,* Westchester, Ill, 1990, Healthcare Financial Management Association.

Tietsort JA: Therapist driven protocols and newer models for patient care delivery, *Respir Care Clin North Am* 2(1):147, 1996.

Glossary

A

abdominal paradox – paradoxical movement of the abdomen during breathing, caused by diaphragm fatigue.

abortion – termination of pregnancy, either spontaneous (natural interruption from abnormalities of the fetus, placenta, uterus, or mother) or therapeutic (induced interruption).

acidemia – an abnormal buildup of hydrogen ions in the blood.

acidosis – a pH less than normal.

acrocyanosis – a bluish discoloration of the digits resulting from inadequate levels of oxygen in the arterial blood.

adenosine triphosphate (ATP) – The body's energy currency molecules.

afterload – the resistance to blood flow out of the ventricle during systole.

ageism – discrimination against older people.

air bronchogram – an abnormal radiographic finding that occurs when the bronchi are surrounded by consolidated alveoli.

airway resistance (Raw) – a measurement defined as the change in pressure in the airway divided by flow: it is the reciprocal of airway conductance.

alkalemia – an abnormal decrease in the hydrogen ion concentration of the blood.

alkalosis – a pH elevated above normal.

alveolar dead space – alveoli that are ventilated but not perfused.

anabolism – the constructive phase of metabolism; making more complex structures out of simple ones.

anatomic dead space – the volume of air in the trachea and other airways not in intimate contact with pulmonary capillaries.

anemia – an abnormal decrease in the circulating red blood cells and/or hemoglobin.

anergy – impaired reaction to antigens administered by skin test.

angina – chest pain associated with inadequate coronary blood flow.

Apgar score – A 10-point score used to evaluate the well-being of infants following delivery.

apical lordotic view – a radiographic technique whereby the patient is positioned at a 45-degree angle in order to better visualize the right middle lobe or the lung apices.

apnea – the cessation of breathing; during sleep the pause in breathing must be at least 10 seconds for apnea to be present.

apparent life-threatening events (ALTEs) – episodes of prolonged apnea in an infant that nearly results in death.

arrhythmias – a disturbance in cardiac conduction.

arterial-mixed venous oxygen content difference $[C(a - \bar{v})O_2]$ – the mathematical difference between the oxygen content of the arterial blood and the oxygen content of the mixed venous sample; normally 3.5 to 5.0 mL/100 mL of blood.

ascites – the accumulation of serous fluid in the abdominal cavity.

atelectasis – a process within lung parenchyma where air is lost and the area collapses; many types of atelectasis are described, depending on the mechanism of air loss (compression, obstruction, or absorption) or amount of lung involved (massive, lobar, segmental, subsegmental, and micro).

atrial kick – the added filling of the ventricles during diastole caused by atrial contraction.

attenuation – The alteration of sounds that travel through the lung.

automaticity – the ability of cardiac tissue to stimulate depolarization spontaneously.

auto-PEEP – the inadvertent application of positive end expiratory pressure; most often resulting from inadequate expiratory time.

B

barrel chest – the abnormal increase in anteroposterior diameter.

basal energy expenditure (BEE) – the measure obtained when a person is at absolute rest with no physical movement.

basophilia – an abnormal elevation of the blood basophil count.

basal metabolic rate (BMR) – rate of oxygen consumption at rest.

blasts – an early cell that produces something.

body mass index (BMI) – the primary method for assessment of the appropriateness of weight for a given height.

bradycardia – a decrease in the heart rate below normal range (< 60/min in adults).

bradypnea – an abnormal decrease in the rate of breathing.

bronchial breath sounds – harsh breath sounds with an expiratory component equal to the inspiratory component.

bronchophony – an increase in intensity and clarity of vocal resonance.

bronchoprovocation testing – a specialized pulmonary function test usually applied to patients with occult asthma that uses substances such as methacholine or histamine in order to "provoke" the airways

into contracting and thus increasing airway resistance.

bronchopulmonary dysplasia (BPD) – chronic lung disease of newborns, usually premature.

bronchoscopes – highly specialized medical devices that allow for examination of the patient's airways: long and thin, with a fiberoptic bundle and with a channel down the entire length, the instruments are used for irrigating distal airways, suctioning, and passing brushes and biopsy forceps. The instruments are used mainly for diagnosis and are rarely used for treatment.

bronchoscopy – the procedure in which the patient's airways are examined with a bronchoscope.

bruit – a cardiovascular term associated with blood passing through a site of obstruction.

bulging – the opposite movement of the skin during exhalation.

C

cachectic – a state of poor health resulting from malnutrition.

capacity – the sum of two lung volumes.

capnography – monitoring the concentration of exhaled CO_2 using a graph.

capnometry – the general process of monitoring exhaled CO_2.

carbon dioxide production ($\dot{V}CO_2$) – the amount of CO_2 produced by metabolism per minute.

cardiac index (CI) – the cardiac output indexed to the size of the patient.

cardiac output – the amount of blood pumped out of the left ventricle in 1 minute.

cardiac work – a measurement of the energy the heart uses to eject blood against the aortic or pulmonary pressures (resistance).

cardiac work index – the work per minute per square meter of body surface area for each ventricle.

catabolism – the destructive phase of metabolism; breaking complex structures into simple ones.

central apnea – pauses in breathing resulting from a temporary loss in the drive to breathe.

central cyanosis – present when the patient's trunk or oral mucosa is cyanotic; occurs when the lungs are not oxygenating the blood adequately or when congenital heart disease causes venous blood to be shunted into the arterial system without passing through the lungs.

central venous pressure (CVP) – the pressure in the right atrium.

chronologic age – the age of an infant in days, weeks, months, or years from birth.

closing volume (CV) – a physiological unit of the lung determined by a specialized nitrogen washout technique that measures the volume of gas remaining in the lung after the small airways close during expiration.

clubbing – painless enlargement of the terminal phalanges of the fingers and toes.

coarctation of the aorta – abnormal narrowing of the internal diameter of the aorta; usually around the ductus arteriosus.

coma – inability to be aroused from a sleeplike state.

compliance – a measure of relative stiffness of the lung; it is defined as volume change per unit change in applied pressure.

computed tomography (CT scanning) – a highly advanced means of imaging where x-ray shadows are enhanced by using a computer.

conscious sedation – the process of sedating a patient using intravenous medications; often used to minimize the patient's discomfort during a bronchoscopy procedure.

contractility – the force of myocardial contractility.

cough – a forceful expiratory maneuver designed to clear the larger airways; a common complaint of patients with lung disease.

crackles – discontinuous adventitious lung sounds.

cranial sutures – the open space between any two of the flat bones of the skull in the newborn and young infant.

creatine phosphate – an energy reserve molecule in muscle.

creatinine – a waste product of metabolism.

creatinine-height index (CHI) – a predictor of muscle mass.

croup – a disorder most often affecting small children that causes inflammation of the upper airway and trachea resulting from viral infection.

crying vital capacity (CVC) – gas volume moved while an infant is crying; this is the closest measurement of vital capacity possible in infants.

cyanosis – a bluish cast to the skin that clinically may be difficult to detect, especially in a poorly lighted room and in patients with dark-pigmented skin.

cytology – the study of cells of the body.

D

dead space – the volume of gas inhaled that does not participate in gas exchange.

dead space-tidal volume ratio (V_D/V_T) – the ratio of the dead space volume to the total amount of gas inhaled.

decerebrate posturing – abnormal posturing seen as extension and internal rotations of the arms and legs, indicative of high brainstem injuries.

decorticate posturing – occurs when the arms, wrists, and fingers flex over the chest while the legs extend and internally rotate.

delta sleep – the deeper stages of NREM sleep.

depolarization – an electrical change in an excitable cell in which the inside becomes positive; associated with contraction of cardiac muscle cells.

diagnostic reasoning – a cognitive activity used to identify the cause of the patient's problem and possible solutions.

diaphoresis – excessive sweating.

diastolic blood pressure – the pressure in the arteries during relaxation of the ventricles.

diffusion capacity (D_L) – the ability of the lung to diffuse gas from the alveoli to the pulmonary capillary blood.

diplopia – blurred or double vision.

direct calorimetry – measures of the heat given off by the body in a carefully designed room.

Doll's eyes – absent oculocephalic reflex is seen as the head is turned from side to side and eyes remain fixed in the head, looking straight ahead; eyes appear immovable just as a doll's eyes that are painted onto the doll's head.

dynamic compliance – represents the total impedance to gas flow into the lungs.

dynamic hyperinflation – a problem seen with severe airway obstruction in which mechanical breaths are stacked upon one another.

dyspnea – shortness of breath as perceived by the patient.

E

ectopic impulse – a heart beat originating outside the SA node.

edema – excessive fluid in tissue.

egophony – when the spoken voice increases in intensity and takes on a nasal or bleating quality.

ejection fraction (EF) – the portion of the end diastolic volume ejected during systole; normally about 60% to 70%.

end-diastolic pressure (EDP) – the pressure in the left ventricle at the end of diastole.

end-diastolic volume (EDV) – the volume of blood in the left ventricle just before systole.

endoscopy – a medical procedure in which a physician looks into the body of the patient using a scope.

end-tidal P_{CO_2} (P_{ETCO2}) – the partial pressure of P_{CO_2} at the end expiratory point.

eosinophilia – an abnormal increase in the presence of eosinophils.

epiglottitis – infection of the upper airway resulting from bacteria; most often seen in children.

erythrocytes – red blood cells.

escape beat – a heart beat that originates outside the sinus node following a period of SA node inactivity.

estimated date of confinement (EDC) – estimated date of a term delivery in a pregnant woman.

expiratory reserve volume (ERV) – a physiologic unit of the lung defined by pulmonary function testing that describes the amount of gas that can be forcefully exhaled after a passive exhalation.

exudate – when used to describe a pleural effusion, it is fluid with a high (more than 3 g/L) protein content.

F

fetal hemoglobin (Hb F) – hemoglobin F, present in the fetus in utero; fetal Hb has a higher affinity for oxygen than does hemoglobin A (adult Hb); it allows the fetus to survive and grow in the relatively low oxygen environment of the uterus.

fever – an increase in the body temperature resulting from disease.

Fick principle – a method for measuring cardiac output using oxygen consumption and the oxygen content difference between arterial and venous blood.

flail chest – the paradoxical motion seen as a sinking inward of the affected region with each spontaneous inspiratory effort and an outward movement with subsequent exhalation.

focus – the site from which the ectopic impulse originates.

forced vital capacity (FVC) – the maximum amount of air the patient exhales after a full, deep inspiration.

fractional saturation – compares the amount of hemoglobin that is saturated with the total amount of hemoglobin present.

functional residual capacity (FRC) – a physiologic unit of the lung that is the mathematical sum of the reserve volume (RV) and the expiratory reserve volume (ERV); it is the point where the expanding chest wall forces are balanced with the contractile rebound forces of the lung.

functional saturation – compares the amount of hemoglobin that is saturated with the amount of hemoglobin that is capable of being saturated.

G

gallop rhythm – an abnormal condition in which a third or fourth heart sound is present.

gestational age – the age of a fetus measured in weeks from the time of conception.

gluconeogenesis – converting protein (amino acids) to sugar.

glucosuria – excessive sugar in the urine.

glycolysis – the process of converting glucose into pyruvic acid.

gravida – number of pregnancies a woman has had.

grunting – the sound made by an infant attempting to increase functional residual capacity by closure of the glottis at end inspiration.

H

harsh breath sounds – breath sounds with increased intensity.

heave – a systolic thrust.

hematemesis – vomiting blood from the stomach.

hemoptysis – coughing up blood from the lungs.

hemostasis – the arrest of bleeding or stagnation of blood flow.

hepatomegaly – enlargement of the liver.

HME – home medical equipment.

home care – prescribed respiratory services provided in a patient's personal residence.

Hoover's sign – abnormal movement of the lateral chest wall during breathing in COPD patients with severe hyperinflation.

hypercapnia – abnormal elevation of $PaCO_2$.

hypercarbia – abnormal elevation of arterial carbon dioxide levels.

hyperchloremia – elevation of the chloride ion concentration in the blood plasma.

hyperdynamic precordium – visible beating of the heart on the chest wall; usually indicates hypertrophy of the left or right ventricles.

hyperglycemia – an abnormal elevation in blood glucose levels.

hyperkalemia – abnormal elevation of plasma potassium.

hypernatremia – abnormal elevation of plasma sodium.

hypertension – abnormal elevation of arterial blood pressure.

hyperthermia – elevation of body temperature.

hypoalbuminemia – reduced blood protein levels.

hypochloremia – abnormal decrease in plasma chloride levels.

hypoglycemia – reduced blood sugar levels.

hypokalemia – abnormal decrease in serum potassium.

hyponatremia – abnormal decrease in serum sodium levels.

hypopnea – a decrease in ventilation during sleep related to elevated upper airway resistance.

hypotension – an abnormal decrease in arterial blood pressure.

hypothermia – an abnormal decrease in body temperature.

hypotonia – loss of muscle tone.

hypoxemia – an abnormal reduction in the partial pressure of oxygen in the arterial blood.

hypoxia – a lack of oxygen.

I

ideal body weight – the optimum weight of the patient as predicted from height and weight charts.

immunosenescence – the age-associated decline in the immune system.

indirect calorimetry – measures respiratory parameters (VO_2 and VCO_2) to determine the energy consumed by the body.

inspiratory capacity (IC) – a physiologic unit of the lung defined by pulmonary function testing which is the sum of the tidal volume and the reserve volume; the maximum amount of air that can be inhaled from resting FRC.

inspiratory reserve volume (IRV) – a physiologic unit of the lung defined by pulmonary function testing, which is the maximum volume of air that can be inhaled following a normal quiet inhalation.

interrupted aortic arch syndrome – a developmental anomaly in which the aortic arch fails to completely form.

intimate space – the area around the patient within 18 inches.

intrapulmonary shunt ($\dot{Q}S/\dot{Q}T$) – blood passing through the lung that is not exposed to ventilated alveoli.

intraventricular hemorrhage (IVH) – bleeding in the lateral ventricles of the brain (grades I-III) or the tissue of the brain (grade IV) in premature infants.

isolated systolic hypertension (ISH) – elevation of only the systolic pressure.

J

Joint Commission on Accreditation of Healthcare Organizations (JCAHO) – an organization designed to inspect and improve hospital patient care.

K

Kerley B Lines – a radiographic finding on a chest x-ray of a patient in congestive heart failure: the lines are short, parallel, and 1 mm thick, and start at the lung base: originating at the pleura, they extend into the lung parenchyma 1 to 2 cm. They are caused by engorged pleural-based lymphatic vessels.

Kilocalories (kcal) – the amount of energy it takes to raise the temperature of 1 kg of water 1° C.

L

lactic acid – the product of anaerobic metabolism.

last menstrual period (LMP) – the date of the beginning of a woman's last menstrual period before pregnancy. This date can be used to calculate the estimated date of confinement (EDC).

lateral decubitus view – a radiographic technique used to demonstrate the presence of a free-flowing pleural effusion: the patient is positioned so that he/she is laying with the side of the hemithorax in question down, allowing for gravity to act on the effusion and layering it out along the dependent lateral chest wall.

lecithin/sphingomyelin (L/S) ratio – ratio of the two phospholipids lecithin and sphingomyelin; as a fetus' lungs mature, the amount of lecithin increases.

left shift – a term used to indicate the presence of immature white cells in the circulating blood.

leukocytes – white blood cells.

leukocytosis – an abnormal increase in the circulating white blood cell count.

leukopenia – an abnormal decrease in the circulating white blood cell count.

long apnea – an apneic episode that lasts longer than 15 to 20 seconds in an infant.

loud P_2 – pulmonary hypertension that increases intensity of S_2 as a result of more forceful closure of the pulmonic valve.

lower inflection point – considered to be the minimal PEEP that should be applied to the lung as determined using a static pressure-volume curve.

lymphocytopenia – an abnormal decrease in the number of circulating lymphocytes.

lymphocytosis – an abnormal increase in the number of circulating lymphocytes.

M

macrocytic – large cell size.

macrophage – a monocyte that has left the circulation and entered tissue.

magnetic resonance (MR) – a high-technology radiographic imaging technique.

maximal voluntary ventilation (MVV) – the volume of gas a patient can move in and out of the lung in 1 minute; value estimate based on patient performance for 15 seconds.

maximum inspiratory pressure (P_{Imax}) – a maximum pressure a patient can generate during a full inspiratory effort.

mean airway pressure – the average pressure recorded during the positive-pressure and spontaneous phases of a respiratory cycle.

mean arterial pressure – the average pressure present in the arterial blood.

meconium – the thick tarry stool that is present in the colon of a fetus in utero.

meconium aspiration syndrome (MAS) – the inhalation of meconium passed into the amniotic fluid by the fetus in utero.

metabolic cart – a computer-controlled unit composed of oxygen and carbon dioxide gas analyzers and flow transducers; used to measure indirect calorimetry.

metabolism – the body's way of transferring energy from food to the body's energy currency molecules: adenosine triphosphate.

microcytic – small cell size.

micrognathia – small lower jaw.

minute volume ($\dot{V}_E$) – the volume of air inhaled or exhaled in 1 minute.

miosis – pinpoint pupils.

mixed venous oxygen saturation [$S\bar{v}O_2$] – the percent saturation of mixed venous blood with oxygen; normally about 75%.

mixed venous oxygen tension [$P\bar{v}O_2$] – the partial pressure of oxygen in the venous blood. Sample obtained from the right atrium or pulmonary artery.

monitoring – repeated or continuous observations or measurements of the patient, his/her physiologic function, and the function of life support equipment, for the purpose of guiding management decisions.

monocytosis – an abnormal increase in circulating monocytes.

multiple sleep latency test (MSLT) – an objective measure of daytime sleepiness. The patient is provided the opportunity to nap multiple times during the day. The average time of sleep latency is measured for each nap. Patients with excessive daytime sleepiness have short sleep latency times during each nap.

mydriasis – dilated and fixed pupils.

N

nasal flaring – the dilation of the ala nasi (the openings of the nose) during inspiration; this is an attempt by the infant to decrease airway resistance and increase tidal volume.

negative inotropic effect – response of the heart in which the contractility is reduced.

negligence – a legal term that refers to a health care professional acting outside the standards of care that causes harm to the patient.

neutral thermal environment (NTE) – the temperature range of an infant's environment (usually an isolette or radiant warmer) where the infant's caloric expenditure is the least.

neutropenia – an abnormal decrease in the circulating neutrophils.

neutrophilia – an abnormal increase in the circulating neutrophils.

night sweats – excessive diaphoresis during sleep.

nitric oxide (NO) – a soluble gas that is normally produced in the body and serves as a powerful vasodilator.

nitrogen balance – when the intake of nitrogen equals excretion of nitrogen.

nitrogen washout – a technique used during pulmonary function testing to determine if there is maldistribution of ventilation of gas within the lung.

non-rapid eye movement (NREM) sleep – a type of sleep composed of four stages: I, II, III, IV; this is the type of sleep in which the sleeper does not dream and makes up the majority of sleep time in the normal sleeper.

normoblasts – immature nucleated red blood cells.

nystagmus – involuntary, cyclic movement of the eyeballs.

O

objective data – information about the patient that can be measured and is not a matter of opinion.

oblique views – the patient is turned 45 degrees to either the right or left, with the anterolateral portion of the chest against the film.

obstructive disease – lung disease characterized by abnormally narrowed airways that cause the expiratory flow measurements to be reduced.

obstructive sleep apnea (OSA) – intermittent pauses in breathing for more than 10 seconds resulting from upper airway blockage during sleep.

oculocephalic reflex – test of brainstem function in which the head is rotated side to side and eye movement is noted.

oncotic pressure – the pressure in the vascular space created by the presence of large protein molecules that draws fluid outside the vessels into the vasculature.

orthodeoxia – hypoxemia associated with sitting upright.

orthopnea – shortness of breath in the reclining position.

orthostatic hypotension – a drop in blood pressure associated with standing or sitting up.

osteopenia of the premature – a bone disease in premature infants that causes weak fragile bones; it is caused by inadequate phosphorous intake.

ototoxicity – a drug that is toxic to the ear.

oxygen consumption – the amount of oxygen consumed per minute by the body tissues.

oxygen content – the amount of oxygen present in the blood; represents the oxygen combined with hemoglobin and dissolved in plasma; expressed as mL/100 mL of blood.

oxygen delivery (Do$_2$) – the amount of oxygen delivered to the body tissues per minute; a function of cardiac output and oxygen content.

oxygen extraction ratio [C(a-$\bar{v}$)O$_2$/CaO$_2$] – the portion of oxygen content in the arterial blood extracted by the tissues.

oxygen transport – the amount of oxygen moved by the blood per unit of time.

oxygen uptake – the amount of oxygen used by the tissues per minute.

oxyhemoglobin dissociation curve (ODC) – graphically depicts the relationship between Pao$_2$ and the oxygen content or hemoglobin saturation.

P

pack years – the number of packs of cigarettes smoked per day multiplied by the number of years smoked. Higher pack years are associated with greater risk of lung cancer and other lung diseases.

Pao$_2$/PAo$_2$ ratio – the arterial-alveolar O$_2$ ratio; the ratio of arterial oxygen level to the alveolar oxygen level; normally > 0.90.

PAOP – pulmonary artery occlusion pressure.

para – the number of delivered infants of a woman.

parenteral – outside of the gastrointestinal tract.

paroxysmal nocturnal dyspnea – the sudden onset of shortness of breath during sleep.

patent ductus arteriosus (PDA) – the vessel that makes the anatomic connection between the pulmonary artery and the aorta during fetal life.

peak expiratory flow (PEF) – the maximum flow rate achieved by the patient during the forced vital capacity maneuver.

peak pressure – the maximum pressure attained during the inspiratory phase of mechanical ventilation.

pedal edema – an accumulation of fluid in the subcutaneous tissues of the ankles.

periodic breathing – an irregular breathing pattern in which periods of apnea are mixed in with periods of normal breathing.

peripheral cyanosis – presence of cyanosis in the digits.

personal space – the zone around the patient from 18 inches to 4 feet.

persistent vegetative state – the inability to be aroused, but the patient's eyes are open.

pertinent negative – a symptom related to the system in question but denied by the patient; for example, if the patient has lung disease but denies shortness of breath, in this case dyspnea would be a pertinent negative.

pertinent positive – a symptom the patient states is present that is related to the primary problem for which the patient is seeking help.

phlegm – mucus from the tracheobronchial tree.

phosphatidylglycerol (PG) – a phospholipid that becomes present with lung maturation in the fetus.

phosphatidylinositol (PI) – a phospholipid that becomes present with lung maturation in the fetus.

physiologic dead space – the conductive airways and alveolar units that are ventilated but not perfused.

plateau pressure – the pressure required to maintain a delivered V$_T$ in a patient's lungs during a period of no gas flow.

platypnea – shortness of breath in the upright position.

pneumoperitoneum – air in the abdomen.

pneumothorax – air in the pleural space.

point of maximal impulse – the thrust of the contracting left ventricle and usually is identified near the midclavicular line in the fifth intercostal space.

polycythemia – an abnormal increase in red blood cell count.

polycythemia vera – an uncontrolled proliferation of hematopoietic cells within the bone marrow.

polysomnogram (PSG) – a sleep study used to diagnose sleep apnea and other sleep-related breathing disorders.

positive inotropic effect – a medication or treatment that increases cardiac contractility.

positron emission tomography (PET) – a high-technology radiographic technique used to determine if a lesion seen on a standard x-ray contains cancer cells.

posteroanterior (PA) view – a radiographic view of the chest where the patient is placed in the upright position and turned so that the x-ray beam travels through the patient from his/her back (posterior) to front (anterior) before striking the x-ray film cassette.

postterm infants – infants born later than 42 weeks' gestational age.

postural hypotension – significant changes in blood pressure associated with changes in position.

precordium – chest wall overlying the heart.

preload – the volume of blood in the ventricle just prior to systole.

presbycusis – the progressive loss of hearing with age.

presbyopia – loss of ability to focus on objects held near the eye with age.

pressure-volume loop – a graph designed to display the relationship between the volume inhaled and the pressure generated.

preterm infants – infants born younger that 37 weeks' gestational age.

protein energy malnutrition – loss of body protein.

pseudohypertension – falsely high blood pressure in older adults because of arterial stiffness.

pseudoneutropenia – a decrease in the neutrophil count associated with cells shifting from the circulatory pool to the marginated pool.

pseudoneutrophilia – elevation of the neutrophil count that is the result of cells

shifting from the marginated pool to the circulatory pool.

ptosis – Drooping of the upper eyelid.

pulmonary angiography – a high-technology radiographic technique used to determine the presence of blood clots (embolisms) in the pulmonary circulation.

pulmonary capillary wedge pressure (PCWP) – the pressure measured at the tip of the pulmonary artery catheter when the balloon is inflated; an estimated of left ventricular filling pressure.

pulmonary vascular resistance (PVR) – the resistance to blood flow through the pulmonary circulation.

pulse oximetry – a monitoring technique used to estimate that oxygen saturation levels in the arterial blood.

pulse pressure – the mathematical difference between the systolic and the diastolic blood pressure measurements.

R

radiolucent – a term used in describing the appearance of a x-ray film where the x-ray beam has gone unimpeded through the patient and has turned that corresponding part of the resultant film black.

radiopaque – a term used in describing the appearance of a x-ray film where the x-ray beam has been absorbed, causing the corresponding part of the resultant film to be white.

rapid eye movement (REM) sleep – the type of sleep in which dreaming is believed to occur.

rapid-shallow breathing index (RSBI) – the ratio of respiratory frequency (f) to V_T.

rate-pressure product – obtained by multiplying the variables of heart rate and systolic blood pressure; used to assess the work load on the heart.

repolarization – the return of a negative charge within the cell; occurs during relaxation of the myocardial cells.

residual volume (RV) – a physiological unit of the lung determined by pulmonary function testing, which describes the volume of gas remaining in the lung after maximal exhalation.

respiratory acidosis – a decrease in pH resulting from elevation of the arterial P_{CO_2}.

respiratory alkalosis – an increase in pH due to a decrease in arterial P_{CO_2}.

respiratory alternans – periods of breathing using only the chest wall muscles alternating with periods of breathing entirely by the diaphragm.

respiratory distress syndrome (RDS) – a lung disease of premature infants characterized by inadequate amounts of lung surfactant.

respiratory disturbance index (RDI) – the number of apneas and hypopneas per hour of sleep.

respiratory quotient (RQ) – the ratio of carbon dioxide produced to oxygen consumed.

resting energy expenditure (REE) – measure of oxygen uptake with patient at rest.

restrictive disease – disease of the chest associated with a loss of lung volume.

reticulocytes – nucleated red blood cells.

retractions – inward movement of the skin around the chest wall during inspiration; retractions are seen in any lung disease where the compliance of the lung is less than the compliance of the chest wall.

retrognathia – a recessed or small lower jaw.

S

serum – the watery fluid portion of the blood.

serum albumin – the major protein fraction of blood.

serum transferrin – the protein that transports iron in the body.

short apnea – a cessation of breathing in infants less than 12 seconds.

signs – physical examination findings consistent with disease.

silhouette sign – a radiographic finding that occurs when the edge of a well-established object (the heart) is obliterated because there is an infiltrate in anatomic contact.

sinus bradycardia – an abnormal drop in heart rate with each beat originating in the SA node.

skinfold measurement – a method for estimating the percent of body fat.

sleep apnea – pauses in breathing of at least 10 seconds during sleep.

sleep continuity theory – the theory that uninterrupted sleep is more restorative.

sleep latency – the amount of time required for the onset of sleep

social space – the space of 4 to 12 feet from the patient.

spirogram – the tracing produced by a spirograph.

spirograph – a piece of equipment that measures a patient's airflows and volumes of gas moved over time and is capable of displaying the information in graphic form.

spirometer – a piece of equipment that measures a patient's airflows and volumes of gas moved over time.

splenomegaly – abnormal enlargement of the spleen.

spontaneous abortion – the physiologic termination of pregnancy because of abnormalities of the fetus, placenta, uterus, or mother.

spurious polycythemia – an increase in the red blood cell count resulting from a decrease in serum (as in dehydration).

sputum – secretions from the tracheobronchial tree that are expectorated through the mouth.

static compliance – the lung volume change per unit of pressure during a period of no gas flow.

stridor – continuous sound heard primarily over the larynx and trachea during inhalation when upper airway obstruction is present.

stroke volume (SV) – the volume of blood ejected from the ventricle during systole.

subcutaneous emphysema – a crackling sound and sensation when fine beads of air are palpated in the tissues.

subjective data – information obtained from the patient that cannot be confirmed with objective testing.

sudden infant death syndrome (SIDS) – a condition of unexplained death of an infant. Usually seen in infants between 6 weeks and 6 months of age. The incidence of this disease is decreased by not letting the young infant sleep in a prone (face down) position.

symptoms – subjective complaints by the patient.

syncope – fainting or dizziness; often resulting from hypotension.

systemic vascular resistance (SVR) – the amount of resistance experienced by the arterial blood as it passes through the peripheral vasculature.

systolic blood pressure – the peak blood pressure in the arteries during ventricular contraction.

T

tachycardia – an abnormal increase in the heart rate.

tachypnea – an abnormal increase in the rate of breathing.

target – a physical structure in the x-ray machine used to direct the x-ray beam.

term infants – infant born between 37 and 42 weeks' gestational age.

territoriality – the patient's sense that items around his/her hospital bed belong to that him/her while admitted.

therapeutic abortion – the medical termination of pregnancy.

thoracocentesis – surgical puncture of the chest wall usually to remove pleural fluid.

thrombocytes – blood platelets.

thrombocytopenia – an abnormal decrease in the circulating platelets.

thrombocytosis – an abnormal increase in the number of circulating blood platelets.

tidal volume (VT) – a physiological unit of the lung, which is the amount of gas moved in and out of the lung during relaxed, at-rest breathing.

tinnitus – an auditory perception not caused by external sounds. It may be described as ringing, buzzing, roaring, or chirping.

total lung capacity (TLC) – a physiological unit of the lung determined during pulmonary function testing, which describes the total amount of gas in the lungs after maximum inspiration.

total parenteral nutrition (TPN) – the feeding of patients by direct infusion of nutrients into either a peripheral or a central vein.

transient tachypnea of the newborn (TTNB) – a lung disease with increased lung water in infants born by cesarean section.

transmural pressure – the net distending pressure within the ventricle; it provides a true estimation of left ventricular end-diastolic filling because the effect of pressure around the heart is considered.

transudate – when used to describe a pleural effusion, it is fluid with a low (less than 3 g/L) protein content.

treopnea – better breathing associated with a certain position.

U

upper airway resistance syndrome (UARS) – a common cause of sleep fragmentation in patients who snore.

upper inflection point – the part of the curve on a static pressure-volume curve that indicates over distention of the lung.

V

venous return – the amount of blood returned to the right side of the heart.

ventricular compliance – the ability of the ventricle to expand as blood enters from the atrium.

ventricular function curves – graphs demonstrating the various stroke volumes achieved at various degrees of filling pressure.

ventricular stroke work – the amount of work performed by the left ventricle during systole.

vesicular breath sound – a soft, muffled sound upon auscultation over the lung parenchyma of a healthy person.

vital capacity (VC) – the maximum amount of air that can be expelled following a full inspiratory effort.

volumes – pulmonary function measurements used to define a portion of the lung capacity.

volutrauma – a lung injury that occurs from overdistention of the terminal respiratory units.

W

wheeze – the musical sounds heard from the chest of the patient with intrathoracic airway obstruction (e.g., asthma).

Answers to Review Questions

CHAPTER 1

1. c
2. c
3. c
4. a
5. b
6. false
7. d
8. true
9. d
10. true
11. true
12. d

CHAPTER 2

1. true
2. true
3. b
4. d
5. d
6. d
7. b
8. a
9. c
10. d
11. a
12. c
13. d
14. b

CHAPTER 3

1. d
2. c
3. d
4. c

5. b
6. true
7. d
8. c
9. true
10. d
11. b
12. d
13. a
14. d

CHAPTER 4

1. true
2. c
3. true
4. b
5. d
6. b
7. false
8. b
9. b
10. c
11. c
12. d
13. true
14. c
15. c
16. d
17. b

CHAPTER 5

1. d
2. d
3. false
4. true
5. b
6. c

7. b
8. b
9. b
10. true
11. b
12. true
13. true
14. b
15. d
16. a
17. c
18. b
19. true
20. a
21. b
22. d
23. false
24. d
25. c
26. c
27. false
28. false
29. d
30. b
31. c
32. true

CHAPTER 6

1. b
2. true
3. false
4. d
5. c
6. a
7. true
8. c
9. d
10. c
11. a
12. c
13. a
14. false
15. true
16. true
17. d
18. b
19. b
20. c
21. b
22. a
23. d
24. d
25. b
26. b

27. c
28. true
29. d
30. d
31. false
32. a
33. c
34. false
35. d
36. b
37. true
38. false
39. d
40. b

CHAPTER 7

1. true
2. c
3. a
4. d
5. a
6. false
7. b
8. b
9. d
10. a
11. c
12. d
13. c
14. true
15. true
16. b
17. b
18. b
19. false
20. false
21. d
22. true
23. false
24. a
25. true
26. b
27. d
28. c
29. false
30. a
31. a
32. c
33. a
34. d
35. a
36. c
37. true
38. false

39. d
40. d
41. c
42. c
43. b

CHAPTER 8

1. false
2. b
3. c
4. d
5. true
6. false
7. a
8. b
9. a
10. d
11. true
12. c
13. d
14. b
15. true
16. true
17. c
18. d
19. a
20. d
21. c
22. d
23. true
24. false
25. false
26. a
27. c
28. true
29. d
30. c
31. a

CHAPTER 9

1. false
2. false
3. c
4. true
5. b
6. d
7. a
8. b
9. d
10. true
11. d
12. c

13. c
14. d
15. true
16. c
17. d
18. true
19. b
20. false
21. c
22. true
23. a
24. true
25. a
26. d
27. b
28. a
29. d
30. a

CHAPTER 10

1. b
2. b
3. b
4. c
5. a
6. c
7. d
8. a
9. b
10. c
11. d
12. a
13. b
14. c
15. e
16. Rate: 80 bpm
    Rhythm: underlying rhythm is regular but irregular with
        PVCs
    P wave: normal
    PR interval: less than 0.2 second
    QRS: less than 0.12 second
    Interpretation: Sinus rhythm with ST segment elevation
        and multifocal PVCs
17. Rate: 60 bpm
    Rhythm: regular
    P wave: absent
    PR interval: absent
    QRS: greater than 0.12 second
    Interpretation: accelerated idioventricular rhythm
18. Rate: 180 bpm
    Rhythm: regular
    P wave: normal, combined with T wave
    PR interval: less than 0.2 second
    QRS: less than 0.12 second

Interpretation: Atrial tachycardia or supraventricular tachycardia

19. Rate: 80 bpm
    Rhythm: regular
    P wave: normal
    PR interval: less than 0.2 second
    QRS: less than 0.12 second
    Interpretation: Normal sinus rhythm with ST segment depression

20. Rate: 80 bpm
    Rhythm: regular
    P wave: sawtooth, more than one per QRS complex, flutter waves
    PR interval: not measurable
    QRS: less than 0.12 second
    Interpretation: Atrial flutter

21. Rate: 80 bpm
    Rhythm: irregular
    P wave: changing configuration, more than one per QRS complex, fibrillatory waves
    PR interval: not measurable
    QRS: less than 0.12 second
    Interpretation: Atrial fibrillation

22. Rate: not measurable
    Rhythm: irregular
    P wave: none
    PR interval: none
    QRS: chaotic, irregular waves
    Interpretation: Ventricular fibrillation

23. Rate: 160 bpm
    Rhythm: regular
    P wave: none
    PR interval: none
    QRS: greater than 0.12 second
    Interpretation: Ventricular tachycardia

24. Rate: 80 bpm
    Rhythm: underlying rhythm is regular but irregular with PVCs
    P wave: normal
    PR interval: less than 0.2 second
    QRS: less than 0.12 second
    Interpretation: Junctional rhythm with ST segment elevation and unifocal PVCs

25. Rate: 60 bpm
    Rhythm: regular
    P wave: normal
    PR interval: greater than 0.2 second
    QRS: less than 0.12 second
    Interpretation: First-degree AV block with ST segment depression

CHAPTER 11

1. d
2. d

3. c
4. true
5. true
6. c
7. a
8. b
9. b
10. c
11. d
12. c
13. a
14. a
15. c
16. c
17. a
18. d
19. b
20. d

CHAPTER 12

1. c
2. b
3. d
4. a
5. a
6. b
7. c
8. d
9. referred pain, syncope, acute confusion, DOE, fatigue, restlessness
10. a
11. d
12. c
13. c
14. b
15. d
16. d
17. a
18. true
19. false
20. true

CHAPTER 13

1. c
2. a
3. c
4. true
5. d
6. b
7. d
8. true
9. d

10. a
11. c
12. false
13. true
14. a
15. e
16. b
17. b
18. true
19. c
20. true
21. d
22. true
23. d
24. b

CHAPTER 14

1. a
2. b
3. true
4. false
5. b
6. c
7. d
8. true
9. a
10. d
11. a
12. true
13. d
14. d
15. false
16. d
17. a
18. b
19. a
20. d

CHAPTER 15

1. true
2. d
3. d
4. b
5. true
6. true
7. d
8. a
9. d
10. d
11. true
12. d
13. b

14. false
15. b
16. true
17. a
18. c
19. d
20. b
21. true
22. c
23. b
24. c
25. d
26. a
27. true
28. d
29. b
30. d

CHAPTER 16

1. d
2. b
3. a
4. c
5. b
6. a
7. b
8. b
9. c
10. d

CHAPTER 17

1. true
2. true
3. d
4. b
5. c
6. a
7. b
8. d
9. d
10. b
11. d
12. a
13. c
14. b
15. b
16. false
17. d
18. d
19. a
20. true

CHAPTER 18

1. b
2. b
3. true
4. false
5. true
6. false
7. a
8. d
9. d
10. b
11. b
12. d
13. b
14. d
15. b

CHAPTER 19

1. a
2. true

3. c
4. b
5. false
6. true
7. a
8. b
9. d
10. d
11. d

CHAPTER 20

1. true
2. true
3. d
4. b
5. c
6. true
7. c
8. c
9. a
10. c

Index